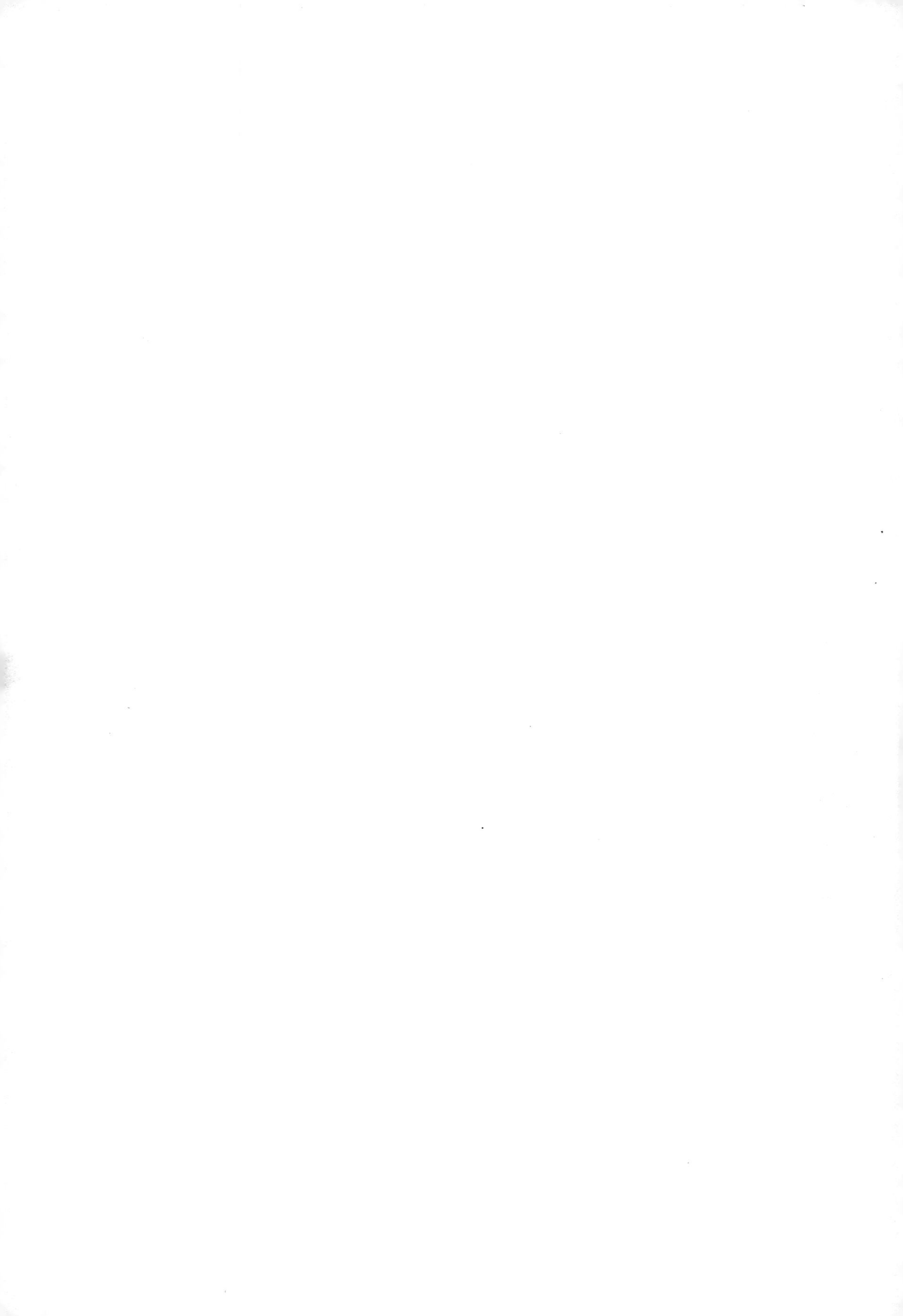

THE ROUTLEDGE COMPANION TO BIOETHICS

The Routledge Companion to Bioethics is a comprehensive reference guide to a wide range of contemporary concerns in bioethics. The volume orients the reader in a changing landscape shaped by globalization, health disparities, and rapidly advancing technologies. Bioethics has begun a turn toward a systematic concern with social justice, population health, and public policy. While also covering more traditional topics, this volume fully captures this recent shift and foreshadows the resulting developments in bioethics. It highlights emerging issues such as climate change, transgender, and medical tourism, and re-examines enduring topics, such as autonomy, end-of-life care, and resource allocation.

John D. Arras is the Porterfield Professor of Biomedical Ethics, and Professor of Philosophy and Public Health Sciences at the University of Virginia. He is a member of the Presidential Commission for the Study of Bioethical Issues.

Elizabeth Fenton is a Research Analyst at the Presidential Commission for the Study of Bioethical Issues. She holds a PhD in Philosophy and an MPH, both from the University of Virginia, and completed a postdoctoral fellowship in the Program in Ethics and Health at Harvard University.

Rebecca Kukla is Professor of Philosophy and Senior Research Scholar at the Kennedy Institute of Ethics at Georgetown University. She is the Editor-in-Chief of the *Kennedy Institute of Ethics Journal* and the former co-coordinator of the Feminist Approaches to Bioethics Network.

Routledge Philosophy Companions

Routledge Philosophy Companions offer thorough, high quality surveys and assessments of the major topics and periods in philosophy. Covering key problems, themes and thinkers, all entries are specially commissioned for each volume and written by leading scholars in the field. Clear, accessible and carefully edited and organised, *Routledge Philosophy Companions* are indispensable for anyone coming to a major topic or period in philosophy, as well as for the more advanced reader.

The Routledge Companion to Aesthetics, Third Edition
Edited by Berys Gaut and Dominic Lopes

The Routledge Companion to Philosophy of Religion, Second Edition
Edited by Chad Meister and Paul Copan

The Routledge Companion to Philosophy of Science, Second Edition
Edited by Martin Curd and Stathis Psillos

The Routledge Companion to Twentieth Century Philosophy
Edited by Dermot Moran

The Routledge Companion to Philosophy and Film
Edited by Paisley Livingston and Carl Plantinga

The Routledge Companion to Philosophy of Psychology
Edited by John Symons and Paco Calvo

The Routledge Companion to Metaphysics
Edited by Robin Le Poidevin, Peter Simons, Andrew McGonigal, and Ross Cameron

The Routledge Companion to Nineteenth Century Philosophy
Edited by Dean Moyar

The Routledge Companion to Ethics
Edited by John Skorupski

The Routledge Companion to Epistemology
Edited by Sven Bernecker and Duncan Pritchard

The Routledge Companion to Philosophy and Music
Edited by Theodore Gracyk and Andrew Kania

The Routledge Companion to Phenomenology
Edited by Søren Overgaard and Sebastian Luft

The Routledge Companion to Philosophy of Language
Edited by Gillian Russell and Delia Graff Fara

The Routledge Companion to Philosophy of Law
Edited by Andrei Marmor

The Routledge Companion to Social and Political Philosophy
Edited by Gerald Gaus and Fred D'Agostino

The Routledge Companion to Ancient Philosophy
Edited by Frisbee Sheffield and James Warren

The Routledge Companion to Eighteenth Century Philosophy
Edited by Aaron Garrett

The Routledge Companion to Bioethics
Edited by John Arras, Elizabeth Fenton, and Rebecca Kukla

Forthcoming:

The Routledge Companion to Sixteenth Century Philosophy
Edited by Benjamin Hill and Henrik Lagerlund

The Routledge Companion to Seventeenth Century Philosophy
Edited by Dan Kaufman

The Routledge Companion to Islamic Philosophy
Edited by Richard C. Taylor and Luis Xavier López-Farjeat

The Routledge Companion to Philosophy of Literature
Edited by Noël Carroll and John Gibson

The Routledge Companion to Medieval Philosophy
Edited by Richard Cross and J.T. Paasch

The Routledge Companion to Hermeneutics
Edited by Jeff Malpas and Hans-Helmuth Gander

The Routledge Companion to Philosophy of Race
Edited by Paul C. Taylor, Linda Martín Alcoff, and Luvell Anderson

The Routledge Companion to Virtue Ethics
Edited by Lorraine Besser-Jones and Michael Slote

The Routledge Companion to Environmental Ethics
Edited by Benjamin Hale and Andrew Light

The Routledge Companion to Free Will
Edited by Meghan Griffith, Neil Levy, and Kevin Timpe

The Routledge Companion to Philosophy of Technology
Edited by Joseph Pitt and Ashley Shew Helfin

The Routledge Companion to Philosophy of Medicine
Edited by Miriam Solomon, Jeremy Simon, and Harold Kincaid

The Routledge Companion to Feminist Philosophy
Edited by Ann Garry, Serene Khader, and Alison Stone

PRAISE FOR THE SERIES

The Routledge Companion to Aesthetics

"This is an immensely useful book that belongs in every college library and on the bookshelves of all serious students of aesthetics." ***—Journal of Aesthetics and Art Criticism***

"The succinctness and clarity of the essays will make this a source that individuals not familiar with aesthetics will find extremely helpful." ***—The Philosophical Quarterly***

"An outstanding resource in aesthetics . . . this text will not only serve as a handy reference source for students and faculty alike, but it could also be used as a text for a course in the philosophy of art." ***—Australasian Journal of Philosophy***

"Attests to the richness of modern aesthetics . . . the essays in central topics—many of which are written by well-known figures—succeed in being informative, balanced and intelligent without being too difficult." ***—British Journal of Aesthetics***

"This handsome reference volume . . . belongs in every library." **—CHOICE**

"The *Routledge Companions* to Philosophy have proved to be a useful series of high quality surveys of major philosophical topics and this volume is worthy enough to sit with the others on a reference library shelf." ***—Philosophy and Religion***

The Routledge Companion to Philosophy of Religion

" . . . a very valuable resource for libraries and serious scholars." **—CHOICE**

"The work is sure to be an academic standard for years to come . . . I shall heartily recommend *The Routledge Companion to Philosophy of Religion* to my students and colleagues and hope that libraries around the country add it to their collections." ***—Philosophia Christi***

The Routledge Companion to Philosophy of Science

A **CHOICE** Outstanding Academic Title 2008

"With a distinguished list of internationally renowned contributors, an excellent choice of topics in the field, and well-written, well-edited essays throughout, this compendium is an excellent resource. Highly recommended." **—CHOICE**

"Highly recommended for history of science and philosophy collections." ***—Library Journal***

"This well conceived companion, which brings together an impressive collection of distinguished authors, will be invaluable to novices and experience readers alike." ***—Metascience***

The Routledge Companion to Twentieth Century Philosophy

"To describe this volume as ambitious would be a serious understatement . . . full of scholarly rigor, including detailed notes and bibliographies of interest to professional philosophers . . . Summing up: Essential." **—*CHOICE***

The Routledge Companion to Philosophy and Film

"A fascinating, rich volume offering dazzling insights and incisive commentary on every page . . . Every serious student of film will want this book . . . Summing Up: Highly recommended." **—*CHOICE***

The Routledge Companion to Philosophy of Psychology

"This work should serve as the standard reference for those interested in gaining a reliable overview of the burgeoning field of philosophical psychology. Summing Up: Essential." **—*CHOICE***

The Routledge Companion to Metaphysics

"The *Routledge Philosophy Companions* series has a deserved reputation for impressive scope and scholarly value. This volume is no exception . . . Summing Up: Highly recommended." **—*CHOICE***

The Routledge Companion to Nineteenth Century Philosophy

A **CHOICE** Outstanding Academic Title 2010

"This is a crucial resource for advanced undergraduates and faculty of any discipline who are interested in the 19th-century roots of contemporary philosophical problems. Summing Up: Essential." **—*CHOICE***

The Routledge Companion to Ethics

"This fine collection merits a place in every university, college, and high school library for its invaluable articles covering a very broad range of topics in ethics[.] . . . With its remarkable clarity of writing and its very highly qualified contributors, this volume is must reading for anyone interested in the latest developments in these important areas of thought and practice. Summing Up: Highly recommended." **—*CHOICE***

The Routledge Companion to Philosophy and Music

"Comprehensive and authoritative . . . readers will discover many excellent articles in this well-organized addition to a growing interdisciplinary field. Summing Up: Highly recommended." **—*CHOICE***

" . . . succeeds well in catching the wide-ranging strands of musical theorising and thinking, and performance, and an understanding of the various contexts in which all this takes place." **—*Reference Reviews***

The Routledge Companion to Phenomenology

"Sebastian Luft and Søren Overgaard, with the help of over sixty contributors, have captured the excitement of this evolving patchwork named 'phenomenology'. *The Routledge Companion to Phenomenology* will serve as an invaluable reference volume for students, teachers, and scholars of phenomenology, as well as an accessible introduction to phenomenology for philosophers from other specialties or scholars from other disciplines." ***—International Journal of Philosophical Studies***

The Routledge Companion to Epistemology

A **CHOICE** Outstanding Academic Title 2011

"As a series, the *Routledge Philosophy Companions* has met with near universal acclaim. The expansive volume not only continues the trend but quite possibly sets a new standard . . . Indeed, this is a definitive resource that will continue to prove its value for a long time to come. Summing Up: Essential." ***—CHOICE***

The Routledge Companion to Philosophy of Language

"This collection presents more than 65 new essays by prominent contemporary figures working in the philosophy of language. Collectively, they represent the cutting edge of philosophical research into issues surrounding the use, understanding, and study of language . . . the book constitutes an invaluable current resource for students and scholars alike. It will appeal to anyone interested in the current state-of-play within this important area of philosophical research. Summing Up: Highly recommended." ***—CHOICE***

The Routledge Companion to Social and Political Philosophy

"This 15th book in the *Routledge Philosophy Companions* series is also the most comprehensive, both chronologically and conceptually . . . The polish and high quality of the essays provide a multifaceted mirror of the passions and interests of contemporary academic Anglophone philosophy. Summing Up: Highly recommended." ***—CHOICE***

THE ROUTLEDGE COMPANION TO BIOETHICS

Edited by
John D. Arras, Elizabeth Fenton,
and Rebecca Kukla

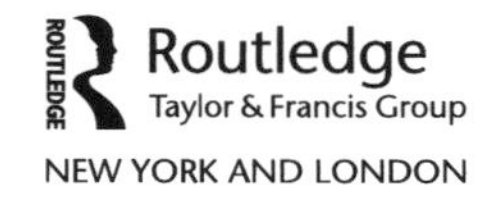

NEW YORK AND LONDON

First published 2015
by Routledge
711 Third Avenue, New York, NY 10017

and by Routledge
2 Park Square, Milton Park, Abingdon, Oxon OX14 4RN

Routledge is an imprint of the Taylor & Francis Group, an informa business

Library of Congress Cataloging in Publication Data
The Routledge companion to bioethics/
[edited by] John D. Arras, Elizabeth Fenton, Rebecca Kukla.
pages cm.—(Routledge philosophy companions)
Includes bibliographical references and index.
1. Bioethics. I. Arras, John D., 1945- editor. II. Fenton, Elizabeth (Elizabeth Mary), editor. III. Kukla, Rebecca, 1969- editor.
QH332.R675 2015
174.2—dc23
2014021150

ISBN: 978-0-415-89666-5 (hbk)
ISBN: 978-0-203-80497-1 (ebk)

Typeset in Goudy Oldstyle Std
by Swales & Willis Ltd, Exeter, Devon, UK

Printed and bound in the United States of America by Publishers Graphics, LLC on sustainably sourced paper.

For Adrienne Asch (1946–2013).

Beloved and devoted friend, pioneering scholar, and tenacious advocate for human rights.

CONTENTS

CONTRIBUTORS

Nicholas Agar is a Reader in Philosophy at Victoria University of Wellington. His research is on the ethics of genetics and technology.

Paul S. Appelbaum is the Dollard Professor of Psychiatry, Medicine, & Law and Director, Division of Law, Ethics, and Psychiatry, Department of Psychiatry, Columbia University College of Physicians and Surgeons, New York. He has written extensively on research ethics and informed consent.

John D. Arras is the Porterfield Professor of Biomedical Ethics, and Professor of Philosophy and Public Health Sciences at the University of Virginia. He is a member of the Presidential Commission for the Study of Bioethical Issues.

Adrienne Asch was a leading bioethics and disability scholar, and, most recently, Director of the Center for Ethics at Yeshiva University. Much of her research and writing concerned the ethics of human reproduction. She died in November, 2013.

Richard Ashcroft is Professor of Bioethics in the School of Law at Queen Mary, University of London. He trained in history and philosophy of science, and has worked mainly in the fields of biomedical research ethics and public health ethics.

Margaret P. Battin, MFA, PhD is Professor of Philosophy and Medical Ethics at the University of Utah. She has authored, co-authored, edited, or co-edited some twenty books, including *Drugs and Justice* and *The Patient as Victim and Vector: Ethics and Infectious Disease*. She has published two collections of essays on end-of-life issues, *The Least Worst Death* and *Ending Life*.

Françoise Baylis is Professor and Canada Research Chair in Bioethics and Philosophy at Dalhousie University, Halifax, Nova Scotia, Canada. She is an elected Fellow of the Royal Society of Canada and the Canadian Academy of Health Sciences.

Tom L. Beauchamp is Professor of Philosophy and Senior Research Scholar, Kennedy Institute of Ethics, Georgetown University. His research interests are in the ethics of human-subjects research, the ethics of animal-subjects research, universal principles and rights, and methods of bioethics.

Jessica Berg, JD, MPH is Professor of Law, Professor of Bioethics, and Professor of Public Health with a joint appointment at Case Western Reserve University's Schools of Law and Medicine. She is first author on the second edition of *Informed Consent: Legal Theory and Clinical Practice*, and has written extensively on capacity and competence.

Justin B. Biddle is Assistant Professor in the School of Public Policy at the Georgia Institute of Technology. His research focuses on the role of values and interests in science and the epistemic and ethical significance of the social organization of research.

Greg Bognar is a Lecturer in Philosophy at La Trobe University in Melbourne, Australia. Formerly he was a Postdoctoral Fellow at the Harvard University Program in Ethics & Health and an Assistant Professor/Faculty Fellow at the Center for Bioethics at New York University. His research interests are in ethics, social and political philosophy, especially bioethics, public health ethics, environmental ethics, and the philosophy of public policy.

Howard Brody, MD, PhD is John P. McGovern Centennial Chair in Family Medicine and the Director of the Institute for the Medical Humanities, University of Texas Medical Branch, Galveston.

Daniel Callahan is President Emeritus of The Hastings Center. He is a graduate of Yale and has a PhD in philosophy from Harvard. He is a member of The Institute of Medicine, The National Academy of Sciences and Co-Director of The Yale-Hastings Program in Ethics and Health Policy. He is the author most recently of *In Search of The Good: A Life In Bioethics*.

James F. Childress is University Professor and the John Allen Hollingsworth Professor of Ethics at the University of Virginia, where he is also Professor of Religious Studies and Director of the Institute for Practical Ethics and Public Life.

Winston Chiong is Assistant Adjunct Professor in Neurology at the University of California, San Francisco. His academic interests lie at the intersection of philosophy, medicine and cognitive science, and his current research focuses on decision-making in aging and disease.

I. Glenn Cohen is Professor at Harvard Law School and Co-Director of the Petrie-Flom Center for Health Law Policy, Biotechnology, and Bioethics. His work has appeared in leading journals in law, medicine, public health, and bioethics, as well as in numerous media outlets. He is the author, editor, or co-editor of three books.

G.K.D. Crozier is the Canada Research Chair of Environment, Culture and Values and an Assistant Professor of Philosophy at Laurentian University, Canada. Dr Crozier's research interests lie in the philosophy of the life sciences and in connections between techno-scientific advancements and global bioethics.

Norman Daniels, formerly at Tufts, is Mary B. Saltonstall Professor and Professor of Ethics and Population Health at Harvard. His most recent books include *Just Health* (Cambridge 2008) and (with Jim Sabin) *Setting Limits Fairly*, second edition (Oxford 2008).

Dena S. Davis, JD, PhD holds the Presidential Endowed Chair in Health at Lehigh University where she is Professor of Religion Studies. She is the author of *Genetic Dilemmas: Reproductive Technology, Parental Choices, and Children's Futures*, second edition (Oxford University Press 2010).

Lisa Eckenwiler is Associate Professor of Philosophy in the Departments of Philosophy and Health Administration and Policy at George Mason University. Her publications include *Long Term Care, Globalization, and Justice* (Johns Hopkins University Press 2012), and *The Ethics of Bioethics: Mapping the Moral Landscape* (co-edited with Felicia Cohn) (Johns Hopkins University Press 2007).

Nir Eyal is Associate Professor of Global Health and Social Medicine (Medical Ethics) at the Harvard Medical School. He works in population-level bioethics, as well as in ethics, bioethics, and political philosophy more generally. Eyal co-edits the Oxford UP series "Population-Level Bioethics."

Elizabeth Fenton is a Research Analyst at the Presidential Commission for the Study of Bioethical Issues. She holds a PhD in Philosophy and an MPH, both from the University of Virginia, and completed a postdoctoral fellowship in the Program in Ethics and Health at Harvard University.

Joseph J. Fins, MD, MACP is the E. William Davis, Jr, MD Professor of Medical Ethics; Chief, Division of Medical Ethics; Professor of Medicine; Professor of Public Health; and Professor of Medicine in Psychiatry at Weill Medical College of Cornell University. He is also Adjunct Faculty and Senior Attending Physician at Rockefeller University and Rockefeller University Hospital.

Chloë FitzGerald is Postdoctoral Fellow at the Institute for Ethics, History, and the Humanities, Geneva University Medical School. She is currently working on the Swiss National Science Foundation project, *Understanding Implicit Bias in Clinical Care*.

Leslie P. Francis, JD, PhD, is Distinguished Professor of Philosophy and Distinguished Alfred C. Emery Professor of Law at the University of Utah. She currently serves as co-chair of the Privacy Subcommittee of the National Committee on Vital and Health Statistics, as a member of the Ethics Committee of the American Society for Reproductive Ethics, as an elected vice president of the International Society for Philosophy of Law and Social Philosophy, and as a regular blogger for HealthLawProf.

Mackenzie Graham is a PhD candidate and member of the Rotman Institute of Philosophy at Western University in London, Ontario. He received his BA in Philosophy from Western in 2009, and his MA in Philosophy from Dalhousie University in 2010.

Ami Harbin is Assistant Professor of Philosophy and Women & Gender Studies at Oakland University (Michigan). Her research interests include feminist philosophy, moral psychology, emotional experience in health care, mental health ethics, and queer bioethics.

Samia A. Hurst is Professor of Bioethics at Geneva University's medical school in Switzerland, and ethics consultant to the Geneva University Hospitals' clinical ethics committee. Her research focuses on fairness in clinical practice, and the protection of vulnerable persons.

Bruce Jennings is Director of Bioethics at the Center for Humans and Nature and is Senior Advisor and Fellow at The Hastings Center, where he served from 1991 through 1999 as Executive Director. He is also on the faculty of the Yale School of Public Health. He has published twenty-five books and numerous articles on bioethics.

Kjell Arne Johansson, MD, PhD is Associate Professor in Bioethics at the Department of Global Public Health and Primary Health Care, University of Bergen. His research emphasizes the integration of equity metrics and fairness concerns into health-economic population models.

Isabel Karpin is Professor of Law at the University of Technology, Sydney. She specializes in feminist legal theory, disability and the law, law and cultural studies and laws regulating the body: specifically, the impact of biotechnological innovations in genetics, and reproductive technology.

Rebecca Kukla is Professor of Philosophy and Senior Research Scholar at the Kennedy Institute of Ethics at Georgetown University. She is the Editor-in-Chief of the *Kennedy Institute of Ethics Journal* and the former co-coordinator of the Feminist Approaches to Bioethics Network.

Keren Ladin, PhD, MSc is Assistant Professor in the Department of Occupational Therapy at Tufts University and the Department of Public Health and Community Medicine at Tufts University Medical School. Dr Ladin is also the Director of Research on Ethics, Aging, and Community Health (REACH Lab) at Tufts University.

Hilde Lindemann is Professor of Philosophy at Michigan State University. A former President of the American Society for Bioethics and Humanities, and a Fellow of the Hastings Center, her published work includes *Damaged Identities, Narrative Repair: An Invitation to Feminist Ethics* and *Holding and Letting Go: The Social Practice of Personal Identities*.

Catriona Mackenzie is Professor of Philosophy, Director of the Research Centre for Agency, Values and Ethics, and Associate Dean (Research) in the Faculty of Arts at Macquarie University, Sydney. She is co-editor of several volumes, including *Relational Autonomy: Feminist Perspectives on Autonomy, Agency, and the Social Self* (Oxford University Press 2000), *Practical Identity and Narrative Agency* (Routledge 2008), *Emotions, Imagination and Moral Reasoning* (Psychology Press 2012), and *Vulnerability: New Essays in Ethics and Feminist Philosophy* (Oxford University Press 2014).

Katherine Shaw Makielski is a May 2014 Juris Doctor candidate at Case Western Reserve University School of Law with a concentration in health law and is currently the Editor-in-Chief of the *Law Review*. She received a bachelor of arts in biology from Washington University in St Louis in 2006.

Sir Michael Marmot is MRC Research Professor of Epidemiology and Public Health at University College London and Director of the UCL Institute for Health Equity. He was Chair of the WHO Commission on the Social Determinants of Health, the Strategic Review of Health Inequalities in England post-2010, and the Review of Social Determinants and the Health Divide in the WHO European Region.

Felice Marshall is a doctoral student at Victoria University of Wellington. Her research is currently on moral enhancement.

Carolyn McLeod is Associate Professor of Philosophy and Affiliate Member of Women's Studies and Feminist Research at the University of Western Ontario. Most recently, she was Principal Investigator on a grant by the Canadian Institutes of Health Research on conscientious refusals in health care. She also, along with Françoise Baylis, edited *Family-Making: Contemporary Ethical Challenges* (Oxford).

Paul B. Miller, JD, PhD is Assistant Professor of Law at the McGill University Faculty of Law. Professor Miller taught previously at the Queen's University Faculty of Law. Professor Miller's research interests include the philosophy of private law, fiduciary law, business law and trusts, and health law. He is the author of several articles on trusts and fiduciary law and co-editor of the forthcoming collection *Philosophical Foundations of Fiduciary Law* (Oxford University Press).

Jonathan D. Moreno is a philosopher and historian. As the David and Lyn Silfen University Professor at the University of Pennsylvania, Moreno is one of fourteen Penn Integrates Knowledge professors. At Penn he is also Professor of Medical Ethics and Health Policy, of History and Sociology of Science, and of Philosophy. Among his books are *The Body Politic*, *Mind Wars* (2012), and *Undue Risk* (2000). His latest book is *Impromptu Man: J.L. Moreno and the Origins of Psychodrama, Encounter Culture, and the Social Network* (2014).

Amy Mullin is Professor of Philosophy at the University of Toronto. She is interested in questions about responsibility in connection with care and vulnerability, and about the responsibilities of those who receive as well as those who provide care.

Jamie Lindemann Nelson is Professor of Philosophy at Michigan State University. Her books include *The Patient in the Family* (with Hilde Lindemann). A Fellow of The Hastings Center, she is also a member of the Consortium on the Ethics of Families in Health and Social Care.

Madison Powers is Professor of Philosophy, Georgetown University, and Senior Research Scholar, Kennedy Institute of Ethics.

David B. Resnik, JD, PhD is a Bioethicist and institutional review board (IRB) chair at the National Institute of Environmental Health Science, National Institutes of Health. He has published eight books and 200 articles on ethical, legal, social, and philosophical issues in science, medicine, and technology and is associate editor of the journal *Accountability in Research*.

Alan Rubel is Assistant Professor in the School of Library and Information Studies and in the Legal Studies program at the University of Wisconsin, Madison. He is a former Greenwall Fellow in Bioethics and Health Policy at Johns Hopkins and Georgetown universities.

Toby Schonfeld, PhD is the Human Subjects Research Review Official and the Director of the Program in Human Research Ethics at the US Environmental Protection Agency (EPA). Her research interests are in ethics education, research ethics, and women in health care.

Alexis Shotwell is Associate Professor at Carleton University, on unceded and unsurrendered Algonquin territory. She is the author of *Knowing Otherwise: Race, Gender, and Implicit Understanding* and has published in *Signs*, *Hypatia*, *IJFAB*, and *Sociological Theory*.

Anita Silvers is Professor and Chair of Philosophy at San Francisco State University, and a longtime member of San Francisco General Hospital's Medical Ethics Committee. Her philosophical research currently focuses on justice and disability. She has been awarded the APA's Quinn Prize (2009) and the Phi Beta Kappa Lebowitz Prize (2013).

Dominic Sisti is Assistant Professor of Medical Ethics & Health Policy and Assistant Professor of Psychiatry at the Perelman School of Medicine at the University of Pennsylvania. He works primarily on the philosophy and ethics of behavioral healthcare and is editor of *Applied Ethics of Mental Health Care: An Interdisciplinary Reader* (2013). He directs a research program supported by the Thomas Scattergood Behavioral Health Foundation.

Nikki Sullivan is Associate Professor of Critical and Cultural Studies in the Department of Media, Music, Communication and Cultural Studies at Macquarie University. She is the author of *Tattooed Bodies: Subjectivity, Textuality, Ethics and Pleasure* (Praeger 2001), and *A Critical Introduction to Queer Theory* (Edinburgh University Press 2003); co-author (with Lisa Downing and Iain Morland) of *Fuckology: Critical Essays on John Money's Diagnostic Concepts* (Chicago University Press 2014); and co-editor (with Samantha Murray) of *Somatechnics: Queering The Technologisation of Bodies* (Ashgate 2009).

Fredrik Svenaeus is Professor at the Centre for Studies in Practical Knowledge, Södertörn University, Sweden. His research areas are philosophy of medicine, bioethics, medical humanities, phenomenology, and philosophical anthropology.

Sridhar Venkatapuram is a Lecturer and Director of the programme in Global Health & Social Justice at King's College London.

Marian A. Verkerk is Full Professor of Ethics of Care at the University of Groningen and the University Medical Centre Groningen, the Netherlands. She received her PhD in Philosophy in 1995 at the University of Utrecht. She is also a member of the Health Council in the Netherlands.

David Wasserman is a visiting scholar in the Department of Bioethics at the National Institutes of Health. He was formerly Director of Research at the Center for Ethics, Yeshiva University. He writes on reproduction, disability, genetics, and the ethical implications of neuroscience.

Charles Weijer, MD, PhD is Professor of Philosophy and Medicine and Canada Research Chair in Bioethics at Western University in London, Canada. He is cofounder of the Rotman Institute of Philosophy, which promotes research and training at the interface of the humanities and sciences.

Alan Wertheimer is Professor Emeritus of political science at the University of Vermont, where he taught from 1968 to 2005. From 2005 to 2013, he was Senior Research Scholar in the Department of Bioethics at the National Institutes of Health. He is the author of *Coercion* (Princeton University Press 1987), *Exploitation* (Princeton University Press 1996), *Consent to Sexual Relations* (Cambridge University Press 2003), and *Rethinking the Ethics of Clinical Research* (Oxford University Press 2011).

ACKNOWLEDGMENTS

The task of preparing a volume of this size and scope is a large and at times daunting one. We are grateful to our editors at Routledge for their support and patience, and to all the contributors to the volume for their high quality and stimulating scholarship, and their ongoing commitment to this project. We are also very grateful to Bryan Cwik, Lisa Kearns, and Joanna Smolenski, who provided extremely able assistance in writing section introductions and helping to meet our deadline for completing the manuscript.

John D. Arras
Elizabeth Fenton
Rebecca Kukla

INTRODUCTION

The term *bioethics* was first used to capture the concerns of life scientists about the human capacity to alter nature and the impact of that capacity on our global future (Potter 1971). With hindsight, and our contemporary understanding of the wide-ranging health impacts of human-caused environmental damage, we can appreciate the prophetic resonance of this original use of the term. Yet the field that went on to shape the evolution of bioethics was not biology but medicine and biomedical research, and bioethics is now firmly established as an integral part of both enterprises.

As traditionally understood, bioethics as an interdisciplinary field has enjoyed exponential growth and has made significant contributions to our public debates about important and fascinating questions, such as the definition of death, the ethics and law of biomedical research, abortion, euthanasia, the ethical deployment of genetic knowledge, the possibility of enhancing human nature, and the nature and limits of an individual's right to health care.

Critics have argued, however, that the limited focus of traditional bioethics upon clinical medicine and research has blinded it to the most pressing moral challenges in public health, in particular vast and unjust global health inequalities, the impact of economic and environmental policies on health, domestic health disparities, and human rights and health (Farmer and Campos 2004). Yet more recently, systematic attention to and engagement with the social and political dimensions of health and health care has begun to transform the field of bioethics (Wikler and Brock 2008; Daniels 2006; Powers and Faden 2006). This transformation, which we believe will and should continue and intensify, is due to at least three interlocking factors.

First, the globalization of our economy, culture, and communications has forced bioethicists to examine how research and care are imported, exported, and delivered across national borders and economic and cultural divides. For example, relatively new key issues in bioethics include research designed and funded by individuals and groups from rich countries and performed in poor countries, duties to provide health care and resources to other countries, international pharmaceutical patenting policy, medical tourism, and the importation of medical values and practices into other countries and the attendant risks of cultural imperialism.

Second, many of the most important, visible, and ethically charged contemporary threats to health can only be understood at the level of populations rather than individuals. The risks of global climate change and pandemics raise key ethical questions, such as resource allocation during a widespread crisis, duties to future generations, and the relationship between health risks and economic and social vulnerability. Tropical diseases such as malaria and sleeping sickness comprise a huge share of the global disease burden yet command a tiny share of our research dollars, raising questions about the social obligations of those who fund and conduct research. New genetic technologies generate questions about indirect eugenics and the long-term effects of manipulating our gene pool.

Third, bioethicists and health care professionals more broadly have become increasingly aware of the social determinants of health and systematic health disparities. We now understand that individual health and access to health care are shaped in complex ways by race, class, education, geography, and cultural conditions such as eating practices and the car-based culture of suburbia. Thus the choices and health status of individual patients, and their relationships to their health professionals, must be situated within a broader social and economic context before their ethical contours can be clearly discerned.

For all of these reasons, bioethics is moving beyond its traditional set of concerns, including the rights of individuals to health care, and embracing an intensified focus on issues of justice more broadly construed, health equity, public and population health, social systems, and incorporating a new sensitivity to social and cultural context into its methods. This more global, systemic vision will not only introduce new issues into the field but should also transform our approach to traditional issues, such as the management of end-of-life care, the appropriate use of reproductive technologies, and the duties of researchers towards research participants. We believe that the tools of social and political philosophy, public health, and economics are now at least as central to bioethics as those of ethics traditionally conceived. *The Routledge Companion to Bioethics* seeks to highlight and advance this new methodology and broadened vision.

John D. Arras
Elizabeth Fenton
Rebecca Kukla

References

Daniels, N. (2006) "Equity and Population Health: Toward a Broader Bioethics Agenda," *Hastings Center Report* 36 (4): 22–35.

Farmer, P. and Campos, N.C. (2004) "Rethinking Medical Ethics: A View from Below," *Developing World Bioethics* 4: 17–41.

Potter, V.R. (1971) *Bioethics: Bridge to the Future*, Englewood Cliffs, NJ: Prentice-Hall.

Powers, M. and Faden, R. (2006) *Social Justice: The Moral Foundations of Public Health and Health Policy*, New York, NY: Oxford University Press.

Wikler, D. and Brock, D.W. (2008) "Population-Level Bioethics: Mapping a New Agenda," in R.M. Green, A. Donovan, and S.A. Jauss (eds.) *Global Bioethics: Issues of Conscience for the Twenty-first Century*, Oxford: Oxford University Press.

Part I

JUSTICE AND HEALTH DISTRIBUTION

Considerations of justice are inseparable from many of the most challenging issues in contemporary bioethics; indeed one of the central aims of this volume is to draw out these considerations in debates in which they may otherwise have been obscured or overlooked. Justice is particularly salient in debates over access to and distribution of health care, and more broadly of the social, economic, and political conditions that make it possible for people to live healthy lives. The chapters in this section explore the general theme of how resources relevant to health can be fairly and justly distributed.

The first chapter in this section explores the contours of the longstanding debate over the right to health care. The debate is complex, including philosophical questions about the nature and function of rights in political and moral discourse; it is also contentious, with significant theoretical commitments on both sides. John Arras examines four leading moral and political theories (libertarianism, utilitarianism, liberal egalitarianism, and communitarianism) and the implications under each for the right to health care. Arras's chapter also importantly situates this debate in the contemporary context of the landmark 2010 U.S. health care law known as the *Affordable Care Act*. In bringing the debate into the current health policy context, Arras pays particular attention to the growing understanding among bioethicists of the role of social, economic, and political factors in creating the conditions necessary for health. He notes that in light of this growing understanding many bioethicists have eschewed the language of a right to health care in favor of a right to *health*, which encompasses access not only to health care services but also to the conditions necessary for health. These conditions, and their relevance to social justice, are the subject of Sridhar Venkatapuram and Michael Marmot's chapter on the social determinants of health and health inequalities. Health inequalities in populations often persist because of unjust distributions of other goods within society, such as income and education. This chapter outlines the increasingly strong evidence for the ways in which social, economic, and political conditions influence health and engender, and sometimes entrench, health inequalities. It also draws attention to the extent to which bioethics as a field (with notable exceptions) has been slow to comprehend the moral significance of the social determinants literature, and is an important reminder that bioethics must be expansive in its disciplinary scope if it is to be a force in addressing health injustice.

A deeper understanding of population-level health trends and the factors that influence them is critical to anyone engaging in contemporary bioethics. No less critical is an understanding of the ways in which health resources are allocated and prioritized in a community. The chapters by Dan Callahan, Greg Bognar, and Norman Daniels and Keren Ladin explore the ways in which health resources can be allocated more or less justly. Callahan discusses the ethics and politics of rationing health resources in an era of increasingly expensive health care and increasingly limited resources. Though many of his examples come from the U.S. context where "rationing" remains a dirty word, they are relevant to all health systems where demand outstrips supply, which is to say all health systems. Bognar's chapter provides an excellent introduction to two concepts widely used in health resource allocation, quality-adjusted life years (QALYs) and disability-adjusted life years (DALYs). These concepts have been criticized for promoting distributions of resources that are insensitive to individual health needs and particularly complex health needs, but they remain fundamental to the strategies of many health systems seeking to spend limited budgets both efficiently and fairly. The final chapter by Norman Daniels and Kerin Ladin unifies the themes of this section by asking what we owe in terms of health resources to people who enter a society as immigrants, whether legally or illegally. The authors ask whether immigration status is morally relevant to the provision of health-related goods, based on considerations of reciprocity and the rights of states.

1
THE RIGHT TO HEALTH CARE

John D. Arras

For many people in the world today, access to health care is unattainable. In the developing (i.e., poor) countries, yearly public expenditure on public health and health care often amounts to less than $10 per person (Pogge 2008). In the U.S. before the *Affordable Care Act* (ACA) took effect in 2010, estimates placed the number of uninsured individuals at roughly 48 million, with another 60 million underinsured (Centers for Disease Control and Prevention 2013). The passage of the ACA promised to place access to health insurance within the reach of just about every citizen, but the weakening of that Act by the Supreme Court and the refusal on the part of many states to implement the expansion of Medicaid under the Act have left millions without access to affordable insurance. Indeed, roughly half of the uninsured in the U.S. reside in states whose political leaders have refused to extend Medicaid to them (Tavernise and Gebeloff 2013). The promise of universal access thus remains unfulfilled for the foreseeable future.

What are we to think of this state of affairs? For those of a libertarian persuasion, premature mortality and untreated morbidity due to a lack of health insurance are viewed as "unfortunate but not unjust" (Engelhardt 1996, 1997). The world might be a better place were everyone's health needs somehow met, but this, libertarians argue, is an issue of charity, not justice. Many others contend that lack of access and its contributions to ill health are indeed an injustice, a wrong perpetrated on the poor that cries out for political redress. For these critics, access to health care is a right, not a privilege underwritten by significant wealth.

These two polar opposite interpretations of the moral valence of lack of access to health insurance framed much of the recent debate in the U.S. regarding health reform. Many proponents of the ACA ("Obamacare") stressed the moral importance of achieving universal access, while many opponents downplayed access in favor of an emphasis on cost containment and limited government. This essay will explore and scrutinize some of the arguments on both sides of this debate. I shall conclude that powerful moral arguments can buttress the case for a right to health care, but I shall also stress the limited (albeit important) role for such a right in debates over health policy.

As we shall see below, the notion of a right to health care is controversial. Some on the political right view it as morally unjustifiable, while others on the political left often view a focus on health care alone as excessively narrow. For these latter critics, a theory of justice in health should consider not just access to health *care*—what Norman Daniels has dubbed "the ambulance waiting at the bottom of a cliff" (Daniels 2008: 79)—but also all those so-called social determinants of health, such as public health provision of clean water and air, safe working conditions, and the social bases of self-respect on the job and in society generally (Wilkinson and Marmot 2003). Following the lead of these critics, I shall focus here on what I call access to health-related goods, not just to health care services.

Some Special Features of "Rights Talk"

First, if someone claims a "right to X," they are saying a lot more than something like "the world would be a better place if everyone had X." Consider this scenario inspired by philosopher Judith Thomson (1971): You are languishing in a New York City hospital, wasting away from some dread, lethal disease. The only prospect for a cure would miraculously require that the actor Matt Damon fly out from Hollywood to place his cool hand on your fevered brow. Since your life depends upon him, wouldn't you have a right to Matt Damon's time and efforts? Thomson's answer is, No. Although it would be "terribly nice" if Matt were to go to all this trouble, you certainly have no right that he do so. It would, however, be a different story had Matt promised you that he'd come, or if he were your father. Hence, the first important defining feature of rights: They are justified claims, demands, or entitlements that we make *vis-à-vis* others. Failure to respect or grant someone's right constitutes an injustice calling for redress; it is not the mere falling short of a social goal or ideal (Buchanan 1984; Wenar 2011).

Second, we must distinguish between moral and legal rights. Some rights—such as the right to be secure in your person or property, or the right of poor people to legal counsel in criminal cases—are carefully articulated and delimited by legal statutes, constitutions, or evolving case law. In the vast majority of cases, if there's any doubt about the existence of such a right, you can just go look it up. By contrast, moral rights are discovered, created, or justified by moral arguments. We say that Joan has a moral right to X if sound and convincing arguments can be given showing that she has a justified entitlement to X. To say that Joan has a moral right to something leaves the legal question open. In many, but not all, cases we say that the existence of a moral right provides us with a good reason for turning that claim into a legal entitlement. So when we debate the existence of health care rights, we are making moral arguments that might later be cashed out as legal arguments.

Another distinction in the topography of rights separates negative from positive rights (Wenar 2011; Holmes and Sunstein 1999). The former are entitlements, *inter alia*, to be let alone, to speak or write freely about political matters in public, to gather with others in voluntary civil and religious associations, all without the interference of others, including the government. Put in a negative mode, these include the right not to be assaulted, not to have our property taken, not to be politically muzzled or imprisoned without good cause, and so on. Putative positive rights, by contrast, are entitlements to certain goods or services, such as legal representation, food, shelter, and, yes, health care.

Just how important this distinction between negative and positive is depends upon one's larger philosophical commitments. Those of a predominantly libertarian persuasion place great stock in this distinction (Cranston 1967). They note that each of us can respect the negative rights of all other persons 24 hours a day, 7 days a week just by refraining from acting upon them in prohibited ways (e.g., stealing their property or killing them). Negative rights thus correlate with the duties of all others to refrain at all times from intervening against them. While negative rights are thus arguably cost free, positive rights obviously require that other people provide the goods and services to which we are allegedly entitled, usually by means of taxation. If we have a right to health care, then someone or some institution must have a corresponding duty to provide it to us, and this raises a fundamental problem: Exactly how are we entitled to the money or labor of others? It is thus often concluded that negative rights are much easier to justify and fulfill than positive rights, which risk encroaching on the negative rights of others to be free to keep or spend their resources as they see fit (Cranston 1967). As we shall see momentarily, non-libertarians place much less weight on this distinction.

A final distinction concerns the weight or demandingness of various rights. Some people claim that some rights, such as the right to life of innocent people, are absolute; they cannot or should not be violated for any reason. Others argue that all or at least most rights are *prima facie* only (or *pro tanto*)—i.e., they hold for the most part or at first blush, but they can be overridden if countervailing rights or interests are sufficiently powerful. Philosopher Ronald Dworkin famously wrote that serious legal rights (e.g., to free speech) function like trumps in the game of bridge—i.e., they are claims that outrank most other claims, such as social utility (Dworkin 1978). Although he argued that most moral and legal rights should function as trumps in political argument, Dworkin conceded that they can occasionally be limited or outweighed by countervailing social considerations of great importance—e.g., shouting "Fire!" falsely in a crowded theater. Thus, if there is a right to health care, the logic of rights would disallow arguments against it merely on grounds of efficiency, social utility, or public opinion. If, however, a putative right claim would have the likely effect of "breaking the bank" or of using up most social resources for the benefit of a few, that right could legitimately be curbed or overridden.

Rights and Correlative Social Duties

We have seen above that rights are justified claims that generate correlative duties in others to either respect our persons and property or provide us with various goods. They are thus said to be "socially guaranteed" (Mill 1863/2001). But guaranteed by whom or what? Skeptics about positive rights often assume that the duties correlating to them must be lodged against individuals, possibly those in the best position to help. This assumption then leads to worries about placing excessively onerous duties upon individuals who would bear the burden of providing food and health care, for example, for all in need—a burden that would supposedly exhaust our resources and preclude our ability to chart the direction of our own lives. One problem with this assumption is that it ignores an important role for social institutions in the securing of rights. According to one influential theory, rights can generate "waves of duty" that might include individuals, to be sure, but also local, state, and regional governments, as well as the United Nations and non-governmental organizations (NGOs) like the World Bank (Shue 1996). Duties spread around such institutions might be much more manageable for individuals to bear.

Contributors to the literature on universal human rights have further specified what these duties linked with rights entail. First, they involve duties to avoid violating negative rights. These duties apply to each of us all the time. Second, they entail a duty to protect vulnerable parties against deprivation of their rights. This is the function of police departments and of military intervention against states that systematically violate the rights of their citizens. Third, there are duties to assist those whose rights have already been violated. This is the function of courts and, for example, of NGOs of health care workers, such as *Médecins Sans Frontières*, who attend to the needs of refugees from state-sponsored tyranny (Shue 1996).

The second and third of the above rights clearly require the investment of resources, and thus tend to blur the distinction between negative and positive rights. Even citizens' negative rights require significant public investments in institutions such as police and courts of law, without which our cherished rights to be let alone would be under constant assault. Viewed from this angle, negative rights can often be just as problematic as positive rights, raising questions about who shall pay, the appropriate level and scope of provision, and so on (Holmes and Sunstein 1999).

Finally, any theory of rights must be attentive to the sorts of burdens that ascriptions of rights might entail for those footing the bill. Failure to attend to such burdens is a common failing of many theories of rights, which consequently often yield "wish lists" with little likelihood of ever moving the great mass of humanity into action. Ruth Macklin once called attention to the claim on the part of Canadian welfare recipients to a "right to own a pet" (Macklin 1976). Not only is such a putative right not exactly high on the list of the most important interests of human beings, but Canadian taxpayers might justifiably be unwilling to make the requisite sacrifice of their own resources to pay for it. Any plausible theory of rights, including a right to health care, would have to seriously consider the "supply side" of rights—i.e., who will bear the burden of paying for them (Lomasky 1981).

The Functions of Rights in Moral Discourse

We can easily imagine a world of political discourse that had no use for the concept of rights (Feinberg 1970). Indeed, rights as we currently deploy them were unknown to the ancient and medieval worlds. What then is the function (or functions) of rights talk within our own political culture? We can make a start on this question by noting that the ascription of rights allows political discourse to "take the victim's side." In contrast to appeals to charity or benevolence, rights allow the individual to speak in his or her own name, to make claims against others without shame or embarrassment. There's no need to beg and scrape for the generosity or beneficence of courtiers and bureaucrats; we can stand up, heads held high, and claim our rights as equal citizens.

More specifically, there are two general approaches to the nature of rights in contemporary political theory: namely, the "will theory" and the "interest theory" (Wenar 2011). The will theory grounds rights in appeals to human dignity. As Kant argued, we human beings derive our dignity or special worth from our capacity for moral agency or ability to make free moral choices. Incursions into our agency—e.g., by means of unjust restrictions on our liberty, property, civil liberties, etc.—threaten our status as free and equal persons. Rights thus help define our social status and opportunities as dignified persons in much the same way as the rules of chess define the roles of the various pieces. As Warren Quinn once put it, rights make us all into "small scale sovereigns" (in Wenar 2011: 30). According to this view, the main function of rights is thus to give us control over our actions and property, and over the actions of others with regard to our person and belongings. In short, rights protect our status as autonomous persons.

The rival interest theory of rights is much more concerned with individual and social consequences. On this view, rights are concerned not with our garden-variety interests—e.g., in maintaining a hobby or pet—but rather with protecting our most important interests (Mill 1863/2001; Buchanan 2010). Many of these interests will map nicely onto the territory protected by the will theory; both will want to protect our person from unjustified physical interference, our liberty to hold and enjoy property, and to enjoy the standard roster of civil liberties. But the interest theory will more naturally want to protect any and all human interests viewed as essential to our flourishing as human beings. Thus, if freedom from chronic pain is crucial to our flourishing, advocates of the interest theory might posit a right to palliative care in our health-related institutions.

What might the will theory and the interest theory of rights say about a right to health care? On the surface, we might imagine these two theories as aligning themselves with opposing stances on the right to health care. The will theory, ostensibly more concerned with external encroachments upon individual moral agency, might tend to side with libertarians who argue, as we shall see shortly, that all positive rights constitute a violation of agency and human dignity. It is unethical, they might claim, to coerce some people to pay for the needs of others. The interest theory, by contrast, easily supports a right to health-related goods insofar as such goods are required for satisfying one of our most important interests in a healthy body and mind.

On closer inspection, however, these two rival conceptions of the function of rights might well agree on the importance of a right to health-related goods. Proponents of the will theory of rights could argue, first, that there are many different kinds of threats to human agency and dignity, of which encroachments upon our liberty by individuals or governments only count for one (Nagel 1975; Sen 1999). How much agency or dignity can we expect from a starving Bangladeshi child whose brain is deprived of nutrients by drought and famine? Second, proponents of the will theory could argue that our dignity as human beings resides in our ability to enjoy all the central human capabilities, including health, so powerfully endorsed by philosophers Martha Nussbaum and A.K. Sen (Nussbaum 2011). Like our capacities for free thought, imagination, and association with others, our capacity for health is central to human flourishing, and thus ultimately to our dignity as human beings.

Finally, a proponent of the will theory of rights might contend that a great deal of individual autonomy is consistent with a moderate amount of state-enforced taxation to support the needs of others. Notwithstanding the inflated, hyperventilating language of some libertarians—"All taxation is theft"—one can lead a perfectly autonomous, self-directed life while at the same time cheerfully paying taxes to support the basic needs of others.

Four Theories of Rights to Health-Related Goods

The literature on rights to health care and health-related goods is both voluminous and highly contentious. I shall content myself here with thumbnail sketches of some of the most influential political theories with relevance for our subject, including libertarianism, utilitarianism, Rawlsian liberal egalitarianism, and some versions of communitarianism. As a pluralist with regard to ethical theory, I believe that each of these accounts should be viewed not, to adapt a phrase from the *Lord of the Rings*, as "one theory to rule them all," but rather as a source of valuable but limited insights into the nature of moral problems. I shall address each theory with two pivotal questions in mind: (1) What kind of good is health care (and other health-related goods)? (2) What does each theory say about a putative right to health care?

Libertarianism

In the context of discussions regarding health care ethics, libertarian political philosophy assumes two somewhat different forms. On one hand, there's what we might call "hard-core" libertarianism, which advances an absolutist conception of negative rights, denies any positive rights, and claims that the right to health care is actually an unjust claim to the resources of others (Nozick 1974). The softer side of this theory is exhibited by "soft-core" libertarians, who focus primarily, not on an absolutist theory of negative rights, but rather upon a policy-level preference for individual choice and free markets in the design and delivery of health services, as opposed to centralized state-sponsored health systems (Lomasky 1981). The focus here will be on the hard-core variant, which is more philosophically fundamental.

The pivotal concept in hard-core libertarianism is the rational agent's right to life, to self-ownership, and to choose values in furtherance of one's own purposes (Sade 2008: 466ff). Sometimes libertarians express their fundamental commitments in terms of Kantian language bearing on the right to be treated as an end in oneself, not as a mere means to the ends of others. For such theorists the supreme value is rational agency, or the ability of rational individuals to make their own decisions. This conception of individual liberty overrides all other considerations. In response to those who would on occasion subordinate individual liberty to other pressing interests, such as forcing taxpayers to feed that starving Bangladeshi child, hard-core libertarians claim that liberty alone can ensure the very possibility of human flourishing (Sade 2008: 468). Libertarians of this stripe thus align themselves against statism or any submersion of the rational individual into the larger social body. Borrowing language they could take from a liberal of a different stripe, John Rawls, libertarians stress the "separateness of persons." There is no over-arching social body or organism whose overall utility or welfare is of any concern to us. There's nobody here but us individuals, and the one life we all have to live.

Hard-core libertarianism thus leads to the conclusion that the only rights we have are negative, and that negative rights take up the entire space of rights. It might be a good, charitable thing for someone to feed that Bangladeshi child, but no one, including the modern state, has the right to coerce some for the benefit of others.

The implications of this view for a putative right to health-related goods are easy to imagine. There simply is no such right because there can be no legitimate positive rights. Health care is not special; it should be treated like any other good—e.g., beer and video games—available on the free market for those willing and able to pay for it. Libertarians do believe, however, that we have negative rights to contract with others to provide for our health care, and they believe we have negative rights to health in the narrow sense that others have duties to refrain from injuring our health. But the key point here is that they view a positive right to health-related goods to be a threat to the negative rights of taxpayers and others.

Utilitarianism

Whereas hard-core libertarianism is all about negative rights, utilitarianism is all about consequences. Utilitarians believe that morality exclusively has to do with improving human welfare; they are not fundamentally interested in agents' motivations, natural rights, or the will of god (Goodin 1995). One theoretical problem with libertarianism, in fact, is its insouciance with regard to consequences. No matter how many Bangladeshi children are starving, hard-core libertarians would condemn any attempt to solve that problem through coercive taxation, even at very low, laughably affordable rates. Many people find this to be an unacceptable result for a moral theory. But utilitarians have the opposite problem: They can easily justify coercion in the name of the greater good, but they have trouble (as we shall see, not insuperable trouble) justifying rights.

The basic structure of utilitarian theory is simple: Figure out what the good is for human beings (and other sentient creatures), then attempt to maximize the amount of that good in our actions and social policies (Mill 1863/2001). For purposes of this drastically truncated discussion, we shall assume that utilitarians focus on maximizing human *welfare*, rather than (mere) pleasure or unfiltered personal preferences. At first glance, then, utilitarianism would seem to have trouble with the concept of rights since, as we've seen above, rights are supposed to function as trumps with regard to the achievement of good social consequences. Even if medical science could advance by leaps and bounds if only researchers were permitted to dragoon unwitting subjects into medical experiments, such violations of freedom are not permitted, at least by our common understanding of morality.

Utilitarians respond to this and other difficulties by stressing the importance of rules and publicity in social policy (Goodin 1995). Were any society to permit this kind of license on the part of researchers to draft unwilling and unwitting subjects into research for the sake of the greater social good, the consequence would be massive social anxiety. It would be hard to plan one's day, let alone one's life, knowing that one could be drafted at any moment into the protracted war against disease. Note that this argument against coercion is based on the likely social consequences, not on some notion of natural human rights. Still, the social rules that utilitarians follow in attempting to maximize the social good often exhibit the same functions as individual rights. Even though in a particular case it might be utility maximizing to dragoon poor Jones into a study of malaria drugs, the long-term welfare of individuals and society will be best served by following publicly promulgated rules that require informed consent and so do not permit this kind of assault on individual liberty. For utilitarians, then, there is room for rights in moral theory, but these rights are equivalent to rules formulated to maximize welfare.

This so-called "rule utilitarian" conception of rights falls neatly into the category of "interest theories" of rights. For utilitarians rights are not mystical emanations from nature or god; they are simply rules erected by humans to protect our most important interests (Mill 1863/2001). One of these paramount interests is good health. In contrast to libertarians, who believe that health care goods are nothing special, utilitarians point to the great importance of access to health-related goods for both individual and social welfare. For individuals, health care can rescue us from premature death, disability, and unrelenting pain. For society, healthy citizens will be more productive workers, soldiers, and participants in democracy.

Because health services are so urgent and special, utilitarians think it makes perfect sense to posit a right to health care. They would, however, insist on an important caveat: We would have a right only to those health-related goods that are instrumental in maximizing human welfare. Some modalities of health care are essential—they produce major improvements in welfare at relatively low cost (e.g., prenatal care)—while others are outrageously expensive and offer only marginal results (e.g., high-tech cancer drugs that cost over $100,000 and yield only a couple of additional months of life). Thus, a utilitarian theory of health care rights would most likely encompass prenatal care while excluding some of those new cancer drugs.

Another way to express this would be to say that the utilitarian right to health-related goods only includes those treatments and diagnostics that pass the test of cost-effectiveness analysis (see Chapter 4 in this volume). Utilitarians sensibly worry constantly about the "opportunity costs" of all proposed medical interventions; they wonder whether more welfare could be achieved by spending our limited health-related dollars on other interventions that yield more bang for the buck. So we are left with a very different approach to health care rights. In contrast to the "will theory" of rights, which views rights as trumps against social utility, the utilitarians' "interest theory" restricts genuine health care rights to those that actually promise to maximize social utility.

Liberal Egalitarianism

Although utilitarianism offers an arguably more satisfying response to the Bangladeshi child than libertarianism, it is notoriously vulnerable to the criticism that it allows for some individuals' rights and welfare to be sacrificed for the greater social good. True, many of these charges can be successfully rebutted by stressing the important role of social rules and publicity within moral theory, but many critics remain skeptical of any theory that would make individual rights dependent upon maximizing social utility. Utilitarianism claims to be a liberal, individualistic theory by insisting that "everyone counts for one, nobody for more than one" (Bentham 1907; Mill 1863/2001: Chapter 5); but critics point out that no sooner does utilitarianism count an individual's welfare than it plunges her into an aggregate social utility function in which her rights may be subjected to political bargaining. Hence the worry that utilitarianism is insufficiently attentive to the "separateness of persons" (Rawls 1971).

The most famous critic of utilitarianism in this vein is the late John Rawls, who was arguably the greatest political theorist of the twentieth century. For Rawls, political morality should be all about fairness—i.e., about what rules and principles free and equal citizens could accept as fair to them—not about achieving a maximal amount of anything. Although Rawls was mostly silent about matters of health, disease, and access to health-related goods, his student, Norman Daniels, has provided us with the most sophisticated and powerful non-utilitarian theory of "just health" available (Daniels 1985, 2008).

Daniels begins by providing an answer to our first guiding question: namely, What kind of good is health care? Is it in some sense special? Whereas utilitarians claimed that the specialness of health-related goods resides in their ability to advance human welfare, Rawlsian liberals like Daniels call attention to the close connections between access to health-related goods, normal human functioning, and opportunity within democratic societies. Daniels argues that health care isn't just some garden-variety good (along with beer and video games) as claimed by some libertarians (Engelhardt 1996); it is rather a special good that can correct for deficiencies in "normal species functioning." If we have an untreated compound fracture of the leg, diabetes, HIV, or frightful dental caries, we and our body parts are not functioning in the normal ways that human organisms function. (For a robust critique of Daniels' account of health and normal species functioning, see Chapter 39 in this volume.)

This shortfall from normal species functioning can have serious implications for the lives we can choose to live. If we have disfiguring dental caries, we won't be able to land a job as a receptionist; if we have an untreated compound fracture of the leg, we won't be able to train for the Olympics; and if we have untreated diabetes or HIV, we won't live much longer. Daniels thus points to the important connection between normal species functioning and equal opportunity. Untreated illness or disability closes the doors of opportunity.

It is noteworthy that even hard-core libertarians could agree with Daniels' analysis thus far. They could concede that people in ill health usually cannot take advantage of all the opportunities their society offers to those who can function within the normal range. However, the next step in his argument is crucial: Whereas libertarians would say that this illness-induced inability to compete is unfortunate but not unfair, Daniels responds that in a democratic society governed by a normative principle of equal opportunity, such inequalities are definitely unfair and cry out for social remediation. In making this key theoretical move, Daniels is rehearsing traditional liberal theory. Each of us has a big stake in being able to chart our own life course, and to change that course from time to time depending upon our capabilities and interests. We will thus want access to the full range of social opportunities compatible with our own natural capabilities.

In addition, Daniels argues that, to a great extent, none of us is personally responsible for our place in either the natural or social lotteries. Just as we are not responsible for being born on the wrong (or right) side of the tracks, so we are largely not responsible for much ill health, especially for that which is caused by our genetic inheritance or industrial pollution. (Accounting for illnesses caused by our own negligent behavior, such as reckless driving or obesity, is, of course, another matter, which I cannot address here; see Segall 2009.) Egalitarian liberals are largely reconciled to significant inequalities of outcome within society, but they insist on fair equality of opportunity in striving for such outcomes. For Daniels, access to health-related goods, like access to education, is crucial for securing equality of opportunity. The function of health-related institutions is thus to help compensate for social disadvantages due to social or medical bad luck. Untreated illness in this theory is thus both unfortunate *and* unjust.

For Daniels, then, a theory of liberal equality gives rise to a theory of rights to health-related goods. These are not natural or God-given rights; they are derived from philosophically prior rights to equal opportunity. Just as utilitarians worry about opportunity costs in health policy debates, Daniels would limit the right to health care by weighing and balancing various claims within the category of equal opportunity. Health-related services aren't the only contributors to opportunity. Some services are more important than others within the sphere of health care, just as some opportunity-based social institutions, such as education and public health, might sometimes take priority over health services.

Communitarianism

All of the political philosophies we've canvassed so far constitute big tents housing lots of individual differences among likeminded scholars. It may be that the political theory of communitarianism can boast the largest, most encompassing tent of all, making room for all sorts of theorists on both the political right (Hegel 1821/1991) and left (Walzer 1984), united only in their common rejection of individualist liberalism of the sort we've seen in Rawls and the libertarians. Communitarians fault liberalism on a number of important grounds, including the latter's alleged disembodied, deracinated conception of the person or moral agent, its alleged "asocial" individualism, its concomitant neglect of important community interests, its aspiration to universalism in moral theory, and, finally, its alleged neutrality concerning the good (Mulhall and Swift 1996). Indeed, the heterogeneity of communitarian thinkers makes placing them all somewhere on a map of health care justice a very daunting undertaking (Kuczewski 2004).

We might begin with communitarians' enthusiasm for a politics of the common good. In contrast to libertarians and Rawlsians, who leave the search for the good up to individuals, and the role of referee among competing visions of the good to the liberal state, communitarians often posit a common good that would function as the wellspring of norms in ethics and social policy. Libertarians and Rawlsians alike, in spite of their vast differences, focus on the individual as the proper subject, the alpha and omega, of political philosophy; communitarians like Daniel Callahan, however, urge us to focus instead on what kind of society we want to live in. As he argues in his aptly titled book, *What Kind of Life?*, Callahan claims that liberals start out in the wrong place, with individual interests and rights, and will therefore end up with a bottomless pit of individual needs and desires, with no available breaking mechanisms or limits to the notion of a right to health care. Instead, Callahan asks us to start with the question of what kind of society we wish to inhabit, and derives answers to health-related questions from that starting point. For example, he claims that the point of health care institutions should be to get everyone to a decent old age (say, 75 years), beyond which point the goals of health care should dramatically shift, away from high-cost, high-tech life-sustaining interventions, and toward more modest goals of palliative care and just plain caring. The contrast with liberalism could not be clearer: Liberals eschew the goal of establishing the "true aims" of health care and how health care should nest within larger, publicly founded conceptions of the good life and good society. Many (but not all) communitarians claim that progress on such issues as the ethics of allocation depends upon a publicly shared conception of the good life.

Another major communitarian thinker, Michael Walzer, proposes a kind of *methodological* approach to communitarianism (Walzer 1984). Instead of searching for political truth in some luminous, transcendent realm of theory in a manner reminiscent of the philosopher in Plato's famous allegory of the cave, Walzer's political thinker examines the actual concrete meanings of various important goods forged by actual historically situated men and women—i.e., the writings on the cave wall. By understanding the meaning of any given good in any given society, we can discern how that good should be properly distributed.

Applied to health-related goods in contemporary well-off Western societies, this approach yields the conclusion that health care should be conceived as a "public need"—right up there with police, fire protection, and education—and distributed universally according to need, not ability to pay. In the middle ages, Walzer notes, physicians' services were regarded as the perquisites of the rich and powerful, but access to the sacraments was regarded as crucially important for each person's salvation—hence, a priest in every parish. By contrast, in the modern era the primacy of the soul has been replaced by the primacy of the body and of good health—hence, the quest for universal health care.

Interestingly, Walzer sees an intimate connection between access to health care and citizenship. Whereas utilitarians stress the contributions of health services to individual (and social) welfare, and whereas Rawlsians stress the connections between health and fair equality of opportunity, Walzer locates the specialness of health care goods in their political symbolism. Lack of access to health services, he claims in a riveting dictum, is not only dangerous, it's degrading, signaling a lack of full citizenship (see also Chesleigh 2004).

Walzer wrote about health care justice in the mid-1980s. A contemporary application of his communitarian method is provided by philosopher Paul Menzel, who eschews high philosophical theory in favor of a careful reading of commitments we have already made as a society that provide, he argues, a compelling justification for the central pillars of President Obama's ACA. In brief, Menzel points to our agreement (1) that there should be universal access to emergency room care; (2) that insurers should not be permitted to deny coverage due to preexisting conditions; (3) that those who get uncompensated care from emergency rooms "free ride" on the rest of society's paying customers; and (4) that the solution to this problem is to bring everyone into the system from the very start via a public policy of insurance mandates and subsidies—also known as the ACA. Space does not permit an adequate fleshing out of this argument here; suffice it to say that Menzel's method is Walzerian and communitarian in spirit, and generates a bounded right to health-related goods (Menzel 2011).

What the Right to Health Care Isn't

Although a great deal of ink has been spilled on the existence or non-existence of a right to health care, the "cash value" of this notion is actually quite limited in our public debates over health policy. Make no mistake, it matters a lot whether we acknowledge such a right in the first place. It matters greatly whether we view access to health services as a mere privilege or an entitlement, and whether we view the uncorrected results of the natural and social lotteries as merely unfortunate or also as unjust. Those who would proclaim a right to health care must, then, grapple seriously with the libertarian challenge.

Importantly, however, the notion of a right to health care does not tell us exactly to what health-related goods and services we are entitled; the right does not yield univocal clues to its substantive content (Brody 1991; Arras and Fenton 2009). In other words, the right to health care tells us that some health-related services are indeed special and should not be subject to the vagaries of the free market, but it does not provide straightforward answers to the hard choices we must make every day in health policy. True, it's easy to predict that some treatments will be included within the ambit of a health care right—e.g., prenatal care and ordinary primary care—but beyond that, it's tough slogging. Simply because some treatments might mean the difference between life and death for some (currently identifiable and unidentifiable) patients doesn't mean that they would have to be covered by an entitlement to health care. Consider again those enormously high-cost, low-benefit cancer treatments that provide constant fodder for heated public debate today (Kolata and Pollack 2008).

Whether society should foot the bill for such treatments cannot simply be read off the surface of a putative right to health care. Among a host of other factors, we need to know the cost-effectiveness ratio of such interventions (see Chapter 4 in this volume), whether they target those who are "medically worst off," whether they should be disseminated in largely urban areas where more people can be reached or in rural areas where people already face significant barriers to care, and so on. One helpful way to think about the proper role of health care rights within the larger ambit of health policy is thus to think of them as establishing for each of us a justifiable claim that certain health-related *institutions* be established within which the tough allocation questions will be debated and resolved in a fair and equitable way (Shue 1996). And this, of course, raises the issue of what a just *process* would be for deciding such questions, an important topic I cannot discuss here (Daniels 2008; Fleck 2006).

One obvious implication of this view of rights needs to be brought out into the open. Some people apparently believe that if there is a right to health care, then any explicit rationing of health care must be morally impermissible. Nothing could be further from the truth. If we define "rationing" as the denial of potentially beneficial care on grounds other than the welfare of the patient—i.e., on grounds of cost, opportunity costs, fairness to others, etc.—then health care rationing is both inevitable and morally justified (Ubel 2001; see Chapter 3 in this volume). Indeed, one philosopher contends that rationing isn't just a necessary evil; it is, rather, morally required of us if everyone is to obtain a just share (Dworkin 2002).

In addition to the libertarian challenge from the political right, the notion of rights to health care is also vulnerable to contestation from the political left. As we saw at the beginning of this essay, the concept of a right to health *care* turns out to be too narrow a claim. If we have learned anything from the burgeoning literature on the social determinants of health during the past two decades (Wilkinson and Marmot 2003; see also Chapter 2 in this volume), it is that health *care* actually plays a relatively minor role in the achievement of health itself, especially at the population level. We've known for a long time that major historical shifts in the health status of populations owe more to various public health interventions—such as safe water systems, better nutrition, and safer working conditions—than to the often admittedly spectacular achievements of modern medicine (McKeown 1980). What we've learned more recently is that factors such as social inequality, lack of status, and stress on the job may also contribute significantly to ill health (Marmot 2005). Conversely, we've learned that if we really want to improve people's health at the population level, we should invest, not necessarily in more, better, and ever more expensive individualized health care, but rather in massive expenditures in education, jobs, the protection of human rights, and the leveling of savage income inequalities.

Related Topics

Chapter 2, "Social Determinants of Health and Health Inequalities," Sridhar Venkatapuram and Michael Marmot

Chapter 6, "Bioethics and Human Rights," Elizabeth Fenton

Chapter 39, "Medicalization, 'Normal Function,' and the Definition of Health," Rebecca Kukla

References

Arras, J.D. and Fenton, E.M. (2009) "Bioethics and Human Rights: Access to Health-Related Goods," *Hastings Center Report* 39 (5): 27–38.

Bentham, J. (1907) *An Introduction to the Principles of Morals and Legislation*, Oxford: Clarendon Press.

Brody, B. (1991) "Why the Right to Health Care Is Not a Useful Concept for Policy Debates," in T.J. Bole and W.B. Bondeson (eds.) *Rights to Health Care*, The Netherlands: Kluwer Publishers.

Buchanan, A. (1984) "The Right to a Decent Minimum of Health Care," *Philosophy & Public Affairs* 13 (1): 55–78.

Buchanan, A. (2010) *Human Rights, Legitimacy, and the Use of Force*, New York: Oxford University Press.

Callahan, D. (1995) *What Kind of Life? The Limits of Medical Progress* (2nd edition), Washington, DC: Georgetown University Press.

Centers for Disease Control and Prevention (2013) *Health Insurance Coverage: Early Release of Estimates from the National Health Interview Survey, January–September 2012*. Available at: http://www.cdc.gov/nchs/data/nhis/earlyrelease/Insur201303.pdf (accessed July 7, 2014).

Chesleigh, F. (2004) "Uninsured, Unwanted, Unworthy?" *Hastings Center Report* 34 (1): 48.

Cranston, M. (1967) "Human Rights, Real and Supposed," in D.D. Raphael (ed.) *Political Theory and the Rights of Man*, London: Macmillan.

Daniels, N. (1985) *Just Health Care*, New York: Cambridge University Press.
Daniels, N. (2008) *Just Health*, New York: Cambridge University Press.
Dworkin, R. (1978) *Taking Rights Seriously*, Cambridge, MA: Harvard University Press.
Dworkin, R. (2002) *Sovereign Virtue: The Theory and Practice of Autonomy*, Cambridge, MA: Harvard University Press.
Engelhardt, H.T., Jr. (1996) *The Foundations of Bioethics* (2nd edition), New York: Oxford University Press.
Engelhardt, H.T., Jr. (1997) "Freedom and Moral Diversity: The Moral Failures of Health Care in the Welfare State," *Social Philosophy and Policy* 14 (2): 180–96.
Feinberg, J. (1970) "The Nature and Value of Rights," *The Journal of Value Inquiry* 4: 243–57.
Fleck, L. (2006) *Just Caring: Health Rationing and Democratic Deliberation*, New York: Oxford University Press.
Goodin, R. (1995) *Utilitarianism as a Public Philosophy*, New York: Cambridge University Press.
Hegel, G.W.F. (1821/1991) *Elements of the Philosophy of Right*, ed. A.W. Wood, trans. H.B. Nisbet, Cambridge: Cambridge University Press.
Holmes, S. and Sunstein, C. (1999) *The Cost of Rights*, New York: Norton.
Kolata, G. and Pollack, A. (2008) "The Evidence Gap: Costly Cancer Drug Offers Hope, But Also a Dilemma," *New York Times*, July 6. Available at: http://www.nytimes.com/2008/07/06/health/06avastin.html?pagewanted=all&_r=0
Kuczewski, M. (2004) "Communitarianism and Bioethics," in S.G. Post (ed.) *Encyclopedia of Bioethics* (3rd edition), New York: Macmillan Reference USA.
Lomasky, L. (1981) "Medical Progress and National Health Care," *Philosophy & Public Affairs* 10 (1): 65–88.
Macklin, R. (1976) "Moral Concerns and Appeals to Rights and Duties," *Hastings Center Report* 6 (5): 31–8.
Marmot, M. (2005) *The Status Syndrome*, New York: Holt Publishers.
McKeown, T. (1980) *The Role of Medicine: Dream, Mirage or Nemesis?* Princeton, NJ: Princeton University Press.
Menzel, P. (2011) "The Cultural Moral Right to a Basic Minimum of Accessible Health Care," *Kennedy Institute of Ethics Journal* 21 (1): 79–120.
Mill, J.S. (1863/2001) *Utilitarianism*, ed. G. Sher, Indianapolis: Hackett Pub. Co.
Mulhall, S. and Swift, A. (1996) *Liberals and Communitarians* (2nd edition), New York: Blackwell.
Nagel, T. (1975) "Rights Without Foundations," *Yale Law Journal* 85: 136–49.
Nozick, R. (1974) *Anarchy, State, and Utopia*, New York: Basic Books.
Nussbaum, M. (2011) *Creating Capabilities: The Human Development Approach*, Cambridge, MA: Harvard University Press.
Pogge, T. (2008) *World Poverty and Human Rights*, Cambridge: Polity Press.
Rawls, J. (1971) *A Theory of Justice*, Cambridge, MA: Harvard University Press.
Sade, R. (2008) "Foundational Ethics of the Health Care System: The Moral and Practical Superiority of Free Market Reforms," *Journal of Medicine and Philosophy* 33 (5): 461–97.
Segall, S. (2009) *Health, Luck and Justice*, Princeton, NJ: Princeton University Press.
Sen, A.K. (1999) *Development as Freedom*, New York: Knopf.
Shue, H. (1996) *Basic Rights* (2nd edition), Princeton, NJ: Princeton University Press.
Tavernise, S. and Gebeloff, R. (2013) "Millions of Poor Are Left Uncovered by Health Law," *New York Times*, October 3: A1.
Thomson, J. (1971) "A Defense of Abortion," *Philosophy & Public Affairs* 1 (1): 47–66.
Ubel, P. (2001) *Pricing Life: Why It's Time for Health Care Rationing*, Cambridge, MA: MIT Press.
Walzer, M. (1984) *Spheres of Justice*, New York: Basic Books.
Wenar, L. (2011) "Rights," in *Stanford Encyclopedia of Philosophy*. Available at: http://plato.stanford.edu/entries/rights/ (accessed July 7, 2014).
Wilkinson, R. and Marmot, M. (2003) "The Social Determinants of Health: The Solid Facts," World Health Organization. Available at: http://books.google.com/books?id=QDFzqNZZHLMC&printsec=frontcover&source=gbs_ge_summary_r&cad=0#v=onepage&q&f=false (accessed July 7, 2014).

2

SOCIAL DETERMINANTS OF HEALTH AND HEALTH INEQUALITIES

Sridhar Venkatapuram and Michael Marmot

Introduction

After a number of years during which bioethics seemed to have become static and was even called boring (Jonsen 2000), various internal and external factors are reshaping its scope and methodologies. Two calls coming from within the field are for bioethics to "broaden" and to "globalize" (Wikler 1997; Brock 2000; Macklin 2001; Benatar et al. 2005; Daniels 2006; Green et al. 2008; Millum and Emanuel 2012). However, either call can be understood narrowly or robustly. A restrained view of broadening could mean expanding the scope of bioethics beyond the clinic and the bio-lab, while remaining confined to particular national borders. And a narrow understanding of globalizing bioethics would mean simply exporting the familiar and possibly staid analyses and methods to other faraway places, namely, less developed countries where the discipline is still nascent.

The present chapter discusses the subject of *social determinants of health* (SDH)—how understanding them and reasoning about their ethical dimensions motivates broadening and globalizing bioethics in the most robust sense possible. The increasing and necessary engagement between, on the one hand, the empirical study of the social determinants of human health and, on the other hand, ethics (and philosophy more generally), should motivate bioethics to expand its scope of analysis far beyond the clinic and bio-lab, and even beyond the healthcare sector. Furthermore, the engagement also motivates expanding the scope of moral concern beyond national borders to include all living human beings, as well as those of future generations. Engaging with SDH literature, and the study of the social context of health more broadly, provides an opportunity for bioethics to truly become the study of the ethics of human life (Rose 2007, 2013).

Over the past few decades, while many bioethicists have focused their attention on ethical issues within the clinic and the bio-lab, a large body of empirical knowledge from a wide variety of disciplines and professional practices has been growing around them about the causes, social distributions (i.e., inequalities), differential experiences, persistence, non-health consequences, and possible social responses to preventable disease, disability, and premature mortality within and across countries. Much of this vast empirical literature and surrounding discussions were considered outside the purview of bioethics, or were simply ignored. A sympathetic reading of the history of bioethics could be that in the face of so many pressing ethical issues related to health within the clinical and lab setting, and being a relatively new area of scholarly inquiry, drawing the discipline's boundaries around the clinic and lab was necessary. It may also be that the traditional philosophical tools and training of bioethicists as well as their lack of grounding in various relevant empirical disciplines limited their abilities to recognize and engage with the numerous ethical issues being raised in the growing corpus of literature on the social context and multiple dimensions of human health (Callahan 1980; Wikler 1997; Schuklenk 2003).

So what has changed? What has happened to motivate bioethicists to begin considering more thoroughly the ethics of health in a broader social and global context? The call to globalize bioethics is surely a consequence of increased globalization across all spheres of social and political life. More specifically, there has been the rise of "global health" as a conceptual framework of analysis, partly as a result of new and resurgent health threats crossing borders more quickly (Birn 2009). This has increased both the recognition of many transnational factors affecting health everywhere and of shared global vulnerability. There has also been an explosion of global public health academic programs and research centers in the United States and Europe that seek to work in or across multiple developing countries. Funding for global health has also significantly increased from about $5.66 billion in 1990 to about $26.87 billion by 2010 (Murray et al. 2011). A globalized bioethics thus seems to be responding to such factors as the increasing awareness of global health interdependence, scale of global health inequalities, the global health concept, and increasing activity in the international dimensions of medicine, public health, and health research.

The second call for broadening the scope for bioethics is primarily coming from bioethicists recently becoming exposed to and engaging with epidemiological research on social determinants of health and social inequalities in health (Marchand et al. 1998; Daniels et al. 1999; Marchand and Wikler 2002; Powers and Faden 2008). A broader bioethics would also aim to integrate a number of substantive ethical arguments about health equity, health justice, and global health justice informed by SDH coming from those working outside of traditional clinical bioethics (Evans et al. 2001; Pogge 2001; Sen 2002b; Farmer 2003; Chatterjee 2004; Barry 2005; Anand et al. 2006; Marmot 2006b; Turner 2006; Segall 2009; Ruger 2010; Venkatapuram 2011; Taket 2012).

Historically, bioethics has largely drawn on moral philosophy to evaluate the dyadic relationship between the physician and patient, or researcher and subject, and advances in health technology (Hope et al. 2008; Beauchamp and Childress 2009). In contrast, SDH directly raise issues about social justice and equity, which requires drawing on political philosophy, because SDH illuminate how multiple dimensions of health, including causes and social patterning, are significantly socially produced. From a justice perspective, health is not only a good that is valuable to people which society may try to provide to some extent, it is also unjust if social conditions are impairing people's health (Peter and Evans 2001; Commission on Social Determinants of Health 2008). An SDH perspective contrasts sharply with the common understanding that health is largely an individual phenomenon; that it is a "natural good" affected by random luck and individual behavior over the life course, and best addressed through behavior modifications and access to preventive and curative healthcare (Rawls 1971: 62; Walzer 1983; Dworkin 1993; Rawls 1993: 20; World Health Organization 2000: 4). Recognizing SDH expands the scope of moral concern for health beyond the individual and healthcare to include social conditions. An ethical perspective on SDH raises questions about the morality of the functioning of diverse social institutions and processes, within and across countries, and over time. Such ethical evaluation of SDH requires engaging with social/global justice philosophy and other branches of philosophy as well as various relevant empirical disciplines—those disciplines that examine the health impacts of the functioning of social institutions and process, within and across countries as well as disciplines that develop, evaluate, and implement social responses (Anand et al. 2006; Wikler and Brock 2008).

"Social determinants of health" is a phrase that emerges from the discipline of epidemiology, the science that identifies the determinants and distribution of morbidity and mortality. However, in the present discussion, the phrase is used broadly to encompass research and activity related to SDH in many disciplines and professional practices. Such broad use of the term is intended to highlight that while epidemiological research on SDH has recently come to the attention of philosophers, many disciplines have been identifying and ethically evaluating SDH and health inequalities, and still continue to do so.

Furthermore, the following discussion reflects a view of bioethics as having disciplinary borders and presents various arguments and individuals as being internal or external to the discipline. Since the birth of academic bioethics, the borders of the discipline or "field" have been constantly shifting, as they are now. What criteria should be used to determine whether a philosophical argument or scholar is within or outside bioethics is an important question. However, that question is not directly addressed here. For ease of discussion on the past and future engagement between bioethics and SDH, bioethics is understood in its mainstream form—the study of the ethics of medical care and biological research. While it is true that bioethics is not exclusively that, the calls to broaden and globalize bioethics are implicitly based on the current scope and other aspects of the discipline being identifiable to some meaningful extent. The following discussion brings these two calls into sharper relief by identifying some disciplinary reasons why bioethics and political philosophy have only recently begun engaging with SDH research. It is a necessary and most welcome engagement. But the initial exchanges have not been as smooth or mutually beneficial as they could be. Interdisciplinary engagements can sometimes be fraught with cross-communication, misunderstandings, or feelings of inequitable benefits. With nothing less than moral judgments about the state of societies and the health of human kind being at stake in the ethical evaluation of SDH, the engagement between bioethicists/philosophers and SDH researchers and policy advocates needs to be carefully undertaken.

A final note on language is that while much of the literature in epidemiology and elsewhere uses the phrase "social determinants of health," in actuality, the language refers to the social determinants of disease, disability, illness, mortality, and other such negative states. Moreover, the concept of health itself is contested and in flux (Nordenfelt et al. 2001; Cribb 2005; Blaxter 2010; Venkatapuram 2011). Important advances in knowledge have also recently occurred about various dimensions of "positive health" (e.g., wellbeing, longevity, resilience, happiness, life satisfaction) (Diener et al. 1999; Ryan and Deci 2001; Huppert et al. 2005). However, despite their profound implications for the present discussion we set aside debates on conceptions of health and research on positive health. Unless stated as otherwise, SDH below refers to the social determinants of ill-health and premature mortality.

The discussion is organized as follows. The second section presents a brief recent history of sources internal and external to mainstream bioethics that have highlighted

SDH and their ethical dimensions. The third section focuses on the science of epidemiology, how SDH research is transforming the prevailing explanatory paradigm in epidemiology, and the insights social epidemiology has so far provided. The fourth section discusses some links between SDH and social justice philosophy. The fifth section concludes.

Bioethics and Health Injustice

At least since the late 1970s researchers and practitioners working outside both bioethics and philosophy have been drawing attention to a wide range of SDH and related ethical issues at the individual, social group, and national population levels. An incomplete list includes epidemiologists researching the social determinants of morbidity and mortality as well as the social gradient in health achievements ("health inequalities"); women's health and HIV/AIDS activists; practitioners of social medicine; international health and development researchers; sociologists; political scientists; anthropologists; and economists. Rather than dilemmas posed by conflicting moral principles, the ethical analyses largely involved claims of inequity and injustice related to such aspects as the causes, distribution patterns, non-health consequences, persistence through generations, experience of illness and mortality, and social responses. Many of the identified injustices related to discrimination, neglect, exploitation, egregious violations of bodily integrity as well as poor reasoning in health policies and other social policies that impact health.

Starting in the late-1980s physicians, HIV/AIDS and health activists, international lawyers, and even academic researchers increasingly expressed their ethical analyses using the language of rights, particularly human rights (Mann et al. 1994). However, some philosophers, including some bioethicists, often found these claims unconvincing and incoherent (Wikler 1997: 187). Outside of rights expressly articulated in law, there has been longstanding philosophical skepticism of the idea of "natural rights," and by extension, human rights. Such skepticism of non-legal rights dates back to at least the eighteenth century, when Jeremy Bentham resolutely criticized the notion of natural rights invoked in the French Declaration of the Rights of Man and the Citizen (Bentham 1843). So, for example, every citizen or human being having a moral right to healthcare was received as empty rhetoric (Fried 1976; Daniels 1985: 4–5; Forman 2010). A popular criticism was derived from Robert Nozick's well known argument that things (i.e., healthcare) just do not appear like "manna from heaven" which then can be distributed among individuals. A physician's labor as well as healthcare goods and services are property that belongs to someone with historical and other legitimate claims. Rights language is seen to ride roughshod over legitimate rules of property ownership. But property ownership has been only one among other worries about a moral or human right to healthcare (Nozick 1974; Fried 1976; Walzer 1983; Daniels 1985: 114–39; Glendon 1991; Human Rights Program, Harvard Law School and Francois-Xavier Bagnoud Center for Health and Human Rights, Harvard School of Public Health 1993).

An argument for a human right to health was dismissed as doubly incoherent for invoking moral rights as well as a claim to be healthy, something that is not plausible for everyone or at all times (Fried 1976; Daniels 1985; Toebes 1999). However, more recently, increasing numbers of philosophers have been identifying the moral foundations for human rights as well as a human right to health. While it seems more plausible than ever that the philosophy of human rights and claims of "real world" health inequity and injustice can be brought together, the debates about the foundations and coherence of a human right to health continues to be vibrant and contentious (Pogge 2002; Farmer 2003; Sen 2004; O'Neill 2005; Vizard 2006; Beyrer and Pizer 2007; Arras and Fenton 2009; Harrington and Stuttaford 2010; Venkatapuram 2011; Preda 2012; Sen 2012; Wolff 2012).

Furthermore, a dominant tradition in liberal political philosophy sees social justice as being centered on a social contract (Kymlicka 2002: 53–101; Nussbaum 2006). And for a theoretical social contract to be formed, there have to be some basic prerequisite "circumstances of justice," including a moderate scarcity of resources (Rawls 1971: 126–30). Where there are few or no material resources, there is seen to be little purpose or possibility for social cooperation, so the concept of justice never gets off the ground. Such theoretical structures and assumptions have meant that discussions about justice in resource poor settings (i.e., poor countries) have been a non-starter; justice simply does not apply in those settings. To try to deal with this particular conceptual architecture in social justice philosophy, some initial theorists of global justice aimed to develop a global social contract where the world's resources are commonly held (Beitz 1975; Pogge 1989; Blake and Smith 2013). In any case, the skepticism of non-legal rights as well as the assumption that justice did not apply in poor countries led many philosophers, including bioethicists, to be skeptical or to dismiss the many varied claims of health injustice. Indeed, they may have been sympathetic to the tragedies motivating the claims, but could not recognize or accept the claims as violations of moral/human rights or instances of injustice (Human Rights Program, Harvard Law School and Francois-Xavier Bagnoud Center for Health and Human Rights, Harvard School of Public Health 1993; Miller 1998; Rawls 1999; Nagel 2005; Risse 2006; Veatch 2006).

Skepticism about moral claims to healthcare and health, especially in places where they are most lacking, may be surprising since justice is one of the four well known principles of bioethics (Beauchamp and Childress 2009). But that principle has often been interpreted to relate to the fair distribution of limited healthcare resources across individuals (within a rich society) rather than encompassing the broader concern for the justness of the many dimensions of health, including the causes, consequences, persistence, distribution, differential experiences, and possible social responses to preventable ill-health and premature mortality in individuals and groups (Wikler 1997). One obvious explanation could be that this principle was narrowly interpreted to mean justice only within healthcare and the lab; that healthcare and research is a special moral domain of justice distinct from other domains (Walzer 1983; Daniels 1985). Another possibility is that the moral concern for health was seen to be wholly dealt with by access to healthcare; the social context and causes of health and its distribution were simply not recognized (Walzer 1983; Daniels 1985; Dworkin 1993; Wikler 1997). Poor countries were hardly considered because there was little healthcare there.

The consequence of the skepticism of rights, theoretical architecture and assumptions in social justice philosophy, and the primary focus on the clinic and bio-lab in bioethics has been that alongside the vocal agitation for health rights even in developed societies since the 1980s and the global movements for human rights, health equity, and health justice, bioethics and philosophy have come to be seen as unsympathetic, largely interested in rich country issues, and possibly impotent in addressing health injustice in the real world (Wikler 1997; Landman and Schüklenl 2001; Macklin 2001; Benatar 2004; Farmer and Campos 2004; Pogge 2005). The visible gulf between the focused and rigorous analysis of ethical issues related to the clinical encounter and biological research mostly in rich countries and the social movements, theories, and empirical evidence about health injustices outside of the clinic and bio-lab and around the world presented a challenge to bioethics and philosophy more generally about their ability to be responsive to the world and its most pressing problems.

Internal Voices

In contrast to traditional focal points, a few bioethicists have been engaging with at least some of the ethics of the broader social contexts of health for some time. For example, the growth of feminist bioethics was a direct effort to integrate concerns about race, class, ethnicity, and gender into the dominant bioethics framework (Donchin 2012). And, starting in the late 1970s, Norman Daniels began to examine how the revitalized philosophical debates about social justice could inform bioethics. His focus was particularly on identifying the moral purpose of healthcare institutions within a just society, and how that would inform fairly distributing limited healthcare resources (Daniels 1985). Onora O'Neill has been arguing for going beyond principlism in bioethics based on a broader understanding of the clinical encounter and health issues (O'Neill 1996). Dan Wikler examined the ethics of coercion in health promotion policies (Wikler 1978) and Solly Benatar wrote about teaching medical ethics in the social context of South Africa (Benatar 1994). Indeed, a more comprehensive review would surely reveal others. Interestingly, even as early as the 1970s, a few philosophers showed interest in the ethics of health of people in other, poor countries. O'Neill and Peter Singer made seminal arguments about the moral obligations to address the health of non-citizens, and specifically, in poor countries (Singer 1972; O'Neill 1975).

So three aspects—the ethical evaluation of social factors and institutions affecting health, using ethical reasoning aside from principles, and expanding the moral concern for the health to include people far away—have been present, though largely on the periphery to the main focus of bioethics. These three efforts have recently become much more prominent, and all come together because awareness of SDH explodes out the scope of moral concern regarding health beyond the individual, healthcare, and health research to include social conditions and social inequalities in health. Those social conditions do not stop at national borders. Reasoning about the ethics of these social conditions requires a different approach than principlism that has been common in bioethics. For example, the international causal pathways to ill-health (e.g., new and resurgent infectious diseases) most immediately raise questions about health-related rights and obligations of people within and across national borders, about the morality of social factors driving the exposures to harmful agents, the ethical underpinnings of global coordination of policies, inequalities in access to benefits of relevant research and available medicines, and so forth.

Outside of clinical bioethics, various philosophers have been considering broader ethical dimensions of health and wellbeing, including SDH. Many of these philosophers are represented in the books, *The Quality of Life* and *Summary Measures of Population Health* (Nussbaum and Sen 1993; Murray et al. 2002). More recently, political philosophers interested in global justice have had to engage with the science and ethics of SDH. The foremost issues of moral concern about the "the distant needy" often turn out to be high premature mortality and high burden of preventable morbidity (Chatterjee 2004). Most notably, Thomas Pogge has caught sight of the global social causal pathways to premature mortality and preventable morbidity of the "global poor." In contrast to viruses moving across borders, the global economic and political order is identified as harming the poor. In response, he and others have been articulating the injustice in, and the required just social response to, many of these pathways (Pogge 2002, 2007).

Development Economics

As previously stated, many disciplines outside of bioethics and philosophy have been making important contributions to the understanding of SDH and social ethics for decades. Among these, two of the most substantive and far-reaching contributions come from the disciplines of epidemiology and economics. What makes these two disciplines worth highlighting is that they identify generalizable pathways between social factors and health. Epidemiology is a central source of information on the subject as it is the science that identifies the determinants of disease and death, and increasingly, positive health. It is discussed in the third section. In the remainder of this section, we discuss development economics. It has provided some of the most directly relevant yet under-recognized insights about SDH and social ethics.

Development economics seeks to understand the causes, processes, and goals of economic development (Ray 1998; Rodrik and Rosenzweig 2010). This includes understanding the nature and causes of poverty and deprivation that, in turn, are most often reflected in high burdens of preventable ill-health and premature mortality. Thus, health is central to the study of economic development. Amartya Sen, the economist and philosopher, is widely recognized as making seminal contributions that have transformed the understanding of the economics of development as well as welfare economics more broadly. In particular, he has been arguing since the 1970s that the health of a population reveals a lot about the functioning of a society's economic and political institutions, and what he calls "public action." This assertion is far less anodyne than it initially seems.

Sen seeks to highlight that health—often using life expectancy as a minimal measure—and its distribution in a population are profoundly socially produced through the actions or neglect of social, economic, and political institutions (Sen 1982a, 1997, 1999, 2002a). Sen's assertion, based on a large body of empirical research, seeks to undermine numerous prominent theories and policy prescriptions related to health and mortality, particularly in developing countries. Sen's targets include the Malthusian thesis and its significant influence on population policies and toleration of famine mortality; development viewed largely as growing gross national incomes (GNIs); the "health follows wealth" thesis propagated by the Preston curve which shows a linear relationship between rising national wealth and rising life expectancy; and many more. Sen's many research projects—including the study of the social causation of modern famines, on the more than 100 million missing women in the world, on the explanation of significant differences in quality of life achievements across developing countries experiencing strong economic growth, on the "outlier" developing countries with high health achievements—all clearly connect health achievements and their distribution to social choices, and thereby, social ethics. For Sen, the functioning of social institutions reflects social choices. What is also worth noting is that the reach of Sen's analysis is extremely wide as it is generalizable to all developing countries where the majority of the world's human beings live and, indeed, experience disease, disability, and die. Moreover, Sen's analyses about the role of social choices or public action in relation to health achievements has also been extended to rich countries, thus giving his analyses a fully global scope (Sen 1993; Marmot 2006a; Stiglitz et al. 2009).

Following Sen, other economists have also presented research findings on the links between health achievements and the role of public action, such as investing in medical coverage, public healthcare, school education, and so forth (Anand and Ravallion 1993; Biggs et al. 2010). These findings interrogate the "strong correlation" between economic growth and improvements in health and longevity, and further undermine the assumption of an automatic relationship. The research increasingly being expanded to include developed countries continues to illuminate the causal role of social choices and health; SDH take the form of macro-economic and other social policies implemented by identifiable actors (Stuckler et al. 2009a, 2009b).

Despite the availability for many decades of development economics research and analyses that clearly identify SDH and link them to social ethics, only very recently have efforts begun to join them up with other analyses of SDH, including those in social epidemiology (Marmot 2006b). In fact, researchers of one prominent line of inquiry in social epidemiology who focus on effects of income inequality on health outcomes conclude that SDH come into play only in countries that are above a $25,000 GNI per capita threshold (Wilkinson and Pickett 2009). Below the threshold (i.e., poor countries), absolute material conditions are said to have a more direct effect on health and longevity. Such a distinction between material conditions versus SDH seems to completely disregard the decades of development economics research on the social determinants of those material conditions which, in turn, impact health.

Perhaps there should be little surprise that awareness or engagement with development economics analyses is largely absent in bioethics. Moreover, it has also been missing in social justice philosophy despite Sen also making seminal contributions in these debates since the late 1970s based directly on his empirical research in developing countries (Sen 1982b). A rare example appears in John Rawls' *The Law of Peoples* where, based on Sen's research on famines, Rawls concludes that famines reflect political failures and indecent governments (Rawls 1999: 9). But even he seems to be unaware of or unable to engage with Sen's broader analyses of social choices and health outcomes. However, the situation seems to be changing. Putting Sen's contributions aside, alongside bioethicists and social justice philosophers engaging with epidemiology, global justice philosophers have recently begun engaging with development economics (Blake and Smith 2013). In both situations there are seen to be various benefits from philosophers engaging with relevant empirical evidence and methods.

The next section discusses how SDH research within epidemiology is challenging the dominant scientific paradigm, partly by attempting to integrate insights from macroeconomics, such as those presented above, and from other social sciences. In fact, there are many interesting parallels between economics and epidemiology. Just as there is a distinction between micro- and macroeconomics, we can distinguish between micro and macro epidemiology. And as there is rich country economics versus poor country economics, there has been a longstanding division between rich country epidemiology and poor country epidemiology. As a result, there is much in common between economists' efforts to show the role of social choice or public action behind the state of health and quality of life of individual human beings in poor *and* rich countries, and the efforts of social epidemiologists seeking to put the health of all human beings on the same plane of analysis—within a single explanatory framework that identifies specific pathways of disease and mortality that include determinants from individual genetics all the way to global institutions and processes. In both these disciplinary efforts, ethical issues have been continually highlighted.

Social Epidemiology

Epidemiology is the informational engine of medicine, public health, health research, and policy. Despite its foundational role in these fields, epidemiologists themselves consider it to be a relatively new discipline still in an early stage of development (Rothman et al. 2008: v) While there has been enormous growth in research and in the understanding of epidemiological concepts starting in the 1960s, there are still some disagreements about fundamental concepts. One of the central controversies is whether epidemiology should include research on social determinants (Rothman et al. 1998; Susser 1999; Zielhuis and Kiemeney 2001; Krieger 2011). To put it simply, there is a debate as to whether epidemiology should strive to be a natural science or a social science. Including the study of social determinants would make epidemiology more like a social science. And in the opinion of some epidemiologists, this would make epidemiology less objective, authoritative, and scientific (Marmot 1976; Rothman et al. 1998; Zielhuis and Kiemeney 2001).

Nevertheless, there is a long history of identifying the role of the social environment in the causal pathways to disease and mortality. It is central to the epidemiological work of Louis-René Villermé and Rudolph Virchow in the nineteenth century (Virchow and Rather 1985; Julia and Valleron 2011). It is very much a visible part of community and social medicine that began to flourish in the mid-twentieth century (Trostle 2004). However, as epidemiology developed into a distinct scientific discipline in the twentieth century, its research paradigm was increasingly narrowed down to individual-level factors (Krieger 1994). In contrast, contemporary social epidemiology harnesses the most current epidemiological tools and methodologies combined with sociological analysis to explicitly identify supra-individual social phenomena that affect both the causation and distribution of ill-health across individuals and social groups, within and across countries, and over time (Marmot and Wilkinson 1999; Berkman and Kawachi 2000; Krieger 2011).

Among the many productive insights from social epidemiology over the last four decades, one discovery has been particularly revolutionary. Initially identified by the Whitehall studies in the late 1970s, epidemiologists have been producing compelling evidence that health outcomes (e.g., life expectancy, mortality rates, obesity, and cognitive development, etc.) are distributed along a social gradient; each socio-economic class—defined by income, occupational grade, educational attainment, etc.—has worse health outcomes than the one above it (Macintyre 1997; Marmot et al. 1997; Kawachi et al. 2002). Health is not simply divided between the haves and have-nots; there is a health/illness gradient from top to bottom of the social hierarchy within all societies. Research also shows that the steeper the socio-economic gradient (i.e., the more social inequality there is in a society), the lower overall health and wellbeing of the entire population. Everyone in a given society is worse off in the domain of health and many other life domains than they could be otherwise if there were less social inequality (Deaton 2003;Wilkinson and Pickett 2009).

Prior to the identification of the health gradient, social epidemiology was largely focused on including social, economic, or cultural factors in the individual-level exposure category and seeing if there was a causal inference to be made with disease. The remarkable findings on the social distribution patterns of ill-health now motivate research that can explain both causation and distribution. Unlike most epidemiological studies that try to identify what causes a disease in one individual rather than another, post-gradient social epidemiology aims to identify what causes disease in certain individuals and in differing amounts in different social groups.

Researchers have so far identified a whole range of social determinants (discrete factors and pathways) to ill-health over the entire life cycle, starting from the social conditions surrounding the mother while the child is still *in utero* all the way to the quality of social relationships in old age. To be clear, healthcare is crucial to treating or mitigating ill-health, but social epidemiologists argue that the more influential *causal* determinants include such things as early infant care and stimulation, safe and secure employment, housing conditions, discrimination, self-respect, personal relationships, community cohesion, and income inequality (Marmot and Wilkinson 1999; Berkman and Kawachi 2000). Along with the rapid growth in knowledge about discrete social factors and pathways, a variety of explanatory theories have been proposed. Keeping in mind that most social epidemiological research has been done in rich countries, Mackenbach presents a good review of the extant theories (Mackenbach 2012). The WHO Commission on the Social Determinants of Health presented an explanatory model for all human beings (Commission on Social Determinants of Health 2008).

For most of the twentieth century, SDH were thought to largely affect the poor through material deprivations, or were perhaps an additional factor to the proximate individual level causal factors of biology, behavior, and exposures to harmful agents. However, in light of the many research findings and the identification of the social gradient in health in every society and across societies, SDH are now argued to be more dominant than proximate factors; SDH in fact shape the proximate causes. And where one stands on the social gradient determines the types and levels of harmful exposures and protective factors in pathways to ill-health and mortality. Social epidemiology, thus, has the potential to produce a more general explanatory paradigm for epidemiology than the current more specific explanatory paradigm that focuses only on individual level factors.

What is currently at play in the field of epidemiology is whether micro-epidemiology, the dominant explanatory paradigm during the second-half of the twentieth century, can continue to survive as a general theory of epidemiology in the twenty-first century. For micro-epidemiology to survive, it must at least be able to integrate macro-analysis. The robustness of SDH research over the last few decades compels both intellectually and ethically pursuing further SDH research and the construction of an explanatory paradigm with less "slippage." As it now stands, the individual-level multi-factorial framework, whether metaphorically described as the web of causation or a causal pie, does not recognize "non-natural" determinants of disease and mortality. The model allocates relative responsibility for the causation of ill-health across three categories of determinants consisting of individual biological factors, individual behaviors, and proximate exposures to harmful substances. While the model does not limit the number of different links in the web of causation or pieces in the causal pie, the directions of interactions, or time scales, all determinants must come from within the three categories. Such a causal model clearly excludes social phenomena that influence the three proximate categories of causal factors, and consequently, cannot evaluate the distribution across social groups within a population, or explain differences across populations.

Furthermore, individual biological endowments, the category that seems to be the most natural of the causal factors, can also be significantly affected by social factors. Prior to an individual's birth, social phenomena can profoundly affect an individual's parents' sexual behavior, reproduction, and the quality of pregnancy, which then directly determine an individual's biological endowments and functioning (Posner 1992; Bauman 2003). So, even individual biological endowments are influenced by social factors, making all three categories in the micro-epidemiology model clearly subject to social influence.

The inability of micro-epidemiology's explanatory framework to recognize the influences of social phenomena on the three individual-level "natural" causal categories yields incomplete explanations. Alternatively, we can say that such explanations are only of specific kinds of causal determinants and pathways. Only when the causal links beyond individual level factors—the causes of proximate causes—are allowed into the frame are we able to perceive other types of proximate natural and social causes as well as social distribution patterns (Rose 1985). If micro-epidemiology cannot integrate macro-analysis, a new general theory or explanatory paradigm for epidemiology must be found that can account for the independent and interactive effects of determinants that work at the molecular level all the way up to the global social environment (March and Susser 2006).

Social Justice

In contemporary domestic and global health policy debates, ethical ideas are often used to justify or critique how limited resources are distributed across individuals or for constraining individual rights for the sake of the greater good. But just beyond these familiar and immediate policy questions, there exist far deeper questions regarding how and why there should be social interventions to address ill-health in the first place. What is it about health or ill-health that compels a social response or makes it a concern for social justice? Is it the types of causes of ill-health, the absolute levels of health achievements, their relative inequalities, or the consequences of ill-health that must be addressed as a matter of social justice? There are good reasons to believe that all of these multiple dimensions of health should matter for realizing social equity and justice (Sen 1998b, 2002b; Daniels 2008; Venkatapuram 2011). Even so, how do we then morally evaluate or prioritize the different dimensions of the types of causes, levels of ill-health, and consequences of ill-health in relation to each other? Which dimension should social action address first, second, and so forth? Furthermore, how does the understanding of what matters about these different dimensions change when the moral concern for individuals is supplemented by concern for groups? These various questions show that the moral concern for health is indeed multi-dimensional.

SDH research complicates these numerous and difficult ethical questions even further by elucidating how improving absolute and/or relative health inequalities requires making changes to a range of basic social practices and institutions. The scope of social intervention to address health concerns is much larger than just providing healthcare or addressing individual-level material causal factors. In fact, SDH research explodes the scope of social intervention to encompass all social/global environments as it strives to identify and address any and all possible social determinants of impairments and mortality. While some social determinants are such things as the social bases of autonomy, freedom, dignity, or respect that impact health through psycho-social pathways, interventions to transform such determinants could mean redistributing economic resources and opportunities, material goods as well as choices and duties of individuals and institutions. What this means is that addressing inequalities in the realm of individual or group health achievements will have to manipulate or, indeed, create inequalities in the other realms of individual lives and societal functioning. For example, stable employment is good for health aside from its income generation, through engendering a sense of self-respect and social relationships. Policies that impede firing people may, however, result in less business growth impacting incomes of all employees and national economic growth. Improving health inequalities could result in lower incomes or larger income inequalities.

In the language of social justice debates, mitigating or manipulating SDH means that there must be a redistribution of some valued "moral goods" in different social spheres. While SDH research, including social epidemiology, has provided information on some social bases of causal pathways to impairments and mortality, the literature has given little attention to the possible consequences in other non-health social spheres that would follow from transforming such causal pathways.

Ideally, transforming or redistributing a particular SDH will improve health achievements which, in turn, will create even more positive SDH. For example, engendering the social bases of dignity through creating opportunities for income and wealth could improve health achievements. Individuals who take advantage of those opportunities could in turn create more opportunities for income and wealth and thus, also, more social bases of dignity for themselves and others. Where such a virtuous circle does not exist, however, what sort of criteria shall we use to evaluate if, when, and how trade-offs are made between improving absolute levels and relative inequalities in health functioning as well as how things function or are distributed in other social domains?

There are a vast number of philosophical and ethical issues that need to be evaluated in light of SDH. What is clear is that health has to be a central component of the theoretical and practical evaluation of social justice. There is perhaps nothing worse to say about a society than that its social institutions, and the social choices behind them, are causing preventable morbidity and premature mortality on a large scale. The practical political implications of SDH research is clearly far-reaching within and across countries. Policies for providing access to healthcare, health insurance, or a minimum package of healthcare goods are a necessary but only small step towards improving health and health equity. Policies designed to address the more egregious SDH and health inequalities would require sweeping social reforms that some societies would find hard to consider let alone implement. However, there are also a number of countries which show that it is possible to implement policies that are directly aimed at SDH and improving health equity (World Health Organization Regional Office for Europe 2013). For example, the government of Finland implemented a national action plan to reduce health inequalities over 2008–11 with noticeable positive results (National Institute for Health and Welfare 2013).

Conclusion

The empirical research of SDH extends the moral scope of the concern for health and health inequalities much wider than healthcare or even the health sector, and deep into the basic structures of domestic and indeed, global society (Sen 1998a; Marmot 2006a; Daniels 2008). Many extant approaches to social justice, and indeed bioethics, are simply ill-equipped to evaluate the ethics of such broad relationships between social and global arrangements and ill-health/health inequalities. The disciplinary boundaries, assumptions, and theoretical structures erase much of the health injustices or push these concerns outside the scope of justice. In contrast, development economics and social epidemiology, among other disciplines, have been able to identify and evaluate such relationships. Greater efforts towards mutually beneficial engagements between philosophers and SDH researchers and policy advocates are essential for progress to be made on the many difficult moral questions about SDH and health inequalities.

For bioethicists and other philosophers, what is relevant to the reasoning about SDH is that the currently identified determinants operate at levels ranging from the micro, such as individual level psychosocial mechanisms, to the macro, such as community cultures, national political regimes, and global processes affecting trade and respect for human rights. The possibility that extra-national, global determinants may also have significant impact on the health and longevity of some individuals and social groups requires that the causal analysis as well as the ethical analysis have a global scope. Health is and has been for at least a century affected by broader global factors.

It is a very exciting time in bioethics and philosophy where careful scholarship and concern for real world justice can come together. Evidence about SDH from social epidemiology, development economics and other disciplines can and should be vital parts of philosophical reasoning about the multiple moral dimensions of health. Just within the past decade, there have been a number of substantial philosophical arguments that make it difficult to dismiss offhand the idea of human rights, the possibility of justice in resource poor countries, or the right to health not just healthcare. These arguments have been motivated or strengthened by engaging with SDH research. Such efforts show that we can and do make progress in ethics. So there is much hope invested in thinking that bioethics, following through on its principle of social justice and expanding its scope and methodologies of inquiry to meaningfully engage with SDH literature and research, will bolster the momentum in progress on reasoning about health and social/global justice even further.

Related Topics

Chapter 1, "The Right to Health Care," John D. Arras
Chapter 6, "Bioethics and Human Rights," Elizabeth Fenton
Chapter 10, "Moral Responsibility for Addressing Climate Change," Madison Powers

References

Anand, S. and Ravallion, M. (1993) "Human Development in Poor Countries: On the Role of Private Incomes and Public Services," *Journal of Economic Perspectives* 7: 133–50.

Anand, S., Peter, F. and Sen, A. (2006) *Public Health, Ethics, and Equity*, Oxford: Oxford University Press.

Arras, J. and Fenton, E. (2009) "Bioethics & Human Rights," *Hastings Center Report* 39: 27–38.

Barry, B. (2005) *Why Social Justice Matters*, Cambridge: Polity.

Bauman, Z. (2003) *Liquid Love: On the Frailty of Human Bonds*, Cambridge: Polity Press.

Beauchamp, T.L. and Childress, J.F. (2009) *Principles of Biomedical Ethics*, New York and Oxford: Oxford University Press.

Beitz, C.R. (1975) "Justice and International Relations," *Philosophy & Public Affairs* 4: 360–89.

Benatar, S.R. (1994) "Teaching Medical-Ethics," *Quarterly Journal of Medicine* 87: 759–67.

Benatar, S.R. (2004) "Blinkered Bioethics," *Journal of Medical Ethics* 30: 291–2.

Benatar, S.R., Daar, A.S. and Singer, P.A. (2005) "Global Health Challenges: The Need for an Expanded Discourse on Bioethics," *PLoS Med* 2: 587–9.

Bentham, J. (1843) "Anarchical Fallacies: Being and Examination of the Declaration of Rights Issues During the French Revolution," in J. Waldron (ed.) *Nonsense Upon Stilts: Bentham, Burke and Marx on the Rights of Man*, New York: Methuen.

Berkman, L.F. and Kawachi, I.O. (2000) *Social Epidemiology*, New York: Oxford University Press.

Beyrer, C. and Pizer, H. (2007) *Public Health and Human Rights: Evidence-Based Approaches*, Baltimore, MD: Johns Hopkins University Press.

Biggs, B., King, L., Basu, S. and Stuckler, D. (2010) "Is Wealthier Always Healthier? The Impact of National Income Level, Inequality, and Poverty on Public Health in Latin America," *Social Science & Medicine* 71: 266–73.

Birn, A.E. (2009) "The Stages of International (Global) Health: Histories of Success or Successes of History?" *Global Public Health* 4: 50–68.

Blake, M. and Smith, P.T. (2013) "International Distributive Justice," in E.N. Zalta (ed.) *The Stanford Encyclopedia of Philosophy*, Stanford University, CA: Stanford University.

Blaxter, M. (2010) *Health*, Cambridge: Polity.

Brock, D.W. (2000) "Broadening the Bioethics Agenda," *Kennedy Institute of Ethics Journal* 10: 21–38.

Callahan, D. (1980) "Shattuck Lecture: Contemporary Biomedical Ethics," *New England Journal of Medicine* 302: 1228–33.

Chatterjee, D.K. (2004) *The Ethics of Assistance: Morality and the Distant Needy*, Cambridge: Cambridge University Press.

Commission on Social Determinants of Health (2008) *Closing the Gap in a Generation: Health Equity Through Action on the Social Determinants of Health.* Final Report of the Commission on Social Determinants of Health, Geneva: World Health Organization.

Cribb, A. (2005) *Health and the Good Society: Setting Healthcare Ethics in Social Context*, Oxford: Clarendon Press.

Daniels, N. (1985) *Just Health Care*, Cambridge and New York: Cambridge University Press.

Daniels, N. (2006) "Equity and Population Health: Toward a Broader Bioethics Agenda," *Hastings Center Report* 36: 22.

Daniels, N. (2008) *Just Health: Meeting Health Needs Fairly*, Cambridge and New York: Cambridge University Press.

Daniels, N., Kennedy, B.P. and Kawachi, I. (1999) "Why Justice Is Good for Our Health: The Social Determinants of Health Inequalities," *Daedalus* 128: 215–51.

Deaton, A. (2003) "Health, Inequality, and Economic Development," *Journal of Economic Literature* 41: 113–58.

Diener, E., Suh, E.M., Lucas, R.E. and Smith, H.L. (1999) "Subjective Well-Being: Three Decades of Progress," *Psychological Bulletin* 125: 276–302.

Donchin, A. (2012) "Feminist Bioethics," in E.N. Zalta (ed.) *The Stanford Encyclopedia of Philosophy*, Stanford University, CA: Stanford University.

Dworkin, R. (1993) "Justice in the Distribution of Health Care," *McGill Law Journal* 38: 883–98.

Evans, T., Whitehead, M., Diderichsen, F., Bhuiya, A. and Wirth, M. (eds.) (2001) *Challenging Inequities in Health: From Ethics to Action*, Oxford and New York: Oxford University Press.

Farmer, P. (2003) *Pathologies of Power: Health, Human Rights, and the New War on the Poor*, Berkeley, CA: University of California Press.

Farmer, P. and Campos, N.G. (2004) "New Malaise: Bioethics and Human Rights in the Global Era," *Journal of Law Medicine & Ethics* 32: 243–51.

Forman, L. (2010) "What Future for the Minimum Core? Contextualising the Implications of South African Socioeconomic Rights Jurisprudence for the International Human Rights to Health," in J. Harrington and M. Stuttaford (eds.) *Global Health and Human Rights: Legal and Philosophical Perspectives*, London: Routledge.

Fried, C. (1976) "Equality and Rights in Medical-Care," *Hastings Center Report* 6: 29–34.

Glendon, M.A. (1991) *Rights Talk: The Impoverishment of Political Discourse*, New York: Free Press.

Green, R.M., Donovan, A. and Jauss, S.A. (2008) *Global Bioethics: Issues of Conscience for the Twenty-first Century*, Oxford and New York: Clarendon Press and Oxford University Press.

Harrington, J. and Stuttaford, M. (2010) *Global Health and Human Rights: Legal and Philosophical Perspectives*, London: Routledge.

Hope, R.A., Savulescu, J. and Hendrick, J. (2008) *Medical Ethics and Law: The Core Curriculum*, Edinburgh: Churchill Livingstone.

Human Rights Program, Harvard Law School and Francois-Xavier Bagnoud Center for Health and Human Rights, Harvard School of Public Health (1993) *Economic and Social Rights and the Right to Health*, Cambridge, MA: Harvard Law School Human Rights Program.

Huppert, F.A., Baylis, N. and Keverne, B. (2005) *The Science of Well-Being*, Oxford: Oxford University Press.

Jonsen, A. (2000) "Why Has Bioethics Become So Boring," *Journal of Medicine and Philosophy* 25: 689–99.

Julia, C. and Valleron, A.J. (2011) "Louis-Rene Villerme (1782–1863), a Pioneer in Social Epidemiology: Re-analysis of His Data on Comparative Mortality in Paris in the Early 19th Century," *Journal of Epidemiology and Community Health* 65: 666–70.

Kawachi, I., Subramanian, S.V. and Almeida-Filho, N. (2002) "A Glossary for Health Inequalities," *Journal of Epidemiology and Community Health* 56: 647–52.

Krieger, N. (1994) "Epidemiology and the Web of Causation: Has Anyone Seen the Spider?" *Social Science & Medicine* 39: 887–903.

Krieger, N. (2011) *Epidemiology and the People's Health: Theory and Context*, New York: Oxford University Press.

Kymlicka, W. (2002) *Contemporary Political Philosophy: An Introduction*, Oxford and New York: Oxford University Press.

Landman, W.A. and Schüklenl, U. (2001) "Why a Developing World Bioethics Journal?" *Developing World Bioethics* 1.

Macintyre, S. (1997) "The Black Report and Beyond: What Are the Issues?" *Social Science & Medicine* 44: 723–45.

Mackenbach, J.P. (2012) "The Persistence of Health Inequalities in Modern Welfare States: The Explanation of a Paradox," *Social Science & Medicine* 75: 761–9.

Macklin, R. (2001) "Bioethics and Public Policy in the Next Millennium: Presidential Address," *Bioethics* 15: 373–81.

Mann, J.M., Gostin, L., Gruskin, S., Brennan, T., Lazzarini, Z. and Fineberg, H.V. (1994) "Health and Human Rights," *Health and Human Rights* 1: 6–23.

March, D. and Susser, E. (2006) "The Eco- in Eco-epidemiology," *International Journal of Epidemiology* 35: 1379–83.

Marchand, S. and Wikler, D. (2002) "Health Inequalities and Justice," in J.L.P. Tao (ed.) *Cross-Cultural Perspectives on the (Im)Possibility of Global Bioethics*, Dordrecht and Boston, MA: Kluwer Academic Publishers.

Marchand, S., Wikler, D. and Landesman, B. (1998) "Class, Health and Justice," *The Milbank Quarterly* 76: 449–67, 305–6.

Marmot, M. (1976) "Facts, Opinions and Affaires du Coeur," *American Journal of Epidemiology* 103: 519–26.

Marmot, M. (2006a) "Health in an Unequal World," *The Lancet* 368: 2081–94.

Marmot, M. (2006b) "Health in an Unequal World: Social Circumstances, Biology and Disease," *Clinical Medicine* 6: 559–72.

Marmot, M., Ryff, C.D., Bumpass, L.L., Shipley, M. and Marks, N.F. (1997) "Social Inequalities in Health: Next Questions and Converging Evidence," *Social Science & Medicine* 44: 901–10.

Marmot, M.G. and Wilkinson, R.G. (1999) *Social Determinants of Health*, Oxford and New York: Oxford University Press.

Miller, D. (1998) "The Limits of Cosmopolitan Justice," in D. Mapel and T. Nardin (eds.) *International Society: Diverse Ethical Perspectives*, Princeton, NJ: Princeton University Press.

Millum, J. and Emanuel, E.J. (2012) *Global Justice and Bioethics*, New York: Oxford University Press.

Murray, C.J., Anderson, B., Burstein, R., Leach-Kemon, K., Schneider, M., Tardif, A. and Zhang, R. (2011) "Development Assistance for Health: Trends and Prospects," *Lancet* 378: 8–10.

Murray, C.J.L., Salomon, J.A., Mathers, C.D. and Lopez, A.D. (eds.) (2002) *Summary Measures of Population Health: Concepts, Ethics, Measurement and Applications*, Geneva: World Health Organization.

Nagel, T. (2005) "The Problem of Global Justice," *Philosophy and Public Affairs* 33: 113–47.

National Institute for Health and Welfare (Thl) (Finland) (2013) *National Programmes and Acts* [online]. Available at: http://www.thl.fi/en_US/web/kaventaja-en/national-programmes (accessed December 11, 2013).

Nordenfelt, L., Khushf, G. and Fulford, K.W.M. (2001) *Health, Science, and Ordinary Language*, Amsterdam: Rodopi.

Nozick, R. (1974) *Anarchy, State, and Utopia*, New York: Basic Books.

Nussbaum, M.C. (2006) *Frontiers of Justice: Disability, Nationality, Species Membership*, Cambridge, MA: Belknap Press, Harvard University Press.

Nussbaum, M.C. and Sen, A.K. (1993) *The Quality of Life*, New York: Clarendon Press, Oxford University Press.

O'Neill, O. (1975) "Lifeboat Earth," *Philosophy & Public Affairs* 4: 273–92.

O'Neill, O. (1996) *Towards Justice and Virtue: A Constructive Account of Practical Reasoning*, Cambridge: Cambridge University Press.

O'Neill, O. (2005) "The Dark Side of Human Rights," *International Affairs* 81: 427–39.
Peter, F. and Evans, T. (2001) "Ethical Dimensions of Health Equity," in T. Evans, M. Whitehead, F. Diderichsen, A. Bhuiya and M. Wirth (eds.) *Challenging Inequities in Health: From Ethics to Action*, Oxford and New York: Oxford University Press.
Pogge, T. (1989) *Realizing Rawls*, Ithaca, NY and London: Cornell University Press.
Pogge, T. (2001) *Global Justice*, Oxford: Blackwell.
Pogge, T. (2002) *World Poverty and Human Rights: Cosmopolitan Responsibilities and Reforms*, Cambridge and Malden, MA: Polity.
Pogge, T. (2005) "Real World Justice," *The Journal of Ethics* 9: 29–53.
Pogge, T. (2007) *Freedom From Poverty as a Human Right: Who Owes What to the Very Poor?* Oxford: Oxford University Press; Paris: UNESCO.
Posner, R.A. (1992) *Sex and Reason*, Cambridge, MA: Harvard University Press.
Powers, M. and Faden, R.R. (2008) *Social Justice: The Moral Foundations of Public Health and Health Policy*, New York and Oxford: Oxford University Press.
Preda, A. (2012) Is There a Human Right to Health? in P.T. Lenard and C. Straehle (eds.) *Health Inequalities and Global Justice*, Edinburgh: Edinburgh University Press.
Rawls, J. (1971) *A Theory of Justice*, Cambridge, MA: Harvard University Press.
Rawls, J. (1993) *Political Liberalism*, New York: Columbia University Press.
Rawls, J. (1999) *The Law of Peoples*, Cambridge, MA: Harvard University Press.
Ray, D. (1998) *Development Economics*, Princeton, NJ and Chichester, Princeton University Press.
Risse, M. (2006) "Do We Owe the Global Poor Assistance or Rectification?" *Ethics & International Affairs* 19: 9–18.
Rodrik, D. and Rosenzweig, M.R. (2010) *Handbook of Development Economics* (Volume 5), Amsterdam: North Holland.
Rose, G. (1985) "Sick Individuals and Sick Populations," *International Journal of Epidemiology* 14: 32–8.
Rose, N. (2007) *Politics of Life Itself: Biomedicine, Power and Subjectivity in the Twenty-first Century*, Princeton, NJ and Oxford: Princeton University Press.
Rose, N. (2013) "The Human Sciences in a Biological Age," *Theory Culture & Society* 30: 3–34.
Rothman, K.J., Adami, H.O. and Trichopoulos, D. (1998) "Should the Mission of Epidemiology Include the Eradication of Poverty?" *Lancet* 352: 810–13.
Rothman, K.J., Greenland, S. and Lash, T.L. (2008) *Modern Epidemiology*, Philadelphia: Wolters Kluwer Health/Lippincott Williams & Wilkins.
Ruger, J.P. (2010) *Health and Social Justice*, Oxford: Oxford University Press.
Ryan, R.M. and Deci, E.L. (2001) "On Happiness and Human Potentials: A Review of Research on Hedonic and Eudaimonic Well-Being," *Annual Review of Psychology* 52: 141–66.
Schuklenk, U. (2003) "AIDS: Bioethics and Public Policy," *New Review of Bioethics* 1: 127–44.
Segall, S. (2009) *Health, Luck, and Justice*, Princeton, NJ and Woodstock: Princeton University Press.
Sen, A. (1982a) *Choice, Welfare, and Measurement*, Cambridge, MA: MIT Press.
Sen, A. (1982b) "Equality of What?" in *Choice, Welfare, and Measurement* (1st MIT Press edition), Cambridge, MA: MIT Press.
Sen, A. (1993) "The Economics of Life and Death," *Scientific American* 268: 40–7.
Sen, A. (1997) *Resources, Values, and Development*, Cambridge, MA: Harvard University Press.
Sen, A. (1998a) "Mortality as an Indicator of Economic Success and Failure," *The Economic Journal* 108: 1–25.
Sen, A. (1998b) "Why Health Equity?" in S. Anand, F. Peter and A.K. Sen (eds.) *Global Health Equity Initiative: Public Health, Ethics and Equity*, Oxford: Oxford University Press.
Sen, A. (1999) *Development as Freedom*, New York: Knopf.
Sen, A. (2002a) *Rationality and Freedom*, Cambridge, MA: Belknap Press.
Sen, A. (2002b) "Why Health Equity?" *Health Economics* 11: 659–66.
Sen, A. (2004) "Elements of a Theory of Human Rights," *Philosophy & Public Affairs* 32: 315–55.
Sen, A. (2012) "The Global Reach of Human Rights," *Journal of Applied Philosophy* 29: 91–100.
Singer, P. (1972) "Famine, Affluence, and Morality," *Philosophy and Public Affairs* 1: 229–43.
Stiglitz, J., Sen, A. and Fitoussi, J.-P. (2009) *Report by the Commission on the Measurement of Economic Performance and Social Progress*. Available at: http://www.stiglitz-sen-fitoussi.fr/en/index.htm (accessed July 1, 2014).
Stuckler, D., Basu, S. Suhrcke, M., Coutts, A. and Mckee, M. (2009a) "The Public Health Effect of Economic Crises and Alternative Policy Responses in Europe: An Empirical Analysis," *Lancet* 374: 315–23.

Stuckler, D., King, L. and Mckee, M. (2009b) "Mass Privatisation and the Post-Communist Mortality Crisis: A Cross-National Analysis," *Lancet* 373: 399–407.
Susser, M. (1999) "Should the Epidemiologist be a Social Scientist or a Molecular Biologist?" *International Journal of Epidemiology* 28: S1019–22.
Taket, A.R. (2012) *Health Equity, Social Justice and Human Rights*, London: Routledge.
Toebes, B.C.A. (1999) *The Right to Health as a Human Right in International Law*, Antwerpen: INTERSENTIA/ HART.
Trostle, J.A. (2004) *Epidemiology and Culture*, Cambridge and New York: Cambridge University Press.
Turner, B.S. (2006) *Vulnerability and Human Rights*, University Park, PA: Pennsylvania State University Press.
Veatch, R. (2006) "Are Human Rights Important in Bioethics?" *Health Affairs* 25: 287–8.
Venkatapuram, S. (2011) *Health Justice. An Argument from the Capabilities Approach*, Cambridge: Polity Press.
Virchow, R.L.K. and Rather, L.J. (1985) *Collected Essays on Public Health and Epidemiology*, Canton, MA: Science History Publications, USA.
Vizard, P. (2006) *Poverty and Human Rights: Sen's "Capability Perspective" Explored*, Oxford: Oxford University Press.
Walzer, M. (1983) *Spheres of Justice: A Defense of Pluralism and Equality*, New York: Basic Books.
Wikler, D. (1978) "Persuasion and Coercion for Health: Ethical Issues in Government Efforts to Change Life-Styles," *The Milbank Quarterly* 56: 303–38.
Wikler, D. (1997) "Presidential Address: Bioethics and Social Responsibility," *Bioethics* 11: 185–92.
Wikler, D. and Brock, D.W. (2008) "Population-Level Bioethics: Mapping a New Agenda," in R.M. Green, A. Donovan and S.A. Jauss (eds.) *Global Bioethics: Issues of Conscience for the Twenty-first Century*, Oxford: Clarendon Press; Oxford and New York: Oxford University Press.
Wilkinson, R.G. and Pickett, K. (2009) *The Spirit Level: Why More Equal Societies Almost Always Do Better*, London: Allen Lane.
Wolff, J. (2012) *The Human Right to Health*, New York: W.W. Norton & Co.
World Health Organization (2000) *Health Systems: Improving Performance*, Geneva: WHO.
World Health Organization Regional Office for Europe (2013) *Review of Social Determinants and the Health Divide in the WHO European Region: Final Report*, Geneva: WHO
Zielhuis, G. and Kiemeney, L. (2001) "Social Epidemiology? No Way," *International Journal of Epidemiology* 30: 43–4.

3
THE ETHICS OF RATIONING
Necessity, Politics, and Fairness

Daniel Callahan

The title of this article is meant to encapsulate the three general problems of rationing health care in the U.S.—but I believe it is relevant for other countries as well. Must we ration health care at all and how might it best be done? Can it be done in a fair way? What are the obstacles—political, medical, and public opinion—that stand in the way of rationing? The combination of those questions, each touching on difficult and controversial issues, have made rationing hard to talk about publicly, evaded by politicians, abhorred by the public, and resisted by physicians. I believe that, however difficult, every health care system, however organized, must ration and that its necessity makes it an ethical requirement. There are no theoretical limits to what human beings can want in the name of their health, but there are many practical limits, cost most notably. The issue with rationing is not whether but how.

Hovering in the background is the nature of our health care system and the values that Americans bring with them into discussions of rationing, few of them helpful. Until very recently—and with the obvious exception of the 50 or more million uninsured—most Americans received good and reasonably affordable care provided either through their employer; or if over 65 through the federal government Medicare program, or if poor by state Medicaid programs. That combination began to change with the beginning of the recession in 2008, putting more people's health care at risk. Steadily, long-term rising costs had become a threat to the entire system, reducing employer-based health care, threatening Medicare and Medicaid, and forcing higher out-of-pocket payments for everyone. The respected and non-partisan Congressional Budget Office put the issue in a direct and succinct way in 2003: "to finance projected spending . . . would require tax increases of an unprecedented magnitude . . . under current policy, future generations will be made worse off by higher taxes or lower benefits" (Congressional Budget Office 2003). If anything, the cost pressures are greater now than when the Congressional Budget Office passed that judgment. Those pressures go against the cultural grain, where expectations about good and indeed always better care (through medical research and technological innovation) have been the norm for many decades.

Defining "Rationing"

While the taxation issue is surely important and will be touched on later, this paper focuses on the cutting of benefits, and particularly that of the most expensive and intimidating program, Medicare. Hardly anyone likes that idea of rationing, even when they agree as a general proposition that it will be necessary. The specter of rationing, and even the open use of the word in the political arena, are the flash point for that debate.

To begin, let me say what I mean by the word "rationing." I define the word in three categories: There is *direct rationing*, by which I mean (a) an open and public policy taken by an agency, public or private, to deny needed or desired health care benefits, and (b) to do so in the name of financial stress or on the grounds that the cost of the benefits exceed the value of those benefits. An important distinction is in order here. In the U.S. there is already one longstanding form of direct rationing, that of organs, heart, kidneys, and lungs in particular. In those cases there is an absolute shortage of organs, with the need far exceeding the available organs. Procedures to choose suitable patients are in place to fairly distribute the available organs and will not be further discussed here.

By contrast, what complicates the problem of rationing in the American health care system is that there is no absolute shortage of money for care—we could politically choose to spend unlimited money on health care, and do so at the expense of all other national needs (education, jobs, national defense, among many others). Such spending would make no sense. Because we do not have a single payer government or fully government-financed system as do European countries (what I call closed systems), we are not forced by them to live within a national health care budget. The American system, which I call an open system, has no firm structure for making priority and rationing decisions. Our private insurance sector can set its own rationing rules company by company. In principle, our Medicare program could do so, but has been forbidden by Congress to do that. Our state Medicaid programs for the poor do have to live within a closed budget but any decision to limit a program or treatment is certain to generate a political struggle, well publicized by the media. Sometimes that pressure succeeds in bringing a change, and sometimes not. But supporting Medicaid benefit cuts can also hurt politicians at election time.

The only known instance of direct rationing in the U.S. was in Seattle, Washington, in 1960. At that time, kidney dialysis was a new technology for treating kidney failure, and advances in its use made it possible to keep patients alive for many years. Yet there was a shortage of those devices; not everyone could be saved. The solution to that problem was to establish two committees. One of them was charged with determining the medical criteria for selecting candidates. The task of the other, called an Admissions and Policy Committee, was to choose, as the prominent journalist Shanal Alexander put it, "who shall live and who shall die" (Jonsen 1998).

But direct rationing is not the only kind of rationing. There is also what I call *indirect rationing*. By that term I mean the use of copayments and deductibles as a way of containing the costs of a health care program. Indirect rationing works by forcing individuals to make financial choices about how much they are willing to spend out-of-pocket for their health care. It is an effective technique for influencing choice and behavior, leading many to forego treatment or diagnosis in some cases, to avoid filling prescriptions with a high copayment, or to take only half a prescribed drug to hold down their personal costs. The result has the impact on many of discouraging those with poor financial resources from getting needed treatment, making them medically worse off.

Then there is *covert rationing*, by which I mean decisions made by physicians to withhold potentially beneficial treatments of patients—and to do so by untruthfully telling patients that nothing can be done for them, or simply telling them nothing. There is, that is, no informed patient consent. The most well known form of covert rationing was in the U.K. in the 1960s and 1970s: There should be no kidney dialysis or expensive heart surgery for those over the age of 55. I call that a *de facto* rule because it was not the result of explicit government regulation but, instead, an informal consensus among physicians forced to make do with tight, fixed budgets, and inadequate funds (Aaron 1984). It seemed self-evident that, given a shortage of money, the most expensive procedures had to be foregone. That practice seems to have faded out in such stark terms by the 1980s, but a distinguished British health policy expert, Rudolf Klein, has observed that it is still going on, though in a more subtle way. As he wrote in 2010:

> the most pervasive form of rationing is the least explicit and least visible: rationing by dilution . . . not to order an expensive diagnostic test, or to reduce ward staffing levels in order to balance the budget . . . decisions can be taken in the name of medical discretion and thus be politically invisible.
>
> (Klein 2010: 389)

Obstacles to Rationing

Of all the inflammatory accusations made during the debate about the 2010 *Affordable Care Act* (ACA), hardly any could top former Vice Presidential candidate Sarah Palin's claim that the ACA would create "death panels." There was nothing whatever in the legislation or even the debate leading up to it that involved the use of panels to make difficult individual life and death decisions. But the fact that her phrase caught on in so many sectors and was well publicized by the media reflected a constant theme in the Republican objections to the ACA: That one way or the other, directly or via a slippery slope, medical decisions would be taken out of the hands of doctors and patients and be put in the hands of faceless bureaucrats interested only in the bottom line.

Three forms of resistance to the 2009 ACA legislation became apparent in the run-up to the legislation:

1. Rejection of any form of cost-effectiveness research, or the use of comparative effectiveness research for devising practice guidelines for physicians; even recommendations to physicians were forbidden.
2. A promised effort by Republicans in the aftermath of the legislation to eliminate the Independent Payment Advisory Board; that Board's task will be to recommend direct across-the-board cuts to the Medicare program if its costs exceed a certain threshold.
3. The further extension of objections (via slippery slope arguments) of that kind to other types of government recommendations, particularly those designed to reduce unnecessary diagnosis and procedures in the name of the quality of care, ostensibly not to control costs but that is thought to be a likely by-product even if not a directly intended result.

More resistance to any kind of rationing came when a 2009 report of the U.S. Preventive Services Task Force (PSTF) recommended that mammography screening of women under the age of 50 should no longer be routinely undertaken (Callahan 2012).

That decision was taken by many critics of the recommendation to be an underhanded and hidden rationing policy to reduce costs. But nothing in the panel's decisions and the reasons given even hinted that its judgment was motivated by cost considerations. But it also fed into a combined physician–industry rejection of government regulation of medical choices. Pressures from industry and physicians were taken to be instrumental in rejecting the first two cost control measures noted above and from physicians in the third case. Why? Industry feared government control of prices of their products and interference with technological innovation. Many physicians feared the replacement of traditional physician discretion and thereby harm to what the American Medical Association called the "sacred doctor–patient relationship." That view was dominant in the ACA debate and its aftermath.

What to Ration

In response to the great pressure against rationing of the direct kind, health policy experts and Democratic legislators fashioning the ACA bill worked hard to find methods that would in fact cut benefits, but in a way that avoided both the reality and the appearance of rationing (save for the Independent Payment Commission). The most common phrase to describe that effort was "bending the cost curve," looking for gradual and incremental improvement in reducing cost escalation over a period of years. The bending is to be accomplished in two ways. One way is by bringing greater efficiency to health care by such mechanisms as better coordinated hospital patient care and the bundling of payments, a number of experimental programs to improve the quality of care, improved information technology, and greater support for primary care medicine (shown by evidence to reduce the use of more costly physician specialists) (Friedberg et al. 2012).

The other method is the reduction of waste, which many experts consider to amount to some 30 percent of costs. Excessive use of expensive diagnostic procedures, poor care of hospital patients resulting in readmissions, and unnecessary bureaucratic procedures top the list of wasteful practices (Berwick and Hackbarth 2012). In the aftermath of the legislation, there have been more claims that the elimination of waste and greater efficiency could itself solve the cost problem (Emanuel 2012). I would only interject here that the call to do just that has been heard for at least 40 years, but without notable success. But it raises no hackles in the medical profession and encounters no patient resistance, making it of great political value.

But if, despite that effort, it is insufficient to control costs, and particularly the high annual overall cost increases (ranging from 3 to 6 percent in recent years), then what? The most common response has been to eliminate diagnostic and therapeutic procedures that are known to have no benefit at all and, beyond that, to go after the "low hanging fruit" where the health gains are minor but come at a high price (itself a form of rationing). No one objects in principle to ridding the system of useless or clearly harmful procedures (even though the ACA legislation bars forcing doctors to do so even in light of good evidence of harm). But the idea of going after the low-hanging fruit runs into trouble in practice. It is the "marginal benefit" issue, where the evidence indicates that little harm (but not no harm) will be done by restricting or discouraging a clinical practice.

Another line of criticism raises a different kind of issue, one going to the heart of technology assessment. Efforts to reduce diagnostic or treatment practices that will be marginal from a population or cost perspective will not necessarily be the case from an individual and physician perspective. And therein lies the moral dilemma of evidence-based medicine: The tension between general statistical evidence based on large groups of patients and the good of individual patients in all their human variety, which can be in conflict. Some small number of women not routinely screened under the age of 50 will come down with breast cancer, and will die of it. Most, but not all, of the screening will be wasteful—and sometimes even harmful—with large amounts of money spent to save a few women, but whose lives are of course important for them and their loved ones. Who, then, is to say that the cost of screening is "not worth it"? In any case, the government backed down in the face of the criticism, saying that doctors and patients only should be the ones to decide on the value of mammography screening. A later report by the PSTF on screening for prostate cancer, also recommending some limits, did not draw a similar response, possibly because there are no organized and outspoken lay advocacy organizations in the same way there are with breast cancer.

Rationing and Chronic Illness

The number of Americans over 65 will grow from 40 million in 2010 to 88 million by 2050. That gain in numbers should be enough to scare anyone. But there is even worse news: The largest proportion of health care costs are incurred by those with one or more chronic illnesses (heart disease, cancer, diabetes, for instance). They are mainly older people, and the fastest growing segment of that cohort are those over 80. The top 1 percent of such patients account for somewhat more than 20 percent of health care costs, and the top 5 percent for almost half of all costs. The average per capita cost of the bottom 50 percent is $236 per capita, the top 5 percent $43,000, and the top 1 percent $90,000 (National Institute for Health Care Management Foundation 2012). It is the success of keeping sick people alive longer than in the past that is at once a great medical triumph and the source of its greatest economic stress. An important part of that problem is costly end-of-life care, not just the few days or weeks while patients are obviously dying but during the often longer preceding time when it is not certain whether a critically ill patient is dying or not. In the latter case they are usually treated vigorously with the hope that they are not at death's door (Callahan 2012).

The care of the elderly critically ill from chronic diseases, and who may or may not be dying, is an obvious—and also a particularly volatile—place to make budget cuts for the Medicare program. No doubt better coordination of that care and a bundling of costs would be helpful, but it is doubtful that they could make a great cost difference. Moreover, as the endlessly debated issue of end-of-life care has made evident, it is by no means easy at present to do that successfully (Callahan 2011: 115). The main tactics have been to encourage people to have a living will and/or to appoint a surrogate to act on their behalf if they are no longer competent; and these practices that assume that many people will not want aggressive efforts to save their lives if the cost is simply more suffering. Yet no more than an estimated 25 percent of the population has a living will and it is not known how many have appointed a surrogate, despite a 40-year effort to bring that about (Donley and Danis 2011).

Doctors are now better trained to deal with dying patients, but when chronically ill patients are in hospitals the default position in practice is to treat then aggressively. Some 50 percent of the dying are now under the care of hospice programs, but most of them come into those programs much too late, on average a week or two before their deaths. This lag is the result of foot-dragging on the part of doctors, of families who do not want to give up hope, and a result most broadly of a strong resistance to open discussions of death. Worst of all perhaps, the magnitude of the costs of caring for the chronically ill would require rationing on a large scale, and accepting as well the likely fact that some, perhaps many, would die as a result of curtailed treatment. If that meant direct rationing, the political reality in that case would predictably lead to a condemnation of it. At the least, therefore, I surmise, legislators and health care administrators would find it necessary to obfuscate that reality, either through shifting more costs to patients or quietly encouraging covert rationing.

If chronic illness in general is an obvious target for rationing, close on its heels (though of much lower aggregate costs) are the high costs of many new cancer drugs and expensive heart disease procedures. The cancer drugs can cost anywhere from $50,000 to $320,000 (Sullivan et al. 2011). In most cases their added survival value is relatively slight, from a few days to a few weeks only, a marginal benefit only from a cost perspective. Yet they are also a perfect example of an imbalance between individual patient needs or desires and their burden on the health care system. Their seemingly small benefit is, in the eyes of many patients and their doctors, well worth the cost—and Medicare cannot, by law, refuse coverage on the grounds of cost alone. There have been no successful efforts over the years to change that law (Fox 2005).

Modes of Rationing

I earlier defined three kinds of rationing: Direct, indirect, and covert. I want to concentrate my attention on direct rationing, but will say a few things about indirect and covert rationing. Indirect rationing by the use of copayments and deductibles has been employed by Medicare and private insurers as a way of lowering their own costs by shifting them to patients. The Medicare program costs its beneficiaries an average of $3,000–5,000 per year in out-of-pocket costs and up to $10,000 in some cases (Komisar et al. 2012: 4). This can be a large burden on those with poor income security, leading them to cut doctor visits and to either not fill prescriptions at all or take less than the recommended dosage to delay getting refills. It is a technique which works to hold down Medicare costs, but comes at the price of increased health risk for vulnerable patients. As for covert rationing, that seems to be undertaken when there is a shortage of resources in systems with constraining budgets, and political realities make it difficult for health care administrators to engage in open and direct rationing. That poses an obvious problem of justice for democratic societies, leaving patients at the mercy of *ad hoc* invisible judgments and the perhaps idiosyncratic values of the physicians who make them.

If there has been any bioethics consensus about direct health care rationing, it is due to the philosopher Norman Daniels and his concept of "accountability for reasonableness" (Daniels 2008: 274). The concept draws upon the work of the late political philosopher John Rawls who stressed the importance of public visibility of decisions taken in the name of justice. Daniels amplifies that premise by specifying that principle and three others as constituting reasonableness: Decisions and their rationales must be publicly accessible; they must appeal to "evidence, reasons and principles that are accepted as relevant by 'fair minded' people who are disposed to finding mutually justifiable terms of cooperation"; they must be open to appeals for revision; and there must be "voluntary or by public regulation of the process to ensure that [the other] conditions are met" (Daniels 2008: 118). Closely related to that set of principles is the work of

Leonard Fleck who speaks in terms of "democratic deliberation." That deliberation encompasses "constitutional principles of health care justice, such as a principle of equality, of liberty, of fair opportunity of opportunity, a principle of publicity, respect for persons, liberal neutrality, and reciprocity" (Fleck 2009: 184).

There is much that could be commented on in the valuable work of Daniels and Fleck, but I want to single out the ideas of "publicly accessible reasons" and "publicity." I will do this in the context of empowering public bodies to make overt rationing decisions, and particularly in a political setting beset by sharp ideological divisions. Sarah Palin's emotionally potent attack on "death panels" reflects that reality, but there are two other interesting cases: One in Seattle and the British National Health Service (NHS) means of controlling costs.

I noted above that a kidney dialysis shortage in Seattle led to the establishment of a committee to decide who would have access to the machine. It ran into considerable criticism. It was for one thing an anonymous committee, and for another its criterion for decision-making was that of "social worth." It is understandable that it was anonymous, protecting the committee members from direct attack for their decisions, but then of course its decisions did not meet the publicity and openness standard. But could the committee have proceeded successfully in any other way? There is no way of answering that question. In any event, Dr Belding Scribner, a research leader on dialysis, later said that "we had been naive" to think that what seemed to be a "reasonable and simple solution" of "letting a committee of responsible members of the community choose patients" would evoke a "serious storm of criticism" (Jonsen 1998: 211). Moreover, it was reported that the committee itself had great difficulty in making decisions: Just what is "social worth" anyway? Some bioethicists entered the fray, with some opting for a simple lottery as the fairest method of choosing, and others supporting a social worth standard. The Seattle experience is not one that other countries are likely to repeat.

The experience in the U.K. of the National Institute for Health and Care Excellence (NICE), established to give advice to the NHS on allowing new (and sometimes old) technologies to be paid for by the government, offers a cautionary tale. One of the main economic tools used by NICE is the use of quality-adjusted life years (QALYs). Since there is another paper in this volume on QALYs (see Chapter 4 in this volume), I will not spell out how it works. But I will note that the decisions of NICE do not escape the eyes of the media. In a few cases, particularly with expensive cancer drugs, the media often turn them into public controversies, typically interviewing the usually anguished cancer victims and their families who might be denied the drugs. In some cases, the NHS backs down or agrees to further studies; and in others the complaints are taken to court (Steinbrook 2008).

Publicity, in a word, is sufficient to create problems for the NHS, which makes the final decision. One criticism of NICE, ironically, is that it does not encompass the views of individual patients, suggesting that it should find ways of doing so—a path that could lead back to individual decision procedures reminiscent of the U.S. Seattle committee (Speight and Reaney 2009). Interestingly, however, NICE approves new therapies in the large majority of cases, thus often increasing costs. Its approvals are automatically accepted by the NHS while its disapprovals are treated as recommendations only, and turn out to be little more than 10 percent of its decisions (Steinbrook 2008).

It is probably no accident that it is hard to find instances anywhere in the world where rationing decision committees have been used and actually adopted the rigorous standards proposed by Daniels and Fleck. Can there be effective and politically acceptable "democratic deliberation" on volatile matters of life and death, with publicly known winners and losers? I have come to doubt it. The fact that Republicans have particularly targeted the Independent Payment Commission, with its capacity for making blunt cuts in the annual Medicare budget, conveys a profound unwillingness to give government agencies that kind of rationing power. And even some of those who favor benefit cuts resist such blunt cuts on the grounds that they could well be unfair to many, systematically indifferent to their variable patient impact. It is hard to imagine, however, what kind of deliberation and decision procedures would work to deal fairly with variable impacts. They would surely be complicated and inherently contentious.

Is Open and Fair Rationing Possible?

I have not painted a bright future for the possibility of open and fair rationing. That the U.K. is now still seeing the covert kind reflects how difficult it can be in practice to make it an open and transparent process. A 2007 study of rationing in four European countries—the U.K., Italy, Norway, Switzerland—found that covert rationing is common, and that the reasons can include patient age and cognitive impairment (Hurst et al. 2007). My own experience over many years in questioning European physicians about rationing in their countries is that I always get vague answers, suggesting that it is a topic that neither they, nor their legislators, like to talk about publicly.

Some years ago two prominent legal scholars wrote a book called *Tragic Choices*, arguing that some delicate and difficult problems in public policy simply could not be treated in a fully open way (Calabresi and Bobbit 1978). They got plenty of criticism for the likely unfairness and other drawbacks of veiled or covert decisions. But they had a point, at least if the experience with open health care rationing shows how hard it is to implement fair and publicly accessible decision-making procedures. Accountability for reasonableness, however theoretically appealing it might be for policy making, may simply be unworkable for health care rationing.

Where might we better look? My own view, in light of that pessimistic judgment, is that modern medicine has created background conditions for the delivery of health care that are the ultimate causes of the cost problems—now experienced by every industrialized country regardless of how its health care system is organized (and they are all different). Some do better than others, and the U.S. has the worst problems, but all have annual health care increases exceeding the annual growth of their gross domestic product. That is the standard most countries aim for, and none succeed. For all countries, rising costs are a source of anxiety and reform efforts. Steadily rising health care costs are simply not sustainable in the long run. Tinkering with the delivery mechanisms of health care with overt rationing is not likely to make a great difference in a way that is politically tolerable.

Changing the Goals of Medicine

There are three main drivers of health care costs, affecting every country's health care system: Aging societies, new and intensified use of medical technologies, and public demand and expectations. Behind all three of them is a model and vision of medicine more or less guaranteed to drive up costs. I call it a progress and innovation model. Its aim everywhere is more and better health for everyone. Medical progress as an ideal has no finite goals: It always seeks more. Technological innovation, its main tool and knowing no inherent limits, is always an open and beckoning frontier with endless vistas of possibility. Patients and would-be patients have come to embrace and expect that kind of medicine. Yet the net result has not been to come anywhere near the conquest of disease. Instead that model has given us a medicine that offers few definitive cures, but can expensively prolong dying bodies, especially from the chronic diseases of aging. What I call "the great tradeoff" is a mixed blessing: We live with much longer lives than our ancestors but with much greater illness in old age; and we are subject to extended suffering, and high costs.

The underlying medical model must be changed if an affordable and sustainable medicine and health care is to be achieved and the need to ration minimized. An important part of that goal will be to understand that we all die. The culturally ingrained medical effort to fight endlessly against death is a losing cause. An aging marked by an extended life with painful and crippling disease is hardly a benefit. To be even more specific, I believe that by 80, people will have achieved most that a human life can give us (if not necessarily everything one might desire): Education, work, travel, and family, for instance.

The goal of medicine should be to keep us alive and in good shape until 80 but should be under no obligation to help us become indefinitely older. I say this as one who is 83. I trust I will be missed when I die by my family and friends, but the country will be able to manage well enough without me. Others will take my place, as they have always done in the passing of the generations.

I propose a model for the future of medicine and the health care system to go with it. Imagine a pyramid. At the broadest bottom level is public health (e.g., sanitation, disease surveillance, prevention), and efforts to improve the socio-economic determinants of good health (income, education, jobs, public and industrial safety). At the next level is primary and emergency care medicine. Still one level up is general hospital care, and at the level above that advanced and ICU care (but the latter only for those who have a reasonably good prognosis). At the top would be the most expensive technological care (e.g., expensive cancer and heart procedures) to be allowed only with an exceptionally good prognosis. The aim of the health care system would be to make care at the top of the pyramid relatively hard to get, aiming to push everyone down the pyramid as far as possible, from the higher to the lower levels.

To be sure, that would be a rationing scheme, but one that will be increasingly plausible if it set more finite goals for medicine, aiming to get a better balance between care and cure, and bringing about a fundamental change in the way people think about health care. It is indeed utopian, but I have provided a variety of reasons why the most conventional ideas about rationing will fail, mainly because rationing is exceedingly hard and filled with traps of one kind or another. Health care systems can attempt to ration health care, but that task becomes insuperable if built on an underlying model of medical progress that has limitless research and curative goals.

What I can imagine emerging is a hybrid system of rationing. It would combine four elements. First, cost-effectiveness and comparative-effectiveness research would be used to generate reliable data assessing the efficacy of technologies, new and old. Second, with that data in hand the government would then lay down some recommended rules and guidelines of a general kind for the treatment of various costly conditions, those at or near the top of the pyramid. Research on prognosis, already underway, would be improved so that it would have reliability with chronically ill patients (Smith 2011; Yourman et al. 2012). Fourth, information technology would be used to keep track of doctor–patient decisions (or at least a good sample of them) in light of the general government guidelines. The assessment standards now used by the U.S. PSTF offer a good model for doing that (categorizing different levels of technology effectiveness).

Adjustments would be made if it became clear that the recommended guidelines were not effective or widely ignored. The principles of "Accountability for Reasonableness" and those offered by Leonard Fleck could be used at the second stage, and that would have to be the work of a committee. But fifth, in taking account of the nature of cost-effectiveness and comparative-effectiveness research, which of necessity is based on population studies, and that of the individual differences among patients, some degree of physician discretion and judgment will in the end always be necessary. And their experience in trying to follow the guidelines can be used to change or improve them.

In sum, this hybrid model is meant to deal with the most common challenge to rationing schemes: That of finding a middle ground between (a) fear of the impersonality and insensitivity to individual patient differences and physician judgments that are widely thought to go with government domination of medical practice, and yet (b) the need to have some central government agency or committee assess the evidence, balance cost benefits and formulate recommended, not commanded, national standards. Each side is given a role, and each side interacts with the other. But the key necessity to make that strategy feasible is that of a finite model of medicine, one that will change the way the goals of medicine are understood in the future.

Related Topics

Chapter 1, "The Right to Health Care," John D. Arras
Chapter 4, "QALYs, DALYs, and Their Critics," Greg Bognar
Chapter 7, "Ethical Challenges of Distributing Limited Health Resources in Low-Income Countries," Kjell Arne Johansson

References

Aaron, H.J. (1984) *The Painful Prescription: Rationing Hospital Care*, Washington, DC: The Brookings Institution.

Berwick, D. and Hackbarth, A. (2012) "Eliminating Waste in U.S Health Care," *Journal of the American Medical Association* 307: 1513–16.

Calabresi, G. and Bobbit, P. (1978) *Tragic Choices*, New York: Norton.

Callahan, D. (2011) "End of Life Care: A Philosophical Or Management Problem?" *The Journal of Law, Medicine & Ethics* 39: 114–20.

Callahan, D. (2012) "Health Technology Assessment Implementation: The Politics of Ethics," *Medical Decision Making* 32: E13–19.

Congressional Budget Office (2003) *Long-Term Budget Outlook*, Washington, DC: Congressional Budget Office.

Daniels N. (2008) *Just Health: Meeting Health Needs Fairly*, Cambridge: Cambridge University Press.

Donley, G. and Danis, M. (2011) "Making the Case for Talking to Patients about the Costs of End-of-Life Care," *Journal of Law, Medicine & Ethics* 39: 183–93.

Emanuel, E. (2012) "A Systemic Approach to Containing Health Care Spending," *New England Journal of Medicine* 312: 949–54.

Fleck, L. (2009) *Just Caring: Health Care Rationing and Democratic Deliberation*, New York: Oxford University Press.

Fox, J. (2005) "Medicare Should, But Cannot, Consider Cost: Legal Impediments to a Sound Policy," *Buffalo Law Review* 53: 577–633.

Friedberg, M., Hussey, P. and Schneider, E. (2012) "Primary Care: A Critical Review of the Evidence on Quality and Costs of Health Care," *Health Affairs* 29 (5): 766–72.

Hurst, S., Reiter-Theil, S., Perrier, A., Forde, R., Slowther, A.M., Pegoraro, R. and Danis, M. (2007) "Physician's Access to Ethics Support Services in Four European Countries," *Health Care Analysis* 15: 321–35.

Jonsen, A. (1998) *The Birth of Bioethics*, New York: Oxford University Press.

Klein, R. (2010) "Rationing in the Fiscal Ice Age," *Health Economics, Policy and Law* 5: 389–96.

Komisar, H.L., Cubanski, J., Dawson, L. and Neuman, P. (2012) *Key Issues in Understanding the Economic and Health Security of Current and Future Generations of Seniors*. Issue Brief, Henry J. Kaiser Family Foundation.

National Institute for Health Care Management Foundation (2012) *The Concentration of Health Care Spending*. NIHCM Data Brief, Washington DC: NIHCM Foundation.

Smith, A.K. (2011) "Discussing Prognosis with the Very Elderly," *New England Journal of Medicine* 365: 2149–50.

Speight, J. and Reaney, M. (2009) "Wouldn't It Be Nice to Consider Patients' Views When Rationing Health Care?" *British Medical Journal* 338: b85.

Steinbrook, R. (2008) "Saying No Isn't NICE: The Travails of Britain's Institute for Health and Clinical Excellence," *Journal of the American Medical Association* 307: 182.

Sullivan, R., Peppercorn, J., Sikora, K., Zalcberg, J., Meropol, N.J., Amir, E. et al. (2011) "Delivering Affordable Cancer Care in High-Income Countries," *Lancet Oncology* 12: 933–80.

Yourman, L.C., Lee, S.J., Schonberg, M.A., Widera, E.W. and Smith, A.K. (2012) "Prognosis Indices for Older Adults," *Journal of the American Medical Association* 182: 182–5.

4

QALYs, DALYs, AND THEIR CRITICS

Greg Bognar

Introduction

Bioethics has its roots in the physician–patient relationship. For a long time, bioethicists mainly focused on ethical issues in clinical practice and medical research. More recently, however, there has been an increasing interest in the health of populations. Some of the factors that have fueled this interest are the heightened awareness of inequalities in health between different groups and populations, the recognition of the health-related causes and consequences of poverty, the aging of societies, and perhaps most importantly, the increasing costs of health care.

There are many ways bioethicists can contribute to the discussion of these issues. For instance, they can work out principles of justice that can be applied to domestic and global health inequalities. They can address ethical questions in public health. And they can help clarify the conceptual and normative questions that arise in the measurement of population health and the allocation of health resources. In this chapter, my focus will be on the last of these contributions.

Measuring the Value of Health

Health policy is concerned with maintaining and promoting the health of the population and with reducing health inequalities. It also has to take into account the fact that resources for health are limited. To achieve its aims, health policy needs to ensure that scarce resources are allocated fairly and efficiently. This requires the measurement of health. In the absence of a measure, it would be impossible to determine which policies are more efficient or fair. A measure of health is needed for identifying health inequalities, for carrying out economic analysis of interventions and health services, for monitoring their impact, and for comparing the health of populations.

The simplest measures of population health include life expectancy, overall mortality rates at different ages, and mortality rates from specific causes. If life expectancy at birth in one country is greater than in another, then its population may be considered healthier. One advantage of expressing population health in terms of life expectancy at birth is that it yields a single, summary value that can be used to represent the overall health of the population.

Life expectancy and mortality rates, however, are very crude measures. They reflect only premature mortality. They do not reflect morbidity at all. But morbidity should obviously be part of any measure of health.

One way to account for morbidity is to calculate the incidence and prevalence rates of different diseases and health conditions within a population. (Incidence is the rate of new cases in the population during a time period. Prevalence is the ratio of the total number of cases to the whole population.) But this approach has at least two limitations. First, it makes it impossible to express population health with a summary value. Health conditions are diverse. Using only incidence or prevalence rates, it is difficult to determine whether a population with a high prevalence of malaria, for instance, is healthier than a population with a high prevalence of diabetic disease.

Second, incidence and prevalence rates do not adequately reflect morbidity. Different diseases cause different functional limitations. They have different impacts on people's physical, psychological, cognitive, and social functioning. A measure of health should reflect these limitations, since ultimately what we care about is the impact of morbidity on quality of life. Thus, health should be measured by its impact on quality of life. In other words, a measure of health should be a measure of the *value* of health.

Any adequate measure of health, therefore, must be evaluative. It must reflect the *badness* of ill-health: The way different health conditions affect quality of life by limiting functioning. An adequate measure of health must combine mortality and morbidity through their impact on quality of life.

Evaluative measures of health come in many forms. The most commonly used are *quality-adjusted life years* (QALYs) and *disability-adjusted life years* (DALYs). They differ with respect to what they try to measure, the way they combine the harms of mortality and morbidity, and the way they establish a summary value for population health.

QALYs

QALYs are derived from *health state descriptions*. A health state is defined by levels of functioning in different aspects of health. A patient who has difficulties with mobility but no pain is in a different health state than a patient who has no difficulties with mobility but has frequent pain. A patient with severe depression is in a different health state than a patient who struggles with substance abuse. By specifying the levels of physical, psychological, cognitive, social or other kinds of functioning, any number of health states can be defined. These can also be used to describe the outcomes of different interventions. For this reason, health states are also called *health outcomes*.

The key step in QALY measurement is the evaluation of health states. This is usually done through empirical surveys, using small samples of the population. Several methods can be used for eliciting evaluations. For instance, respondents may be asked to indicate their valuation of particular health states on a visual scale. Alternatively, the value of health states can be established indirectly, by asking respondents to answer trade-off questions. One method requires respondents to indicate their preferences in situations where they have to sacrifice some time spent in good health for the sake of avoiding some health outcome with functional limitations. For instance, suppose respondents would be indifferent between 7 years in full health and 10 years with a particular health outcome. In this case, the value of the health outcome is set at 0.7. (This method is called the time trade-off method.) In another method, respondents have to determine the probability of death they would be willing to risk to avoid some health outcome. They are asked to consider a choice in which they can either live with a particular health outcome for a certain amount of time, or undergo a risky treatment that can either return them to full health for the same amount of time with probability p, or lead to instant death with probability $(1 - p)$. The value of the health outcome is determined by the value of p at which respondents would be indifferent between the treatment and living with the health outcome. For instance, if $p = 0.7$, then the value of the health outcome is set at 0.7. (This is known as the standard gamble method.)

The evaluations that emerge from using these methods are on a numerical scale between 1 and 0, where 1 represents perfect health and 0 represents a health outcome that is no better than death. All health outcomes are assigned values along the scale. The values are interpreted as the *health-related quality of life* associated with health outcomes. They represent how bad (or good) different health outcomes are.

The health-related quality of life scale is an interval scale. This means that the differences between pairs of values can be compared. Hence it becomes possible to compare changes in health-related quality of life. For instance, a treatment that increases health-related quality of life from 0.4 to 0.6 and another that increases it from 0.8 to 1 result in improvements of the same magnitude. Thus, it can be determined which alternative treatment results in the greatest improvement. Interventions that target different conditions can be compared by their impact on health-related quality of life.

A QALY is a combination of the health-related quality of life associated with health outcomes and the time spent with those health outcomes. For convenience, years are used as the unit of time. The numbers on the health-related quality of life scale are used as quality adjustment factors. Thus, 1 year in full health has the QALY value of 1; 1 year at the health-related quality of life level of 0.5 has a QALY value of 0.5. Consequently, 1 QALY can represent a year in full health, or 2 years with a health outcome whose value is 0.5, or 4 years of life with a health outcome whose value is 0.25, and so on.

For example, suppose a cancer treatment provides, on average, a remission of 5 years, but it is accompanied by severe functional limitations. The health-related quality of life during these years is 0.3. An alternative treatment provides, on average, 4 years of remission, but it is accompanied by less severe functional limitations, so that the health-related quality of life during these years is 0.4. The first treatment results, on average, in 1.5 QALYs (5×0.3) per patient, and the second treatment results in 1.6 QALYs (4×0.4). Since the second treatment results in more QALYs, it brings about a greater health improvement. Other things being equal, it can be considered better—that is, it offers a greater benefit for patients.

QALYs are usually calculated for alternative treatments and interventions, but they can also be used as a summary measure of population health. To take an obviously oversimplified example, suppose that people in a population have a life expectancy of 75 years at birth. They typically spend 65 years in full health, then 5 years at the health-related quality of life level 0.8 and another 5 years at 0.6. Their *health-adjusted life expectancy* (also known as HALE) is 72 years. Compared with another population, people in this population may have a lower life expectancy, but a higher HALE. Taking into account both mortality and morbidity, this population may be considered healthier.

Needless to say, things are much more complicated in practice. Life expectancies change with age and time. Health outcomes differ across patient groups. For estimating QALYs, researchers must use standard life tables for calculating life expectancies, observational studies of cohorts, epidemiological data, mathematical models based on the outcomes of clinical research, and other sources of information.

QALYs have been used since the late 1960s in health economics and health policy. Their primary use has been in *cost-effectiveness analysis*, a method for evaluating the aggregate health benefits of different interventions and health services, taking into account their costs. Health economists calculate cost-effectiveness ratios for interventions by dividing their costs by their health benefits, expressed in QALYs. The smaller this ratio, the more cost-effective the intervention is.

Suppose two interventions have the same outcomes in terms of QALYs. One of them, however, costs more than the other. The cheaper intervention, therefore, is more cost-effective, since it realizes the same health benefits for a lower cost. More often, however, interventions differ both in terms of costs and benefits. One intervention may require fewer resources, but result in fewer QALYs; another intervention may be more costly but result in more QALYs. Cost-effectiveness analysis can determine which of these interventions is "better value for money." The one with the lower cost-effectiveness ratio yields greater benefits per unit of cost.

Interventions and health services can be ranked according to their cost-effectiveness ratios, and policy makers can use these rankings to decide how to allocate resources by excluding interventions and services with unfavorable ratios. They can use cost-effectiveness analysis to determine which interventions should be funded publicly or covered in a health insurance package. In practice, policy makers are usually interested in *incremental cost-effectiveness*—comparing the benefits of a new intervention, with the additional resources it requires, to the costs and benefits of interventions already in place.

In the United Kingdom, for instance, the National Institute for Health and Care Excellence (NICE) advises the National Health Service (NHS) on cost-effectiveness. It considers new interventions and services to be worth providing in the health care system when their incremental cost-effectiveness ratio is lower than approximately £20,000–30,000 per QALY (Rawlins and Culyer 2004).

The idea that resources for health should be allocated by using cost-effectiveness analysis is often characterized by its critics as the simple view that the maximization of QALYs should be the only objective of health resource allocation (e.g., Harris 1987). This is both imprecise and somewhat unfair. It is imprecise because, as we have just seen, QALYs are used in a more complex way in cost-effectiveness analysis. It is also unfair because very few health economists and policy experts would argue that cost-effectiveness should be the *only* morally relevant consideration in health resource allocation.

In the last two decades, a second evaluative measure has also become prevalent. I will briefly present its methodology before returning to the ethical issues of using QALYs for setting priorities in health care.

DALYs

The Global Burden of Disease (GBD) project began in the early 1990s with the support of the World Health Organization (WHO) and the World Bank. Its aim is to quantify the burden of mortality and morbidity from disease and injury in different regions of the world. The GBD studies use DALYs as their measure of the value of health. DALYs are designed to compare the health of different populations, to assist in international health and development policy, and to be used in cost-effectiveness analysis.

As new data became available in the last two decades, the GBD project has published a number of updates. The most recent is the 2010 update, which also introduces a number of methodological revisions (*The Global Burden of Disease Study 2010*). Some of the revisions were prompted by ethical objections. The overview below reflects the most recent methodology, but it also traces some of the debates.

Originally, DALYs were designed to represent the badness of particular diseases and injuries. Disability weights were assigned to conditions such as HIV, malaria, ischemic heart disease, and so on. In the early GBD studies, approximately 800 conditions were included, many of them in both treated and untreated forms (Murray and Lopez 1996).

The 2010 version takes a somewhat different approach. It begins by identifying slightly less than 300 general causes of disease and injury. They include such diverse causes as cancers, different forms of heart disease, malaria, rheumatoid arthritis, Down's syndrome, road injuries, falls, and so on. Of course, these causes may lead to different pathological conditions. Thus, each cause is associated with a number of pathological conditions—called *sequelae*. Altogether, the cause sequelae list has 1,160 pathological conditions. Therefore, at the most general level, there are causes of disease and injury. At the next level, there are different conditions as the consequences of those causes. For instance, anemia is associated with 19 items on the cause list, including malaria, maternal hemorrhage, iron deficiency, peptic ulcer disease, and sickle cell disorder.

Anemia, of course, can be more or less severe. Thus, from the perspective of the burden of different pathological conditions, what matters is the level of disability that anemia from malaria or iron deficiency or sickle cell disorder may lead to. Within each form of anemia, therefore, mild, moderate, and severe forms are distinguished. They are treated as different *health states*. Altogether, 220 different health states are defined. Each of the 1,160 pathological conditions is associated with one health state. Thus, mild anemia due to malaria leads to the same health state as mild anemia due to iron deficiency or sickle cell disorder. The associated health state represents the same disability.

The 220 health states each have their separate disability weights. The disability weights in DALYs are assigned on a numerical scale from 0 to 1. This scale is inverted from the one that is used for QALYs: 0 represents full health (absence of any disease or injury) and 1 represents loss of life. Thus, on this scale, the *smaller* its disability weight, the *less* of a burden a health state is. The scale is inverted between QALYs and DALYs because QALYs represent health benefit and DALYs represent harm.

For instance, the disability weight associated with mild anemia is 0.005; the weight associated with moderate anemia is 0.058; and with severe anemia it is 0.164. This procedure makes it possible to determine the burden associated with mild, moderate, or severe anemia in a population. In addition, it also makes it possible to determine how much of that burden can be attributed to malaria, iron deficiency, or other causes.

DALYs are a *gap measure*: They represent the shortfall in health in a population. Like QALYs, they combine the time spent in a health state with its disability weight. Thus, for instance, the burden of severe anemia for 1 year is 0.164 DALYs, for 2 years it is 0.328 DALYs, and so on. If there is only one patient in a population who has severe anemia for a year, then the overall burden of severe anemia is 0.164 DALYs; if there are a thousand, it is 164 DALYs. These values represent the gap between actual population health and the health that the population would have if it were free of a particular disability.

This is, however, only one part of the calculation of DALYs. It reflects only the harm of morbidity. This component of DALYs is called *years lived with disability*, since it is determined by the weights of disabilities and the time spent with those disabilities. But diseases and injuries also kill people. Thus, DALYs have another component: *Years of life lost due to premature mortality*. This component reflects the harm of early death due to disease and injury. In summary, DALYs are the sum of two components: Years lived with disability and years of life lost due to premature mortality.

Years of life lost due to premature mortality is simply the number of years that a person loses due to premature death. But how many years does a person lose when he or she dies? People in different countries and regions of the world have different life expectancies. Years of life lost could be calculated on their basis. But if the prevailing life expectancies were used, a death in Sub-Saharan Africa would represent a smaller harm than a death at the same age in Western Europe. This would be an objectionable implication, since a death in Sub-Saharan Africa should not matter any less morally. The developers of the DALY, therefore, chose to measure years of life lost on the basis of an *ideal* life expectancy: Years of life lost due to premature mortality is the gap, in years, between the actual age of death and the ideal life expectancy.

The idea behind using ideal life expectancies is that all populations should be able to reach the highest life expectancy in the world. It is a harm if they cannot do this, and the burden of that harm should be reflected in DALYs. This, of course, is a normative consideration. Thus, it should not be considered a harm if a population cannot reach a life expectancy of 100 years, but it should be considered a harm if it cannot reach what is possible for others. The burden of premature mortality, therefore, should be determined by the shortfall from what the longest-living population can achieve. The country with the longest-living population is currently Japan.

Originally, the ideal life expectancy was set at 80 years for men and 82.5 years for women, reflecting life expectancies at birth in Japan in the early 1990s. One argument for different life expectancies for men and women was that women have a greater biologically determined "survival potential" (Murray 1996). In addition, men tend to take greater risks with their health. The consequence of this discrimination is that the death of a man counts for less than the death of a woman at the same age. This is morally problematic. In the *2010 Update*, therefore, the ideal age for both men and women was set at 86 years. This also reflects the gains in life expectancy in the last two decades, and the narrowing of the gap between male and female life expectancies (Murray et al. 2012).

A summary measure of population health can be calculated by aggregating DALYs for different diseases and injuries. A disease can cause a health loss for a person for a certain amount of time. This part of its burden is represented by years lived with disability. The disease might also kill the person prematurely. This part of its burden is represented by years of life lost. The sum of these two components determines the burden of the particular disease in DALYs. DALYs associated with different disabilities can be added up, and the aggregated number of DALYs represent the overall disease burden in a population.

Ethical Issues

The use of QALYs and DALYs in health policy raises a number of ethical issues. One set of issues concerns measurement. How should the quality adjustment factors be determined? Another set of issues concerns the use of QALYs and DALYs in health resource allocation. Does their use in cost-effectiveness analysis lead to unfair discrimination against some patient groups? A third set of issues concerns their social or moral value: Do all QALYs and DALYs have the same value regardless of their distribution?

Whom to Ask?

Researchers customarily use a small sample of the general population for determining the quality adjustment factors in QALYs. The developers of the DALY originally used the responses of an international group of health professionals to assign disability weights. In the latest revision of the GBD studies, they used household surveys in several countries and a general, web-based population survey. Questions have been raised about the use of different preference elicitation methods as well as the cross-cultural applicability of the quality adjustment factors and disability weights.

Broadly speaking, there is a fair degree of convergence in the evaluation of health outcomes across different methodological approaches and socio-economic and cultural settings. There remains, however, an important source of discrepancy. When health outcomes are evaluated by members of the general population, their responses often imply *lower* quality adjustment factors than those that result from the evaluations of people who have direct or indirect experience of those health outcomes. It appears that the general population considers many health outcomes worse than health professionals do, who in turn consider them worse than patients who live with those outcomes.

Some critics argue that this raises a fundamental problem. Why should health outcomes be evaluated by those who have less experience of them? Shouldn't QALYs and DALYs reflect the values of those who have the best knowledge of health outcomes and health conditions?

The problem is not merely lack of knowledge and experience. People living with chronic conditions and permanent disabilities tend to consider their conditions less bad when they have *adapted* to them. Faced with long-term illness, people tend to change their activities, aims, and values in light of their functional limitations. Adaptation is often a healthy way of coping with adverse conditions. People with chronic conditions and disabilities can compensate for their health loss by adjusting their pursuits and life plan. As a result, their *overall* quality of life need not be lower. Critics point out that QALYs and DALYs that are not based on "patient values" do not reflect this (see Menzel *et al.* 2002; Brock 2004).

Yet using evaluations that reflect adaptation leads to a problem. QALYs and DALYs are used in cost-effectiveness analysis to determine how scarce social resources should be allocated. When the patients' evaluations are used, the prevention and treatment of their conditions can turn out to be less urgent. Because the evaluations of health professionals and members of the general population generate lower QALY values—reflecting a greater impact on quality of life—using their values makes the prevention, treatment, and rehabilitation of these conditions more important.

Some health economists also argue that using the responses of a sample of the general population reflects "community values"—the value that society places on the prevention and treatment of different conditions. Using community values may confer legitimacy on health resource allocation choices, which they would lack if only patient values were used.

Finally, adaptation to disability is not always desirable or admirable. A patient can adapt to her functional limitations by substituting her aims and activities with worthwhile alternatives. Sometimes, however, adaptation can take the form of giving up worthwhile aims and activities, and finding satisfaction with the limited opportunities that remain. It would be problematic if health outcomes and health conditions were considered less bad just because patients become resigned to the limitations imposed by them. A practical proposal is to use the lowest QALY values in order to avoid neglecting any health needs: It is worse to fail to address a health problem that is more severe than empirical surveys suggest than to address one that is less severe than it appears (Wolff *et al.* 2012).

Disability Discrimination

The most persistent moral debate associated with QALYs and DALYs is their use in the allocation of health resources. In one form or another, scarcity is always present in health care systems. Whether explicitly or implicitly, "rationing" decisions are routinely made by politicians, health policy makers, insurance providers, health care administrators, and many other actors in the health care system.

Cost-effectiveness analysis is one of the most important tools for evaluating health resource allocations. According to its critics, however, if cost-effectiveness analysis is used for setting priorities in health care, lower priority will be given to those whose capacity to benefit from interventions is limited (see Brock 2009). Some patient groups, including people living with disabilities and chronic health conditions, may have a limited capacity to benefit compared with those who can be returned to full health. Thus, their treatment will be given lower priority. They will be unfairly discriminated against.

This problem is most acute when it comes to life-saving interventions. It seems that patients who can be returned to full health will always be favored by the cost-effectiveness calculus. Suppose that two patients suffer from the same life-threatening disease. The costs of treatment are equal, but only one of them can be treated. The first patient can be returned to full health for another 10 years; treating her will result in 10 QALYs. The second patient would also survive for another 10 years, but she cannot be returned to full health—her health-related quality of life would be 0.8. Saving her would result in only 8 QALYs. Thus, according to the cost-effectiveness calculus, the first patient should get the treatment. But this is unfair towards the second patient who would not receive the treatment because of her preexisting disability.

There are several possible replies to this objection. One is to deny that people with disabilities and chronic conditions would be discriminated against on account of their condition. The objection misunderstands the way QALYs, DALYs, and cost-effectiveness analysis are used in practice. Another reply concedes the possibility of discrimination, but argues that not all forms of it are unfair. When people with disabilities are treated unequally, it is either not an instance of unfairness or, all things considered, the unfairness can be justified. The third reply is simply to point out that cost-effectiveness should not be the only consideration in health resource allocation. It should be used along with other moral principles to avoid unfairly discriminating against anyone (for a fuller account of these replies, see Bognar and Hirose 2014).

I will return to the third reply in the next section. Here I will focus on the first and the second.

Consider again the example of the two patients, where treating the first one would result in 10 QALYs and treating the second would result only in 8 QALYs. When only cost-effectiveness is taken into account, the judgment that the first patient should be saved is simply a matter of arithmetic. It would be pointless to debate arithmetic. Thus, if resources for health are allocated in the way described, people with limited capacity to benefit will indeed be disadvantaged. But the example is misleading. It does not represent the way cost-effectiveness analysis is used in practice.

To begin, note that cost-effectiveness analysis ranks those interventions and health services the highest whose *relative* benefits are greatest (given their costs). If some patients have a low health-related quality of life, their treatment can potentially realize the greatest relative benefit. Thus, the treatment of people with disabilities and chronic health conditions will often have a favorable cost-effectiveness ratio, since the treatment and rehabilitation of disabling conditions have both immediate and long-term benefits. To be sure, the treatment of disabling conditions can be costly or uncertain, and chronic conditions might require long-term management. Nevertheless, the point is that the use of cost-effectiveness analysis does not *inherently* discriminate against anyone: Its rankings depend on how costs and benefits work out in particular cases.

Critics will point out that this is not the case in the example of life-saving interventions, when the person with the preexisting disability can only be returned to the level of 0.8. But in practice, QALYs are not assigned to specific patients or patient groups, but to treatments and interventions. Cost-effectiveness analysis is used to rank alternative *resource uses*, not to rank patients. When NICE in the UK recommends a new treatment or medical technology to the NHS, it calculates its benefits in QALYs. It does not calculate different QALY values for different patient groups. There are no separate cost-effectiveness ratios for patients with and without disabilities. An intervention is recommended if it has a favorable cost-effectiveness ratio. When it does, its use is recommended for all patients who need it, regardless of their other characteristics.

Therefore, it is misleading to object to the use of QALYs and DALYs on the basis of examples like the one above. Cost-effectiveness analysis is not used to ration treatments for specific patients. A patient with a preexisting disability or chronic condition is just as eligible for treatments and life-saving interventions as anyone else, once it is determined that the intervention should be provided by the health care system because of its favorable cost-effectiveness ratio.

Nevertheless, critics might insist that it is sometimes an inevitable consequence of the use of QALYs and DALYs that some groups of patients will be disadvantaged. For instance, some health care systems do not provide certain cancer treatments due to their high costs and limited benefits. Patients who need these treatments but are unable to pay for them themselves will be left untreated. These patients are "rationed out" as a consequence of using cost-effectiveness analysis (Bognar 2010).

This point leads to the second reply to the discrimination objection. Priority setting in health care is about the use of common resources, pooled from the contributions of many people. This is as true of private health insurance as of publicly funded health care. Scarcity requires putting limits on what can be provided. The objection in its present form amounts to denying that considerations of costs and benefits can ever be used in setting limits. It argues that it is unfair to use them when they lead to the unequal treatment of some groups. But not all unequal treatment is unfair. If costs and benefits are ignored, there will inevitably be others whose health needs cannot be met because of the inefficient allocation of the available resources. Ultimately, the health care system becomes a "bottomless pit," in which resources are spent on providing small benefits to a few and neglecting the greater benefits of the many. In order to avoid this, some inequalities can be justified. They are not unfair (Fenton 2010).

Alternatively, it could be argued that ignoring the greater benefits of others is in itself a form of unfairness. Refusing to fund an intervention with an unfavorable cost-effectiveness ratio is not unfair. It may be unfortunate that some patients cannot have free or subsidized access to a beneficial treatment, but when resources are scarce, it would be even more unfair to deny treatments that bring greater benefits to others at lower costs. Refusing to take into account costs and benefits in conditions of scarcity is morally more problematic than not funding a particular intervention because of its limited effectiveness or high costs.

Cancer treatments are a case in point. Many cancer drugs offer limited benefits for very high costs. For instance, Provenge, a prostate cancer drug, extends life by an average of 4 months, but it costs $93,000 per patient. Yervoy, a melanoma drug, costs $120,000 and extends life by an average of 3 and a half months (*The Economist* 2011). NICE was widely criticized when it did not recommend to the NHS the use of Avastin for advanced bowel cancer, arguing that the £21,000 that it cost for each patient was not worth the six weeks of extra life that it provided (*The Guardian* 2010).

Setting priorities among alternative resource uses requires a complex balancing of harms and benefits. It will often be impossible to provide benefits to some groups without foregoing benefits for others. Critics who worry about patients with limited capacity to benefit may in the end be troubled by the assumption that all QALYs and DALYs have the same value in cost-effectiveness analysis, regardless of their distribution. Perhaps the solution is to give different weights to the QALYs and DALYs of different groups of people.

Weighting QALYs and DALYs

DALYs are used for calculating the burden of disease. Before the *2010 Update*, their calculation in the GBD studies had a unique feature: DALYs were given different weights depending on the age of the person who suffered from disability. DALYs were age weighted.

The age-weighting function that represented the relative weights of DALYs at different ages started from a low value at birth, increased until young adulthood, and steadily diminished afterward. Thus, a disease or injury was considered worst when a person was 25 or 30. It was considered less bad at age 5 or 65.

The researchers in the GBD project justified age weighting the following way. People are more productive in their young adulthood. They are more likely to be employed. They also contribute to social productivity in other ways: They often take care of their children and elderly parents. Hence the welfare of children and older people depends, to a large extent, on their contributions. This sort of *welfare interdependence* has a crucial role in society. In particular, the illness of a young adult is likely to negatively affect the welfare of others. Therefore, it should have more weight when the burden of disease is calculated. Age weighting was introduced to take welfare interdependence into account (Murray 1996).

Age weighting in the GBD studies became very controversial, and not only because the idea of welfare interdependence may be a form of cultural bias. As I explained above, DALYs are an evaluative measure of health. When the DALYs of young adults are given more weight, considerations that should be irrelevant to measuring the burden of disease are introduced—namely, considerations about the *social* value of health. Disability in a young adult is considered worse not because it is worse for him or her, but because it is worse *for others*. Arguably, that sort of consideration should have no place in a measure of health. Moreover, even if the burden of disease is interpreted in the broad way that the argument from welfare interdependence suggests, age weighting leads to double counting, since the care that some people provide to others is already reflected in the measure of the burden of those who receive care (see, e.g., Bognar 2008).

Because of the objections, age weighting was abandoned in the *2010 Update*. Nevertheless, some philosophers and health economists argue that giving different weights to QALYs and DALYs at different ages can be justified in other ways.

One proposal is to age weight QALYs according to socio-economic group. In all societies, people lower down the socio-economic ladder have shorter life expectancies and worse health outcomes than people who are better educated, do less hazardous work, and have higher incomes. These inequalities can be mitigated if the QALYs of people from disadvantaged socio-economic groups are given greater weight. On this proposal, extra resources should be spent on extending healthy life for disadvantaged groups. This would necessitate trade-offs between overall population health and equality in life prospects, but the trade-offs could be made explicit by the weighting (Williams 1997).

A more general extension of the use of QALYs in health resource allocation is the introduction of *equity weights*. Equity weighting is proposed to reflect the idea that health improvements for people who have a lower health-related quality of life should have greater moral weight. Giving more weight to their QALYs would lead to more equal outcomes. Societies are concerned with the fair distribution of health benefits. There is a lot of empirical evidence showing that people prefer to give more weight to the treatment of those who are more severely ill and to those who have a limited capacity to benefit from treatment. People also believe that life-saving interventions are more important than health-improving interventions. Equity weights have been suggested as a method for taking these moral concerns into account (Nord 1999).

Nevertheless, equity weighting has not been used in practice, in part because many questions remain as to whether this method can capture all of the moral considerations that should be taken into account in health resource allocation.

Conclusion

This chapter has presented only some of the many challenging ethical issues in the measurement of population health and the allocation of health resources. The intersection of ethics and health policy remains a largely uncharted area, and so it is a fertile ground for new questions and challenges for bioethicists.

Related Topics

Chapter 1, "The Right to Health Care," John D. Arras
Chapter 2, "Social Determinants of Health and Health Inequalities," Sridhar Venkatapuram and Michael Marmot
Chapter 3, "The Ethics of Rationing," Daniel Callahan

References

Bognar, G. (2008) "Age-Weighting," *Economics and Philosophy* 24: 167–89.

Bognar, G. (2010) "Does Cost-Effectiveness Analysis Unfairly Discriminate against People with Disabilities?" *Journal of Applied Philosophy* 27: 394–408.

Bognar, G. and Hirose, I. (2014) *The Ethics of Health Care Rationing: An Introduction*, New York: Routledge.

Brock, D.W. (2004) "Ethical Issues in the Use of Cost Effectiveness Analysis for the Prioritisation of Health Care Resources," in S. Anand, F. Peter and A. Sen (eds.) *Public Health, Ethics, and Equity*, Oxford: Oxford University Press.

Brock, D.W. (2009) "Cost-Effectiveness and Disability Discrimination," *Economics and Philosophy* 25: 27–47.
Fenton, E. (2010) "Making Fair Funding Decisions for High Cost Cancer Care: The Case of Herceptin in New Zealand," *Public Health Ethics* 3: 137–46.
Harris, J. (1987) "QALYfying the Value of Life," *Journal of Medical Ethics* 13: 117–23.
Menzel, P., Dolan, P., Richardson, J. and Olsen, J.A. (2002) "The Role of Adaptation to Disability and Disease in Health State Evaluation: A Preliminary Normative Analysis," *Social Science and Medicine* 55: 2149–58.
Murray, C.J.L. (1996) "Rethinking DALYs," in C.J.L. Murray and A.D. Lopez (eds.) *The Global Burden of Disease: A Comprehensive Assessment of Mortality and Disability from Diseases, Injuries, and Risk Factors in 1990 and Projected to 2020*, Cambridge, MA: Harvard School of Public Health.
Murray, C.J.L. and Lopez, A.D. (eds.) (1996) *The Global Burden of Disease: A Comprehensive Assessment of Mortality and Disability from Diseases, Injuries, and Risk Factors in 1990 and Projected to 2020*, Cambridge: Harvard School of Public Health.
Murray, C.J.L. et al. (2012) "Comprehensive Systematic Analysis of Global Epidemiology: Definitions, Methods, Simplification of DALYs, and Comparative Results from the Global Burden of Disease Study 2010," web supplement to Murray, C.J.L. et al. (2012) "GBD 2010: Design, Definitions, and Metrics," *The Lancet* 380 (9859): 2063–6. Available with free registration at: http://www.thelancet.com/journals/lancet/article/PIIS0140-6736%2812%2961899-6/fulltext (accessed July 7, 2014).
Nord, E. (1999) *Cost–Value Analysis in Health Care: Making Sense out of QALYs*, Cambridge: Cambridge University Press.
Rawlins, M.D. and Culyer, A.J. (2004) "National Institute for Clinical Excellence and Its Value Judgments," *British Medical Journal* 329 (7459): 224–7.
The Economist (2011) "The Costly War on Cancer," May 26.
The Guardian (2010) "Avastin Prolongs Life But Drug Is Too Expensive for NHS Patients, Says NICE," August 24.
The Global Burden of Disease Study 2010 (2012) *The Lancet* 380 (9859): 2053–260.
Williams, A. (1997) "Intergenerational Equity: An Exploration of the 'Fair Innings' Argument," *Health Economics* 6: 117–32.
Wolff, J., Edwards, S., Richmond, S., Orr, S. and Rees, G. (2012) "Evaluating Interventions in Health: A Reconciliatory Approach," *Bioethics* 26: 455–63.

Further Reading

Useful collections include:

Anand, S., Peter, F. and Sen, A. (eds.) (2004) *Public Health, Ethics, and Equity*, Oxford: Oxford University Press
Bell, J.M. and Mendus, S. (eds.) (1988) *Philosophy and Medical Welfare*, Cambridge: Cambridge University Press.
Murray, C.J.L., Salomon, J.A., Mathers, C.D. and Lopez, A.D. (eds.) (2002) *Summary Measures of Population Health: Concepts, Ethics, Measurement and Applications*, Geneva: World Health Organization.

For a broader treatment of the issues in this chapter, see Bognar, G. and Hirose, I. (2014) *The Ethics of Health Care Rationing*, New York: Routledge.

5

IMMIGRATION AND ACCESS TO HEALTH CARE

Norman Daniels and Keren Ladin

Overview

Health insurance is important because it improves access to health care, which protects health, and provides needed financial protection, both of which are objectives of a just system (Saloner and Daniels 2011). In a system that ensures universal coverage—whether it includes private insurance or not—the term "universal" suggests that *all* people have insurance coverage. Despite this, in most such systems, unauthorized immigrants are excluded from coverage. In the United States, unauthorized immigrants number in the millions and form a significant part of the uninsured population, even under the 2010 *Patient Protection and Affordable Care Act* (PPACA). Is such exclusion justified? To be sure, unauthorized immigrants have access to some medical care and are guaranteed access to emergency medical care (*Emergency Medical Treatment and Active Labor Act* (EMTALA) 1996). Still, exclusion of unauthorized immigrants from PPACA begs the question: Is it ethically justifiable to exclude unauthorized immigrants from the comprehensive non-acute care provided by most insurance policies?

Our main conclusion is that there is a strong presumption in favor of including unauthorized immigrants, and that this presumption is not defeated by arguments against including them. In this chapter, we first consider claims of global justice and human rights, which insist on inclusion either because they claim that open borders are a requirement of global justice or because they claim that human rights to health care preclude such exclusion. We shall argue that these claims fail to mark out supportable claims of justice regarding unauthorized immigrants. Specifically, the global justice claims fail a relevant requirement of feasibility on all principles of justice, and the human rights claims are inconclusive. We also reject the opposing stance that grants states the unconstrained authority (right) to regulate the flow of immigrants into them, making the exclusion of unauthorized immigrants a clear state prerogative.

Instead, we take a middle course. Specifically, we believe that any state authority to regulate borders is constrained by conditions on the justification of such regulations (although space prevents the development of a comprehensive account of here). We consider the specific arguments offered in the U.S. context for inclusion, as well as the counter arguments for exclusion. We propose two main arguments for inclusion: First, that health care is a benefit owed as a matter of reciprocity for contributions made by unauthorized immigrants; and second, that unauthorized immigrants are entrenched and contributing members of the community and all members of the community must have the opportunity to have their health protected. These arguments succeed in establishing a presumption in favor of inclusion that is not defeated by the arguments for exclusion. We conclude that unauthorized immigrants should be included in efforts to establish universal coverage, such as the PPACA. The general theory of justice that we appeal to in our claim that members of a community have entitlements to social benefits also claims they should also have a political voice about their fair share of those benefits. One route to providing political voice, namely a route citizenship, is a task for immigration reform that is beyond the scope of this chapter.

Before taking up the arguments in favor of exclusion or inclusion, we begin with some background to the coverage issue and to American immigration policy.

Background

We contend that the very large unauthorized immigrant issue in the United States is the result of an immigration policy that ignores longstanding patterns of demand for low-skilled workers in certain American industries. For many decades, lower-skilled immigrant workers coming to the United States, especially from Latin America, have responded both to push factors, such as low wages and poor job opportunities in their home countries, and pull factors, such as economic opportunities and policy changes (Rosenblum and Brick 2011). The Braceros program, instituted during WWII (but later criticized for the exploitation of migrant farm workers), authorized hundreds of thousands of low-skilled Mexican workers for temporary employment until 1964. Even after quotas were imposed in 1965, employment opportunities still provided significant incentives for workers from Latin America, leading to both authorized and unauthorized immigration. Unauthorized immigration increased with the economic expansion in the U.S. in the 1990s, particularly following the North American Free Trade Agreement (NAFTA) of 1993. NAFTA displaced many Mexican farmers who then sought work in the United States. At the same time, the militarization of the U.S. border effectively trapped millions of these immigrant workers by raising the costs and risks of border crossings (Massey 2007). Such immigrant workers in previous decades had often returned to their home countries but now they could not easily do so, increasing the numbers of unauthorized immigrants from fewer than 4 million to nearly 12 million in the decade after the militarization of the border. The flow of these immigrants stopped by 2012 because of poor job opportunities in the U.S. and intensified enforcement of borders, including increased deportation (Passel et al. 2012)

At the same time that the numbers of unauthorized immigrants swelled, they were made ineligible for many welfare benefits. In 1996, the passage of the *Personal Responsibility Work Opportunity Reconciliation Act* (PRWORA) disrupted the existing federal equality in access between authorized and unauthorized immigrants to public benefits, which had been the norm in the U.S. (Fix and Tumlin 1997; Viladrich 2012). PRWORA banned federal funding of health care for unauthorized immigrants, eliminated a cash-assistance program for unauthorized immigrants, and reduced funding for the uncompensated care pool, shifting the financing burden and oversight of immigrant health care in particular, to states. The law also barred "legal" (authorized) immigrants from means-tested benefits and public programs during a five-year waiting period.

PRWORA reflected an increase in anti-immigrant sentiment and legislation; such sentiment heightened in 2001 after the 9/11 terrorist attacks and increased further during the Great Recession that began in 2008. At the federal level, the Department of Homeland Security instituted the Secure Communities program (2008), a new deportation program aimed at identifying and deporting criminal aliens. At the state level, Arizona's SB 1070 (*Support Our Law Enforcement and Safe Neighborhoods Act* 2010), and Alabama's HB 56 (*Hammon-Beason Alabama Taxpayer and Citizen Protection Act* 2011) require public officials (police officers and public school personal) to verify and detain persons suspected of being unauthorized.

The PPACA reinforces the difference established by PRWORA between authorized and unauthorized immigrants. Authorized immigrants can participate in the high-risk pools, health benefit exchanges, and cost-sharing subsidies that the PPACA establishes without a five-year waiting period, although it does not overturn the waiting period for eligibility for public programs. Unauthorized immigrants are not eligible for any of these benefits.

Cosmopolitan Claims of Global Justice

One way to argue that unauthorized immigrants should not be singled out for exclusion from benefits available to other residents is to claim that global justice denies states the authority or general right to exclude immigrants (Cole 2000). States would then lack the authority to distinguish those who obey immigration rules from those who do not. Individuals would then have a right to immigrate and not just to emigrate. This claim goes beyond the standard interpretation of the human right to migrate, affirmed in international covenants, which restricts state authority to prevent residents from departing their homeland but does not challenge the rights of states to regulate immigrant flows into their borders. Another line of argument from global justice is that the exclusion of immigrants is coercive, and this coercion requires a justification that would be agreed to, at least ex ante, by those who may turn out to be immigrants (Blake 2002; Carens 1987; Risse 2002).

A different global justice perspective that supports significant restrictions on state authority to regulate immigrant flow argues that a principle assuring equality of opportunity has global scope and is not just a principle governing cooperative terms within a state (Butt 2012). Some strong ethical intuitions support such a view: If we believe that certain social contingencies should not shape what counts as just, then the contingency of birth in a poor, developing country as opposed to a developed country, like the United States, should not determine the opportunities open to people. Such views suggest that globally individuals are the subjects of justice and that we can know what justice requires for people regardless of their situation in the institutions that states construct or maintain. (A variant on this version of cosmopolitan justice suggests that there exists a global basic structure of institutions that function in the ways state-specific institutions do. Therefore, "fair terms of cooperation" of the sort that John Rawls articulated in justice as fairness should be understood globally and not just within states (Beitz 1979, 2000)).

Pursuit of greater opportunities across state boundaries in a world of unequal opportunities no doubt underlies the decision to migrate made by millions of people globally. One philosopher proposes operationalizing this concern for equality of opportunity globally through a measure of the "immigration pressure" opportunity-rich countries face from people in opportunity-poor ones (Cavallero 2006). Specifically, either countries should admit immigrants until there is equilibrium between immigrants and emigrants, or they should offset the immigration pressure through appropriate development aid to opportunity-poor countries. (We shall not discuss weaker versions of such claims, which may be referred to as "more open borders" since they still allow for the distinction between unauthorized and authorized immigrants.)

In the next section, we argue that these claims of global justice fail an important criterion that claims of justice must meet, namely that it is feasible for people to sustain a regime in which compliance with them generally obtains. If we are right, this argument implies that states, under some conditions, may regulate immigration in a way that excludes some people and distinguishes between authorized and unauthorized immigrants (although we do not go as far as Weiner (1996) in affirming complete state authority to regulate immigrant flows).

Justice and Feasibility

Is such a view of open borders feasible? We argue that if open borders are infeasible in an appropriate sense, then this policy is not a requirement of justice. This insistence on feasibility is a way of making sense of the ethical maxim that "ought implies can." For something to be an obligation of justice it must be feasible for people (or for states) to meet that obligation.

Sometimes lack of feasibility can block a requirement of justice by leading us to abandon or modify a view about what justice requires (Estland 2011). When is a lack of feasibility requirement-blocking? We propose that if a requirement of justice is not feasible because we cannot *sustain* an institution or practice conforming to it (feasibility as sustainability), then the infeasibility blocks the requirement of justice, but the mere fact that we do not know how to *achieve* it (feasibility as achievability) is not sufficient to block it as a requirement of justice. Of course, something might never be achievable because it is beyond human ability—and then it is requirement-blocking (and also clearly unsustainable). Consider, for example, a racist or gender-biased practice. We may not know how to eliminate the racism or the gender bias in this context, perhaps because the group imposing the practice is too powerful to overcome. That lack of achievability should not stop us from denouncing the racism or gender bias, since we know that societies can sustain (at least in important ways) non-racist and non-gender-biased institutions and practices. We know the requirement of justice is feasible in the relevant sense even if we do not know how to achieve justice in this context. Sustainable feasibility is arguably what Rawls (1971) thought relevant when he claimed that a principle of justice that imposes less strain of commitment than an alternative on people raised to conform to it is a more acceptable principle.

Is the open borders claim part of a sustainable order? Is it sustainably feasible? To be sure, we may not know just what some of those stable features of persons or institutions are, and so some of our arguments about sustainability may be speculative. Still, if we have reason to believe that a practice is not sustainable and thus not feasible, we have reason to question whether there is a clear requirement of justice to do what we have reason to believe we cannot do.

To test for the sustainable feasibility of the open borders view, we would have to consider these scenarios: (1) a welfare benefit in a particular country is jeopardized by an inflow of immigrants seeking it, so that longer-term residents (citizens, for example) face the prospect of losing some benefits; (2) the influx of immigrants into a nation results in constrained economic opportunities and lower wages for many vulnerable citizens due to increased competition; (3) a local economy needs additions to its labor force to promote economic growth, but only in some areas that require specialized training; (4) among a significant immigrant flow are those that seek radical, perhaps even violent, change to local institutions, and these immigrants are identifiable and could be excluded. All of these scenarios involve economic or political threats to the wellbeing of existing residents and social institutions, and therefore they may provide sufficient grounds for regulating immigration. Though it would take us beyond the scope of this discussion to debate the more controversial sorts of threats to the ethnic or religious composition of the existing state—"they are culturally different from us"—and thus develop a comprehensive account, we view attempts to exclude people who would form an ethnic or religious minority as unjust. In the absence of such a comprehensive account, we must consider matters case by case. The cases listed in 1–4 are all ones to which there might be legitimate opposition from the non-immigrant population; such opposition will render open borders infeasible.

Perhaps a world government could enforce open borders, on the model of the federal system such as the U.S. (or perhaps the weaker system of the EU). Then the discussion of what is needed to convert our global order based on sovereign states into such a federal system with a global government becomes central. We cannot address here the desirability or feasibility of such a global government; we note only that we lack any examples of even regional federal systems that have proven sustainability.

If open borders lack feasibility as sustainability, then the same problem faces a global version of fair equality of opportunity. Arguably, long-term residents of states facing large-scale immigration of people seeking greater opportunity will organize to oppose that immigration and make reasonable complaints about the threat to their interests, and this opposition will undercut the redistribution of opportunity globally through open borders. Even if we can sustain a fair distribution of opportunity and power within a state through checks and balances against undue power concentration, globally we lack the means to prevent such accumulation within states that will undermine global equalization efforts. In the absence of institutions that operate globally or even regionally to assure fair equality of opportunity, including the protection it affords through the provision of health care, we have good reason to believe that global equality of opportunity is not feasible in the way that we may believe it is feasible within a state. If we are right, and the appeal to open borders is blocked, then a global appeal to access health care through a claim that opportunity must be protected as a matter of global justice is blocked as well.

Human Rights Claims

Human rights focus on individual claims to certain kinds of protections or goods that all states should respect or provide. In this regard, the human rights framework shares elements with many prominent cosmopolitan views of global justice according to which individuals are the subjects of these claims regardless of who or where they are, and some duties or obligations are imposed on states to assure the provision of these protections or goods (Miller 2008; United Nations 2000). We might then think that if all individual humans have a human right to health care, then it does not matter morally if they are authorized or not, but this conclusion about human rights is drawn too quickly.

Though the cosmopolitan views we have considered challenge state powers to regulate immigration, human rights views do not, at least not so extensively. We can see this difference in the way the right to migrate is understood. The human right to migrate is only a right to leave a home country. There is no correlative duty on any state to accept the émigré as an immigrant. Indeed, a human right to immigrate to any country one wished to enter would abridge existing powers (rights) of states to regulate the flow of immigrants, contrary to human rights covenants and treaties. Only with regard to some kinds of refugees are states under an obligation to consider whether their claims for refuge meet international standards and whether they should be admitted under international agreements on asylum. Most immigrants are not asylum seekers, and the rights of asylum seekers are not to be confused with what a human right to immigration would entail.

Is the human right to health care that implies that all residents of a country, whether unauthorized or not, have a right to the more comprehensive kinds of health care included in the PPACA? No such entitlement is explicit in the judgments of the Committee on Economic, Social, and Cultural Rights. Human rights covenants and the international law based on them give states considerable leeway to determine policy with regard to welfare rights, such as a right to health care. Other states are obliged to contribute toward improvements in the ability of developing countries to progressively realize a right to health or health care, which means developing countries are not the sole states responsible for improving health care in their jurisdictions. But developing country governments, and other states, remain the primary bearers of duties to deliver health care that progressively satisfies this right, and this leaves the duty primarily to them, including what policy to follow regarding undocumented immigrants. In the U.S., as in almost all European universal coverage systems, emergency medical care is provided to all individuals, authorized or not. It is not clear from the human rights doctrine that unauthorized immigrants are entitled to more than that.

Conditional State Authority to Regulate Borders

"Open borders" cannot be a requirement of global justice because it violates the "feasibility as sustainability" constraint on what counts as just. A human rights framework does not support an open borders view either, and if it were modified to do so it would become merely aspirational, while violating the same feasibility condition. Our conclusion is that states may regulate the flow of immigrants—at least under some conditions—and this means that the distinction between unauthorized and authorized immigrants will sometimes be defensible in that it is not itself unjust.

These conclusions, however, do not mean that states have a general authority or right to regulate immigrant flow for any reason it sees appropriate. Whether such regulation is justifiable depends on the reasons for it. Similarly, the reasons for allowing or prohibiting unauthorized immigrants to have access to insurance for comprehensive health care must justify those policies regarding them.

We cannot offer a comprehensive account of which reasons for regulating immigrant flow are sufficient and which are not. We instead rely on examining the arguments on a case-by-case basis. Earlier, for example, we rejected arguably discriminatory exclusions, but we noted that some reasons for constraining open borders, such as those involved in scenarios 1–4 on pp. 59–60, might prove compelling. Pursuing the same strategy, we turn to the reasons that have played a role in the debate about coverage for unauthorized immigrants in the U.S.

Arguments for Providing Comprehensive Health Insurance to Immigrants

Two distinct lines of argument about distributive justice support the view that unauthorized immigrants should have access to the kinds of health insurance that are provided by the

PPACA. One argument is that, since unauthorized immigrants contribute to a collective product that benefits the community, reciprocity requires that they should share in the benefits they help produce. The second argument is that longstanding unauthorized immigrants should be viewed as rooted, contributing members of a society, unlike residents of other countries or temporary visitors (e.g., visiting students, businessmen, and tourists), which means they should be included under universal health insurance coverage, at least if there are no reasons strong enough to exclude them.

Reciprocity

People who contribute to society, in the form of paid and unpaid labor, taxes, and other aspects of community membership, ought to be eligible for the benefits their contributions make possible. That is what reciprocity requires. Contrary to exclusionary rhetoric, unauthorized immigrants should be credited with such contributions. The majority of unauthorized immigrants work for employers who withhold taxes (Passel and Cohn 2011). At the federal level, unauthorized immigrants contribute through their taxes to Social Security and Medicaid and Medicare, services they are unable to consume (Porter 2005; Ortega 2009). At the local level, unauthorized immigrants pay sales tax and property tax on rent.

Beyond their economic contributions, unauthorized immigrants contribute to the social fabric of their communities. Many immigrants pursue home ownership, a hallmark of assimilation, and strong community ties; their affiliation with religious and civic groups also strengthens communities. Younger, working immigrant families reduce demographic challenges to society from an aging population with low birth rates. Because a concern for reciprocity undergirds public programs, all of these contributions to society should earn all immigrants the right to participate in public benefits (assuming they meet other eligibility requirements, e.g., means testing).

Fair Equality of Opportunity, Health, and Fair Terms of Cooperation

John Rawls' contractarian view of social justice seeks fair terms of cooperation for all "free and equal citizens" of a society (Rawls 1971). Specifically, Rawls argues that such fair terms require protecting the fair equality of opportunity of all citizens, meaning that we need institutions that correct for inequalities in the development of talents and skills, so that equally capable individuals have equal chances of occupying jobs and offices they seek. Protecting health, including through coverage for health care, contributes to protecting opportunity (Daniels 1981; Rawls 1995).

Should we take Rawls' reference to "citizens" literally? Do we have justification only for protecting citizens' opportunities through protection of their health?

Since unauthorized immigrants are not citizens, taking Rawls literally would imply they are not included in the argument. But the spirit of his account includes them as members of the society in a relevant sense because they cooperate with others in it. Unlike residents of other nations, unauthorized immigrants, especially those who live and work for considerable periods among other members of society, are present as cooperating members of that society and they should be treated fairly according to fair terms of cooperation for all of its members. This difference from members of other societies should count heavily in favor of Rawls including them. In addition, interpreted generously,

Rawls' contractarian view requires that we consider, inclusively, all moral agents who are contributing members of society and who should cooperate on fair terms acceptable to them. Visitors, such as temporary students, business people, and tourists, for example, should not count as members, but most longstanding unauthorized immigrants should be considered members of society by virtue of their working, paying taxes, and being active members of local communities. The distinction between citizenship and informal membership is undeniably important since it demarcates some important special rights, such as voting and political participation generally, but many aspects of social justice require the same treatment for all members, whether people are citizens or not. As James Dwyer argues, "although they are not citizens or legal residents, they may be diligent workers, good neighbors, concerned parents, and active participants in community life. They are workers, involved in complex schemes of social cooperation" (Dwyer 2004: 40).

Rawls' theory also provides for protection of basic liberties, including political participation rights. So the "fair terms of cooperation" include having a voice in the implementation of those terms. We believe that the link between having health protection and having political voice is important, but we cannot here consider the ways in which immigration reform should provide a route to obtaining that voice.

The protection of health, we also note, should be viewed from a lifespan perspective. This implies that denial of health care services beyond emergency medical care to unauthorized immigrants should be assessed for its impact over a lifespan, not simply as a temporary denial of benefits. Depriving immigrants of access to more comprehensive health care presents a significant harm to their ability to live a functional life and pursue and revise their plans of life. The obligation of society is to keep all cooperating members as close to normal functioning as possible over their lifespan, so denials of needed health care to some cooperating members requires strong reasons for exclusion.

We argue next that the reasons for exclusion do not justify ignoring this presumption in favor of inclusion.

Arguments Against Including Unauthorized Immigrants in PPACA

Are there adequate reasons for excluding unauthorized immigrants from the kinds of health protections they presumably ought to have? We think not. We consider six arguments for exclusion.

No Legal Obligation to Provide Health Care

Some argue that unauthorized immigrants do not have legitimate claims to public benefits because the law does not provide them with such benefits. For them, because there is no legal duty to provide benefits, denying benefits is justified. Furthermore, formal exceptions to the law are "an affront to the democratic process of representative government" and to fairness in procedural justice (Sen. Charles Grassley quoted in Welsh 2012).

We disagree. This line of argument presents a legal, not a moral, justification and rests upon the belief that the law as it stands is just and reflects the will of the people. Accepting this appeal to what is law at the time implies that no one should have objected to Jim Crow laws in the U.S. or apartheid laws in South Africa, for they too were the laws of the land in their time and place. Obviously, laws may be unjust, and unjust ones should be opposed.

Criminality of Illegal Immigration

Since the rule of law is vital to maintaining civil society and promoting trust in its institutions, some argue that persons residing unlawfully in the U.S. do so knowingly and voluntarily, thereby forfeiting rights to coverage. Some also argue that immigrants pose a public health threat by increasing crime rates in their communities.

But, illegal activity by itself does not justify the denial of health care benefits. Many Americans commit crimes, ranging from misdemeanors to aggravated felonies, without losing access to health care. Even in the most egregious cases of those convicted and incarcerated for criminal offenses, offenders maintain their entitlement to health care, both emergent and continuous. Undocumented presence is generally not a criminal offense but a misdemeanor. Misdemeanors generally result in the loss of privileges not civil rights. Ruth Faden argues that, "People who are in this country illegally have broken our laws, but the magnitude of their crime does not justify depriving them of the basic right to health care coverage while they are in our midst" (Faden 2009). Our point is not to presuppose that unauthorized immigrants have a right to health care, but to note that we do not deprive real criminals of entitlements to health care, so claiming the lesser offense warrants denial of health care through the ACA is unjustified.

Further, there is no conclusive evidence that immigrants increase crime rates or that they are more likely to commit crimes than those who are native born (Sampson 2008). Finally, punitive measures aimed at punishing illegal immigration should be addressed by immigration policy, not health policy. Immigrants convicted of criminal acts are subject to deportation, regardless of their legal status. This is an appropriate punishment that serves to both punish the offender and protect the community.

Avoiding Incentives

Does providing unauthorized immigrants with health care benefits act as an incentive for illegal immigration? Both sides of the vitriolic debate about immigration agree that policies incentivizing illegal border crossing should be avoided.

The facts suggest there is no incentive. As we noted earlier, the reduction in benefits following PRWORA was not associated with a corresponding decline in immigration, contrary to expectations if incentives were present (Fix et al. 2011). Immigration trends show that, after a decline in legal immigration from 1996 to 1999, immigration increased through 2006, confirming that reductions in welfare benefits do not have a dramatic effect on immigration. Even in states that provide benefits to immigrants, enrollment among immigrants is low relative to enrollment among native born, likely due to the "chilling effect" and fear of being deported (Kaushal and Kaestner 2005). There is little evidence that welfare benefits resulted in moral hazard, neither in greater dependence on welfare nor in swaying immigrants towards states with more generous benefits.

One reason for the lack of incentives is that immigrants are generally healthier and demand fewer services than the domestic-born population (Abraido-Lanza et al. 1999). Indeed, even when in need, eligible immigrants are less likely to enroll in Medicaid and less likely to seek treatment. A study examining foreign-born adults in Los Angeles County demonstrated that while immigrants constituted 45 percent of the population aged 18–64, they accounted for only 33 percent of health spending (Goldman et al. 2006). Even relative to other Latinos, unauthorized immigrants underutilize health care and contribute less to costs relative to their population share (Capps et al. 2004).

Depriving immigrants of health care coverage is not effective in regulating illegal immigration, but is likely to harm the health of immigrant households (Berk et al. 2000).

Cost of Providing Health Care to Immigrants

Since feasibility is a condition of justice, would it be infeasible, in the sense of unsustainable, to include unauthorized immigrants in the PPACA, or would that place an undue burden on taxpayers? No doubt, there may be an increased cost in covering more people, but covering immigrants may not be prohibitive as some suggest. In fact, recent evidence suggests that immigrants contribute more to health care than they use (Zallman et al. 2013). As we remarked above, immigrants are generally healthier than non-immigrants and utilize fewer health services. Even for those enrolled in public programs such as Medicaid and the State Children's Health Insurance Program (SCHIP), a state–federal entitlement program that expands access to services for families with modest incomes who do not qualify for Medicaid, expenditures are much less for immigrants than non-immigrants. In these programs, 21 percent of total medical costs were paid through public sources for native-born citizens, compared with only 16 percent for documented and undocumented immigrants (Capps et al. 2004). The cost of providing care to immigrants is similar to or lower than providing care to citizens.

Emergency Care Is Sufficient

Some may argue that the need for universal coverage for the uninsured is met through emergency care. EMTALA requires that hospitals treat all patients, including unauthorized immigrants, in an emergency. Emergency care alone, however, is not enough to preserve health and normal functioning. Lack of insurance is associated with severe health deficits. Uninsured persons are more likely to delay care and present with more severe symptoms (Mohanty et al. 2005). Despite lower utilization, expenditures associated with emergency room use by immigrant children were more than three times higher than those for native-born children using emergency services, suggesting worse health upon admission. Among unauthorized immigrants, an estimated one-fifth of day laborers suffer work-related injury, but less than half received medical care for their injuries (Valenzuela et al. 2006). Purchasing private health insurance is not feasible for many migrants because the cost of premiums exceeds their annual earnings. Continued access to primary and preventive care could mitigate these harms and likely reduce costs to the health system overall.

In addition, the boundary between emergent and non-emergency care is often vague, placing a burden on clinicians who cannot provide adequate quality of care and are forced, in the absence of coverage, to pursue discharge plans that go against their conscience and duty to provide care (Hacker et al. 2012). Because hospitals are often not reimbursed for care provided to unauthorized immigrants, medical deportations and discharge plans that harm patients have become commonplace. The tradeoff between the hospitals' financial burden and providing poor quality of care for immigrants could be avoided if immigrants were covered by insurance.

Avoiding Harms to the Most Vulnerable

Some argue that admitting too many immigrants, and not eliminating the flow of unauthorized immigrants, increases competition for jobs and hurts the most vulnerable parts of the American population—low-skilled workers with limited education—and so we should do everything possible to discourage the competition such immigrants bring with them, including denying access to the benefits of the PPACA.

This argument for exclusion combines a claim about immigration effects with a conclusion about health care benefits, thus combining two issues we believe should be kept distinct for reasons of social justice. Any increase in competition for jobs that lowers wages in general (no evidence shows this) or that lowers wages for the most vulnerable parts of the U.S. workforce (there is limited evidence that shows this) should be dealt with through immigration policy generally, not by restricting health care for people who are members of the society.

We conclude that none of these arguments for exclusion is sufficient to constitute adequate grounds for excluding unauthorized immigrants from the kinds of health insurance provided by the PPACA.

Should Unauthorized Immigrants Be Included in Comprehensive Coverage?

We have argued that there is a presumption in favor of including unauthorized immigrants in health care coverage because there are no compelling arguments justifying exclusion. This presumption does not derive from either cosmopolitan global justice or human rights arguments. Specifically, the global justice claims for open borders fail as a requirement of justice because they demand something that is not sustainably feasible. We do not support the claim that states should regulate their borders as they see fit. We believe that such regulation is justifiable only for certain kinds of reasons, for example, avoiding certain kinds of security threats, or economic and social harms, though we have not tried to offer a comprehensive account of those reasons. The human rights arguments do not yield a clear claim for inclusion because states still retain the discretion to determine who is a member entitled to the health benefits the PPACA provides.

The presumption in favor of inclusion rests on strong reasons to view most longstanding unauthorized immigrants as members of a society. As contributing members of society, reciprocity requires that they share in its benefits. As members of society, as a matter of justice, their opportunities should be protected, including those affected by access to health care. This presumption in favor of inclusion is not overridden by the arguments that have been made for their exclusion. Our view allows states to regulate the flow of immigrants under certain conditions, though we have not given a comprehensive account of these conditions. It also permits higher standards for citizenship and the rights and privileges that accompany it, but addressing that issue also takes us beyond the scope of this paper (though we note that the entitlement to a fair share of benefits should carry with it a route to acquiring political voice, and this should be incorporated in immigration policy).

Our conclusion is that the PPACA should have included all immigrants, unauthorized or not. There may well be some conditions where inclusion would not be justified—say because there is evidence that doing so brings some kind of harm to the rest of the population—but there is currently no evidence for these conditions.

Related Topics

Chapter 1, "The Right to Health Care," John D. Arras
Chapter 6, "Bioethics and Human Rights," Elizabeth Fenton
Chapter 34, "Family Caregivers, Long-Term Care, and Global Justice," Lisa Eckenwiler

References

Abraido-Lanza, A.F., Dohrenwend, B.P., Ng-Mak, D.S. and Turner, J.B. (1999) "The Latino Mortality Paradox: A Test of the 'Salmon Bias' and Healthy Migrant Hypotheses," *American Journal of Public Health* 89 (10): 1543–8.

Beitz, C.R. (1979) *Political Theory and International Relations*, Princeton, NJ: Princeton University Press.

Beitz, C.R. (2000) "Rawls's Law of Peoples," *Ethics* 110: 669–96.

Berk, M., Schur, C., Chavez, L. and Frankel, M. (2000) "Health Care Use Among Undocumented Latino Immigrants," *Health Affairs* 19 (4): 51–64.

Blake, M. (2002) "Distributive Justice, State Coercion, and Autonomy," *Philosophy and Public Affairs* 30 (3): 257–96.

Butt, D. (2012) *Global Equality of Opportunity as an Institutional Standard of Distributive Justice*, Bristol: University of Bristol.

Capps, R., Fix, M., Ost, J., Reardon-Anderson, J. and Passel, J. (2004) *The Health and Well-Being of Young Children of Immigrants*, Washington, DC: The Urban Institute.

Carens, J.H.C. (1987) "Aliens and Citizens: The Case for Open Borders," *Review of Politics* 49: 251–73.

Cavallero, E. (2006) "An Immigration-Pressure Model of Global Distributive Justice," *Politics, Philosophy and Economics* 5 (1): 97–127.

Cole, P. (2000) *Philosophies of Exclusion: Liberal Political Theory and Immigration*, Edinburgh: Edinburgh University Press.

Daniels, N. (1981) "Health-Care Needs and Distributive Justice," *Philosophy and Public Affairs* 10 (2): 146–79.

Dwyer, J. (2004) "Illegal Immigrants, Health Care, and Social Responsibility," *Hastings Center Report* 34 (1): 34–41.

Estland, D. (2011) "Human Nature and the Limits (If Any) of Political Philosophy," *Philosophy and Public Affairs* 39 (3): 207–37.

Faden, R. (2009) "Denying Care to Illegal Immigrants Raises Ethical Concerns," *Kaiser Health News*. Available at: http://www.kaiserhealthnews.org/columns/2009/December/123109Faden.aspx (accessed July 7, 2014).

Fix, M. and Tumlin, K. (1997) *Welfare Reform and the Devolution of Immigrant Policy*, Washington, DC: The Urban Institute.

Fix, M., Capps, R. and Kaushal, N. (2011) "Immigrants and Welfare: Overview," in M.E. Fix (ed.) *Immigration and Welfare: The Impact of Welfare Reform on America's Newcomers*, New York: Russell Sage Foundation.

Goldman, D., Smith, J. and Sood, N. (2006) "Immigrants and the Cost of Medical Care," *Health Affairs* 25 (6): 1700–11.

Hacker, K., Chu, J., Arsenault, L. and Marlin, R. (2012) "Provider's Perspectives on the Impact of Immigration and Customs Enforcement (ICE) Activity on Immigrant Health," *Journal of Health Care for the Poor and Underserved* 23 (2): 651–65.

Kaushal, N. and Kaestner, R. (2005) "Welfare Reform and Health Insurance of Immigrants," *Health Services Research* 40 (3): 697–722.

Massey, D.S. (2007) "Understanding America's Immigration 'Crisis'," *Proceedings of the American Philosophical Society* 151 (3): 309–27.

Miller, D. (2008) "National Responsibility and Global Justice," *Critical Review of International Social and Political Philosophy* 11 (4): 383–99.

Mohanty, S.A., Woolhandler, S., Himmelstein, D.U., Pati, S., Carrasquillo, O. and Bor, D.H. (2005) "Health Care Expenditures of Immigrants in the United States: A Nationally Representative Analysis," *American Journal of Public Health* 95 (8): 1431–8.

Ortega, A. (2009) ". . . And Health Care for All: Immigrants in the Shadow of the Promise of Health Care," *American Journal of Law and Medicine* 35 (1): 185–204.

Passel, J.S. and Cohn, D.V. (2011) "Unauthorized Immigrant Population: National and State Trends, 2010," Washington DC: Pew Hispanic Center.

Passel, J., Cohn, D.V. and Gonzalez-Barrera, A. (2012) *Net Migration from Mexico Falls to Zero—and Perhaps Less*, Washington DC: Pew Hispanic Center.

Porter, E. (2005) "Illegal Immigrants Are Bolstering Social Security With Billions," *The New York Times* April 5.

Rawls, J. (1971) *A Theory of Justice*, Cambridge, MA: Belknap Press of Harvard University Press.

Rawls, J. (1995) *Political Liberalism*, New York: Columbia University Press.

Risse, M. (2002) "What Equality of Opportunity Could Not Be," *Ethics* 112: 720–47.

Rosenblum, M.R. and Brick, K. (2011) *US Immigration Policy and Mexican/Central American Migration Flows: Then and Now*, Washington, DC: Migration Policy Institute.
Saloner, B. and Daniels, N. (2011) "The Ethics and Affordability of Health Insurance," *Journal of Health Politics, Policy and Law* 36 (5): 815–27.
Sampson, R. J. (2008) "Rethinking Crime and Immigration," *Contexts* 7 (1): 28–33.
United Nations (2000) *The Right to the Highest Attainable Standard of Health*, Geneva: United Nations, Committee on Environment, Social and Cultural Rights.
Valenzuela Jr, A., Theodore, N., Melendez, E. and Gonzalez, A.L. (2006) *On the Corner: Day Labor in the United States*. Available at http://www.sscnet.ucla.edu/issr/csup/uploaded_files/Natl_DayLabor-On_the_Corner1.pdf (accessed July 16, 2014).
Viladrich, A. (2012) "Beyond Welfare Reform: Reframing Undocumented Immigrants' Entitlement to Health Care in the United States, A Critical Review," *Social Science and Medicine* 74 (6): 822–9.
Weiner, M. (1996) "Ethics, National Sovereignty and the Control of Immigration," *International Migration Review* 30 (1): 171–97.
Welsh, T. (2012) "Is Obama's Plan for Young Illegal Immigrants Right?" *U.S. News*.
Zallman, L., Woolhandler, S., Himmelstein, D., Bor, D. and McCormick, D. (2013) "Immigrants Contributed an Estimated $115.2 Billion More to the Medicare Trust Fund Than They Took Out in 2002–09," *Health Affairs* 32 (6): 1–7.

Part II

BIOETHICS ACROSS BORDERS

Throughout much of its history bioethics teaching and scholarship has focused on the domains of the clinic, hospital, or research protocol, often in a domestic or national context. More recently, however, and reflecting the trend of globalization more broadly, bioethics has become a global field as human health and the myriad factors that influence it increasingly transcend national borders. Some direct threats to health, such as infectious diseases or bioterrorism, can only be addressed through international cooperation; indirect threats to health are also now distinctly global, as the world's economies are intertwined in a complex web of global economic policies that influence quality of life along many dimensions. International multi-site clinical trials bring into play ethical considerations that often vary widely from country to country. The health care industry is now a global enterprise, as patients from wealthy nations seek cheaper care in less wealthy countries seeking new ways of generating tourist revenue. Health care workers migrate for better-paid employment, often leaving significant gaps in the health systems of their home countries. In keeping with this volume's emphasis on social justice the chapters in this section highlight the influence of massive global inequality on individual and population health.

The first chapter explores the relationship between bioethics and human rights, the most powerful and universal movement for global social justice. Elizabeth Fenton examines the arguments both of those who call for human rights to be the "lingua franca" of global bioethics, and those more circumspect about whether these two distinct domains can or should merge. Fenton lays out the philosophical and practical arguments on both sides of this debate, which serves as a useful entry point into considering other issues that arise when health, health care, and bioethics cross borders.

Fenton draws attention to a criticism sometimes leveled at bioethics, that it has focused largely on the problems of the wealthy and advantaged, and has devoted a shamefully small amount of space to health needs, concerns, and challenges in resource-poor settings. Kjell Arne Johansson's chapter confronts some of these challenges in the context of priority setting in resource-poor settings. Prioritization of scarce health resources is difficult and complex even in wealthy settings, but in low-income countries, where health expenditures are as low as 1/180th of those in high-income countries, the problems are even more acute. Johansson argues that while access to and quality of health care in these settings is important, the distribution of other social goods, such as income and education, has a substantial impact on population health. This chapter highlights the issues of justice at the heart of priority setting in health and its impact on health at the population level, and in so doing exemplifies the broader bioethics scholarship that is critical to the future of the field.

The movement of both patients and health workers around the globe shines a light on a number of complex problems in global health delivery. I. Glenn Cohen provides insight into the legal and ethical challenges of patients seeking and receiving health care in foreign countries. These challenges are not limited to the individual patient, though issues such as safety, liability, and follow-up care are significant, but extend much more broadly to include the ways in which medical tourism depletes already impoverished local health systems, and the inequitable distribution of access to health care in home countries that pushes patients to travel overseas for needed medical care. The other side of the medical tourism coin is the global movement of health care workers, often from low- to high-income countries, and often facilitated by health systems in high-income settings. Nir Eyal and Samia Hurst's discussion of health worker migration lies at the intersection of global health policy and global justice, highlighting the often detrimental impact of health worker migration on population health while acknowledging its appeal for health workers from low-income countries. The authors explore competing ethical considerations, including whether health workers have a moral responsibility to remain in their home countries when need is great, whether they can be required to remain by more or less coercive policies, whether the individual liberty interests of health workers trump any obligation to remain, and the responsibilities of recruiting health systems to the countries whose workers they are recruiting.

The final chapter in this section addresses one of the most truly global contemporary problems of health and social justice. The phenomenon of climate change has not escaped serious moral analysis, but is less often couched in terms of bioethical concerns. Yet as Madison Powers argues, climate change poses some of the most significant contemporary threats to human health and wellbeing, ranging from disruption of agriculture and food production, to expansion of geographic zones at high risk for infectious diseases, and the differential impact of climate change on poorer nations. Implicit in the debate over climate change are issues that arise again and again in global bioethics, namely health and social justice, and moral responsibility. Powers' contribution shows the complexity of the debate over who should bear that responsibility and take the necessary steps to mitigate the injustices of climate change, injustices that are likely to have a significant impact on population health in the future.

6

BIOETHICS AND HUMAN RIGHTS

Elizabeth Fenton[1]

Bioethics and human rights are deeply intertwined, not least because of their common origins in the horrors of war—both emerging from the post-World War II International Military Tribunal in Nuremberg, including the trial of "Nazi doctors"—but also because of their common desire to reduce human suffering and protect human health and wellbeing.

As bioethics increasingly turns its attention to issues of global health and social justice, the intersections with human rights are more numerous and more profound. Bioethics has most notably encountered human rights in terms of the human right to health care (see Chapter 1 in this volume), but the scope of the relationship is much broader. Some have argued, for example, that debates over human genetic engineering engage human rights at the deepest level, raising questions about what it is to be human and what forms of change might endanger the notion of humanity at the core of human rights (Annas 2005; Andorno 2002; Fukuyama 2002). And as our understanding grows of the many and varied factors that influence health, the human right to health care has been eclipsed by the more expansive human right to health (or "health-related goods"), that encompasses the social, economic, and political contexts in which we live. As others in this volume point out, bioethics has been somewhat slow to recognize the moral significance of these broader contextual factors (see Chapter 2 in this volume), but as it does so it is increasingly pulled into the powerful force field of human rights, particularly social and economic rights.

This chapter explores the relationship between bioethics and human rights from two perspectives. The first perspective is broadly enthusiastic about an intimate relationship between bioethics and human rights, with some authors considering human rights to be an important common ground or *lingua franca* for global bioethics, and others imagining a merger between these two fields. Also included in this perspective are critics of bioethics who urge the field to adopt a stronger human rights focus, paying greater attention to the social and economic contexts in which bioethical issues arise.

The second perspective is more circumspect about the relationship between bioethics and human rights. This circumspection is justified in part by philosophical problems raised by human rights themselves, and in part by resistance to the notion that the ethical analysis characteristic of bioethics might be exhausted by the moral concepts and language of human rights. Those who view the notion of a merger between bioethics and human rights with caution argue that a rights-based framework is just one lens through which to view issues of social justice in bioethics, and while sometimes critical, it can also be unhelpful or inhibit other forms of moral reasoning. I will begin with a brief discussion of the "globalization" of bioethics, and note some important historical landmarks in the development of the relationship between bioethics and human rights.

Bioethics Goes "Global"

Bioethics has gone global in one obvious sense. As a response to threats to health, bioethics must now consider pandemics that cross national boundaries; the doctor–patient relationship may involve doctors in India or Thailand treating "medical tourists" from the United States and Europe; health workers trot the globe seeking better pay and working conditions, leaving health care in resource-poor settings to the vagaries of the philanthropic and non-governmental organization sectors; drug trials take place all over the world, funded by vast transnational corporations, testing drugs that will be distributed under a range of complex international aid and trade agreements; biotechnology and climate change are truly global phenomena that will, at some point, challenge the health of every human being on the planet.

Bioethics has also gone global in a less obvious sense. Its concerns have moved beyond the individual patient and medical professional to the health of groups and populations, beyond health *care* to encompass all of human health and its relationship to "global" wellbeing, beyond justice for this or that patient to justice across a growing health gap between rich and poor, advantaged and disadvantaged.

Human rights are a natural fit with globalized bioethics in both of these senses. On the one hand, human rights provide a ready-made language and framework for navigating complex cultural and religious differences that arise when ethical issues cross borders; thus Lori Knowles describes human rights as a "lingua franca that can both facilitate and broaden international bioethics discourse" (Knowles 2001: 253). They also provide a legal framework that transcends domestic law and regulatory regimes; thus Roberto Andorno describes human rights as "the best, if not the only available grounds for the development of international legal standards for biomedicine" (Andorno 2009: 224). In the second sense, human rights are a powerful force of social justice, setting out the conditions of human wellbeing and flourishing. When serious attempts are made to ensure that all human rights, and particularly social and economic rights, are fulfilled, health and health equity are improved. Thus the failure to fulfill these rights is, as Paul Farmer and others have argued, one of the most pressing ethical issues for contemporary bioethics (Farmer and Campos 2004a).

In many respects the origin stories of bioethics and the modern human rights movement are inseparable. In a succinct summary of their history, Robert Baker highlights the argument made by an American physician at Nuremberg, employed by the prosecution, that unconsented human experimentation of the sort practiced by Nazi doctors was impermissible as a violation of ethical principles *and* human rights—he argued, in effect, that the ethical principles of the medical profession are mechanisms for protecting human rights (Baker 2001: 244). But this argument, that "transcultural" medical ethics could be grounded in human rights, was ignored in favor of "the myth of converging civilized opinion" condemning the Nazi doctors' actions. The ethical principles of the Nuremberg Code were thus not grounded in human rights, and in spite of many parallels in the development of the two fields, Baker argues that "American bioethics has been ill at ease with the idea of human rights" ever since (Baker 2001: 247). Baker and others have called for bioethics and human rights to be reconciled; George Annas argues that "it is time to reunite the estranged twins who can work much more effectively together in the global health arena than they can separately" (Annas 2010: 135).

In the last several decades a series of international bioethics documents invoking human rights suggests that a reconciliation between these two fields is indeed occurring. In 1997 the Council of Europe adopted the Convention on Human Rights and Biomedicine, which aims to protect individuals from the misuse of biology and medicine. This document echoes the emphasis of the Universal Declaration of Human Rights (UDHR) on human dignity, endorses certain principles, for example that "the interests and welfare of the human being shall prevail over the sole interest of society or science," and issues substantive prescriptions, for example prohibiting the creation of human embryos for research, or human genetic modifications for anything other than preventive, diagnostic, or therapeutic purposes (Council of Europe 1997). Also in 1997 the United Nations Educational, Scientific, and Cultural Organization (UNESCO) adopted the Universal Declaration on the Human Genome and Human Rights, which again echoes the UDHR in emphasizing that human genetic research must "fully respect human dignity, freedom, and human rights" (UNESCO 1997). In addition to this document, UNESCO adopted the International Declaration on Human Genetic Data in 2003, which aims to protect individuals from the risks posed by collecting, storing, and using genetic data in the service of "human rights, fundamental freedoms, and respect for human dignity" (UNESCO 2003).

Most recent in this series of documents is UNESCO's 2005 Universal Declaration on Bioethics and Human Rights (UDBHR). The aim of the UDBHR is to "determine those principles in the field of bioethics that are universally acceptable, in conformity with human rights as ensured by international law," and, as far as possible, to "inscribe scientific decisions and practices within the framework of a certain number of general principles common to all" (ten Have 2006: 341). The UDBHR is significant, first, because it can be viewed as an achievement to have garnered agreement among virtually all states in the "sensitive area" of bioethics, and second because as a legal (though non-binding) document it encourages states to commit to common standards without forcing them to do so (Andorno 2007). A strong advocate of the UDBHR, Roberto Andorno is careful to note that its purpose is not to "invent new bioethical principles or to provide the definitive solution to the growing list of bioethical dilemmas." Rather, it aims to provide one-stop guidance to states in the form of "basic standards" for responsible biomedical research and clinical practice that conform to international human rights law (Andorno 2007: 153).

Merging Human Rights and Bioethics

The controversy surrounding the UDBHR (some of which will be explored further below) suggests that the document has achieved at least one of its aims, namely to open "a new agenda for international bioethics" (Ashcroft 2008: 38). I set aside this controversy for the moment in order to focus on the argument that the Declaration, and the related documents that preceded it, are part of a much-needed reconciliation or merger between bioethics and human rights.

A number of reasons have been given in support of such a merger. First is the notion that bioethics (particularly "American" bioethics) needs human rights to escape its limited domestic preoccupations; human rights can "enhance American bioethics by helping to move it from a self-absorbed and self-referential worldview to a global one that reaches outward rather than inward" (Annas 2010: 134). Human rights are a global language, in comparison to the parochial or ethnocentric languages of bioethics as practiced in different national or cultural contexts. The term "lingua franca" is used frequently, and Baker describes human rights as having "transcultural scope" that can "dissipate problems of moral parochialism" and free global bioethics from "the feckless dispute over whose principles are preferable" (Baker 2001: 250). In a similar vein, it is often argued that the success of the human rights movement is due in large part to the fact that adherents leave their philosophical commitments at the door; questions of deeper moral foundations for human rights are simply bracketed in favor of an "overlapping consensus" on the identification of the rights themselves. Principles of bioethics, treated similarly, may have the same success on the global stage. Of course these claims about human rights as the locus of consensus, sitting above the petty squabbles that muddy the foundational waters beneath, gloss over lingering and not insignificant disputes about human rights principles, but I take up this issue in more detail below.

Another reason in favor of a merger is that human rights give bioethics a broader and more socialized context in which to situate its traditional concerns, since they carry a greater emphasis on justice, social structure and social power (Ashcroft 2008). Human rights also have "great rhetorical, moral, and popular force" that can only enhance the power and reach of bioethics, and imposing the framework of international law on bioethics will produce tangible effects of this enhanced power, in the form of national action and the passage of national laws (Knowles 2001: 254). Moreover, as Thomas Faunce points out, the use of human rights law in cases relevant to bioethics, such as end-of-life decisions, reproductive technology, privacy, and informed consent, has established a body of interpretations of bioethics principles that can provide important guidance in difficult cases. Perhaps most significantly, human rights law lends credibility to the principles of bioethics, without which they can easily be ignored by the range of multinational organizations and corporations that increasingly control or influence the medical profession and delivery of health services (Faunce 2004).

Faunce explores other ways in which the assimilation of bioethics and human rights may advance bioethics, noting that human rights may be a more powerful mechanism for motivating a concern for social justice among physicians and medical students than bioethics alone. He goes on to argue that consensus documents that impose a human rights framework on bioethics, like the UDBHR, are the first steps in a process in which "the moral, political, and international law aspects of human rights begin to *subsume* medical ethics" (Faunce 2004: 177, emphasis added). His enthusiasm for this outcome is evident in his speculation that in the future an international bioethics convention will create "binding obligations on states under international law," obligations to ensure that domestic legislation "on bioethics, public health, or the doctor/patient relationship conforms to international norms" (Faunce 2004: 177).

Although it is important not to become mired in linguistic differences, it is noteworthy that other proponents of merging bioethics and human rights have rejected Faunce's notion that human rights will *subsume* bioethics. The term *subsume* connotes the loss of bioethics as an independently identifiable field, whereas Andorno and Baker, for example, view human rights as a necessary foundation or grounding for global bioethics (Baker 2001; Andorno 2009). Andorno argues that bioethics must be understood broadly, as both an ethical and a legal discipline; the UNESCO declarations and other similar documents are "*an extension of international human rights law into the field of biomedicine*" (Andorno 2009: 225, emphasis in original). Far from losing its identity, then, on this view human rights bolsters bioethics, giving the field a stronger global presence and legal heft.

The Human Rights Critique of Bioethics

In addition to arguments from within bioethics for a reconciliation with human rights, those in the human rights community, including activists and advocates of a human rights framework for health, have criticized bioethics in at least two ways for a lack of engagement with human rights. First, they argue that as a field deeply rooted in philosophy, problems in bioethics are too often approached through abstractions rather than through concrete realities; problems are analyzed in terms of the "mythical figure of the autonomous subject" and individual values and preferences, abstracted from the social context in which those individuals actually live (Ashcroft 2008: 43). Rejecting the biological individualism that views health and disease as "ascertainable in isolation from the broader context in which people live," advocates of a rights-based approach to health argue that health is deeply tied to social, political, historical, and economic contexts, and suffering arises not only from biological causes but from "human choices about policies, priorities, and cultural norms, about how we treat each other and what we owe each other" (Yamin 2008: 47). Physician and anthropologist Paul Farmer argues that in its detachment from social context, bioethics has failed to appreciate the most challenging ethical problem in health, namely the large and growing health outcome gap between rich and poor. He calls for "resocialising" bioethics to draw more from relevant social science disciplines, such as economics, anthropology, and history (and perhaps less from philosophy) in order to fully understand the ways in which poverty, racism, and gender inequality impact on people's choices, their vulnerability, and their access to equitable health care (Farmer and Campos 2004a: 27). Farmer's chief concern, and that of the health and human rights community more broadly, is with the health of the world's poorest and most marginalized, whom bioethics has failed "on numerous occasions, be it from lack of influence or failure to consider social justice." Farmer urges bioethics to adopt a new focus on human rights, through which it can "engage other disciplines to ensure that social and economic rights for the poor are realized" (Farmer and Campos 2004b: 245).

The second, related, human rights criticism of bioethics is that it is too often detached from real human suffering in its analysis of health and human rights, and too often unengaged from the political struggles waged by human rights activists. Although Farmer's criticisms extend to those working in human rights as well as in bioethics, his call for a more pragmatic and less theoretical approach to addressing social injustices is particularly powerful for disciplines like bioethics that are often more intellectual than practical. Treating the poorest of the poor in the world's most under-resourced health systems, Farmer loses patience with endless theorizing or philosophizing about human rights, hand-wringing about cost-effectiveness, and repetitive data collection ("let's just say no to more surveys sure to reveal the same problems already revealed by previous surveys"). He insists that the "traditional exhortatory role" of health and human rights be replaced by a focus on "prosaic" issues like supply chains for basic medical equipment, and immediate, short-term action to address the most egregious resource shortages that inhibit progress in areas such as maternal mortality: "We will need gloves. We will need sutures and antihemorrhagics. We will need drapes and hot, clean water" (Farmer 2008: 10). The call to action extends to bioethicists as well, whom Farmer argues should be prepared to engage actively with problem solving on the ground, becoming "part of teams seeking to lessen the outcome gap by remediating access to effective medical care" (Farmer and Campos 2004a: 39).

Whether Farmer and other proponents of a human rights focus in bioethics view formal documents such as the UDBHR as progress is unclear. Critics of this document in particular have argued that its emphasis on individual liberty indicates a failure to take seriously issues of substantial inequality and collective action in efforts to promote health equity (Selgelid 2005), suggesting that Farmer and others would find little reassurance in this latest explicit "reconciliation" of human rights and bioethics. Other developments in the field may offer more hope, for example, a growing body of work in public and population health ethics, where the social determinants of health and health inequalities are given more attention than in traditional bioethics. Nevertheless, many in bioethics remain skeptical about human rights and their role in bioethics, both practically and theoretically, and this skepticism is the topic of the next section.

Resisting a Merger Between Bioethics and Human Rights

Richard Ashcroft has provided a pithy summary of the sometimes "troubled" relationship between human rights and bioethics: "There is a bioethical critique of human rights; and a human rights critique of bioethics" (Ashcroft 2008: 38). Whereas Farmer's challenge to bioethics is indicative of the latter, in this section I explore the criticisms bioethics has leveled at human rights theory and practice, and the extent to which it has resisted engagement with human rights. These criticisms can broadly be categorized as philosophical and practical.

Philosophical Problems

A striking and much discussed feature of the development of the Universal Declaration of Human Rights is the fact that the drafters reached any agreement at all on such moral principles, given the vastly different moral, religious, cultural, and ethnic commitments that they brought to the table. Famously, one of the drafters reported that "we agree on these rights, *provided we are not asked why*" (Maritain 1949: 9, emphasis in original). This form of agreement on principles, where foundational commitments or justifications on which there is likely to be substantial disagreement are bracketed, is often referred to as an "overlapping consensus," following political philosopher John Rawls' use of the term to describe agreement on principles of justice in a pluralistic society (Rawls 1993, 1999 [1971]). Not surprisingly, this term has also been used in reference to the UDBHR, where again foundational issues are bracketed in order to arrive at "general principles common to all" (ten Have 2006). While there is much to be said for seeking common ground and consensus around principles of justice, there are substantial and difficult questions about whether such general principles are ever either "common to all," or devoid of the sorts of theoretical commitments that undermine the claim of an "overlapping consensus" to have successfully bracketed foundational issues.

One of the central philosophical problems raised by both the UDBHR and the imposition of a human rights framework on bioethics more generally is the concern that human rights, far from being "neutral" with respect to foundational issues, are in fact rife with presumptions and theoretical commitments that many find objectionable. For example, a number of commentators have noted the emphasis placed in the UDBHR on individual autonomy and liberty, which is viewed by some as a bias inherited from the Western Enlightenment tradition (of which human rights are a legacy) that ignores the strongly relational nature of individual lives and the extent to which family and social networks "ground and sustain individual identity" (Rawlinson and Donchin 2005: 262). Another criticism is that the UDBHR fails to give any indication of how conflicts between individual liberty and social welfare should be adjudicated; Michael Selgelid, for example, argues that it fails to recognize that in the health care context individual liberty must sometimes be sacrificed to achieve the common good (Selgelid 2005). Yet another criticism highlights the document's somewhat clumsy attempt to show respect for cultural diversity by stating that cultural diversity and pluralism "are not to be invoked to infringe upon human dignity, human rights and fundamental freedoms" (UDBHR Article 12). Jing-Bao Nie argues that this statement sets up a false sense of antagonism between the notions of human dignity, human rights, and fundamental freedoms on the one hand, and non-Western cultures on the other, whereas in fact these notions are deeply rooted in many such cultures. The UDBHR thus perpetuates a myth that universal ethical ideals, such as human dignity and human rights, are incompatible with moral values in non-Western cultures (Nie 2005).

These criticisms of the UDBHR mirror criticisms of the notion of *universal* human rights more broadly. The notion of whether there can be universally shared moral principles is a perplexing one, but the extent to which human rights have been embraced globally lends it considerable support. Nevertheless, philosophers worry that even if universal or widespread support can be gained for a limited set of basic moral principles, the more these principles attempt to cover complex issues that implicate deep moral and political disagreement—issues that are the bread and butter of global bioethics—the less likely it is that they can be described as "universal." Moreover, it is debatable whether supplanting local norms with the supposedly universal norms codified in the principles of the UDBHR is always a good thing. The cloak of universality lends the principles a higher moral status than may be warranted when they come into conflict with legitimate moral values at the local level.

Perhaps the most notoriously controversial aspect of human rights documents such as the UDBHR for philosophers is their grounding in the concept of human dignity, a concept that, despite receiving considerable attention in the literature, remains nebulous. Dignity is something of a lightning rod in the debate over human rights and bioethics, with passions running high on both sides. Defenders of the importance of dignity have described it as the "overarching principle" of international bioethics and biolaw, which is placed first on the list of principles in the UDBHR because it "embodies the central aim of the whole instrument" (Andorno 2009: 227). Detractors argue that dignity is a "useless" concept (Macklin 2003), or at least a slippery one, meaning very different things to different people and in different contexts. As such, it is deeply philosophically problematic to declare that certain practices, such as reproductive cloning, germ-line modifications, or the creation of embryos for research are or could be "contrary to human dignity" (such claims are made in the Universal Declaration on the Human Genome and Human Rights and the Convention on Human Rights and Biomedicine; dignity also plays a central role in the work conducted on human cloning by the United States President's Council on Bioethics under Leon Kass (Kass 2002)). Without a clearer idea of what human dignity is, such statements are difficult to comprehend.

The extent to which the language of human rights and human dignity has been used to justify prohibitions in these areas constitutes one of the central reasons why many philosopher-bioethicists are critical of the importation of human rights into bioethics. To claim that germ-line interventions or genetic enhancements, for example, are necessarily contrary to human dignity and therefore a violation of human rights is not only a weak argument, since dignity is always under-defined, but also a short-sighted and potentially destructive one. Given the power of human rights, grounding a prohibition on an action in human rights terms takes that action off the table. But future enhancements may have the capacity to *improve* human health and wellbeing: Do these potentially beneficial enhancements also endanger human dignity and violate human rights? Critics of the use of human rights to prohibit human enhancement argue that dignity is too imprecise a concept to ground blanket bans on complex technologies of this sort. Appeals to human dignity and human rights are no substitute for a more fine-grained moral analysis of the moral issues at stake (Fenton and Arras 2010).

Arguments about the foundational or philosophical commitments of human rights are sometimes dismissed as, at best, examples of the "harmless entertainment" produced by philosophers, "which if taken too seriously would look ridiculous" (Churchill 1999: 255), or at worst, as a way of postponing the protection of human rights in practice (Annas 2010), or undermining "the force of rights claims and instruments in practice," by giving rights-abusing governments a reason to argue that supposedly universal and non-derogable rights may, according to the intellectual ditherings of philosophers, be neither of those things (Ashcroft 2008: 44). But concerns about the foundations of human rights are not so easily dismissed. Whether germ-line genetic interventions, for example, are or ought to be considered a violation of human rights is a significant question, but one that cannot be answered without a deeper and more precise understanding of what it is that human rights seek to protect. The standard answer "human dignity" is insufficient, since whether enhanced memory, intelligence or athleticism are contrary to human dignity is far from obvious. Moreover, to claim that human rights rest straightforwardly on the foundation of human dignity, with all its myriad interpretations, or any other singular notion of what it is to be human, can undermine the doctrine's claims both to universality and political legitimacy. As Amy Gutmann observes:

> If human rights necessarily rest on a moral or metaphysical foundation that is not in any meaningful sense universal or publicly defensible in the international arena . . . then the political legitimacy of human rights talk, human rights covenants, and human rights enforcement is called into question.
>
> (Gutmann 2001: xvii)

Of course, it is precisely for this reason that questions of foundations are typically set aside in favor of overlapping consensus, but as the case of genetic enhancement shows, there are instances in which we cannot know whether something violates human rights simply by looking to the documents on which the consensus has been achieved. Similarly for questions about balancing individual liberty against social goods, on which there is no guidance in human rights documents. Unless we are willing to engage deeper foundational issues we have no way to answer these important questions; the notion that philosophical commitments can be checked at the door is a convenient, but ultimately unhelpful fiction.

Clearly the overlapping consensus on both human rights and the UDBHR is an imperfect one; and as Jonathan Wolff has pointed out, one response to "residual differences" in understanding and interpreting human rights is simply to "acknowledge the limits of philosophical argument" and allow disputes to be resolved through democratic processes and legal doctrine (Wolff 2012a: 20). But the fact of disagreement about the foundations of human rights should not preclude further discussion. The literature in this area is rich with suggestions for what the foundations of human rights might be, including human agency, fundamental human interests, and basic human capabilities. A discussion of each of these arguments is beyond the scope of this chapter, but suffice it to say here that however we choose to understand the foundations of human rights, that understanding is highly relevant to the way in which human rights are practiced, interpreted, protected, and promoted in global health and bioethics.

Practical Problems

Just as Paul Farmer has urged bioethicists to take up a more practical attitude with respect to human rights and social justice, so many bioethicists have argued that it is in the detail of practical ethical problems that a human rights approach in bioethics shows its limitations.

Over a decade ago Dan Brock drew bioethicists' attention to the need for bioethics to broaden its purview beyond health care and establishing a right to it (Brock 2000). This limited focus is problematic, Brock argued, for two reasons. First, it fails to recognize the fact that differential access to health care is only one factor in persistent health inequities, and in many cases not the primary factor. The other factors, the social and economic determinants of health, should be as familiar to and of as much concern to bioethicists as access to health care. Second, the focus on a right to health care left most bioethicists, with prominent exceptions, silent on the complex moral problem of prioritizing limited resources for health. Recognizing that advocates of a human rights approach to bioethics view this approach as much broader than just the right to health care, Brock's concerns about the failure to address prioritization problems under the human rights framework continue to be borne out.

To put this problem most simply, consider the government of a poor country trying to lower its rate of maternal mortality. Even accepting that all women have a right to the conditions necessary for healthy pregnancies and safe deliveries, a government with a small health budget faces numerous policy options that may all advance a right to health, but may benefit some women more than others. Exploring this problem in detail, Norman Daniels suggests that in such a case the policy options might include improving access to services for rural women, investing in expensive facilities in urban or population-dense areas, or investing in education for girls in secondary schools (Daniels 2008: 320). The problem in this case is that the notion of a human right to health justifies and perhaps demands each of these options, but where resources are limited to pursuing only one strategy, the human rights approach cannot tell us which to choose. While the human rights framework (both rhetoric and law) is essential for the mammoth task of getting governments to recognize their responsibility for creating social structures and institutions, and implementing policies that will advance the human right to health, it stops short of specifying how limited resources should be allocated so as to begin to realize that right. Limited resources mean that not all needs can be met; determining which needs will be met and which will not is a complex moral problem for which tools of analysis other than human rights are required. Discussing the role of human rights in the analysis of the determinants of health Venkatapuram, Bell, and Marmot argue that the power of the human rights framework is best used as a supplement to rather than as a substitute for the analysis of the causes of ill health and mortality (Venkatapuram et al. 2010). Bioethicists might argue similarly that human rights should be viewed as a supplement to and not a substitute for a *moral* analysis of the prioritization of resources for health, which should include a concern for equality, for the worst off, for the victims of prior discrimination, for the results of cost-effectiveness analyses, and so on.

One of the most prominent and challenging areas in which the prioritization issue remains at the forefront is in the management of resources for the treatment and prevention of HIV disease. The health and human rights framework was forged in the early days of the HIV/AIDS pandemic, in which human rights were a bulwark against discrimination, prejudice, and ignorance. In spite of an early focus on prevention and the underlying social determinants of HIV transmission, with the advent of better and cheaper treatments for the disease the human rights agenda on HIV shifted from prevention to treatment, "driven by advocacy to respond to the dying individual regardless of the broader public health impact" (Mason-Meier et al. 2012: 264). While global policy on HIV continues to emphasize both treatment and prevention, the realities of limited health budgets, falling levels of donor funds, and increasing HIV incidence have led some to argue that universal life-long treatment efforts are unsustainable, and that a focus on prevention rather than treatment is a more cost-effective and morally justifiable strategy (Brock and Wikler 2009; Mason-Meier et al. 2012). From the perspective of the health and human rights framework this is a controversial argument. In de-prioritizing treatment in favor of prevention, what becomes of the right to health of those patients who are already sick and in need of treatment? Even if it is true that prevention saves more lives, and that, all things being equal, we should save more lives than fewer, are not those whose lives cannot be saved by prevention *entitled* to treatment under the human right to health?

This question demonstrates the shortcomings of the unmodified human rights framework. In their "ideal" form—i.e., as aspirational statements—human rights operate outside the limitations of budgets and "donor fatigue." Talk of cost-effectiveness and saving the most lives is anathema to human rights advocates, who argue that cost ought not to stand in the way of meeting core human rights obligations; they argue that we should either shame drug companies, governments, and donors into lowering costs and funding essential health services, or impose duties on the international community to assist countries who cannot meet core human rights obligations on their own (Wolff 2012b). It is true that adding more money could solve many global health problems, and human rights advocacy has often shown that what is accepted as hard economic fact is actually a matter of social choice, thus broadening the scope of what is possible in global health. On the other hand, funds will *always* be limited relative to need, and there is a moral responsibility to allocate them carefully, human rights notwithstanding. In a South African case in which a man argued that his right to life and right to health entitled him to kidney dialysis at public expense, the court ruled that so long as a fair procedure had been followed, the denial of access to dialysis machines (which were insufficient to meet demand) did not violate those rights. Emphasizing the fact that even the right to health cannot overcome resource shortages, the court stated: "The state has to manage its limited resources in order to address all these claims. There will be times when this requires it to adopt a holistic approach to the larger needs of society rather than to focus on the specific needs of a particular individual within society" (Constitutional Court of South Africa 1997: 19).

Health resource allocation requires complex and morally challenging tradeoffs, tradeoffs for which human rights offer little substantive guidance. Filling this gap is the role of moral analysis of the sort offered by Brock and Wikler, who build a case for prevention over treatment from careful consideration of the justifications for different moral principles. The answer to such questions requires substantive moral analysis, and cannot simply be read off the notion of the right to health (Arras and Fenton 2009).

This is not to say that human rights do not have an important place in a global HIV policy focused on prevention rather than treatment. As Mason-Meier et al. argue, the notion of *collective* rights provides a sounder foundation for large-scale public health efforts than do individual human rights (Mason-Meier et al. 2012). Under a collective rights framework the needs of the group or population are considered, thus balancing the rights of the sick to receive treatment against the rights of the well to be protected from disease. This is a significant shift that captures the complexities of prioritization problems, in which, under ubiquitous resource constraints, not all health needs can be met.

Conclusion

In discussing his skepticism regarding the notion of a moral right to health, Gopal Sreenivasan articulates some important areas of common ground with advocates of that same right, including the moral importance of health for every human being and the moral importance of preserving or restoring health through social action (Sreenivasan 2012). Sreenivasan's argument is significant because it demonstrates the fact that skeptical questions about rights are not incompatible with endorsement of the moral values inherent in those rights. Critics of a human rights framework for bioethics are sometimes assumed to be anti-human rights (Annas 2010), but this is generally far from the truth. Many critics are broadly supportive of human rights yet seek greater clarification about what those rights are and how they should operate within a field such as bioethics. Ashcroft raises a number of questions about the UDBHR, for example, that might be on the lips of skeptics more generally: "Does the Declaration codify best practice? Or reflect international consensus only? Or interpret higher order norms for this specific context? Or declare a new agenda somewhat ahead of current policy and state context?" (Ashcroft 2008: 35). These and many other questions signify a need for further discussion and careful reflection; in this respect the UDBHR is best viewed as the beginning, not the end, of a complex conversation about bioethics and human rights.

There can be no doubt of the moral, political, and legal importance of human rights to the improvement of global health. Since making these improvements in health, in particular for those who are worst off, is a pressing and perhaps defining ethical issue for contemporary bioethics, human rights are a critical tool in the bioethicist's toolbox. But the limitations of the human rights framework must be recognized alongside its legal and political power. In response to shameful resource shortages in maternity care in developing countries, Paul Farmer has asked, "Should there be a right to sutures? To sterile drapes? To anesthesia?" (Farmer 2008: 9). When the lack of these resources leads directly to high rates of maternal morality, it is reasonable to try to locate such rights in the law, but fixing global health problems is not as simple as defining ever more specific human rights. As Venkatapuram et al. argue, the human rights framework is not capable of doing all of the work we want it to do; it is "only one of many instruments of advancing health and health equity" (Venkatapuram et al. 2010: 12). In arguing that it is unacceptable *both* to ignore the social causes of morbidity and mortality simply because they are not "explicitly identified in existing law" *and* to "opportunistically stretch the meaning of rights so much that the term 'human rights' risks becoming an empty concept," these authors identify precisely the balance that bioethics ought to seek between endorsement of and skepticism about the human rights framework.

Related Topics

Chapter 1, "The Right to Health Care," John D. Arras
Chapter 2, "Social Determinants of Health and Health Inequalities," Sridhar Venkatapuram and Michael Marmot

Note

1 This chapter was written by Elizabeth Fenton in her private capacity. No official support or endorsement by the Presidential Commission for the Study of Bioethical Issues or the Department of Health and Human Services is intended, nor should be inferred.

References

Andorno, R. (2002) "Biomedicine and International Human Rights Law: In Search of a Global Consensus," *Bulletin of the World Health Organization* 80 (12): 959–63.

Andorno, R. (2007) "Global Bioethics at UNESCO: In Defense of the Universal Declaration on Bioethics and Human Rights," *Journal of Medical Ethics* 33: 150–4.

Andorno, R. (2009) "Human Dignity and Human Rights as a Common Ground for a Global Bioethics," *Journal of Medicine and Philosophy* 34: 223–40.

Annas, G.J. (2005) *American Bioethics: Crossing Human Rights and Health Law Boundaries*, New York: Oxford University Press.

Annas, G.J. (2010) "Human Rights and American Bioethics: Resistance is Futile," *Cambridge Quarterly of Healthcare Ethics* 19: 133–41.

Arras, J.D. and Fenton, E.M. (2009) "Bioethics and Human Rights: Access to Health-Related Goods," *Hastings Center Report* 39: 27–38.

Ashcroft, R. (2008) "The Troubled Relationship Between Bioethics and Human Rights," in M. Freeman (ed.) *Law and Bioethics*, Oxford: Oxford University Press, pp. 31–51.

Baker, R. (2001) "Bioethics and Human Rights: A Historical Perspective," *Cambridge Quarterly of Healthcare Ethics* 10: 241–52.

Brock, D.W. (2000) "Broadening the Bioethics Agenda," *Kennedy Institute of Ethics Journal* 10: 21–38.

Brock, D.W. and Wikler, D. (2009) "Ethical Challenges in Long-Term Funding for HIV/AIDS," *Health Affairs* 28: 1666–76.

Churchill, L.R. (1999) "Are We Professionals? A Critical Look at the Social Role of Bioethicists," *Daedalus* 128 (4): 253–74.

Constitutional Court of South Africa (1997) *Thiagraj Soobramoney* v. *Minister of Health (Kwazulu-Natal)* CCT 32/97. Available at: http://www.constitutionalcourt.org.za/Archimages/1617.pdf (accessed October 29, 2013).

Council of Europe (1997) *Convention for the Protection of Human Rights and Dignity of the Human Being with Regard to the Application of Biology and Medicine: Convention on Human Rights and Biomedicine*. Available at: http://conventions.coe.int/Treaty/en/Treaties/Html/164.htm (accessed October 28, 2013).

Daniels, N. (2008) *Just Health: Meeting Health Needs Fairly*, Cambridge: Cambridge University Press.

Farmer, P. (2008) "Challenging Orthodoxies: The Road Ahead for Health and Human Rights," *Health and Human Rights* 10: 5–19.

Farmer, P. and Campos, N.C. (2004a) "Rethinking Medical Ethics: A View from Below," *Developing World Bioethics* 4: 1–41.

Farmer, P. and Campos, N.C. (2004b) "New Malaise: Bioethics and Human Rights in the Global Era," *Journal of Law, Medicine and Ethics* 32: 243–51.

Faunce, T.A. (2004) "Will International Human Rights Subsume Medical Ethics? Intersections in the UNESCO *Universal Bioethics Declaration*," *Journal of Medical Ethics* 31: 173–8.

Fenton, E. and Arras, J.D. (2010) "Bioethics and Human Rights: Curb Your Enthusiasm," *Cambridge Quarterly of Healthcare Ethics* 19: 127–33.

Fukuyama, F. (2002) *Our Posthuman Future*, New York: Farrar, Straus, Giroux.
Gutmann, A. (2001) Introduction, in M. Ignatieff (ed. A. Gutmann) *Human Rights as Politics and Idolatry*, Princeton, NJ: Princeton University Press.
Kass, L.R. (2002) *Human Cloning and Human Dignity: The Report of the President's Council on Bioethics*, New York: PublicAffairs.
Knowles, LP. (2001) "The Lingua Franca of Human Rights and the Rise of a Global Bioethic," *Cambridge Quarterly of Healthcare Ethics* 10: 253–63.
Macklin, R. (2003) "Dignity Is a Useless Concept: It Means No More Than Respect for Persons or Their Autonomy," *British Medical Journal* 327 (7429): 1419–20.
Maritain, J. (1949) Introduction, in UNESCO (ed.) *Human Rights: Comments and Interpretations*, New York: Columbia University Press.
Mason-Meier, B., Brugh, K. and Halima, Y. (2012) "Conceptualizing a Human Right to Prevention in Global HIV/AIDS Policy," *Public Health Ethics* 5: 263–82.
Nie, J. (2005) "Cultural Values Embodying Universal Norms: A Critique of a Popular Assumption About Cultures and Human Rights," *Developing World Bioethics* 5: 251–7.
Rawlinson, M.C. and Donchin, A. (2005) "The Quest for Universality: Reflections on the *Universal Draft Declaration on Bioethics and Human Rights*," *Developing World Bioethics* 5 (3): 258–66.
Rawls, J. (1993) *Political Liberalism*, New York: Columbia University Press.
Rawls, J. (1999) [1971] *A Theory of Justice*, Cambridge, MA: Belknap Press.
Selgelid, M. (2005) "Universal Norms and Conflicting Values," *Developing World Bioethics* 5: 267–73.
Sreenivasan, G. (2012) "A Human Right to Health? Some Inconclusive Scepticism," *Proceedings of the Aristotelian Society Supplementary Volume* 86: 239–65.
ten Have, H. (2006) "The Activities of UNESCO in the Area of Ethics," *Kennedy Institute of Ethics Journal* 16: 333–51.
UNESCO (1997) *Universal Declaration on the Human Genome and Human Rights*, United Nations Educational, Scientific and Cultural Organization. Available at: http://portal.unesco.org/en/ev.php-URL_ID=13177&URL_DO=DO_TOPIC&URL_SECTION=201.html (accessed October 28, 2013).
UNESCO (2003) *International Declaration on Human Genetic Data*, United Nations Educational, Scientific and Cultural Organization. Available at: http://portal.unesco.org/en/ev.php-URL_ID=17720&URL_DO=DO_TOPIC&URL_SECTION=201.html (accessed October 28, 2013).
UNESCO (2005) *Universal Declaration on Bioethics and Human Rights*, United Nations Educational, Scientific and Cultural Organization. Available at: http://www.unesco.org/new/en/social-and-human-sciences/themes/bioethics/bioethics-and-human-rights/ (accessed October 28, 2013).
Venkatapuram, S., Bell, R. and Marmot, M. (2010) "The Right to Sutures: Social Epidemiology, Human Rights, and Social Justice," *Health and Human Rights* 12: 3–16.
Wolff, J. (2012a) *The Human Right to Health*, New York: W.W. Norton.
Wolff, J. (2012b) "The Demands of the Human Right to Health," *Proceedings of the Aristotelian Society Supplementary Volume* 86: 217–37.
Yamin, A.E. (2008) "Will We Take Suffering Seriously? Reflections on What Applying a Human Rights Framework to Health Means and Why We Should Care," *Health and Human Rights* 10: 45–63.

Further Reading

Ashcroft, R.E. (2010) "Could Human Rights Supersede Bioethics?" *Human Rights Law Review* 10 (4): 639–60. (An analysis of the thesis that human rights law will subsume bioethics.)
Sen, A. (2012) "The Global Reach of Human Rights," *Journal of Applied Philosophy* 29 (2): 91–100. (A reflection on the idea of human rights and the concern that it is lacking in foundation.)
Thomasma, D. (2001) "Proposing a New Agenda: Bioethics and International Human Rights," *Cambridge Quarterly of Healthcare Ethics* 10: 299–310. (Argues that human rights provide the basis for international and intercultural bioethics discourse.)

7

ETHICAL CHALLENGES OF DISTRIBUTING LIMITED HEALTH RESOURCES IN LOW-INCOME COUNTRIES

Kjell Arne Johansson

Introduction

Children born in low-income countries (LICs) can on average expect to live 20.1 life years less and are 16 times more likely to die before their fifth birthday than children born in high-income countries (see Table 7.1). Is this inequality in life prospects acceptable? Many people live in poverty; 74 percent of the people in LICs live on less than U.S.$2 per day. Low-income populations are growing due to high fertility rates and there is a high burden of disease; in addition, the majority of people in LICs live in rural regions and are hard to reach with health care services. Health care expenditures in LICs are on average 1/180th of high-income country expenditures. This scarcity of resources raises the justice issue: Whom should governments and charity organizations favor in allocating these limited resources? And what can theories of justice tell us about the moral grounds for making fair decisions? Policy decisions on access, availability, and quality of medical and public health services influence both the overall level of health in a population and the distribution of health between individuals. But access and quality of medical services do not solve the whole problem. Improving the position of the worst off in other, non-health domains of justice, such as liberty, income, education or capabilities, will have a substantial impact on population health. It is thus urgent to establish legitimate and practical procedures for making fair priority decisions and involving key stakeholders in an impartial and reasonable way. What should such legitimate priority setting procedures look like?

Many new and expensive health care technologies have been developed over the last several decades. However, few countries have universal coverage of even basic health care. The health gap, meaning the difference between the *potential* improvements in population health that could be achieved with universal coverage of all the health technology that is currently available, and the more *realistic* health improvements that are actually affordable, gives rise to many difficult problems. The scale of the gap problem is larger in LICs. Three methods can be used to narrow the health-gap: (1) Improve

Table 7.1 Key numbers that illustrate inequalities in global health (UN Population Division 2011)

Region	*Population size*	*Life expectancy at birth*	*GDP per capita (I$-PPP)*	*Health expenditures per capita (US$)*	*% living <2$ a day (PPP)*	*Rural pop. (% of total)*	*Fertility rate (births per woman)*	*<5 mortality (per 1,000 live births)*
High income	1 135 003 957	79.8	38 572	4 877	–	20	1.8	6.0
Upper middle income	2 489 098 440	72.6	10 705	380	20	40	1.8	20.0
Lower middle income	2 532 825 559	65.5	3 833	71	59	62	2.9	62.9
Low income	816 810 477	58.8	1 383	27	74	72	4.1	95.3
World	6 973 738 433	69.6	11 574	950	–	49	2.5	52.5

GDP = gross domestic product, PPP = purchasing power parity.

health care system efficiency; (2) increase health budgets; or (3) set priorities. All three approaches may narrow the health gap and influence distribution of health. Priority setting is crucial since it seems unrealistic that (1) and (2) are able to close the health gap sufficiently to make priority setting superfluous in any society. Methods (1)–(3) are not mutually exclusive options in any society, where for example the level of resources available and the efficiency of the health system have an impact on the urgency of making priorities between patient groups and interventions.

Because of the potential for different resource distributions to dramatically alter the health of populations, either positively or negatively, setting priorities for limited health resources is a significant concern of population-level bioethics and distributive justice (Wikler and Brock 2007). In a LIC where demand for health care vastly outstrips supply, the cost of making a poor allocation decision could amount to millions of lives. So how can these decisions be made? We cannot simply use our intuition to tell us who in the population is the most needy or will derive the greatest benefit from an intervention, since intuitions are a notoriously unreliable means of judging health and health-care allocation problems at the population level. Our intuitions need to be guided by ethical arguments and principles; and by rigorous health statistical information containing as little uncertainty as possible (Broome 1991).

As I will go on to show, however, there is no agreement on which of the available ethical principles should be used to solve difficult allocation problems. Moreover, there is no agreement on whether distributive principles should be applied globally, creating obligations for wealthier countries to assist LICs, or whether they should be limited to the distribution of resources within a single state. It is not my concern to engage these issues of global justice in this chapter, but it is worth mentioning that some argue that justice is only relevant domestically and appeal to weaker duties of humanitarianism and charity beyond borders (Nagel 2005). Others argue for more demanding commitments across borders, claiming that individual persons, not borders, are the appropriate objects of moral thought, and that principles of distributive justice should therefore operate globally (Caney 2005).

This chapter focuses on moral challenges concerning access to health care and health-related goods, such as the social determinants of health (Arras and Fenton 2009), at the population level. In the first section I introduce general priority setting issues that are relevant in many resource-poor settings. Second, I describe substantive distributive principles and show how they conflict on who should get what and which diseases or treatment groups should be prioritized. Third, I discuss how principled and reasonable disagreement about health care priorities can be addressed, and procedures for legitimate decision-making on those priorities.

Multi-Level Priority Setting Across Patient Groups

Priority setting occurs at different levels of health systems. At the international level, the Millennium Development Goals (MDGs) are a very influential priority setting mechanism. The MDGs were set by all government leaders at the United Nations Millennium Summit in 2000, and represent a united action to increase development aid to LICs. The goals give concrete priority guidance and serve as input to many key performance indicators for national health systems. For example, reductions in child and maternal mortality, treatment and prevention of HIV, tuberculosis, and malaria. Improvements in key social determinants of health (poverty, education, and gender equality) are considered more important than other health improvement interventions.

The goals are intuitively appealing. Nevertheless, they lack a coherent ethical justification. It is not clear what guiding ethical principles justify scale-up of the included MDG interventions rather than other plausible paths to better health and wellbeing.

Priority setting at the more concrete level of policy involves practical decisions on which *health services* to fund (e.g., should vaccines or treatment be scaled up to reduce the burden of diarrhea and pneumonia among children?) and *indications* for treatment and testing (e.g., when should one start antiretroviral treatment for HIV?). In addition, another set of priority decisions is health policies on *financing mechanisms* (e.g., user fees, partial or universal public finance), *infrastructure* (e.g., how many doctors to hire, health worker training programs, siting and quality of facilities, roads), *regulatory interventions* (e.g., curtailing smoking and alcohol consumption), or *education and communication programs* to improve healthy behaviors. Priority setting in health potentially involves the intentional or non-intentional withholding of some such useful services from individuals who could directly or indirectly benefit from them (Norheim 1996; Ham and Roberts 2003). Policy decisions of this kind, made either explicitly or implicitly, will all have an impact on who receives health benefits and on the size of health budgets.

In addition to these general priority setting challenges, there are particular and unique problems in health systems of LICs. Structural bottlenecks such as shortages of qualified health personnel, large rural populations that are hard to reach, and cultural barriers make scale-up of interventions more difficult. In addition, there is a large three-tiered burden of disease from communicable diseases, non-communicable diseases, and injuries (World Health Organization 2008). Often, there is a lack of financial protection and well functioning welfare systems for the many poor people in these countries. Moreover, a large proportion of health care funding in LICs comes from multiple international donors and many stakeholders with potentially different agendas. Donor-dependent health programs are also somewhat insecure and unstable due to the fact that financing always faces a risk of drying up if donors stop donating. The global economic crisis has for example created an additional pressure for many HIV programs, where treatment and prevention scale-up has flattened or slowed down due to shortfalls in HIV funding (Brock and Wikler 2009).

To appreciate these challenges, imagine that you are a Minister of Health in a LIC with extremely scarce resources and extremely large unmet health needs in the population. How would you decide which groups in the population will receive needed health-related goods and which will have to go without? To make these decisions you would need measures and information on baseline levels of the burden of disease and current coverage of services, and expected impacts and costs of available health interventions. Such estimates require large amounts of high-quality data and detailed population models, none of which your government may be able to acquire. Because such data are difficult to accumulate even when resources are available, your priority decisions would in many cases rest on imperfect information. Normative problems might be even more difficult than these technical difficulties. Just priority decisions and legitimate processes must be impartial and respect the interests of each individual in the society. As a rational, ethically motivated Minister of Health, you would want to deliberate on which distributive principles are relevant and on the relative importance of each one.

Distributive Principles

The distributive justice literature yields four distributive principles. First, the traditional utilitarian *greater-benefit principle* aims at maximizing outcomes (e.g., welfare, resources, capabilities, wellbeing, goods) to the highest aggregated level for the lowest cost (Sen 1979; Coast 2009). Second, an *egalitarian principle* is more sensitive to the way in which outcomes are distributed within a population and favors strict equality in outcomes or chances between individuals (Temkin 2003). Third, a *prioritarian principle* represents something of a middle ground between egalitarianism and utility maximization. It views crude equality as insufficiently sensitive to total gains, and maximization as insufficiently sensitive to distributions. Prioritarianism instead opts for less demanding distributions where the worst off are given absolute priority (Parfit 2000). Inequality between individuals is acceptable on this view as long as the distribution raises the absolute level of the worst off in the society. Fourth, the *sufficency principle* is a special form of prioritarianism and defends raising the worst off above a certain threshold level (Crisp 2003). Distributions above the threshold then matter less. Below, I explore disagreements and agreements between the first three general principles when applied to priority setting in health. For reasons of space I will not discuss the sufficiency principle any further below. A useful discussion of this threshold principle applied to a LIC setting can be found in Alvarez (2007).

Health Maximization

It is widely accepted that a principle of health maximization is important in the allocation of limited health care resources (Brock and Wikler 2006). Limited health resources should not be wasted; the population and individuals should attain the greatest achievable health level at the lowest cost possible (Weinstein and Stason 1977).

The most common method for determining how resources should be allocated to achieve the greatest benefit for the lowest cost is cost-effectiveness analysis or CEA. Standard CEAs rank interventions according to their efficiency, i.e., those interventions that generate the highest aggregated health benefits for the lowest costs are considered to be most efficient. The ratio between *incremental cost* (e.g., the marginal cost by going from health intervention A to B) and *incremental effectiveness* (e.g., marginal increase in any health metric by introducing health intervention A rather than B) determines the rank order of interventions (Weinstein and Stason 1977). Interventions with low cost-effectiveness ratios have high efficiency, and vice versa. Such efficiency rankings are typically done in the Disease Control Priorities Project (DCP) (see Figure 7.1) and WHO-CHOICE (Jamison et al. 2006; World Health Organisation and WHO-CHOICE 2012).

Life years lost or gained, with or without disability (DALY) or quality (QALY) adjustments, are common outcome metrics in CEA rankings. QALY and DALY metrics assess effectiveness over a lifetime and they allow for comparisons across life-saving treatments or preventions and interventions that only improve quality or disability (for a full discussion of QALYs and DALYs, see Chapter 4 in this volume).

CEAs are important decision-making tools for preventing waste in health systems (Weinstein and Stason 1977; Williams 1985). We see clearly from the DCP2 sum ranking in Figure 7.1 that there are large opportunity costs involved by choosing a less-efficient use of resources. For example, if U.S.$1,000,000 were spent on a less cost-effective intervention like antiretroviral therapy (ART) for HIV rather than on a very cost-effective intervention like deworming (albendazole for soil-transmitted helminthic infections), around 300,000 fewer DALYs would be averted according to DCP2 estimates. However, patients who need interventions with the least favorable incremental cost-effectiveness ratio will be excluded according to a crude health-maximizing principle.

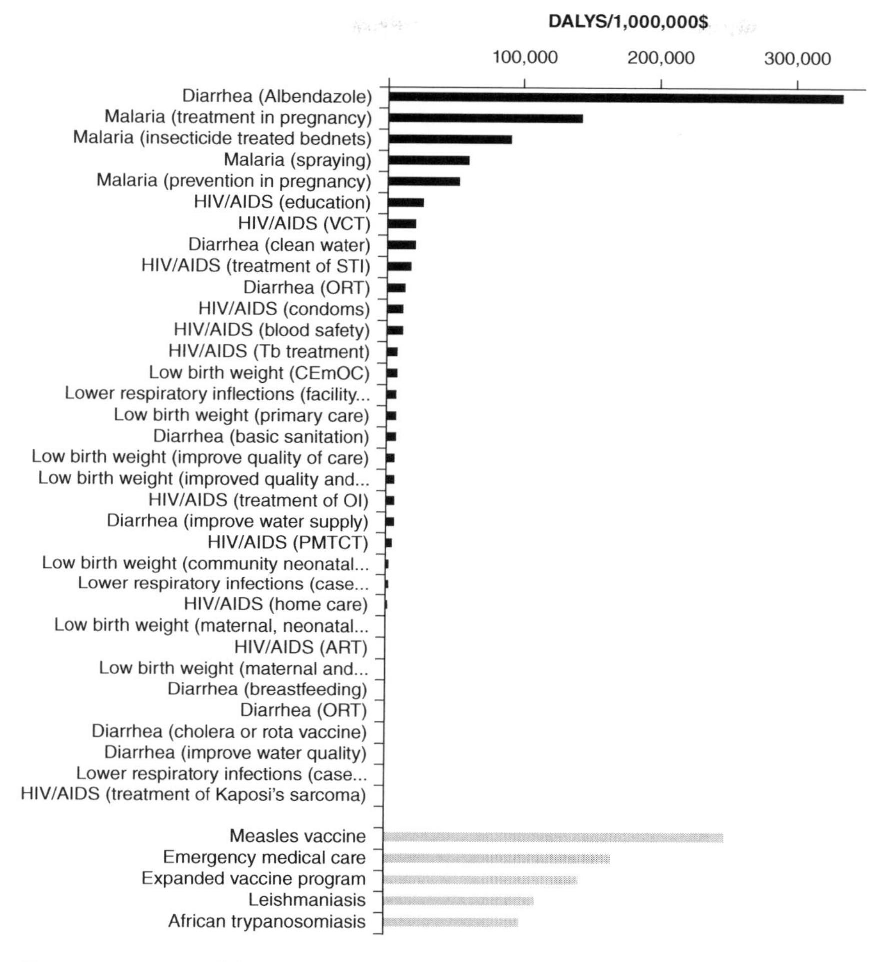

Figure 7.1 Huge differences in potential health gains from investments in health: DCP2 ranking according to the cost-effectiveness of interventions targeted to the five disease categories with the highest disease burden in LICs (black). The five most cost-effective interventions that do not target the top disease burdens (gray) are ranked at the bottom. For a complete list of interventions see the DCP2 web page (http://www.dcp-3.org/dcp2). ART = antiretroviral therapy, CEmOC = comprehensive emergency obstetric care, OI = opportunistic infections, ORT = oral rehydration therapy, PMTCT = prevention of mother to child transmission, STI = sexually transmitted infection, TB = tuberculosis, VCT = voluntary counselling and testing.

There are several moral problems with crude health maximization, which I will discuss further below. In addition to many of the moral problems, cost-effectiveness estimates also involve considerable uncertainty. Models with a high degree of transparency on calculations and underlying assumptions are more likely to avoid errors and arrive at better estimates. This is because if more people examine the details of the models, a better validation of methods and assumptions will result. This is important since incorrect estimates can lead to incorrect conclusions, and the resulting recommendations will thus not maximize population health. The deworming case provides a useful example of this problem. GiveWell, a charity evaluator, found an error in the DCP2 estimates on deworming when they recalculated the DCP2 model. GiveWell experts reran the DCP2 model and estimated, after correcting for what they claim were errors in the model, that deworming is likely to be 100 times less cost-effective than what was previously reported (GiveWell 2012). If this is correct, investments in deworming rather than more cost-effective interventions will hinder the achievement of potentially larger health gains from more cost-effective interventions.

Standard CEAs have also been criticized for ignoring *distributive concerns* and *non-health benefits* (Brock 2003). Distributive concerns are raised by the fact that CEAs typically do not produce favorable results for persons with long-lasting disabilities, or lethal conditions of the young, or diseases among the poor. They also do not take into account non-health benefits, such as the financial protection gained from health care interventions. For example, scaling up less cost-effective interventions may be considered acceptable if doing so prevents catastrophic health expenditures among poor groups. The neglect of distributive concerns and non-health benefits in standard CEAs has diminished the perceived relevance of CEAs and hindered uptake of results from applied cost-effectiveness studies. For this reason, WHO-CHOICE recently developed broad multidimensional guidance for priority setting in resource-poor settings that emphasizes relevant normative criteria that are inadequately considered by CEA (World Health Organisation 2012). Three categories of normative criteria were singled out by WHO-CHOICE as reasons for deviating from CEA rankings: Disease related criteria (e.g., less cost-effective interventions are favorable if they target a severe health condition or patient groups with a poor capacity to benefit from treatment); criteria related to characteristics of social groups (e.g., less cost-effective interventions should be favored when they reduce disparities in health between geographic regions, genders, or socioeconomic groups if they act on upstream factors like social determinants of health, prevention, and health promotion); criteria related to protection against the financial and social effects of ill health (e.g., less cost-effective interventions have special value when they protect against catastrophic health expenditures or enhance the target population's productivity and ability to take care of others).

It can be argued that diseases with high aggregated burden should be given more priority than those with a low aggregated burden. The five diseases that cause the highest burden of disease in LICs (black columns in Figure 7.1)—lower respiratory infections, diarrheal diseases, HIV/AIDS, malaria, and prematurity and low birth weight—together cause approximately 30 percent of the burden of disease in LICs (World Health Organization 2008). The gray columns show other very cost-effective interventions for diseases with a lower disease burden. Investments in the most cost-effective interventions will then maximize health, relative to cost, but will do less for those with diseases imposing greater burden to the society. The normative issue, then, is whether we are willing to sacrifice potentially large health gains in order to target those diseases that cause the highest aggregated disease burden.

Complicating this issue is the fact that a disease with an aggregated large disease burden is not necessarily a severe disease, and large aggregated benefits do not necessarily give large individual benefits. Deworming children with albendazole, for example, is the best aggregated buy because its use leads to a large reduction of aggregated disabilities. This antiparasitic medicine improves cognitive functioning for children due to fewer symptoms of abdominal pain and less malnutrition from helminths. On an individual level, however, disabilities caused by helmintic infections are minor to moderate compared with other diseases, and few children die as a result of them. Decision-makers thus have to make a normative choice about whether it is acceptable to *aggregate* (i.e., add up) all of the benefits and burdens associated with this disease and its treatment, since only when they are aggregated do they amount to a significant health burden. Improved cognitive functioning from albendazole is also likely to improve school results and the productivity of millions of children. Decision-makers must therefore make a second normative choice on whether to take into account these *indirect non-health* benefits, or whether to restrict the relevant outcome to direct health benefits (Brock 2003).

Equality

Principles of equality in health aim at "leveling up" those members of the population with less health to the level of the healthy. Interventions targeted to diseases that are severe and cause a high burden would be given priority on an egalitarian view, regardless of how cost-effective they are. A principle of relative equality judges how bad a situation is by evaluating the health gap between groups in a population (Temkin 2003). Egalitarians view it as intrinsically bad that some persons are in an unfavorable position compared with others. A principle of equality in health would favor interventions that give equal health outcomes or equal chances to receive health benefits between groups (e.g., socio-economic groups, disease groups, geographic groups, ethnic groups, gender, age groups).

Equality of health outcomes is important because it secures equality in opportunity (Temkin 1993). However, equality is a contested concept with many controversies. First, given differences in individual choices, natural genetic profiles, health behavior skills, and available technology, it can be technically impossible to equalize actual and potential health attainments (Sen 1992). Second, egalitarianism appears to allow "leveling down" the better off groups as means to narrow the gap between groups (Temkin 2002). In health this would mean lowering the level of health for some members of the population to achieve equality, which many find intuitively unacceptable (Parfit 2000).

In addition to this difficult "leveling down" problem, there is the third problem that raising up the sickest members of the population to the level of health of the healthiest members can require a "bottomless pit" of resources (Daniels 1994). If health systems always give absolute priority to the worst off and relative equality, this may open up unlimited channeling of resources to patient groups that need vast resources to gain minor marginal benefits. The best-off groups may as a consequence of implementing egalitarian principles sacrifice potential large health gains.

Other controversies make it problematic to adhere fully to a principle of equality in health outcomes. One problem with strict outcome-based equality is that personal freedom may be restricted to a large extent if the distribution of end results is judged without concerns about how the results came about. Examples could be lifestyle choices, where inequalities that are caused by lifestyle choices may be perceived as legitimate (Fleurbaey and Schokkaert 2009). Another example is the case with user fees, where such financing mechanisms may "level up" the health of worse off groups. However, they may also result in catastrophic health expenditures for poor households. Even if such policies reduce health gaps between groups, they may be seen as illegitimate if they would exacerbate inequality in other social goods, such as welfare, income, education, or liberty.

Another central problem for health egalitarians is that health is a product not only of access to health care but also of a myriad of social conditions. Because of the influence of these social determinants of health, there is actually a limited amount that improved access to health care can do to improve health outcomes. As Michael Marmot (2008) puts it, what good does it do to treat people's illnesses, then send them back to the conditions that made them sick? Socio-economic inequalities in health are present within a range of diseases across contexts, even in countries with universal access to health care (World Health Organization and Commission on Social Determinants of Health 2008; World Health Organization 2010). Canada, for example, has an almost six-year difference in life expectancy between wealthy and poor groups. The wealthiest families in India have an under 5 mortality rate of 32.8 per 1,000 live births while the poorest families have a rate three times as high (92.1) (International Institute for Population Sciences 2007). Health egalitarians face a difficult question: If the goal is to equalize health outcomes, should limited health resources be invested in correcting existing social inequalities and improving social conditions, such as housing, education, and public transport, or should they instead be invested only in improving access to health care?

Prioritarianism

Prioritarianism represents a "middle way" between strict equality and strict health maximization. A principle of priority is understood to give some (absolute or weighted) priority to the worst-off persons (Parfit 2000, 2003). Principles of prioritarianism require us to organize social institutions so as to make the worst off as well off as possible and not to reduce the steepness of the inequality gradient. The first priority, according to prioritarianism, should be to elevate the position of the worst-off person as much as possible; the second priority should be to elevate the position of the second worst-off person as much as possible and so on up to the best-off person. A diminishing weight is assigned to benefits as recipients become better off and "benefiting people matters more the worse off these people are" (Parfit 2000).

Prioritarianism is a blend of a health-maximizing principle and an egalitarian principle, and it has wide support. However, some of the problems and controversies as discussed with a principle of equality in health outcomes are also relevant for prioritarianism. Perhaps the most difficult question for this view is who are worst off? Are they the sickest patients, or the youngest, or the most disadvantaged? It is also extremely difficult to determine priority weights in situations where the health level of a person is uncorrelated with their level in other justice domains, such as welfare, income, education, or liberty. Is it worse to be poor with good health than rich with poor health? The problems with social determinants of health are also just as intractable for prioritiarianism as for a principle of equality in health. Should limited health resources give higher weights to correcting existing social inequalities and improving social conditions, or should they instead give weight to improving access to health care?

Nevertheless, prioritarians avoid some of the controversies that egalitarians face. The objections that genetic incurable diseases could be given too much weight, the "leveling down" objection, and the "bottomless pit" problem are less problematic for prioritarianism since the size of the expected health benefits are taken into account by assigning diminishing weights to health benefits as persons become better off. However, it is not clear how much weight the worse off should have compared with those who are better off. In other words, the sizes of the priority weights are not clear. In the next section I therefore focus on the balance between giving weight to equality (or the worse off) and health maximization.

Balancing Equality and Maximization

To begin this discussion a case from the HIV program in the Iringa region in Tanzania is illustrative (Johansson et al. 2011; Johansson and Norheim 2011). The HIV program in this region was structured so as to give more weight to providing treatment to a large number of patients with HIV than to providing accessible services for poor patients in rural parts of the region, which would have gone some way towards reducing the gap in health outcomes between urban and poorer rural populations. Patients living in many of these rural areas had low access to facilities, and they were in a sense the worst off due to the high burden of HIV in the population (a severe disease that causes high rates of disability and kills young people), many HIV orphans, and high rates of extreme poverty. However, investing in programs to overcome rural barriers to health services, such as long distances and low population density, poor road conditions, and inability to pay for transport, would be very costly. Investments to enhance rural health outcomes would in this context give fewer health benefits compared with scale-up of services in the urban setting. There was already an existing health system in the cities and more patients with HIV lived in the urban catchment area. Larger health gains were therefore expected for fewer resources with an urban HIV treatment rollout.

A strict health-maximizing principle would clearly favor urban HIV treatment rollout since this would save a larger number of persons and more life years. A strict egalitarian principle would consider it important to narrow the geographical gap in health outcomes and therefore favor equal rollout of HIV treatment in urban and rural settings. This dilemma invokes legitimate disagreement and hard trade-offs (Daniels 1994). Anand frames the trade-off question as follows: What amount of healthy life years, if enjoyed equally by everybody, would have equivalent value to a greater average healthy life expectancy (Anand 2002: 485)? This question is relevant for all societies that have resource constraints on interventions that can influence the population health in a positive direction. General theories of distributive justice give inadequate guidance about what the right balance is between distributing health outcomes equally and maximizing health outcomes.

Social welfare functions could be useful in making such trade-offs explicit and they are typically used in welfare economics to operationalize the social value of welfare distributions. Such welfare functions could also be used in evaluations of health policies. Inequality measures like the Gini index and the Atkinson index are traditional welfare economic measures of inequality that handle trade-offs between efficiency and equity (Wagstaff 2002; Bleichrodt and van Doorslaer 2006; Norheim 2009). Such equity-sensitive measures evaluate the magnitude of inequality aversion that is needed to favor, for example, urban versus rural scale-up of HIV treatment.

Elsewhere, we tested the Atkinson index as an index for evaluation of a hypothetical case similar to the urban versus rural case above (Johansson and Norheim 2011). The Atkinson index can be seen as an inequality-sensitive summary measure of average health (Atkinson 1970). Inequality aversion, when applied to health policies, expresses the strength of preference for a concern for those who are worse off that is needed in

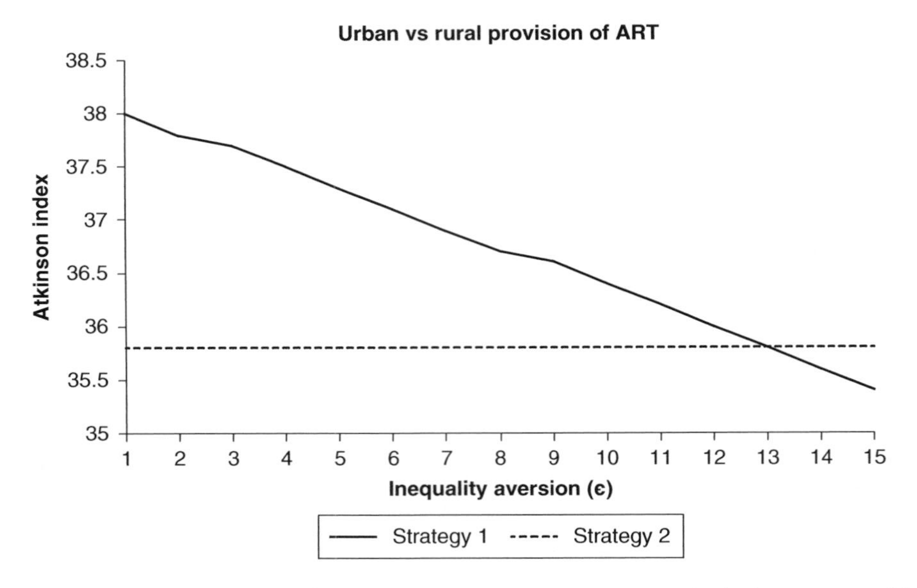

Figure 7.2 Atkinson index estimates from a previous study (Johansson and Norheim 2011) where we evaluated scale-up of HIV treatment only in urban settings (strategy 1) or 50/50 scale-up in both urban and rural settings (strategy 2). Fewer lives are saved and a more equal distribution is the result with strategy 2. ART = antiretroviral therapy.

order to favor, e.g., urban versus rural scale-up of HIV treatment. A parameter (ε) represents the magnitude of inequality aversion. High levels of ε indicate a large inequality aversion (when $\varepsilon = 0$ there is no aversion to inequality and when $\varepsilon = \infty$ there is absolute aversion to inequality). People's intuitions and preferences are often somewhere in between absolute and no aversion to inequality. See Figure 7.2 for the magnitude of inequality aversion that was needed in our evaluation of a similar case to the one above (Johansson and Norheim 2011). Urban scale-up of HIV treatment was favored for all $\varepsilon < 12.9$, which indicates that a relatively large inequality aversion is needed in order to favor rural scale-up of HIV treatment (see Johansson and Norheim (2011) for more details on these calculations).

However, measures such as the Atkinson index have until recently been unexplored as normative analytical tools in distributive conflicts of health interventions (Anand 2002, 2004; Norheim 2010). Many different variables are relevant for the distribution of health care resources, including how severely ill persons are, the cost-effectiveness of interventions, and how effective an intervention is for the individual patient. Because these variables can come into conflict, however, trade-offs such as those in the urban versus rural case must be made between the value of equality and maximization of health (Norheim and Asada 2009).

Procedural Justice

How can societies respond fairly to the gap between available and affordable health care when resource limitations mean that some people will be denied substantial improvements in health? Reasonable people disagree on many of the substantive principles discussed above, and we may suspect similar disagreements to occur in actual health care priority settings. It seems that we lack a supreme distributive principle that no one could reasonably reject, and therefore health allocation decisions will often be morally problematic, one way or another.

In the absence of agreement on substantive principled solutions, Daniels and Sabin have developed "accountability for reasonableness," a theory of procedural justice in health care priority setting (Daniels and Sabin 2002). The goal of this theory is to ensure that the *process* of allocating resources is fair and just, so that even those who disagree with the final decisions can accept them as legitimate. Accountability for reasonableness has become a well known procedural framework internationally and was adopted in the 2004 WHO/UNAIDS guidance on ethics of HIV care and treatment roll-out (Holm 1998; Daniels 2004; World Health Organization 2004). Accountability for reasonableness specifies four conditions of a fair health care priority setting process (Daniels 2004):

1. *Publicity condition*: The process must be transparent and involve publicly available rationales for the priorities that are set. People have a basic interest in knowing the grounds for decisions that fundamentally affect their wellbeing.
2. *Relevance condition*: Stakeholders affected by these decisions must agree that the rationales rest on reasons, principles, and evidence that stakeholders view as relevant to making fair decisions about priorities.
3. *Revisability and appeals condition*: The process allows for revisiting and revising decisions in light of new evidence and arguments, and allows for an appeals process that protects those who have legitimate reasons for being an exception to policies adopted.
4. *Enforcement or regulation condition*: There is a mechanism in place that ensures the previous three conditions are met.

Private or public priority setting bodies that adhere to all four procedural requirements are accepted as legitimate moral authorities. The decisions will be legitimate (seen as acceptable by all parties) because, first, none of the four conditions specifies what the right distributions are, and second, the conditions ensure impartiality and include the perspective of all affected parties, including those being denied potentially beneficial health care (Daniels and Sabin 2002; Daniels 2008). The idea is to ground decision-making in a legitimizing process that is supported or bounded by substantive principles of justice, an idea that is based on theories of deliberative democracy and democratic decision-making (Gutman and Thompson 1996; Bohman and Rehg 1997).

Sabik and Lie argue that a shift from substantive principles to a fair process will not entirely solve the legitimacy problem, since problems of substantive justice are implicated in the choice of various processes (Sabik and Lie 2008). Even if a fair process ensures a more legitimate decision-making process, the end result may still be considered unjust if the outcome is in conflict with one particular view on justice. Friedman argues that the four conditions in accountability for reasonableness are inadequate and that there is a need for greater public involvement in a legitimate decision-making process. In addition, Friedman argues, democratic processes should allow for all kinds of reasons to enter the discussion, and that they should instead be judged by their consistency, plausibility, and explanatory power after they have entered the discussion (Friedman 2008).

Countries differ in how they set health priorities and assign relative weights to the substantive priority setting criteria, which is a good reason for having fair decision-making processes. Norheim and Kapiriri differentiate priority criteria into (a) acceptable, (b) unacceptable, and (c) contested criteria. *Acceptable criteria* are the following: (1) Severity of disease, i.e., prognosis without intervention; (2) effectiveness, i.e., prognosis with intervention; (3) cost-effectiveness, i.e., cost per QALY/DALY/life-year gained; and (4) the quality of evidence supporting criteria 1–3 (Norheim 1999; Kapiriri and Norheim 2004). There seems to be general consensus that these serve as an important basis of many of the health care priorities. The Norwegian health care priority setting guidelines, for example, are grounded on these acceptable rationing criteria (Norges Offentlige Utredninger 1997: 18). Other countries, such as Israel, New Zealand, the Netherlands, Sweden, Denmark, and the U.K. have applied different versions of these acceptable rationing criteria (Sabik and Lie 2008). Sabik and Lie found that some countries tend to focus more on severity of disease, while others emphasize cost-effectiveness and level of evidence behind the health technology. *Unacceptable criteria* are those reasons that are not relevant for all affected parties, which might include gender, sexual orientation, religion, race, tribe, social status, and educational level (Kapiriri and Norheim 2004). Rationing based on these criteria will not treat all people in the society with equal respect and lead to discrimination.

There are theoretical discussions about the acceptability of some hotly *contested criteria*, which sometimes figure in practical contexts (Kapiriri et al. 2007). The contested criteria include age, prioritizing the younger before the older, economic status (whether it is fair to prioritize the poorest), individual responsibility for one's own health status, and the individual's productivity for the family or the society (Kapiriri and Norheim 2004). Examples of uses described in the literature include the denial of organs for alcoholic liver failure (formulated in guidelines) and queue jumping in waiting lists (informal clinical decisions) (McGough et al. 2005).

Concluding Remarks

Our intuitions tell us that it is unfair and unjust when children die of diarrhea, when mothers bleed to death during childbirth, or when young people do not get access to health information and condoms. Policy-makers, donors, and health personnel face huge ethical challenges when dealing with these unmet health needs in distributing limited and often extremely scarce health resources. Through this sketch of moral reasons, substantive principles, and what legitimate priority setting procedures should look like, I have tried to show that there is no straightforward way to get priority setting decisions right. Legitimate decision-making demands that reasons for decisions be given and that the process is transparent. Reasonable disagreement exists about which principles and reasons are just, and how much weight should be assigned to each of them. I hope this introduction will motivate others to participate in the further exploration of these important issues.

Related Topics

Chapter 2, "Social Determinants of Health and Health Inequalities," Sridhar Venkatapuram and Michael Marmot

Chapter 3, "The Ethics of Rationing: Necessity, Politics, and Fairness," Daniel Callahan

Chapter 4, "QALYs, DALYs, and Their Critics," Greg Bognar

References

Alvarez, A.A. (2007) "Threshold Considerations in Fair Allocation of Health Resources: Justice Beyond Scarcity," *Bioethics* 21 (8): 426–38.

Anand, S. (2002) "The Concern for Equity in Health," *Journal of Epidemiology and Community Health* 56 (7): 485–7.

Anand, S. (2004) "The Concern for Equity in Health," in S. Anand, F. Peter and A. Sen (eds.) *Public Health Ethics, and Equity*, New York: Oxford University Press.

Arras, J.D. and Fenton, E.M. (2009) "Bioethics & Human Rights: Access to Health-Related Goods," *Hastings Center Report* 39 (5): 27–38.

Atkinson, A.B. (1970) "On the Measurement of Inequality," *Journal of Economic Theory* 2 (3): 244–63.

Bleichrodt, H. and van Doorslaer, E. (2006) "A Welfare Economics Foundation for Health Inequality Measurement," *Journal of Health Economics* 25 (5): 945–7.

Bohman, J. and Rehg, W. (1997) *Deliberative Democracy: Essays on Reason and Politics*, Cambridge, MA: MIT Press.

Brock, D.W. (2003) "Separate Spheres and Indirect Benefits," *Cost Effectiveness and Resource Allocation* 1 (1): 4.

Brock, D. and Wikler, D. (2006) "Ethical Issues in Resource Allocation, Research, and New Product Development," in D.T. Jamison, J.G. Breman, A.R. Measham et al. (eds.) *Disease Control Priorities in Developing Countries* (2nd edition), Washington, DC: Oxford University Press and The World Bank, pp. 259–70.

Brock, D.W. and Wikler, D. (2009) "Ethical Challenges in Long-Term Funding for HIV/AIDS," *Health Affairs (Millwood)* 28 (6): 1666–76.

Broome, J. (1991) *Weighing Goods*, Oxford: Basil Blackwell.

Caney, S. (2005) *Justice Beyond Borders: A Global Political Theory*, Oxford: Oxford University Press.

Coast, J. (2009) "Maximisation in Extra-welfarism: A Critique of the Current Position in Health Economics," *Social Science & Medicine* 69 (5): 786–92.

Crisp, R. (2003) "Equality, Priority, and Compassion," *Ethics* 113 (4): 745–63.

Daniels, N. (1994) "Four Unsolved Rationing Problems: A Challenge," *Hastings Center Report* 24 (4): 27–9.

Daniels, N. (2004) "How to Achieve Fair Distribution of ARTs in '3 by 5': Fair Process and Legitimacy in Patient Selection," Background Paper for a WHO/UNAIDS consultation on equity in 3 by 5.

Daniels, N. (2008) *Just Health*, Boston, MA: Cambridge University Press.

Daniels, N. and Sabin, J.E. (2002) *Setting Limits Fairly: Can We Learn to Share Medical Resources?* Oxford: Oxford University Press.

Fleurbaey, M. and Schokkaert, E. (2009) "Unfair Inequalities in Health and Health Care," *Journal of Health Economics* 28 (1): 73–90.

Friedman, A. (2008) "Beyond Accountability for Reasonableness," *Bioethics* 22 (2): 101–12.

GiveWell (2012) http://www.givewell.org/ (accessed July 7, 2014).

Gutman, A. and Thompson, D. (1996) *Democracy and Disagreement*, Cambridge, MA: The Belknap Press of Harvard University Press.

Ham, C. and Roberts G. (2003) *Reasonable Rationing: International Experience of Priority Setting in Health Care*, Philadephia, PA: Open University Press.

Holm, S. (1998) "Goodbye to the Simple Solutions: The Second Phase of Priority Setting in Health Care," *BMJ* 317 (7164): 1000–2.

International Institute for Population Sciences (2007) *National Family Health Survey (NFHS-3) 2005–06*, Ministry of Health and Family Welfare Government of India.

Jamison, D.T., Breman, J.G., Measham, A.R., Alleyne, G., Claeson, M., Evans, D.B., Jha, P., Mills, A. and Musgrove, P. (eds.) (2006) *Disease Control Priorities in Developing Countries* (2nd edition), Washington DC: Oxford University Press and The World Bank.

Johansson, K.A. and Norheim, O.F. (2011) "Problems with Prioritization: Exploring Ethical Solutions to Inequalities in HIV Care," *American Journal of Bioethics* 11 (12): 32–40.

Johansson, K.A., Miljeteig, I., Kigwangalla, H. and Norheim, O.F. (2011) "HIV Priorities and Health Distributions in a Rural Region in Tanzania: A Qualitative Study," *Journal of Medical Ethics* 37 (4): 221–6.

Kapiriri, L. and Norheim, O.F. (2004) "Criteria for Priority-Setting in Health Care in Uganda: Exploration of Stakeholders' Values," *Bulletin of the World Health Organization* 82 (3): 172–9.

Kapiriri, L., Norheim, O.F. and Martin, D.K. (2007) "Priority Setting at the Micro-, Meso- and Macro-levels in Canada, Norway and Uganda," *Health Policy* 82 (1): 78–94.

Marmot, M. (2008) http://www.who.int/social_determinants/final_report/media/csdh_report_wrs_en.pdf (accessed August 20, 2014).

McGough, L.J., Reynolds, S.J., Quinn, T.C. and Zenilman, J.M. (2005) "Which Patients First? Setting Priorities for Antiretroviral Therapy Where Resources Are Limited," *American Journal of Public Health* 95 (7): 1173–80.
Nagel, T. (2005) "The Problem of Global Justice," *Philosophy & Public Affairs* 33 (2): 112–47.
Norges Offentlige Utredninger (1997) *Priority Setting Revisited* [in Norwegian], Oslo: Statens forvaltningstjeneste, Statens trykking.
Norheim, O.F. (1996) *Limiting Access to Health Care: A Contractualist Approach to Fair Rationing*, PhD Dissertation, University of Oslo.
Norheim, O.F. (1999) "Healthcare Rationing: Are Additional Criteria Needed for Assessing Evidence Based Clinical Practice Guidelines?" *BMJ* 319 (7222): 1426–9.
Norheim, O.F. (2009) "A Note on Brock: Prioritarianism, Egalitarianism and the Distribution of Life Years," *Journal of Medical Ethics* 35 (9): 565–9.
Norheim, O.F. (2010) "Gini Impact Analysis: Measuring Pure Health Inequity Before and After Interventions," *Public Health Ethics*, August.
Norheim, O.F. and Asada, Y. (2009) "The Ideal of Equal Health Revisited: Definitions and Measures of Inequity in Health Should Be Better Integrated with Theories of Distributive Justice," *International Journal of Equity and Health* 8: 40.
Parfit, D. (2000) *Equality or Priority? Lindley Lectures Delivered at the University of Kansas* (Lawrence, Kansas, 1991). Reprinted in M. Clayton and A. Williams *The Ideal of Equality*, New York: Palgrave Macmillan.
Parfit, D. (2003) "Justifiability to Each Person (Scanlon, 'On What We Owe to Each Other')," *Ratio-New Series* 16 (4): 368–90.
Sabik, L.M. and Lie, R.K. (2008) "Priority Setting in Health Care: Lessons from the Experiences of Eight Countries," *International Journal of Equity and Health* 7: 4.
Sen, A. (1979) "Utilitarianism and Welfarism," *Journal of Philosophy* 76 (9): 463–89.
Sen, A.K. (1992) *Inequality Reexamined*, Oxford: Clarendon Press.
Temkin, L. (2002) "Equality, Priority, and the Leveling Down Objection," in M. Clayton and A. Williams *The Ideal of Equality*, New York: Palgrave Macmillan.
Temkin, L.S. (1993) *Inequality*, New York: Oxford University Press.
Temkin, L.S. (2003) "Egalitarianism Defended," *Ethics* 113 (4): 764–82.
UN Population Division (2011) http://www.un.org/esa/population/unpop.htm (accessed September 4, 2012).
Wagstaff, A. (2002) "Inequality Aversion, Health Inequalities and Health Achievement," *Journal of Health Economics* 21 (4): 627–41.
Weinstein, M.C. and Stason, W.B. (1977) "Foundations of Cost-Effectiveness Analysis for Health and Medical Practices," *New England Journal of Medicine* 296: 716–21.
Wikler, D. and Brock, D. (2007) "Population-Level Bioethics: Mapping a New Agenda," in A. Dawson and M. Verweij (eds.) *Ethics, Prevention and Public Health*, Oxford: Clarendon Press Oxford University Press, pp. 78–94.
Williams, A. (1985) "Economics of Coronary Artery Bypass Grafting," *BMJ* 291: 326–9.
World Health Organization (2004) *Guidance on Ethics and Equitable Access to HIV Treatment and Care*, Geneva.
World Health Organization (2008) *The Global Burden of Disease: 2004 Update*, Geneva.
World Health Organization (2010) *Equity, Social Determinants and Public Health Programmes*, E. Blas and A.S. Kurup, Geneva.
World Health Organization (2012) *Guidance on Priority Setting in Health (GPS Health)*, Geneva, draft.
World Health Organization and Commission on Social Determinants of Health (2008) *Closing the Gap in a Generation: Health Equity Through Action on the Social Determinants of Health*, Final Report of the Commission on Social Determinants of Health, Geneva.
World Health Organization and WHO-CHOICE (2012) http://www.who.int/choice/en/ (accessed July 7, 2014).

Further Reading

Bognar, G. and Hirose, I. (2014) *The Ethics of Health Care Rationing: An Introduction*, London: Routledge.
Millum, J. and Emanuel, E.J. (eds.) (2012) *Global Justice and Bioethics*, Oxford: Oxford University Press.
Ruger, J. (2009) *Health and Social Justice*, Oxford: Oxford University Press.
The Lancet Commission on Investing in Health (2013) *Global Health 2035: A World Converging within a Generation*.
The Lancet-University of Oslo Commission on Global Governance for Health (2014) *Global Governance Gaps Propagate Health Inequities: Political Determinants of Health*.

8
MEDICAL TOURISM

I. Glenn Cohen

Health care has ceased to be a set of goods and services delivered only locally; it is now a truly globalized phenomenon, including medical migration—the "brain drain" of health care practitioners, largely from the developing to the developed world; telemedicine; multi-regional clinical trials; the global intellectual property regime that both facilitates innovation and stymies access to drugs; and the flow of tissues, including pandemic influenza vaccine strains. This chapter focuses on one part of this globalization: Medical tourism.

The Growth of Medical Tourism

Medical tourism involves the travel of patients from their home country to a foreign country in order to save on costs, receive insurance coverage, or access services unavailable or illegal in their home country. Although studies have come to widely different conclusions about the exact size of the current medical tourism trade, there is no doubt it is significant (Cohen 2013b; Cortez 2011: 878). According to one estimate 750,000 U.S. patients traveled abroad in 2007 for medical procedures, with the total number rising to six million by 2010 (Cortez 2011: 878, n. 119; Murphy 2009; Ehrbeck et al. 2008: 2, 3, 6). In one year alone, 952,000 California residents traveled to Mexico for medical care or prescription drugs, and medical tourism along this border has been consistent and longstanding (Wallace et al. 2009: 662). In 2004, more than 150,000 foreigners sought medical treatment in India, and that number was projected to increase by 15 percent per year (Lancaster 2004). In 2005, Bumrungrad International Hospital in Bangkok saw 400,000 foreign patients (Milstein and Smith 2006: 1638). The revenues generated by this trade are staggering: Some claim that medical tourism will generate in India $2.2 billion in revenues this year, and $8 billion in Thailand between 2010 and 2014 (Cohen 2010b: 1472). This market is likely to expand significantly with the development of robust insurer-prompted medical tourism plans that each of the four largest insurer plans in the U.S. have introduced or are considering (Cohen 2010b: 1486–8; Cortez 2011: 882–4). The European market for medical tourism is poised to continue growing as well (Cohen 2014; European Parliament 2011). These estimates do not include harder-to-quantify forms of medical tourism, such as traveling to obtain abortions, assisted suicide, stem cell treatments, and reproductive technology services (Cohen 2012c).

This chapter considers the bioethical and legal issues raised by medical tourism.

Types of Medical Tourism

It is useful to categorize medical tourism in two separate ways (Cohen 2012a). The first division is by patient population, of which there are three broad categories. First, there are patients paying out-of-pocket. In the U.S., this population includes uninsured or underinsured patients using medical tourism to achieve substantial cost savings, and those seeking to use services unavailable at home in universal health care systems; this group also includes patients seeking to queue jump (Cohen 2010b). A second group consists of patients engaged in private insurer-prompted medical tourism. In its weakest form, insurers simply cover the service abroad without any incentive, but more commonly insurers offer "tourism-incentivized plans," in which individuals are offered rebates, waived deductibles, or other payment incentives for receiving treatment abroad (Cohen 2010b; Einhorn 2008). A final group consists of patients engaged in government-prompted medical tourism. For example, there have been recent proposals in the U.S. to give Medicare and Medicaid patients incentives to use medical tourism; another version is already in place in the European Union (Cohen 2010b, 2014; Baker and Rho 2009; Terry 2007).

The second division is by the legality of the type of service sought. First, there is medical tourism for services that are illegal in both the patient's home and destination countries (such as organ purchase in the Philippines). Second, there is "circumvention tourism": Medical tourism for services that are illegal or unapproved in the patient's home country but legal in the destination country (such as travel abroad for fertility services, abortion, assisted suicide, experimental drugs, and stem cell therapies). Finally, there is medical tourism for services legal in both the home and destination countries—where medical tourism is used because of lower prices or higher expertise abroad, high domestic queuing time, or domestic unavailability (Cohen 2010a). Typically, government-prompted and insurer-prompted medical tourism will only involve the last category, while medical tourism by those paying out-of-pocket can involve any of these categories.

Ethical Issues

When considering the ethical problems raised by medical tourism it is useful to keep *both* these divisions in mind. For example, paternalistic concerns regarding individuals choosing poorer quality health care may vary depending on whether individuals are making choices in a global marketplace for health services or choosing only amongst medical facilities approved by their home country government, as is the case in some parts of the European Union. Also, in cases where medical tourism is thought to cause negative effects on the health care available to poor destination country residents, whether or not the medical tourism is government sponsored may matter a great deal for determining who has what obligations (Cohen 2011a).

I will explicitly put to one side organ tourism, the main kind of medical tourism for services illegal in both the patient's home and destination country, as it is covered in more depth elsewhere in my work and raises fairly distinct issues (Cohen 2013a; France and Francis 2010: 287; Scheper-Hughes 2000; Transplantation Society 2008).

Medical Tourism for Services Legal in Both Home and Destination Countries

This kind of medical tourism represents the largest share of the existing market for services, with patients frequently traveling abroad for cardiac bypass, hip replacements, cosmetic surgery, and reproductive services, often motivated by huge price savings of 80 percent or more off the cost of their surgery, or the ability to jump queues (Cohen 2010b; Cortez 2008: 74, 91).

Quality

One ethical issue here concerns the quality of health care provided to traveling patients. In the U.S. there are several interlocking regulatory and tort mechanisms designed to protect patients in the health care setting. These include the accreditation, certification, and professional self-regulation of health care providers; the medical-malpractice system; the reporting of malpractice suits to the National Malpractice Database; the licensure and accreditation of hospitals; medical staff bylaws; hospital privileges regulation; conflict of interest regulation; and anti-kickback statutes (Cohen 2010b). Many other home countries have similar safeguards, but many foreign countries lack them or have versions that do not neatly correspond to the home country versions. As a result, some worry that a U.S. patient traveling abroad will receive poorer medical care and argue that this justifies some kind of governmental intervention.

We lack good systematic data on this issue. A few small-scale empirical studies of specific therapies and hospitals suggest high-quality care abroad. Arnold Milstein and Mark Smith (2006: 1639) "doubt" that the average U.S. hospital can "offer better outcomes for common complex operations such as coronary-artery bypass grafting, for which several JCI-accredited offshore hospitals report gross mortality rates of less than 1 percent." Aaditya Mattoo and Randeep Rathindran (2006: 359) single out Bumrungrand Hospital in Bangkok, Apollo Hospital in New Delhi, and Crossroads Center in Antigua as "examples of reputable medical facilities in developing countries that are comparable to the best in industrial countries" and note that the Apollo hospital chain has maintained a 99 percent success rate in more than 50,000 cardiac surgeries performed, which is "on par with surgical success rates of the best U.S. cardiac surgery centers." However, Leigh Turner (2013) has recently compiled a list of several reports of death or serious injury connected to poor quality of care at destination hospitals.

Suppose, however, that a foreign facility really did provide poorer care than that available to a well insured patient in the home country. This would not settle the ethical or legal issues.

To begin with, what baseline should we use in evaluating this issue? The counterfactual care that this particular patient would likely receive at home (including any inability to access the service because of inability to pay domestic prices) or a moral baseline based on that to which the patient is entitled? In particular, in countries without universal health care such as the U.S., where some uninsured patients will not have access to many non-emergency forms of health care, a focus on the counterfactual care baseline will lead us to have a more positive view of medical tourism as expanding their choice set in positive ways.

Further, in shaping regulatory policy, what are the limits of justified paternalism? Providing information is a very easy to justify intervention that even anti-paternalists support. Unfortunately, given what we know about domestic health care markets, such interventions are unlikely to make major headway in guiding patients to make better choices; the evidence shows that when presented with information relevant to choosing physicians or insurers, patients often ignore it in favor of word of mouth and in some instances make objectively irrational decisions (Cohen 2010b). So-called "libertarian paternalists" are also open to the creation of default rules of various levels of "stickiness"—in this approach policy is set at a default that paternalists would favor with individuals free to opt for a different choice, but regulators know that individuals are unlikely to change the default (e.g., opt-out rather than opt-in), especially as the transaction costs of making such changes will increase (Sunstein and Thaler 2003). As default rules become "stickier" these interventions are more likely to succeed, but also more likely to offend anti-paternalists.

The regulatory difficulties may be both better and worse when it comes to insurer-prompted medical tourism. On the one hand, insurers may be able to make better quality, more rational determinations than would individual consumers buying for themselves. On the other hand, insurer incentives may not align well with patient desires given the fact that many patients change insurers annually such that insurers do not fully internalize the benefits of higher-cost higher-quality care. Moreover, the empirical evidence shows that patients have difficulty in choosing insurance products, which suggests that patients will have great difficulty choosing between plans incorporating various forms of medical tourism at various price points in a way that furthers their self-interest (Cohen 2010b).

To the extent that patients believe price-to-quality ratio improves their welfare, should the state simply leave patients alone to make their own decisions about where they receive health care? One middle course is what I have called "channeling" regimes, wherein the state attaches penalties or mandates incentives (such as insurance reimbursement) to use facilities that disclose pertinent information, adopt quality control mechanisms, have lower mortality and morbidity rates, achieve accreditation, etc. (Cohen 2010b). A similar approach can be taken to regulate health insurance incorporation of medical tourism. However, creating the necessary regulatory infrastructure would be costly and challenging (Cohen 2010b, 2012a). Finally, as I have argued elsewhere, for uninsured and underinsured Americans in particular, who lack good health care options at home, even if the care provided is not ideal, medical tourism services may prove a necessary way of improving their health care access and too strong an anti-paternalist set of regulations may make these patients even worse off and "protect" them out of their only good option (Cohen 2010b).

Poor quality of care may harm not only tourist patients—the patient protective concern—but it may also lead to substantial externalities. Numerous authors have worried about the propensity for medical tourists to bring back antibiotic superbugs (Hodges and Kimball 2012). Moreover, poorly performed surgeries will often require costly and extensive follow-up care, which in universal health care systems will be paid for by fellow taxpayers and even in the U.S. will indirectly increase costs through uncompensated care pools for the uninsured (Cohen 2014; Crooks et al. 2013). These externalities give home countries another reason to regulate.

Liability

Separate from concerns about quality of care is the question of recovery when medical tourism leads to medical errors or malpractice. The two issues are not entirely separate to the extent that liability rules deter medical error, something that is contested in the domestic medical malpractice literature (Frakes 2012; Currie and MacLeod 2008; Greenberg et al. 2010).

U.S. medical tourists (as well as those from many other home countries) will face a series of difficulties in recovering from medical errors that occur abroad: Difficulties in establishing personal jurisdiction over the defendants, in enforcing judgments patients are granted by courts, and in getting around the fact that much less remunerative foreign laws will often apply to an action even if it can be brought in a U.S. court. If patients are unable to bring suit and must fight in the destination country to recover, the delays and expenses are still discouraging and likely to render a lawsuit non-viable (Cohen 2010b; Cortez 2010: 10).

In the U.S., and in many home countries, we prohibit individuals from contracting with their domestic physician to waive medical malpractice recovery in exchange for a better price. Medical tourism allows patients to circumvent this prohibition. That might seem problematic, but as I have argued elsewhere (Cohen 2010b) there may be some good reasons to distinguish opting into a less remunerative regime through travel versus through contract. In any event, if worried about the lack of recovery, a home country could attempt more muscular "channeling" regimes that required foreign facilities to, for instance, engage in agreements to arbitrate, consent to jurisdiction, or offer medical malpractice insurance.

Effects on Health Care Access for the Destination Country Poor

Even as medical tourism may be a boon for home country patients, it threatens to make things worse for the poor in the destination country. From their perspective, medical tourism presents a host of cruel ironies. Vast medico-industrial complexes replete with the newest technologies provide wealthy medical tourists hip replacements and facelifts, while large swaths of the population die from malaria, AIDS, and a lack of clean water (Cohen 2011a).

These kinds of stark disparities have prompted discomfort and academic and policy critiques (Cohen 2011a; Hopkins et al. 2010; Johnston et al. 2010; Gupta 2008; Bookman and Bookman 2007; Benavides 2002: 55; Chanda 2002: 160; Janjaroen and Supakankunti 2002: 87, 98). As Leigh Turner suggests, "the greatest risk for inhabitants of destination countries is that increased volume of international patients will have adverse effects upon local patients, health care facilities and economies" (2007: 320). This worry has been expressed in discussions regarding Thailand, Cuba, India, and even Israel (Cohen 2011a).

Behind this worry are three fundamental questions. First, how likely is it that medical tourism will cause negative consequences on health care access in less developed countries? Second, do home countries (or international bodies) have an obligation to discourage or regulate medical tourism to prevent such consequences? Finally, how might governments do so?

Despite prominent expressions of concern, there currently exists little empirical evidence as to whether medical tourism has adverse effects on health care access in destination countries (for a review of the best data suggesting it might, see Chen and Flood 2013). As is often the case in bioethics, then, we are judging under conditions of uncertainty and lack of pertinent information, and it is unclear if that argues in favor of or against the status quo (Cohen 2011a; Chen and Flood 2013). I have drawn on health development literature to suggest that increased medical tourism is likely to reduce access to health care in the destination country for its poor citizens when some combination of six triggering conditions obtains, and others have attempted to show these dynamics occurring in some destination countries (Cohen 2011a; Chen and Flood 2013):

1. The health care services consumed by tourists come from the same pool of health care resources available to the destination country poor.
2. Health care providers are "captured" by the medical tourist patient population, rather than serving a mix of tourist clientele and the local population.
3. The supply of health care professionals, facilities, and technologies in the destination country is inelastic, in the sense that it cannot easily be scaled up when there is increased demand.
4. The positive effects of medical tourism in counteracting the "brain drain" of health care practitioners from developing to developed countries are outweighed by the negative effects of medical tourism on availability of health care.
5. Medical tourism prompts destination countries to redirect resources away from basic health care services in a way that outweighs positive health care spillovers.
6. Profits from medical tourism are unlikely to "trickle down" to the destination country poor.

This list is not exhaustive, and assessments can only be done on a country-by-country basis, but there is sufficient support for such negative effects to put the following issue on the radar: Assuming that medical tourism reduces health care access in destination countries for local populations, under what conditions should such a reduction trigger obligations to regulate medical tourism and/or mitigate its effects?

Identifying and weighing the moral claim is not easy. Medical tourism appears to involve willing providers of services (destination country physicians and facilities) and willing consumers (home country patients, insurers, and governments) pursuing an ordinarily morally unproblematic activity (medical services). Moreover, unlike cases such as organ sale or clinical trials in sub-Saharan Africa of drugs that will not readily be available there, there is no plausible claim that the seller (or buyer) is being exploited. Instead, the moral problem, if any, with medical tourism must stem from the negative externality of reduced care for poor patients in the destination country. There may be separate problems with existing health care disparities in destination countries, but, at least on some theories of global justice (especially more statist and some intermediate theories), if not caused by medical tourism then they are not strictly speaking moral problems *with* medical tourism.

The claim that such negative effects of medical tourism are the moral responsibility of home countries or their citizens is best understood as a claim that might be made under either a theory of enlightened self-interest or based on a theory of global justice, which might take a cosmopolitan, statist, or intermediate form. Elsewhere (Cohen 2011a) I have tried to synthesize the work of the most prominent theorists in this area in the last 50 years (e.g., Daniels 2008; Nussbaum 2006; Nagel 2005; Pogge 2002, 2005; Rawls 1999; Beitz 1975, 1979) and then move from political theory to applied ethics by asking what these theories should tell us about the concrete case of medical tourism. I myself favor intermediate approaches that impose obligations when there are mediating institutions with coercive or rule-making authority connecting home and destination countries. These theories concede to statist theories the importance of "joint authors[hip] of the coercively imposed system" for full-blown duties of distributive justice, but are prepared to find lesser duties of inclusion—wherein the interests of those outside the nation state count for something—under less demanding circumstances (2011a). While I have defended this view in my own work, what one should think about home country responsibility in the context of medical tourism is deeply entwined with one's views of these theories more generally.

While an overlapping consensus on medical tourism between these different theories currently eludes us, it is fair to say that as to medical tourism we can identify two "central tendencies" among them. I have argued that (2011a) private insurer-prompted medical tourism and government-prompted medical tourism are areas where the argument that states and international bodies have a moral obligation to intervene is the strongest, though for different reasons. More robust curbs on insurer-prompted medical tourism are easier to justify because the patients who use this form of medical tourism (as opposed to the uninsured or underinsured) at least typically have access to non-emergency insured medical services in the home country, such that losing the option of traveling abroad puts them in a less perilous situation. The case for intervening in government-prompted medical tourism is stronger because there is a fairly direct causal tie between the state's action and the deficits caused by medical tourism (which matter on intermediate theories). Claims of an obligation on the part of the home country government or international bodies to do something about medical tourism by those purchasing essential services out-of-pocket seem correspondingly weaker. Beyond these central tendencies, however, there is a fair amount of divergence among the theories in picking out which circumstances give rise to obligations (Cohen 2011a).

Home Country Physician Obligations, Follow-Up Care, and Dynamic Effects of Medical Tourism

There are a series of other ethical issues raised by this kind of medical tourism. First, what are the obligations of home country physicians regarding patients who want to go abroad for treatment? If physicians have a preexisting relationship with a patient, they may face moral or legal obligations not to abandon that patient when the patient returns for follow-up care merely because the patient wants to go abroad. However, physicians may subject themselves to significant liability if a patient suffers medical error during medical tourism but the results become manifest only when the patient returns to their care. While in theory the home country physician is not legally responsible for injuries he did not cause, in practice the medical malpractice system may have difficulty disentangling which physician caused the injury, and there is always significant pressure to settle such cases. To mitigate these problems, home countries may want to consider establishing non-tort compensation schemes for medical tourists, similar to worker's compensation funding (Cohen 2010a; Cohen 2014).

More generally, follow-up care for poorly performed medical tourism procedures may generate significant externalities for the home country's health care system. Health care records detailing what transpired abroad may not be available or readily recognizable (Crooks et al. 2013). Many patients may be embarrassed to notify their home country physician that they went abroad, thus compounding the injury and attendant costs. Despite legal obligations not to abandon patients, many physicians may prove unwilling to assist returning patients—for example, a general practitioner or cardiologist seeing a patient who has gone abroad for cardiac bypass surgery. Medical tourism paid for through insurance schemes, with their robust regulation of home and destination country physicians through insurance authorization, may be better poised to deal with these challenges than will medical tourism for patients paying out-of-pocket, but there remain significant questions about how best to ensure continuity of care and about who should pay for follow-up care.

Finally, ethical issues may arise from the effect, hard to predict, that competition from medical tourism offerings might have on home country health care industries. Thus far the volume of medical tourism has been too small to have anything but local competition effects (Cohen 2010b). But if the volume were to significantly increase, especially in privatized health care systems, physicians may face pressure to price-match their much cheaper foreign "competitors." Some fear this would lead to "cutting corners," arguing that protectionist measures are needed to avoid the problem, while others welcome such competition because they think that this competition will drive down prices but not quality (Cohen 2014).

Medical Tourism for Services Illegal in the Home Country But Legal in the Destination Country ("Circumvention Tourism")

In "circumvention tourism," patients travel abroad to access a treatment that is illegal/unavailable in their home country, but legal/available in their destination country. It can take many forms. Here are a few hypotheticals (adapted from Cohen 2012b, 2012c, 2014):

- Nawal is a 2-year-old U.S. citizen whose parents emigrated from Sudan 20 years earlier and want to have female genital cutting (FGC) performed on her. The procedure is illegal in the U.S., so Nawal's parents take her to Sudan, where a local doctor legally performs the surgery. Could/should the U.S. apply the criminal prohibition extraterritorially to her parents?
- Andrea, a 21-year-old Irish woman, experiences an unwanted pregnancy. Abortion is illegal in Ireland. She travels to "Women on Waves," a floating abortion clinic in international waters. Ships in international waters are governed by the law of the country whose flag they fly, so this ship flies the flag of the Netherlands, where abortion is legal. Nevertheless, on Andrea's return, the Irish government initiates criminal process against her. Can/should Ireland be able to do so?
- Susan is a 50-year-old Connecticut woman diagnosed with Lou Gehrig's disease with very few months to live. Because of the disease, Susan has difficulty speaking, chewing, and swallowing. Assisted suicide is illegal in Connecticut. Her brother Jon helps her travel to Switzerland, where a clinic assists in ending her life. Upon his return, can/should the state prosecute Jon for assisting Susan's suicide?
- Jason and his partner Jonathan are having difficulty securing a surrogate in Canada, where paid surrogacy is criminalized. They turn to a clinic in the village of Anand, India, where the practice is legal. Can/should Canada prosecute them?
- Rea and Mark are considering taking their 6-year-old son, Noah, from their home in Minneapolis to a stem cell clinic in China for stem cell therapy. Noah suffers

from a rare and severely disabling neurological disorder called ataxia telangiectasia that causes, *inter alia*, decreased mental development. The therapy, involving the injection of adult stem cells into the child's cerebrospinal fluid is unapproved in the U.S. In the one case of treatment that has been documented, the child gained no benefit and instead experienced headaches caused by tumors in the brain and spinal cord that developed from the stem-cell-based injections (DeRenzo 2011: 889; Amariglio et al. 2009). Nevertheless, Noah's parents are adamant that they are willing to take a chance. Does their home country physician have an obligation to report them? Is this procedure a form of child abuse and neglect? Should child and protective services become involved?

All of these hypotheticals are based on real world cases. Fertility tourism is dealt with elsewhere in this volume (see Chapter 30), so I will concentrate on the other examples.

Extraterritoriality and Pluralism

The first set of issues concerns attempts by a home country to extend its domestic prohibitions to activities by its citizens abroad, or in legal terms "extraterritorial application of domestic law." More specifically, I am referring to "prescriptive jurisdiction" for criminal law, which involves the power to render a particular offense criminal, as opposed to, for example, the power to extradite (Cohen 2012c; Lowe 2006: 337–40). As a matter of international law, home countries clearly have the *power* to criminalize these activities (although in some cases, the home country's *own domestic* law may prevent it from criminalizing extraterritorially) (Cohen 2012b, 2012c).

Even if a home country does have the power to criminalize the medical tourism activities of its patients abroad, should it use that power? One way of answering the question would be to consider the legality and morality of the activities domestically. If the U.S. permitted abortion on its own soil, it would have no obvious reason to forbid it abroad, except for the kind of patient-protective concerns discussed earlier for medical tourism for legal services. The more interesting and difficult case, though, is where the home country *prohibits* a practice on its home soil. If the home country conceives of these prohibitions as not only lawful but morally well grounded, under what circumstances does it have the moral prerogative or obligation to extend that prohibition to its citizens abroad?

The key question here is the meaning of "citizenship" and whether, on either communitarian or social contractarian theories of the state's power to punish, the location of the conduct and the fact that the conduct is not prohibited under the law of the foreign sovereign matters (Cohen 2012b). One way of framing the issue is to ask whether the sovereignty of the home country and its power to make people answer to it through criminal law is primarily based on territoriality (the presence of a person in the boundaries of the home country), citizenship (the person's "ties" to the home country), or both. The more citizenship is thought of as a justifiable basis for the sovereign to exercise its criminal jurisdiction, the less problematic criminalizing circumvention tourism becomes.

One also needs to develop a way of weighing the destination country's interest in enabling the circumvention tourist to engage in the domestically prohibited activity within its territory. This interest might be economic, as in fertility tourism, which can be a substantial boon to an economy, or it might be moral, as when the destination country aims to serve as a refuge for those governed by what it perceives to be unjust laws. Because a home country's criminalization of the conduct of its own citizens abroad is minimally disruptive to the destination country—the provision of services by destination country doctors and the design of its health care system are otherwise unaffected—it is easier to justify than, for example, criminalizing the activity of destination country citizen providers.

Beyond this balancing of potentially conflicting interests of the two countries, one must examine a constellation of questions involving "cost of exit," "accommodation," and "cultural defense." Circumvention tourism offers the citizen a middle ground between the political-theoretical Hobson's choice of either being bound by the domestic law or "exiting"—renouncing one's citizenship and presence in the home country. On this view, circumvention tourism is "exit light": The citizen need only temporarily leave the country in order to avoid its criminal laws (Cohen 2012c). Guido Pennings has been the most staunch proponent of this approach in relation to abortion or assisted suicide, claiming that "[a]llowing people to look abroad demonstrates the absolute minimum of respect for their moral autonomy" (Pennings 2002: 337–41). In the case of something like FGC with strong religious or cultural origins, the accommodation may be to "cultural defense" claims by minority groups within the society (Minow 2008: 252).

However, this middle position is not without problems. First, it would result in a kind of masking of what some (especially the home country legislators that prohibit it domestically) might think of as murder or child abuse, whereby we allow ourselves to avoid confronting evils by making sure they happen outside our view. Second, the accommodation privilege seems to be distributed in a morally arbitrary way since it correlates with an individual's ability to afford to travel. If we were serious about accommodation of the views of home country citizens by allowing them to perform these acts abroad, it seems fairer instead to hold a lottery for those who want to perform the service in the home country and grant them a fixed number of permits, or at least pay for the expense of traveling abroad for those who want to circumvent, so that not only the rich have access to the accommodation, although this would introduce an additional level of complicity. If we are uncomfortable with such suggestions, this may indicate that there is something wrong with accommodation through circumvention tourism. Finally, and most importantly, when the interest is preventing harm to a home country citizen who has not meaningfully consented (e.g., a child, and on some views that are especially likely to be subscribed to in home countries banning abortion domestically, a fetus (Cohen 2012c)), it seems irrelevant to the "victim" that the injury took place outside of the territory; it is, at least on some understandings, still a home country citizen (or at least a "stateless person") who has been harmed by another home country citizen, and the "victim" is not in the destination country voluntarily in a robust sense (Cohen 2012c).

The push and pull of these considerations cannot be resolved in a one-size-fits-all way that generates a single answer for all forms of circumvention tourism. Instead, one should evaluate the propriety of extraterritorial criminalization in light of the reasons that underlie the home country's domestic prohibition along with a determination of who is the "victim" (Cohen 2012c). Putting these two criteria together—type of justification and victim citizenship—can help us sort through these and other case studies.

On communitarian and social contractarian grounds, the permissibility or obligation of the home country to criminalize the activities of its citizens engaged in circumvention tourism is at its zenith when there is a "double coincidence of citizenship"—when both the "perpetrator" and "victim" are citizens of the same home country that has a domestic criminal prohibition of the act. In such cases, excusing the perpetrator-citizen from criminal liability forces the victim-citizen to forego the protection of the country's criminal law. Extraterritorial criminalization is particularly appropriate when the "victim's" presence in the destination country is not voluntary in a meaningful sense: This is certainly the case with abortion (for home countries that view the fetus as a person, of course) and, given the infancy of the "victim," FGC. For reproductive technology, the issue depends on a specification of who the "victim" is, and for assisted suicide, on whether the home country is willing to accept consent to the killing as negating its criminality.

Where the justification for the domestic prohibition is preventing serious bodily harm and the "victim" is also a home country citizen—e.g., fetuses in abortion, children in FGC, and on some accounts (though I am skeptical (2011b)) some reproductive technology use—the state has very good reasons to extend its prohibition extraterritorially, and the claim for accommodation is at its weakest. This is because under criminal law theory the sovereign is most justified in criminalizing in order to prevent serious bodily injury by one citizen against another, the core of the Harm Principle. By contrast, the state's justification for extraterritorial prohibition is more complex when it comes to "corruption" or "attitude-modification" concerns, exploitation of destination country citizen "victims," and paternalistic protections of patients (justifications often at work in the context of travel for assisted suicide, stem cell therapies, and reproductive technology). In sum, only under some conceptions of why the domestic prohibition is in place may the home country have a prerogative or obligation to criminalize extraterritorially (Cohen 2012c).

Paternalism, Child Abuse, and Home Country Physicians as Double Agents

Medical tourism for stem cells or other experimental therapies raises some distinct issues.

The existing literature paints a sobering picture of the quality, effectiveness, and safety of stem cell therapies currently offered to medical tourists, particularly in China. Clinics often overpromise, given that few existing therapies have peer-review data supporting them; are not always forthright about the type of stem cells they use; and rarely mention the serious risks associated with these therapies (Cohen 2014; Levine and Wolf 2012: 122; Chen and Gottweis 2011; DeRenzo 2011: 889; Ryan et al. 2010; Lau et al. 2008). Yet despite these risks and lack of benefits, many patients are desperate to try stem cell therapies and even report gains afterwards and a desire to pursue further treatments (Chen and Gottweis 2011; Ryan et al. 2010).

The key ethical question here is how to balance patient autonomy and patient protection. One approach again focuses on providing information. The International Society for Stem Cell Research (ISSCR), a leading voice in stem cell research regulation, has developed "Guidelines for the Clinical Translation of Stem Cells" and proposed developing a web-based resource wherein individuals can "submit an entity to the ISSCR for formal inquiry," whereby the ISSCR would then perform an evaluation of the clinic for each of the diseases for which it advertises therapies (Cohen 2014; ISSCR 2008, 2010). Unfortunately, this proposal was never implemented, in part due to legal threats by clinics worried about bad reviews. There is a clear opportunity for home country governments or intergovernmental organizations to step in and fill this informational gap (Cohen 2014).

The bigger question is whether such informational interventions would go far enough. For stem cell therapies specifically, one focus group study concluded that even when individuals were exposed to "cautionary information . . . most remained receptive to obtaining (unproven) treatments under desperate circumstances" (Einsendel and Adamson 2012). Other studies show that these patients are deeply skeptical of the motives or attitudes of naysaying home country authorities (Chen and Gottweis 2011: 11, 13).

Another possibility would be to extend domestic criminal prohibitions extraterritorially, but even if this were possible, it is not clear that it is desirable, at least for adult patients. A long libertarian tradition, for instance, rejects the use of criminal law sanctions to protect individuals from their own bad decisions, and the experimental drug case for terminally ill patients seems a particularly hard one on such views because there is (at least in the patient's own mind) some chance of benefit for which they may be prepared to accept the risk (Stein and Savulescu 2011; Volokh 2007; Feinberg 1986). Indeed at least one author has analogized the right involved to be one of "medical self-defense" (Volokh 2007). Moreover, some patients might prefer hope (even if false) with risks, to no hope and no risks (Murdoch and Scott 2010: 18).

The situation is quite different, though, when it comes to parents transporting their children for stem cell therapies, which makes up a significant portion of this type of medical tourism. Such cases raise two related questions. First, can and should the state try to prevent parents from taking their children abroad for these therapies? Second, what is the role of home country pediatricians in advising parents and potentially reporting them to authorities if they fear for the child's health and safety because of the parents' desire to seek such therapies in destination countries?

On the first issue, parents who opt for stem cell therapies are arguably engaging in acts that might constitute child abuse or neglect, at least in the U.S. and Canada (Cohen 2014; Zarzezcny and Caulfield 2010: 5). Existing case law in both countries has mostly focused on parents who decline conventional cancer therapies for their child in favor of experimental ones, a scenario that offers a compelling analogy with states assuming medical or other guardianship in the case of parents who seek to have their kids use stem cell therapies (Re M.M. 2007; Children's Society of Peel Region v. B. (C.) 1988; Custody of a Minor 1978). While stem cell therapy is a somewhat harder case because it involves more unknown risks, in general more muscular application of child protection laws in this sphere is arguably appropriate (Cohen 2014).

Usually, however, the state will not even know that a parent intends to take the child abroad for a stem cell therapy. Health care providers thus play a crucial role in activating child protective service mechanisms, but placing such obligations on providers also forces them into the uncomfortable position of a double agent. The best approach to this problem may be multi-step, for providers to first provide information and an assessment of the risks, then seek to actively dissuade parents from choosing stem cell tourism, and only then consider reporting the parents to protective services (Cohen 2014; Zarczeny and Caulfield 2010; AAPCCD 2001: 600). However, given robust reporting requirements relating to child abuse in the U.S. and other jurisdictions, when attempts to dissuade fail, providers should face real legal and ethical duties to report parents if the safety of the therapy has not been established. The fact that these parents love their children and are only trying to help makes the situation particularly poignant, but it does not change the underlying legal or ethical rules that should apply (Cohen 2014).

Conclusion

Medical tourism poses varied and difficult ethical questions, and the analysis provided in this chapter merely scratches the surface. Governments, physicians, hospital administrators, and others are already facing these issues in day-to-day decisions, and as the trade grows so will its problems. It is exciting to see bioethics increasingly shaping the landscape of this complex and challenging area.

Related Topics

Chapter 9, "Do Health Workers Have a Duty to Work in Underserved Areas?" Nir Eyal and Samia Hurst
Chapter 30, "Reproductive Travel and Tourism," G.K.D. Crozier

References

AAPCCD (American Academy of Pediatrics' Committee on Children With Disabilities) (2001) "Counseling Families who Choose Complementary and Alternative Medicine for Their Child with Chronic Illness or Disability," *Pediatrics* 107: 598–601.

Amariglio, N. et al. (2009) "Donor-Derived Brain Tumor Following Neural Stem Cell Transplantation in an Ataxia Telangiectasia Patient," *PLOS Medicine* 6: 221–31.

Baker, D. and Rho, H.J. (2009) "Free Trade in Health Care: The Gains from Globalized Medicare and Medicaid," *Center for Economic Policy and Research*. Available at: http://www.cepr.net/documents/publications/free-trade-hc-2009-09.pdf (accessed July 7, 2014).

Beitz, C. (1975) "Justice and International Relations," *Philosophy and Public Affairs* 4: 360–89.

Beitz, C. (1979) *Political Theory and International Relations*, Princeton, NJ: Princeton University Press.

Benavides, D. (2002) "Trade Policies and Export of Health Services: A Development Perspective," in N. Drager and C. Vieira (eds.) *Trade in Health Services: Global, Regional, and Country Perspectives*, Washington, DC: Pan American Health Organization.

Bookman, M. and Bookman, K. (2007) *Medical Tourism in Developing Countries*, New York: Palgrave Macmillan.

Chanda, R. (2002) "Trade in Health Services," *Bulletin of the World Health Organization* 80: 158–63.

Chen, H. and Gottweis, H. (2011) "Stem Cell Treatments in China: Rethinking the Patient Role in the Global Bio-Economy," *Bioethics* [online], November 17.

Chen, Y.Y.B. and Flood, C.M. (2013) "Medical Tourism's Impact on Health Care Equity and Access in Low- and Middle-Income Countries: Making the Case for Regulation," *Journal of Law, Medicine and Ethics* 41: 286–300.

Children's Society of Peel Region v. B. (C.) (1988) W.D.F.L. 794 (Ont. Prov. Ct. Fm. Ct. Div.).

Cohen, I.G. (2010a) "Medical Tourism: The View from Ten Thousand Feet," *Hastings Center Report* 40 (2): 11–12.

Cohen, I.G. (2010b) "Protecting Patients with Passports: Medical Tourism and the Patient-Protective Argument," *Iowa Law Review* 95: 1467–567.

Cohen, I.G. (2011a) "Medical Tourism, Access to Health Care, and Global Justice," *Virginia Journal of International Law* 52: 1–56.

Cohen, I.G. (2011b) "Regulating Reproduction: The Problem with Best Interests," *Minnesota Law Review* 96: 423–519.

Cohen, I.G. (2012a) "How to Regulate Medical Tourism (and Why Bioethicists Should Care)," *Journal of Developing World Bioethics* 12: 9–20.

Cohen, I.G. (2012b) "Medical Outlaws or Medical Refugees? An Examination of Circumvention Tourism" in J. Hodges et al. (eds.) *Risks and Challenges in Medical Tourism: Understanding the Global Market for Health Services Controversies in the Exploding Industry of Global Medicine*, Santa Barbara, CA: Praeger, pp. 207–29.

Cohen, I.G. (2012c) "Circumvention Tourism," *Cornell Law Review* 97: 1309.

Cohen, I.G. (2013a) "Transplant Tourism: The Ethics and Regulation of International Markets for Organs," *Journal of Law, Medicine and Ethics* 41: 269–85.

Cohen, I.G. (2013b) "Introduction," in I.G. Cohen (ed.) *The Globalization of Health Care: Legal and Ethical Challenges*, Oxford: Oxford University Press, pp. xvi–xxiv. Available at: http://global.oup.com/academic/product/the-globalization-of-health-care-9780199917907;jsessionid=3793130A801EABC477E59E8E911B9F86?cc=us&lang=en& (accessed August 15, 2014).

Cohen, I.G. (2014) *Patients with Passports: Medical Tourism, Law and Ethics*, Oxford: Oxford University Press. Available at: http://www.amazon.com/Patients-Passports-Medical-Tourism-Ethics/dp/0190218185/ref=tmm_pap_title_0?_encoding=UTF8&sr=&qid= (accessed August 15, 2014).

Cortez, N. (2008) "Patients Without Borders: The Emerging Global Market for Patients and the Evolution of Modern Health Care," *Indiana Law Journal* 83: 71–132.

Cortez, N. (2010) "Recalibrating the Legal Risks of Cross-Border Health Care," *Yale Journal of Health Policy, Law, and Ethics* 10: 1–89.

Cortez, N. (2011) "Embracing the New Geography of Health Care: A Novel Way to Cover Those Left Out of Health Reform," *Southern California Law Review* 84: 859–931.

Crooks, V., Turner, L., Cohen, I.G., Bristeir, J., Snyder, J., Casey, V. and Whitmore, R. (2013) "Ethical and Legal Implications of the Risks of Medical Tourism for Patients: A Qualitative Study of Canadian Health and Safety Representatives' Perspectives," *BMJ Open* 3: e002302.

Currie, J. and MacLeod, W.B. (2008) "First Do No Harm? Tort Reform and Birth Outcomes," *Quarterly Journal of Economics* 123: 795–830.

Custody of a Minor (1978) 379 N.E.2d 1053 (Mass.).

Daniels, N. (2008) *Just Health: Meeting Health Needs Fairly*, Cambridge: Cambridge University Press.

DeRenzo, L. (2011) "Stem Cell Tourism: The Challenge and Promise of International Regulation of Embryonic Stem Cell-Based Therapies," *Case Western Reserve Journal of International Law* 43: 877–918.

Ehrbeck, T., Guevara, C. and Mango, P. (2008) "Mapping the Market for Medical Travel," *McKinsey Quarterly*, May.

Einhorn, B. (2008) "Hannaford's Medical-Tourism Experiment," *Business Week*, November 9.

Einsiedel, E. and Adamson, H. (2012) "Stem Cell Tourism and Future Stem Cell Tourists: Policy and Ethical Implications, *Developing World Bioethics* 12: 35–44.

European Parliament (2011) "Directive 2011/24 of the European Parliament and of the Council of 9 March 2011 on the Application of Patients' Rights in Cross-Border Healthcare," *Official Journal of the European Union* L 88/45.

Feinberg, J. (1986) *The Moral Limits of the Criminal Law, Volume 3: Harm to Self*, Oxford: Oxford University Press.

Frakes, M. (2012) "Does Medical Malpractice Deter? The Impact of Tort Reforms and Malpractice Standard Reforms on Healthcare Quality," *Cornell Legal Studies Research Paper* No. 12–29.

France, L. and Francis, J. (2010) "Stateless Crimes, Legitimacy, and International Criminal Law: The Case of Organ Trafficking," *Criminal Law and Philosophy* 4: 283–95.

Greenberg, M., Haviland, A., Ashwood, J.S. and Main, R. (2010) "Is Better Patient Safety Associated with Less Malpractice Activity? Evidence from California," *RAND Institute for Civil Justice*. Available at: http://www.rand.org/pubs/technical_reports/TR824.html (accessed July 7, 2014).

Gupta, A. (2008) "Medical Tourism in India: Winners and Losers," *Indian Journal of Medical Ethics* 5: 4–5.

Hodges, J. and Kimball, A. (2012) "Unseen Travelers: Medical Tourism and the Spread of Infectious Disease," in J. Hodges et al. (eds.) *Risks and Challenges in Medical Tourism: Understanding the Global Market for Health Services Controversies in the Exploding Industry of Global Medicine*, Santa Barbara, CA: Praeger, pp. 111–37.

Hopkins, L., Labonté, R., Runnels, V. and Packer, C. (2010) "Medical Tourism Today: What is the State of Existing Knowledge?" *Journal of Public Health Policy* 31: 185–98.

ISSCR (International Society for Stem Cell Research) (2008) "Guidelines for the Clinical Translation of Stem Cells." Available at: http://www.isscr.org/home/publications/ClinTransGuide (accessed August 14, 2014).

ISSCR (International Society for Stem Cell Research) (2010) "Patients Beware: Commercialized Stem Cell Treatments on the Web," *Cell Stem Cell* 7: 43–9.

Janjaroen, W. and Supakankunti, S. (2002) "International Trade in Health Services in the Millennium: The Case of Thailand," in N. Drager and C. Vieira (eds.) *Trade in Health Services: Global, Regional, and Country Perspectives*, Washington, DC: Pan American Health Organization, pp. 87–106.

Johnston, R., Crooks, V., Snyder, J. and Kingsbury, P. (2010) "What Is Known About the Effects of Medical Tourism in Destination and Departure Countries? A Scoping Review," *International Journal for Equity in Health* 9: 1–13.

Lancaster, J. (2004) "Surgeries, Side Trips for 'Medical Tourists,'" *Washington Post*, October 23: A1.
Lau, D., Ogbogu, U., Taylor, B., Stanfinski, T., Menon, D. and Caulfield, T. (2008) "Stem Cell Clinics Online: The Direct-to-Consumer Portrayal of Stem Cell Medicine," *Cell Stem Cell* 3: 591–4.
Levine, A. and Wolf, L. (2012) "The Roles and Responsibilities of Physicians in Patients' Decisions about Unproven Stem Cell Therapies," *Journal of Law, Medicine, and Ethics* 40: 122–34.
Lowe, V. (2006) "Jurisdiction," in M. Evans (ed.) *International Law* (2nd edition), Oxford: Oxford University Press, pp. 335–60.
Mattoo, A. and Rathindran, R. (2006) "How Health Insurance Inhibits Trade in Health Care," *Health Affairs* 25: 358–68.
Milstein, A. and Smith, M. (2006) "America's New Refugees: Seeking Affordable Surgery Offshore," *New England Journal of Medicine* 355: 1637–40.
Minow M. (2008) "About Women, About Culture: About Them, About Us," in R.A. Shweder, M. Minow and H.R. Markus (eds.) *Engaging Cultural Differences: The Multicultural Challenges in Liberal Democracies*, New York: Russell Sage Foundation.
Murdoch, C. and Scott, C. (2010) "Stem Cell Tourism and the Power of Hope," *The American Journal of Bioethics* 10: 16–23.
Murphy, T. (2009) "Health Insurers Explore Savings in Overseas Care," *Associated Press*, August 23.
Nagel, T. (2005) "The Problem of Global Justice," *Philosophy and Public Affairs* 33: 113–47.
Nussbaum, M. (2006) *Frontiers of Justice*, Cambridge, MA: Harvard University Press.
Pennings, G. (2002) "Reproductive Tourism as Moral Pluralism in Motion," *Journal of Medical Ethics* 28: 337–41.
Pogge, T. (2002) *World Poverty and Human Rights*, Cambridge: Polity Press.
Pogge, T. (2005) "Human Rights and Global Health: A Research Program," *Metaphilosophy* 36: 182–209.
Rawls, J. (1999) *The Law of Peoples*, Cambridge, MA: Harvard University Press.
Re M.M. (2007) ABPC 6.
Ryan, K., Sanders, A., Wang, D. and Levine, A. (2010) "Tracking the Rise of Stem Cell Tourism," *Regenerative Medicine* 5: 27–33.
Scheper-Hughes, N. (2000) "The Global Traffic in Human Organs," *Current Anthropology* 41: 191–224.
Stein, M. and Savulescu, J. (2011) "Welfare Versus Autonomy in Human Subjects Research," *Florida State University Law Review* 38: 303–43.
Sunstein, C. and Thaler, R. (2003) "Libertarian Paternalism Is Not an Oxymoron," *The University of Chicago Law Review* 70: 1159–202.
Terry, N.P. (2007) "Under-Regulated Health Care Phenomena in a Flat World: Medical Tourism and Outsourcing," *Western New England Law Review* 29: 421–72.
Transplantation Society (2008) "The Declaration of Istanbul on Organ Trafficking and Transplant Tourism," *Nephrology Dialysis Transplantation* 23: 3375–80.
Turner, L. (2007) "'First World Health Care at Third World Prices': Globalization, Bioethics and Medical Tourism," *Biosciences* 2: 303–25.
Turner, L. (2013) "Patient Mortality in Medical Tourism: Examining News Media Reports of Deaths Following Travel for Cosmetic Surgery and Bariatric Surgery," in I.G. Cohen (ed.) *The Globalization of Health Care: Legal and Ethical Challenges*, Oxford: Oxford University Press.
Volokh, E. (2007) "Medical Self-Defense, Prohibited Experimental Therapies, and Payment for Organs," *Harvard Law Review* 120: 1813–46.
Wallace, S., Mendez-Luck, C. and Castañeda, X. (2009) "Heading South: Why Mexican Immigrants in California Seek Health Services in Mexico," *Medical Care* 47: 662–9.
Zarzezcny, A. and Caulfield, T. (2010) "Stem Cell Tourism and Doctors' Duties to Minors: A View from Canada," *The American Journal of Bioethics* 10: 3–15.

9

DO HEALTH WORKERS HAVE A DUTY TO WORK IN UNDERSERVED AREAS?

Nir Eyal and Samia A. Hurst

Background

Health worker shortages are a crucial obstacle to relieving the burden of disease in many countries. Their impact is most concentrated in the remote, rural areas of sub-Saharan Africa and South Asia, where a great number of the world's poorest, sickest, and most vulnerable populations reside. Local health workers are often reluctant to work in these critically underserved areas, preferring instead to work in cities and the private sector. Exacerbating this problem, some of the wealthiest countries allow in, and often actively recruit, health workers from these poorer countries. Large differences in the availability of health workers result. According to the most recent WHO data available, the ratio of physicians per 1,000 population in Malawi is 0.019, whereas in the U.S. it is 2.42, for 2008 and 2009 respectively (WHO 2012a: 14–15). Disparities in the availability of physicians and other health workers inside countries are also extreme.

As a result, basic medical procedures including HIV care, mental health services, and vaccinations are not delivered, setting back infant, child, and maternal survival, and the overall health status of these communities (WHO 2006; but see Clemens 2007). Health worker migration to so-called "destination countries" also translates into loss of potential employers, teachers, and role models in migrants' "source countries" (Aluwihare 2005). Especially when unplanned, such migration can wreak havoc in medical delivery systems (Martineau et al. 2004). Moreover, because in many developing countries medical education is publicly funded, global medical "brain drain" amounts to absurd humanitarian aid by poorer nations to richer ones (Alkire and Chen 2006: 113).

The option to migrate is good for health workers. Many compatriots can only dream of this opportunity. It is also good for patients in rich countries, who can improve their access to care through better-staffed health systems. But the patient populations from whom these doctors are taken often need them much more.

Several options exist for attempting to secure healthcare for underserved populations even when health workers leave. One is to train many physicians and nurses to replace those who leave, hoping that not all replacements will leave. Another is to train different cadres of health workers with cheaper training and employment. Thus far, these workers have proven less likely to leave resource-poor settings (WHO 2012b). With

WHO backing, African countries already delegate tasks including screening, management of most first-line HIV care, mental health treatment, and Caesarian sections to such non-traditional health workers (WHO 2006, 2008, 2010b, 2012b). Finally, some healthcare services can be provided through telemedicine, which usually involves a highly skilled worker consulting patients over the phone or video from afar, with assistance from a local, less skilled worker (Mars 2010). Each of these options to replace migrating physicians has its limitations, however (Eyal and Hurst 2008). For example, while less-trained health workers can safely perform a range of tasks, physicians currently remain necessary for many referral, supervision, and even clinical tasks (Hirschhorn et al. 2006; WHO 2008; Chu et al. 2009), and less-trained health workers are also increasingly likely to move to well served settings (Dugger 2004).

Several claims have been made about the potential benefits of physician migration. First, it is sometimes claimed that remittances, or money sent home by migrants, offset any loss from professionals' emigration (Clemens 2011). But remittances may be small in the specific case of physicians (our focus in this chapter), whose families are typically middle class and urban; usually such families do not need or feel comfortable asking emigrating relatives for money. Nor do transfers to urban families greatly assist the rural needy. Another potential benefit is that lucrative migration options for physicians create some incentive to study and excel in the profession (Clemens 2011). While this is true, these incentives might be too weak to restore the supply of physicians to their home countries, and may perpetuate the vicious cycle of expensive training and professional flight (Kangasniemi et al. 2007). A third alleged benefit, skill-sharing upon a physician's return to his or her country (Ana 2005), is largely a pipedream: The vast majority of migrants never return to enable such sharing to take place (Mullan 2005).

One proposal for a coordinated political intervention to improve the balance of benefits and harms from physician migration is for source countries to impose a so-called "Bhagwati" tax on migrant workers' foreign incomes (Hannum 1987: 39; Bhagwati 2012; see also Brock and Blake forthcoming). That tax on emigrants would be imposed by the source country and collected for it by the receiving country. Bhagwati originally proposed a progressive tax, or flat 10 percent tax, on emigrant earnings for 10 years (Bhagwati and Dellalfar 1973). Even if such a tax were practically enforceable abroad (Alkire and Chen 2006: 113), tax revenues might fail to reach source countries' underserved and often disenfranchised populations. Nor is it clear that it is the most efficient or ethical solution for migrants to be forced to pay source countries, as opposed to the institutions or countries that recruit and employ them (Ypi 2008: 414; Clemens 2011: 92–3; Dumitru 2012).

The global crisis in human resources for health was the focus of the 2006 World Health Report. This canonical document argues that on balance the domestic or international flight of health personnel from areas of critical shortage vastly undermines public health and welfare in those areas—and this chapter operates on a similar assumption. Furthermore, in 2010 the World Health Assembly unanimously adopted the *Global Code of Practice on the International Recruitment of Health Personnel.* This document strikes a balance between the rights of underserved patients, those of health workers, and the prerogatives of Member States, with a more extensive monitoring process than that of earlier WHO codes and conventions.

The next section of this chapter introduces some of the most important, and often underexplored, ethical questions about the crisis in human resources for health. The final section explores one such question in depth: Whether health workers have either a moral duty, or a morally defensible legal duty, to work in underserved areas rather than, for instance, migrate to countries where their services are less critically needed.

Ethical Questions about the Distribution of Human Resources for Health

When we think of resource allocation in health care, we typically think about distributing pills, procedures, or access to facilities among patients. Much less attention has been paid to the skilled health professionals without whom these other resources lie unused or misused. How should these "resources" be "allocated"?

The concepts and methods used in economic, medical, and ethical reflection on the allocation of ordinary health resources do not straightforwardly govern this area. "Human resources for health" are special. Antiretroviral pills do not have a will of their own. They lack rights. We lack responsibilities toward them. We cannot "disadvantage," "coerce," or "exploit" them. Nor do pills have duties toward patients. No pill has ever taken the Hippocratic Oath.

A full theory of the ethical distribution of human resources for health must heed the fact that the "resources" here are persons. It should also clarify what remains constant in comparison with non-human resources like drugs or surgeries.

This section explores some central questions in the ethics of allocating human resources for health, especially in light of the challenges associated with medical migration. Our hope is to elicit more scholarship on these often neglected questions.

Responsibility for the Harm of Insufficient Access to Health Services

According to Norman Daniels, when rich countries lure health workers away from underserved patient populations in poor countries, this is paradigmatic of the active harm perpetuated on the poor at the global level—the sort of harm that Thomas Pogge often argues is such a wrong for rich countries to perpetuate (Pogge 2002; Daniels 2008: 337–9, 353). But this claim faces three challenges. First, when rich country employers recruit doctors from underserved areas, rich country governments may be involved only passively, by failing to meddle with that interaction. How does that count as *active* harm?

Second, even when active harm takes place, when it is the result of market competition, commonsense morality often holds that no wrong was done. For example, market competitors are not wronging me by opening a nearby shop that drives mine out of business—although that actively harms me. And rich universities are not wronging other rich universities and their typically privileged students by actively recruiting their star professors. Even if it is morally wrong for a rich university to recruit professors from struggling public universities that serve the less well-off, what makes it wrong is not simply the fact of active harm—or the same action would have been wrong between rich institutions as well. The wrong consists of something else.

A final challenge is the agency of health workers. Does the fact that workers are persons whose consent and collaboration are necessary for uptake affect the recruiters' moral responsibility for downstream effects on patients from source countries at all? And can we call it "poaching," as many do, although these workers are individuals with free will and not the property of others to poach (Snyder 2009)?

Source versus Destination Country Patients

Global health worker migration often increases access to services in destination countries while thwarting it in source countries. This casts new light on the universal coverage schemes found in rich countries. Following the 2010 *Patient Protection and Affordable Care Act* (ACA, or "Obamacare"), the U.S., for example, offers coverage and services to many more Americans. This expansion of services is excellent for many uninsured and underinsured Americans, but unless U.S. doctors flock to primary care, which is unlikely (Schwartz 2012), or the U.S. trains enough additional doctors and physician assistants to treat everyone, it may lead to increased demand for foreign-trained health workers. One result could be fewer physicians available in rural India and other developing countries. Broadly stated, when greater health workforce availability in a developed country has a detrimental impact on its availability in source countries, how much is that developed country ethically permitted to prioritize its patients over those in the source country?

This broad question may also play out beyond the borders of the developed country. In the future, the U.S. may send many patients as "medical tourists" to India or Thailand to receive surgeries and other treatments that are much less expensive there than at home (see Chapter 8 in this volume). Such medical tourism may lure Indian health workers to their home country's private hospitals, thereby undermining service availability in rural sectors. Is the U.S. government obligated to prevent these prospects from materializing, even at the expense of Americans' health?

Self-Sufficiency

The World Health Assembly's *Code of Practice on the International Recruitment of Health Personnel* calls on destination countries to take serious measures to be self-sufficient, for example, by training more physicians and nurses of their own. But *shouldn't* some countries focus on producing what they produce best, rather than doctors? Some countries, like the Philippines and India, seem to deliberately train health workers as an "export industry," hoping to benefit from taxed foreign income and remittances. These doctors are then available to supplement the pool of available doctors in other countries that have produced fewer doctors than they require (Alkire and Chen 2006: 113; Dimaya et al. 2012). However, the human cost on migrants' families and on underserved patients in these countries is tremendous. Should these workers be barred from moving, or should their movement persist?

Medical School Intervention

By training physicians, medical schools help their countries address physician shortages. But many other things that medical schools can do to help address these shortages are less clearly legitimate. For example, is it morally permissible for medical school faculty to let students understand that they would greatly disappoint them unless they work with the underserved—which might be considered emotional blackmail or an implicit threat to breach entitlements to future support? Is it permissible for schools intentionally not to teach some essential aspects of care in rich countries precisely in order to delimit graduates' "marketability" abroad (Eyal and Hurst 2011)? Is it permissible for schools to admit preferentially applicants who are relatively likely to choose later to work in underserved areas—say, residents of underserved rural areas (WHO 2010a), or applicants with suboptimal academic performance—who are more likely to work in such areas than the academically best (Zimmerman et al. 2012)? Is it permissible for schools to offer applicants scholarships conditional on a very long commitment to later rural service (Eyal and Bärnighausen 2012)?

Intra-societal Wage Inequality

One way to increase health worker retention is to make their salaries at home more competitive with salaries abroad. This strategy is rarely criticized, but for local salaries to be genuinely competitive, they may have to be grossly disproportional to those of other local public workers. Would "overpayment" to health workers not violate social equality? When such competitive salaries follow a bargaining process and raise the specter of threats to emigrate without the guarantee of disproportional salaries, don't the bargaining health workers thereby exploit their patients' desperate needs in order to secure unfair privileges from employers (Cohen 1992)? However, can high salaries really compensate health workers fairly for disadvantages such as stunted professional development ladders, inadequate personal safety, or lack of social respect?

When Is Compensation Enough?

Recently it has become popular to demand that destination countries or workers compensate source countries for lost workers. Such resources could for example facilitate future efforts to train and potentially retain the next generation of health workers. Some authors defend this demand, for example, as a matter of internalizing externalities or reparation (Brock 2009; Brock and Blake forthcoming; Wellman 2010).

This demand, however, raises questions about specification and justification. First, what should determine the scale of compensation? Is it how much the destination country's population benefits from the migration? How much the source country had spent on the migrant's studies, upbringing, and conditions enabling them to become physicians, such as functioning infrastructure (Brock and Blake forthcoming)? How much the source country or its underserved populations stand to lose from the migration (under the ideal assumption that the migrant would work with underserved populations if he or she could not migrate, or under realistic assumptions)? And who should pay that compensation—migrant health workers, destination country employers and recruiters, or destination country governments? Who should receive the money—the source country government, its health ministry, its medical schools, its underserved communities, or charities working for the latter? Questions also arise as to whether such compensation is in fact appropriate. In normal market transactions, when one employer lures workers from another company, usually we do not think that compensation is due absent special contractual arrangements that make that the case. And aren't remittances from individual migrant workers to their families compensation enough?

Doctors' Liberties versus Patients' Health

After this necessarily brief survey of the central ethical issues raised by physician migration, let us focus on one set of these questions. Some policies to draw health workers to work in underserved areas seem coercive. Consider several cases:

1. In Ghana, physicians are in short supply in rural areas, and temporary district hospital and rural clinic postings and training are often compulsory preconditions for obtaining medical degrees or entering residency and specialization programs (Appiah-Denkyira et al. 2012).
2. Many countries and schools expect medical graduates who received a special stipend to stay and work in underserved areas in return. The current expectation is typically that they would stay for the same number of years that they received funding, but in principle, commitment periods could last much longer (Eyal and Bärnighausen 2012).
3. Since 2008, the UK has almost completely stopped issuing work visas to doctors and nurses from countries outside the European Union, including ones with critical shortages (Travis 2008). If and when many more Western countries adopt similar policies, international employment options for health workers from countries with critical shortages would be severely curtailed.
4. Until recently, Norway determined by lottery which newly minted physicians would do their residency in which areas (Skinningsrud 2011). In spring 2011, the European Union banned this practice. Now the best students pick residency locations first, the second-best, second, and so forth. The new arrangement offers the best graduates greater autonomy and liberty; but it might saddle underserved remote populations with less well qualified physicians.

These cases highlight the potential tension between underserved populations' health needs and physicians' liberties. To what extent, if any, do physicians and other health workers have a moral duty to work for patients in underserved (home country) areas? And if this moral duty exists, is it a legitimately enforceable legal duty?

Traditional liberals devoted to both liberty and equality tend to give two responses to this question: Health workers have a moral responsibility to prioritize the underserved, but it remains morally illegitimate to force them to do so. Their moral duty, in other words, is non-enforceable.

This twin message figures in related codes of practice. The *WHO Global Code of Practice on the International Recruitment of Health Personnel* says, on the one hand, "The health of all people is fundamental to the attainment of peace and security and is dependent upon the fullest cooperation of individuals and states." But it also states, "nothing in this Code should be interpreted as limiting the freedom of health personnel, in accordance with applicable laws, to migrate to countries that wish to admit and employ them" (WHO 2010c). Similar duality is present in the American Medical Association's *Code of Medical Ethics*. One of the Code's opening principles reads, "A physician shall recognize a responsibility to participate in activities contributing to the improvement of the community and the betterment of public health . . . A physician shall support access to medical care for all people." But another principle warns, "A physician shall, in the provision of appropriate patient care, except in emergencies, be free to choose whom to serve, with whom to associate, and the environment in which to provide medical care" (American Medical Association 2012). Political theorists have shared this dual stance (Carens 1992: 33, 34; Cohen 2011: 129–30; Brock and Blake forthcoming; and others). Kieran Oberman, for example, agrees that "a skilled worker has a [moral] duty to assist her poor compatriots," but "finds that justifying immigration restrictions on brain drain grounds is far from straightforward" (Oberman 2013: 430).

Most policy proposals to decrease migration likewise consider access to health for all people very important, and recognize its dependence on individual practitioners, but remain emphatically non-compulsory. Formal limits on doctors' immigration and emigration, for example, are rejected outright on grounds of doctors' basic freedoms of movement, occupation, and education (Hannum 1987: 34–40; Physicians for Human Rights 2004; Hunt 2005, par. 46–49, 60ff.). The following statement, backed by no further argument, is typical:

> Protective strategies cannot be coercive. Slowing the pace of emigration cannot be done through prohibition of the human right to movement . . . Potential source country policies must address directly the disincentives to health personnel in the form of remuneration, working environments, and security concerns.
>
> (Alkire and Chen 2006: 112)

In the next two sections we argue a rather different position. It is far from clear that choosing not to work for the underserved is necessarily wrong for physicians. Nevertheless, when other interventions fail, compelling physicians to work for the underserved can remain perfectly legitimate.

The Moral Permissibility of Failure to Work in Underserved Areas

Do health workers, and especially physicians, have a moral duty to work in severely or critically underserved areas? Accepting offers to work in cities, in the private sector, or abroad is not illegal, but many writers believe that it is morally wrong.

Assistance?

It is clear that patients in critically underserved areas would benefit from medical assistance, often far more so than patients in well served areas. It is also clear that physicians are often best placed and best qualified to provide this assistance. On this basis physicians can be said to have general moral reasons to respond to the needs of the underserved. Moreover, many patients in critically underserved areas are disadvantaged in terms of socio-economic *and* health status; they are often far worse off than either typical physicians or well served patients. Many come from the world's poorest and sickest populations. From a utilitarian standpoint, but also from an egalitarian, prioritarian, and sufficientarian standpoint (that is, one that minds inequalities, failure to prioritize the worse off, or failure to bring everyone above some minimum threshold), physicians typically have very good reasons to dedicate their finite ability to helping them. This implicates physicians' duty of beneficence and, at least for compatriot physicians, it is also a matter of distributive and social justice (Dwyer 2007: 39).

General duties to promote basic needs, utility, and distributive justice are not usually viewed as limitless. Common sense morality grants individuals moral "prerogatives" to prioritize their own basic commitments over optimizing good (Slote 1977; Scheffler 1992). While some thinkers insist that these duties admit of no limits (Kagan 1989; Unger 1996; Ashford 2003), their position would equally suggest that intelligent non-physicians must sacrifice whatever life plans *they* might have, study medicine, and treat underserved patients whenever that would help the underserved. Indeed, because all physicians tend to have reasonable salaries, for many non-physicians, the opportunity cost of becoming a physician for the underserved is economically *smaller* than for a high-earning physician for the well served. But no existing legal or political system endorses such a suggestion. Usually we assume that the stringency of general duties of assistance or beneficence depends *inter alia* on the size of burden one would incur in meeting them—we have duties of assistance, but only if they can be discharged without being "too burdensome"—and that this remains the case even when the assistance is needed for medical reasons (Beauchamp and Childress 2009: 202, note condition 4; Akabayashi et al. 2012). This, at least, is what the political and legal *status quo* recognizes. Work in medically underserved areas will often limit physicians' life choices, comfort, professional development options, safety, and access to quality health care and education, for themselves and for their families. Such burdens would appear to preclude (*status quo* recognition of) any limitless duty to assist the underserved.

Reciprocity?

Do physicians have special duties, then, to work in underserved areas? Several authors cite reciprocity as the kernel of such special duties (Oberman 2013: 435; Brock and Blake forthcoming; de Lora and Ferracioli fortcoming). For one thing, physicians have benefited from elite education, often fully state funded, and bear a special obligation to "give back," or simply "repay" (Oberman 2013: 430), rather than "free ride" (Ypi 2008). The point here is that physicians have enjoyed benefits that the state made available through the cooperative work of their fellow citizens. Physicians who then refuse to share their efforts with them in return unfairly exploit the work of others for their unilateral advantage (Ypi 2008: 408). Former Tanzanian President Julius Nyerere dubbed such physicians "traitors" (quoted in Dumitru 2012).

In fact, a special duty of reciprocity should not be narrowly construed around financial investment in students. For one thing, "If social responsibility is merely a matter of paying off debts incurred by individuals, those receiving private training are morally off the hook to their communities" (Snyder 2009; de Lora and Ferracioli forthcoming). Physicians will also have benefited from earlier public education, from public safety that facilitates studies, from mentors' good advice, from patients who undertook risks during physicians' training, from later exclusive license to practice medicine, and so forth (Ypi 2008; Brock and Blake forthcoming; de Lora and Ferracioli forthcoming).

Put generally, medicine is a collective endeavor, which none of us could sustain on our own. Every step of it, from basic research to the development of clinical strategies, training of health professionals and delivery of care, requires not only many different people but also some form of coordination of their efforts and collective support. To become a health professional is to benefit from the assistance of many, usually on the understanding that one would thereby become able to contribute to a collective good.

This reciprocity account only works to a limited extent. One complication is that health workers will rarely be needed for the specific individuals who had benefited them—most clearly, the taxpayers who funded medical education, public safety and so forth. Health workers are needed for impoverished patient populations, and they only rarely contribute to their education. While advocates of the reciprocity account have responded that their model of reciprocity is "transitive"—because I received good mentoring from my teachers, I should be a good mentor to my *students* (de Lora and Ferracioli forthcoming)—it remains difficult to see how even transitive duties of reciprocity would call on medical graduates to work in underserved areas. When the underserved are unpopular, disenfranchised minorities, they are rarely taxpayers' or mentors' first priority, and it is hard to see how helping the underserved does anything for taxpayers or for aloof mentors. Student training may place some underserved urban patients who receive care in academic hospitals at risk, but how can that account for graduates' duties to remote rural populations?

Any duty of reciprocity must count just as much against a South African doctor moving to richer New Zealand without helping South Africans, and also against her moving to poorer Malawi without helping South Africans. Either way she fails to reciprocate for her South African training. It even counts against New Zealand doctors who leave upon graduation to volunteer in Malawi (except perhaps if their volunteering pleases Kiwi taxpayers and professors). Indeed, several sub-Saharan countries have no medical school, and on this logic of reciprocity, they might have ended up with no graduates who owe "their" patients care. All that seems absurd. For most doctors there are no significant moral reasons against moving to less-served countries—whether they be reasons of reciprocity or any other moral reasons.

Similar responses threaten attempts to ground obligations to assist the medically underserved as a matter of special duty toward compatriots. They also threaten Jeremy Snyder's relational theory of the duty of health workers to serve the underserved. For Snyder, that duty comes from encountering (coming into contact with) people in great need, which medical students do during externships in their country of study (Snyder 2009). Despite Snyder's account, however, medical students do not come into contact with more vulnerable populations elsewhere. So a Snyderian obligation would also—absurdly—count against fresh medical graduates moving from South Africa to Malawi.

A Professional Obligation?

Physicians are also thought to have special or role-based obligations to treat the sick simply because they are physicians. As for firefighters and lifeguards, becoming a health professional involves accepting a duty to provide services even at significant personal risk (Emanuel 2003). At least some health workers must show up for work during Ebola or severe acute respiratory syndrome (SARS) outbreaks and treat patients who might give them a fatal infection. Or so, at least, we shall assume here. If so, one may argue that physicians are also obligated to forego some options and remain working in the communities that need them the most, at least once it becomes clear that their colleagues will not go there. Whether or not we have the political power to force them to stay in the profession, in the country, and in such communities, we can agree that morally, they should do so.

Or so the argument goes. This rationale cannot fully ground moral duties to find jobs and remain in underserved communities. No one would say that a lifeguard has a special professional duty to find a job in an understaffed beach. As we shall put it, highly demanding *internal* professional duties (to enter tumultuous waters to rescue the drowning child once you work there, *or* to show up and work at your ward during a SARS outbreak) do not always give rise to equally demanding *external* professional duties (to seek work in an understaffed beach *or* clinic). We can therefore accept that duties to treat one's patients are very stringent while denying that the duty to make them into one's patients is remotely as stringent.

Admittedly this is not the case for all professions. Priests, for example, may have not *only* internal professional duties toward their flock (to show up at their church every Sunday), but also external professional duties (to seek a community in need of pastoral guidance, assigning little weight to compensation). Still, their external duties remain far weaker and less clear than the simple duty to be in church for their own sermon on Sunday. And it is not clear—not without an argument—that physicians are more like priests than they are like lifeguards.

We are not making the extreme and to our minds implausible claim that (assuming that professional obligations exist) physicians have unique obligations only to their own active patients. That extreme claim was recently made in defense of physicians who might have dreaded radiation and refused to serve in nuclear disaster zones following the accident in Fukushima, Japan (Akabayashi et al. 2012). In our view, physicians have special obligations not only once they meet, obtain consent, and establish an *active* doctor–patient relationship with determinate patients (call the latter obligations "super-internal" because they are even more closely linked to a clinical encounter than the obligations that above we call "internal"). In our middle-of-the-road approach, physicians may encounter special obligations to remain in workplaces and develop new therapeutic relationships at some personal sacrifice even earlier than the establishment of these active relationships. What we question are the moral obligations physicians allegedly have to seek work in such workplaces in the first instance. In the terms just introduced, we question physicians' external special obligations while recognizing both their super-internal and internal special obligations.

America's *Emergency Medical Treatment and Active Labor Act* (EMTALA) might be seen as a counter-example to this argument: As proof that health providers have external obligations to help even people who are not their patients as yet, when they lack other sources of care. EMTALA allows hospitals to reject patients in emergent conditions only after having stabilized them or transferred them elsewhere (42 U.S.C. § 1395dd 1986). However, even if health providers have a moral obligation not to abandon patients, this obligation might not apply outside strict medical emergencies and to each individual practitioner (as opposed to hospitals). Consider again the case of lifeguards. Are chronically overworked and underpaid individual lifeguards morally prohibited, absent any active emergency, from leaving their jobs when their contract ends but the replacement is not there? At least when no identified patient has an emergent need of a doctor, it is hard to argue that the doctor cannot move to another job.

Our analogy between physicians' external duties and those of lifeguards might be questioned on grounds of a difference in terms of service-seekers' personal responsibility for their need of service. When a lifeguard leaves a job and the beach is unguarded, a black flag is flying. People who later come to need a lifeguard there could have simply chosen to swim in a guarded beach instead. Patients usually have no parallel way to avoid disease. While we have reservations about applying considerations of personal responsibility to health practice (Eyal 2011), some readers may take this difference to show that physicians' external duties are somewhat stronger than those of lifeguards. Even so, it would not show that physicians' external duties are limitless.

Avoiding Harm

As discussed above, for Daniels physician migration is a case of developed nations *causing* harm, and not merely one of allowing harm to take place. He argues that international institutions like the World Bank and the International Monetary Fund have in fact forced many poor countries to trim their public sectors, drying up potential budgets for health worker positions. Given these austerity-inducing interventions, international institutions bear responsibility for the absence of health workers in these countries. As

Daniels puts it, this is an instance in which Thomas Pogge's concerns about causing harm in the international sphere hold strong (Daniels 2008).

Similarly, James Dwyer highlights the responsibility of migrants' receiving countries for ensuing medical harm in source countries:

> The problem of medical migration [arises] because the destination countries are . . . restricting immigration in a highly selective way. They seem only too willing to accept highly qualified health care workers while trying to keep out less skilled workers. It is this approach to immigration that raises issues of justice.
>
> (Dwyer 2007: 39)

If the wrongful active harm and injustice that Daniels and Dwyer stress were always the reason behind critical physician shortages, that might have made it physicians' moral duty to stay, or destination countries' duty to stop luring them over. Why? Because if harmful shortages stemmed entirely from wrongful agency by international monetary institutions, recruiting agencies, destination countries, or physicians themselves, that would cancel out any moral prerogatives on the parts of physicians or destination countries to prioritize their own plans. They would be under a moral duty to address critically unmet needs that they have caused. As Thomas Pogge writes, we have no prerogative to do harm to others, not even if the cost to us of refraining is steep (Pogge 2002).

But what Daniels and Dwyer describe are only contingent phenomena, not general characteristics of all physician shortages and migration in the world. Not all physician failure to help the critically underserved stems from wrongful active or selective agency. Some of it does not. Critical scarcity in health workers also arises in countries that have not seen devastating structural reforms. Some physicians don't need agencies' coaxing in order to want to move. Physicians' own *failure* to help the neediest patients is not an action but a failure to act in a certain way. Even if what precipitates and forces it is action on the part of the physician (moving abroad), the failure to help remains inaction.

Moreover, recall the case of one rich university luring workers from another. Free market transactions that selectively do harm are not always wrongful. They do not always encounter special prophylactic or reparatory obligations. So even if Daniels and Dwyer captured a universal characteristic of critical physician shortages, it would remain unclear that it is morally wrong for physicians to leave. The case against physicians who leave critically underserved areas rests then on something else—perhaps on the especially devastating nature of the resulting harm to vulnerable populations, as opposed to the sheer fact that harm takes place. Dwyer himself notes that the wrongness of medical migration does not depend solely on the fact that migration has taken place, but on the health status of the relevant communities:

> I am troubled by the emigration of 30 percent of Ghana's physicians because life expectancy in Ghana is about fifty-seven years. I am less troubled by medical migration out of Ireland. About 40 percent of Irish physicians have emigrated, yet in spite of this high rate, life expectancy in Ireland is about seventy-six years. Of course, the high rate of Irish medical emigration still raises questions about international fairness, postcolonial exploitation, and national policies, but the questions lack the moral salience and urgency that they have when we think about Ghana.
>
> (Dwyer 2007: 40)

Let us recapitulate our discussions of assistance, reciprocity, professional obligations, and avoiding active harm. Despite the arguments of several authors, it is *not* clear, and contemporary political, legal, and professional institutions cannot consistently assume, that it is the moral duty of all physicians, all things considered, to work for critically underserved patient populations or to compensate them, either as a matter of general duty, or as a matter of special duty.

The Moral Permissibility of Forcing Physicians to Work in Underserved Areas

Despite serious doubts about a moral duty to work in underserved areas, might forcing health workers, and especially physicians, to work in underserved areas remain legitimate, under certain conditions and in certain forms? This section defends an affirmative answer to this question, a position further developed elsewhere (Eyal and Hurst 2010).

Although restricting medical migration carries some costs for physicians—namely, being barred from working (or living) where they please—the stakes are much higher for underserved patients. As one author explained, "To be prevented from entering a foreign state is one thing; to die from an easily curable disease for lack of medical attention is quite another" (Oberman 2013: 429). Given these high stakes for patients, there are humanitarian and distributive justice reasons for compulsory measures to keep physicians working for the underserved—whether or not it is their personal moral duty to do so.

Obviously that does not settle the debate about compulsory measures, because there are also considerations pushing in the other direction, against coercion. For example, forcing health workers to work in specific underserved areas for life would surely be wrong; indeed, it would constitute outright enslavement. It would grossly violate any freedoms of movement and occupation of these workers, exposing them to exploitation and arbitrary power in their workplaces. It would defeat virtually any personal project that these health workers might have formed earlier in life, and would probably alienate them both from the health care system and their own identities, further decreasing already low workforce morale.

And yet, in other areas of life, some policies that seem compulsory at first glance can be decisively morally justified. For example, forcing doctors who harbor prejudices against patients with HIV to treat them is legitimate. Inserting fluoride into communal drinking water despite the opposition of some is legitimate. Forcing the rich to pay redistributive taxes is legitimate. Forcing medical residents to work more hours than is necessary for their professional training to help care for local patients is legitimate. The fact that a policy seems compulsory or coercive is far from a conclusive reason against it. Some seemingly coercive policies are morally justifiable, either because they are not really coercive, or because the coercion they involve is not problematic, or because overriding factors make that policy legitimate on balance (Eyal and Hurst 2010).

The level of coercion or compulsion that a policy to reduce the brain drain involves affects its overall justification. Coercing doctors to work in rural areas for one or two years post-graduation may be legitimate, even if coercing them to work there for 25 years would not be morally permissible. Issuing migrant doctors only temporary work visas (Kupfer et al. 2004) may be legitimate, even if denying them entry visas and asylum is not. To treat *any* seemingly compulsive measure as a categorically forbidden encroachment of self-ownership is highly implausible for all but the staunchest libertarians (Tesón 2008; Dumitru 2012).

These intrusions into physicians' option sets are small relative to the stakes for patients. Many medical students have acceptable alternatives to studying medicine; for example, they can study biology or engineering, which also lead to comfortable lives. Furthermore, any coercion against them typically affects social elites with relatively robust social and economic standing, whose option sets remain on balance far better than those of the patient populations who need them. What coercion *not* to take up lucrative jobs abroad forces them to give up is a privilege that is (unfairly) unavailable for their poor patients and for most other compatriots. There is no injustice to speak of when the price of substantially more universal access to basic care is blocking access to a lucrative job that is itself an unfair privilege (Eyal and Hurst 2010).

For some writers, the notions of coercion and involuntary measures conjure up images of arbitrary border officers or even work camps. But far from defending any of these draconian measures, we support fairly benign ways to encourage or even compel physicians to work for the underserved: Measures such as short compulsory service, or somewhat longer service in return for prior funding of physicians' education (Eyal and Bärnighausen 2012); deliberately *not* starting or funding "concierge" medical services and training targeted at the needs of the wealthy; focusing medical training on skills that are relevant in underserved settings and less relevant elsewhere, which can make physicians' skills less portable (Eyal and Hurst 2008).

We shall now address several potential responses to this defense of apparently compulsory measures to counteract physician shortages.

Inefficiency?

Coercion and compulsion are often counterproductive. Do physicians working under duress make for good caretakers? Physicians' many judgment calls are notoriously difficult to monitor. Making them work for the needy *or else* could increase burn-out and absenteeism that already exacerbate shortages (Dovlo 2005).

The question whether coercive or compulsive measures actually work is empirical. The answer may vary for different measures and different settings. But recent reviews of compulsory service and conditional scholarship programs are telling (Bärnighausen and Bloom 2009; Frehywot et al. 2010). Compulsory service and conditional scholarship programs, at least, are rather compulsory measures but they usually work when done properly and promote health worker availability in underserved areas.

Disrespect?

Even if coercion increases net utility, Kantians and many other thinkers may oppose it. According to legal thinker Fernando Tesón, for example, coercive measures assume that physicians are "mere resources" of the state, and that assumption "fails to treat persons as autonomous agents." Most fundamentally, "For the state to decide what I am supposed to do with my talents is to debase my humanity" (Tesón 2008: 906, 917; see also Dumitru 2012: 14–15).

Tesón probably assumes that, no matter how worthy the cause, to promote it through coercion is to treat people wrongfully as mere resources (at least when it is not their independent duty to do so). Coercion violates at least Lockean self-ownership, which Tesón, following Robert Nozick, associates with Kantian rights (Tesón 2008: 908–11).

Tesón's Nozickian libertarianism is, however, a minority position. Not only has it been philosophically refuted (Cohen 1979, 1995; Murphy and Nagel 2002), but states use coercion all the time, and most people rightly think nothing of it. The examples of distributive taxation and medical residency remain telling. Generous welfare states legitimately coerce the rich to pay more in redistributive tax than it would have been their moral duty to donate to the poor, absent a generous welfare state, and most people think that is highly justified. Medical residency programs put pressure on physicians to use their bodies and minds to perform actions that help others, and they remain legitimate (even libertarians do not object to them), so long as the actions expected and the coercive means being used remain limited. The same could be true of measures to address critical health worker shortages.

Violation of Basic Rights?

How can these measures be defended in the face of fundamental rights to free association and free movement that some coercive or compulsive measures might violate (Dumitru 2012)?

These rights, while fundamental, are not absolute. Lucas Stanczyk explains that liberal rights such as the right to free movement, employment, or association cannot be seen as fundamental constraints that apply in every environment, regardless of any devastating impact on social welfare and on proper positive rights to healthcare. Instead, we should view all rights as derivative from society's proper goals. And on that view, any rights to emigrate or to work in an area of one's choosing are likely to give way when what is at stake is the fundamental health interests of some of the world's worst-off populations—a very important social goal (Stanczyk 2012). In Dwyer's succinct summary,

> the right to emigrate is . . . certainly an important right. Still, like all rights, it needs to be specified, qualified, and balanced against other rights and concerns . . . The right to emigrate should be qualified by and balanced against the social responsibility of health care professionals.
>
> (Dwyer 2007: 38)

Does our approach lead to extreme violation of the person's moral agency? Some theories ascribe to people rights to conscientious objection to perfectly legitimate social goals, when complicity in promoting these goals would violate deep personal commitments, misguided though these commitments may be. Nevertheless, several years of communal work rarely violates anyone's deep moral commitments (Fabre 2006: ch. 3), especially not those of physicians, whose prevailing ethos valorizes helping the needy (Eyal and Hurst 2010). Further, a physician's claim to conscientious objection would be questionable when she cannot be easily replaced (Brock 2008). Part of the reason why is that physicians had the liberty to pick another profession in the first instance (Eyal and Gosseries 2013).

Inequality?

Carens' rationale for the freedom of movement is not only that such freedom is good in itself, but also that it is "essential for equality of opportunity," and that it "contributes to reduction of political, social, and economic inequalities" (Carens 1992: 26; see also Dumitru 2012).

However, surely physician shortages pose a major threat to global equality—in health resources and in every real opportunity that depends on living and remaining healthy and independent. Fully free movement for health workers maximizes protection of opportunities for them, but it comes at a major cost to the protection of opportunities for patient populations with far fewer opportunities. Restrictions of that movement would then seem typically to increase equality of opportunity (Caney 2012). And limited restrictions upon free movement would seem easy to justify.

Even Carens admits that "restrictions may sometimes be justified because they promote liberty and equality in the long run" (Carens 1992: 25). When it comes to restrictions of medical migration from certain settings and against certain background conditions, promoting long-term liberty and equality might be the rule, not the exception.

Hypocrisy?

Oberman reasons that sometimes physicians might have a duty to stay and assist their poor compatriots, but this is not a duty that the rich state "has the legitimacy to enforce." Such cases arise because the hypocrisy involved is particularly strong—for example, when "skilled workers only have a secondary duty to stay and assist their poor compatriots because a rich state has failed in its own primary duties towards people in that country." Here, Oberman holds, "in the absence of reparative steps, rich states do not have the legitimacy to enforce counter-brain-drain immigration restrictions." Non-enforcement may lead to worse consequences but, he answers, "why should we think that it is the consequences alone which matter?" (Oberman 2013: 450–1).

On Oberman's implicit approach to hypocrisy, it may follow that just because an agent has wronged someone, that agent must, to avoid hypocrisy, continue to wrong her. That can't be true. It may also follow on his implicit approach that when an agent's only way to right a wrong to a population would involve placing pressure on a third party to treat them right—in our case, placing pressure on physicians to work with underserved compatriots—the agent mustn't do so. And she mustn't do so even if placing that pressure would have otherwise been perfectly legitimate. Oberman, recall, agrees that treating the underserved could be an *otherwise* enforceable duty of these physicians.

It is especially remarkable that Oberman presses his point regardless of consequences, catastrophic as they might be—in absolutist fashion. Whatever stance one may take on the moral import of hypocrisy, absolutism seems implausible. Reassuringly, on the practical matter of barriers to health worker migration, Oberman concedes that "Perhaps in most ordinary cases rich states will retain the right to enforce restrictions despite their own failures" (Oberman 2013: 450).

Carens also warns about what he calls "hypocrisy." We would surely oppose barriers to workers' movement as ways to reduce intra-country regional inequalities. We would insist that workers have a basic freedom of movement. Therefore, we should not stop workers from moving across national borders simply in order to reduce international inequalities. Their freedom of movement is no less basic in the international context (Carens 1992: 27–8, 33).

Carens' warning about hypocrisy is unwarranted. The regional inequalities inside (developed) countries that fuel his argument rarely create critical worker shortages. Health worker shortages in sub-Saharan Africa and South Asia are critical. It is true that existing border controls provide the opportunity to implement these legitimate restrictions and protect public health. But is it evil to use arrangements (bound to remain in place in the foreseeable future) to address the critical health needs of some of the world's most vulnerable populations?

Leah Ypi, who is friendly to some migration restrictions, decries what she nevertheless sees as inconsistency. For her, "if R provides a valid reason for restricting incoming freedom of movement, R also provides a valid reason for restricting outgoing freedom of movement." She complains that those who worry about the public health consequences of medical brain drain typically approve of limitations on immigration while opposing limitations on emigration (Ypi 2008: 391, 402–5).

But there is at least one big difference between typical restrictions of immigration and restrictions against emigration. That difference may make the former more palatable in the fight against critical health worker shortages. When physicians are completely denied entry to a given developed country, or even to all *developed* countries, they retain their ability to flee persecution in a hostile home country. That is not so when physicians are completely denied exit rights from their home country. As we have already mentioned, to say that some coercive or compulsive-looking measures (in this case, denial of entry rights) are permissible vehicles of health promotion, is not to prejudge any and all such measures.

In conclusion, then, despite continuing doubt about a moral duty to work in critically underserved areas, some policies that compel physicians to work in such areas could be legitimate and morally justifiable. Leaders and policy-makers should not rule out seemingly coercive responses to critical physician shortages in underserved areas. They could complement existing policies in the fight to provide access to basic care for all people.

Acknowledgments

The authors would like to thank John Arras, Elizabeth Fenton, Luara Ferracioli, and Pablo de Lora for their comments, and Dan Wikler for comments on earlier related work. We are also grateful to students at the Harvard Program in Health Policy and Harvard's Petrie-Flom Center, who attended a related presentation. This work was funded by the Harvard Medical School, the Institute for Biomedical Ethics at the Geneva University Medical School, and the Swiss National Science Foundation (grant PP00P3_123340).

Related Topics

Chapter 8, "Medical Tourism," I. Glenn Cohen
Chapter 30, "Reproductive Travel and Tourism," G.K.D. Crozier

References

Akabayashi, A., Takimoto, Y. and Hayashi, Y. (2012) "Physician Obligation to Provide Care During Disasters: Should Physicians Have Been Required to Go to Fukushima?" *Journal of Medical Ethics* 38 (11): 697–8.

Alkire, S. and Chen, L. (2006) "'Medical Exceptionalism' in International Migration: Should Doctors and Nurses be Treated Differently?" in J. Palme and K. Tamas (eds.) *Globalizing Migration Regimes: New Challenges to Transnational Cooperation*, Farnham: Ashgate, pp. 100–18.

Aluwihare, A.P. (2005) "Physician Migration: Donor Country Impact," *Journal of Continuing Education in the Health Professions* 25 (1): 15–21.

American Medical Association (2012) "AMA's Code of Medical Ethics." Available at: http://www.ama-assn.org/ama/pub/physician-resources/medical-ethics/code-medical-ethics.page? (accessed December 25, 2012).

Ana, J.N. (2005) "Africa's Medical Brain Drain: Brain Gain and Brain Circulation Result When Drain Is Reversed," *British Medical Journal* 331 (7519): 780; discussion 780–1.

Appiah-Denkyira, E. et al. (2012) *Annual Report, Human Resources for Health Development*, Accra: Ghana Ministry of Health.

Ashford, E. (2003) "The Demandingness of Scanlon's Contractualism," *Ethics* 113 (2): 273–302.

Bärnighausen, T. and Bloom, D.E. (2009) "Financial Incentives for Return of Service in Underserved Areas: A Systematic Review," *BMC Health Services Research* 9 (1): 86.

Beauchamp, T.L. and Childress, J.F. (2009) *Principles of Biomedical Ethics*, Oxford: Oxford University Press.

Bhagwati, J. (2012) "The Brain-Drain Panic Returns," Project Syndicate. Available at: http://www.project-syndicate.org/commentary/the-brain-drain-panic-returns (accessed July 5, 2014).

Bhagwati, J. and Dellalfar, W. (1973) "The Brain Drain and Income Taxation," *World Development* 1 (1–2): 94–101.

Brock, D.W. (2008) "Conscientious Refusal by Physicians and Pharmacists: Who Is Obligated to Do What, and Why?" *Theoretical Medicine and Bioethics* 29: 187–200.

Brock, G. (2009) *Global Justice: A Cosmopolitan Account*, New York: Oxford University Press.

Brock, G. and Blake, M. (eds.) (forthcoming 2015) *Debating Brain Drain*, New York: Oxford University Press.

Caney, S. (2012) "When, If Ever, May Destination States Limit Migration: Minimizing Injustice in a Radically Non-ideal World," *Brocher Summer Academy in Population-Level Bioethics: Distributing Human Resources for Health—Ethics and Health Policy*, Hermance, Switzerland.

Carens, J. (1992) "Migration and Morality: A Liberal Egalitarian Perspective," in B. Barry and R. E. Goodin (eds.) *Free Movement: Ethical Issues in the Transnational Migration of People and of Money*, University Park, PA: Pennsylvania State University Press, pp. 25–47.

Chu, K., Rosseel, P., Gielis, P. and Ford, N. (2009) "Surgical Task Shifting in Sub-Saharan Africa," *PLoS Med* 6 (5): e1000078.

Clemens, M.A. (2007) "Do Visas Kill? Health Effects of African Health Professional Emigration," Working Paper no. 114, Washington DC: Center for Global Development.

Clemens, M.A. (2011) "Economics and Emigration: Trillion-Dollar Bills on the Sidewalk?" *Journal of Economic Perspectives* 25 (3): 83–106.

Cohen, G.A. (1979) "Capitalism, Freedom and the Proletariat," in A. Ryan (ed.) *The Idea of Freedom Essays in Honour of Isaiah Berlin*, Oxford: Oxford University Press, pp. 7–25.

Cohen, G.A. (1992) "Incentives, Inequality, and Community," in G. Peterson (ed.) *The Tanner Lectures on Human Values, Volume 13*, Salt Lake City: Utah University Press, pp. 262–329.

Cohen, G.A. (1995) *Self-Ownership, Freedom, and Equality*, Cambridge: Cambridge University Press.

Cohen, G.A. (2011) "Fairness and Legitimacy in Justice, and: Does Option Luck Ever Preserve Justice?" in G.A. Cohen and M. Otsuka (eds.) *On the Currency of Egalitarian Justice, and Other Essays in Political Philosophy*, Princeton, NJ: Princeton University Press, pp. 127–43.

Daniels, N. (2008) *Just Health: Meeting Health Needs Fairly*, Cambridge: Cambridge University Press.

de Lora, P. and Ferracioli, L. (forthcoming) "Primum Nocere: Medical Brain Drain and the Duty to Remain," *Journal of Medicine and Philosophy*.

Dimaya, R.M., McEwen, M.K., Curry, L.A. and Bradley, E.H. (2012) "Managing Health Worker Migration: A Qualitative Study of the Philippine Response to Nurse Brain Drain," *Human Resources for Health* 10 (1): 47.

Dovlo, D. (2005) "Wastage in the Health Workforce: Some Perspectives from African Countries," *Human Resources for Health* 3: 6.

Dugger, C.W. (2004) Lacking Doctors, Africa is Training Substitutes, *New York Times*, November 23.

Dumitru, S. (2012) "Skilled Migration: Who Should Pay for What? A Critique of the Bhagwati Tax," *Diversities* 14 (1): 9–23.

Dwyer, J. (2007) "What's Wrong with the Global Migration of Health Care Professionals? Individual Rights and International Justice," *Hastings Center Report* 37 (5): 36–43.

Emanuel, E.J. (2003) "The Lessons of SARS," *Annals of Internal Medicine* 139 (7): 589–91.

Eyal, N. (2011) "Why Treat Noncompliant Patients? Beyond the Decent Minimum Account," *Journal of Medicine and Philosophy* 36 (6): 572–88.

Eyal, N. and Bärnighausen, T. (2012) "Precommitting to Serve the Underserved," *American Journal of Bioethics* 12 (5): 23–34.

Eyal, N. and Gosseries, A. (2013) "Obamacare and Conscientious Objection: Some Introductory Thoughts," *Ethical Perspectives* 20 (1): 109–17.

Eyal, N. and Hurst, S.A. (2008) "Physician Brain Drain: Can Nothing be Done?" *Public Health Ethics* 1 (2): 180–92.

Eyal, N. and Hurst, S.A. (2010) Coercion in the Fight Against Medical Brain Drain, in R. Shah (ed.) *Global Health, Justice and the Brain Drain*, New York: Palgrave Macmillan, pp. 137–58.

Eyal, N. and Hurst, S.A. (2011) "Scaling Up Changes in Doctors' Education for Rural Retention: A Comment on World Health Organization Recommendations," *Bulletin of the World Health Organization* 89 (2): 83.

Fabre, C. (2006) *Whose Body Is It Anyway? Justice and the Integrity of the Person*, Oxford and New York: Oxford University Press.

Frehywot, S., Mullan, F., Payne, P.W. and Ross, H. (2010) "Compulsory Service Programmes for Recruiting Health Workers in Remote and Rural Areas: Do They Work?" *Bulletin of the World Health Organization* 88 (5): 364–70.

Hannum, H. (1987) *The Right to Leave and Return in International Law and Practice*, Dordrecht: Martinus Nijhoff.

Hirschhorn, L.R., Oguda, L., Fullem, A., Dreesch, N. and Wilson, P. (2006) "Estimating Health Workforce Needs for Antiretroviral Therapy in Resource-Limited Settings," *Human Resources for Health* 4: 1.

Hunt, P. (2005) *The Right of Everyone to the Enjoyment of the Highest Attainable Standard of Physical and Mental Health*, Commission on Human Rights.

Kagan, S. (1989) *The Limits of Morality*, Oxford: Clarendon Press.

Kangasniemi, M., Winters, L.A. and Commander, S. (2007) "Is the Medical Brain Drain Beneficial? Evidence from Overseas Doctors in the UK," *Social Science & Medicine* 65 (5): 915–23.

Kupfer, L., Hofman, K., Jarawan, R., McDermott, J. and Bridbord, K. (2004) "Roundtable: Strategies to Discourage Brain Drain," *Bulletin of the World Health Organization* 82 (8): 616–19.

Mars, M. (2010) "Health Capacity Development Through Telemedicine in Africa," *Yearbook of Medical Informatics* 87–93.

Martineau, T., Decker, K. and Bundred, P. (2004) "'Brain Drain' of Health Professionals: From Rhetoric to Responsible Action," *Health Policy* 70 (1): 1–10.

Mullan, F. (2005) "The Metrics of the Physician Brain Drain," *New England Journal of Medicine* 353 (17): 1810–18.

Murphy, L.B. and Nagel, T. (2002) *The Myth of Ownership: Taxes and Justice*, Oxford and New York: Oxford University Press.

Oberman, K. (2013) "Can Brain Drain Justify Immigration Restrictions?" *Ethics* 123 (3): 427–55.

Physicians for Human Rights (2004) "An Action Plan to Prevent Brain Drain: Building Equitable Health Systems in Africa," New York.

Pogge, T. (2002) *Global Justice*, Oxford: Wiley-Blackwell.

Scheffler, S. (1992) "Prerogatives Without Restrictions," *Philosophical Perspectives* 6: 377–97.

Schwartz, M.D. (2012) "The US Primary Care Workforce and Graduate Medical Education Policy," *JAMA* 308 (21): 2252–3.

Skinningsrud, K. (2011) "Norway's Plan to Change Placement Scheme for Trainee Doctors Proves Controversial," *British Medical Journal* 342.

Slote, M. (1977) "The Morality of Wealth," in W. Aiken and H. LaFollette (eds.) *World Hunger and Moral Obligation*, Englewood Cliffs, NJ: Prentice-Hall, pp. 124–47.

Snyder, J. (2009) "Is Health Worker Migration a Case of Poaching?" *American Journal of Bioethics* 9 (3): 3–7.

Stanczyk, L. (2012) "Productive Justice," *Philosophy and Public Affairs* 40 (2): 144–64.

Tesón, F.R. (2008) "Brain Drain," *San Diego Law Review* 45 (4): 899–932.

Travis, A. (2008) "200,000 Jobs Barred to Non-European Migrants," *The Guardian*, November 11.

Unger, P.K. (1996) *Living High and Letting Die: Our Illusion of Innocence*, New York: Oxford University Press.

Wellman, C.H. (2010) "Immigration," in E.N. Zalta (ed.) *Stanford Encyclopedia of Philosophy*, Stanford, CA.

WHO (2006) *The World Health Report 2006: Working Together for Health*, Geneva: WHO.

WHO (2008) *Treat Train Retain. Task Shifting: Global Recommendations and Guidelines*, Geneva: World Health Organization.

WHO (2010a) *Increasing Access to Health Workers in Remote and Rural Areas Through Improved Retention*, Global Policy Recommendations, Geneva, WHO.

WHO (2010b) *mhGAP Intervention Guide. For Mental, Neurological, and Substance Use Disorders in Non-specialized Health Settings*, Geneva: WHO.

WHO (2010c) *WHO Global Code of Practice on the International Recruitment of Health Personnel. WHA*. 63.16, Geneva: WHO.

WHO (2012a) "Global Health Observatory Data Repository—Aggregated Data: Density per 1000." Available at: http://apps.who.int/ghodata/?vid=92000 (accessed November 26, 2012).

WHO (2012b) *WHO Recommendations for Optimizing Health Worker Roles to Improve Access to Key Maternal and Newborn Health Interventions Through Task Shifting*, Geneva: WHO.
Ypi, L. (2008) "Justice in Migration: A Closed Borders Utopia?" *Journal of Political Philosophy* 16 (4): 391–418.
Zimmerman, M., Shakya, R., Pokhrel, B.M., Eyal, N., Rijal, B.P., Shrestha, R.N. and Sayami, A. (2012) "Medical Students' Characteristics as Predictors of Career Practice Location: Retrospective Cohort Study Tracking Graduates of Nepal's First Medical College," *British Medical Journal* 345: e4826.

10

MORAL RESPONSIBILITY FOR ADDRESSING CLIMATE CHANGE

Madison Powers

The United Nations Framework Convention on Climate Change (UNFCCC 1992) grew out of the 1992 United Nations Conference on Environment and Development in Rio. The agreement (hereafter, the Convention) became the internationally recognized basis for creating legally binding treaty obligations that were to be developed in subsequent rounds of negotiations, thus far unsuccessful. However, the Convention is more than a legal document of interest only to international lawyers and diplomats. It is an explicitly moral framework designed as a guide for assignment of responsibility for addressing global warming under a comprehensive treaty agreement that would bind an overwhelming majority of the world's nations. Two of the Convention's key elements have provoked the most discussion and they are the focus of this chapter.

Two Persistent Issues

The first element is the ultimate objective of a comprehensive treaty and it is described in Article 2 of the Convention as the "stabilization of greenhouse gas concentrations in the atmosphere at a level that would *prevent dangerous anthropogenic interference with the climate system*." Left open in this statement of objective are the appropriate scientific benchmarks by which dangerous climate change should be judged. Subsequent negotiations among parties to the Convention led to the adoption of a target of 2°C above pre-industrialization levels. The Intergovernmental Panel on Climate Change (IPCC) estimates that the 2° target corresponds to an atmospheric concentration of greenhouse gases (GHGs) at roughly 450 parts per million (ppm) (Solomon et al. 2007; Parry et al. 2007). While other influential bodies, including the World Bank (WDR 2010) also endorse the 2° target, many leading scientists set the threshold much lower at 1.5°C, or roughly 350 ppm, because of the irreparable damage a 2° increase will cause to the most vulnerable regions of the world (Hansen 2008).

There is a broad scientific consensus, however, that what makes climate change "dangerous" is a constellation of effects on human health and wellbeing, other species, and the capacity of the planet to sustain life. The list of adverse impacts of even a 2° increase is lengthy, widely documented, and highly consequential (Solomon et al.

2007; Parry et al. 2007; WDR 2010; UNDP 2008; Samson et al. 2011). They include species extinction and decline of plant and animal populations; sea-level rise threatening island nations and low-lying coastal areas; increased frequency and intensity of extreme weather events; excess rain and cold weather during growing seasons, leading to crop loss, flooding, and freshwater runoff; decreases in annual rainfall, resulting in drought, desertification, and disruption of the hydrologic cycle processes; and expansion of the geographic zones at high risk for infectious diseases.

Moreover, the consequences of a failure to mitigate the production of GHGs are dramatically portrayed in estimates of the differential impact of climate change at the 350 ppm level and above on poorer, less developed nations, especially in the global South, the less developed regions of Asia, and island nations (Parry et al. 2007; WDR 2010; UNDP 2008). The effects are already being felt by, and will be greatest for, the nations that are the poorest, hottest, agriculturally most vulnerable to weather pattern disruption, economically most dependent on agriculture, most vulnerable to vector borne diseases that are expected to increase dramatically, and least able to adapt by virtue of both disadvantaging geography and fewer economic resources.

The second key element of the Convention consists of twin assumptions regarding the distribution of responsibility. Article 3.1 of the Convention endorses a principle of "*common but differentiated responsibilities*." While the UNFCCC concept is highly abstract, its major premise is that the locus of moral responsibility rests with nation-states, rather than with individual persons or corporate entities. In addition, Article 3.2 states that the primary treaty objective should be promoted within the limits set by other goals, such as food production, the need for time for adjustment of national economies, and especially, the energy needs of developing nations for the alleviation of poverty.

Critics of the Convention argue that the focus on development of a treaty among nation-states misses the mark morally, for it fails to pin the primary moral responsibility for addressing climate change on the specific persons and firms who bear the greatest and most direct causal responsibility for creating the problem (Baer et al. 2010: 219; Gardiner 2011: 48). While disagreements over the appropriate target influence debates over assignment of moral responsibility, the full significance of the choice of target comes into view only after surveying the moral responsibility debates. The issue of whether the appropriate locus of moral responsibility is the nation-state is therefore examined first.

The Shape of the Moral Responsibility Problem

Two of the main types of climate-related moral responsibilities (Shue 2010a) should be distinguished at the outset. The first type of duty involves *mitigation* efforts designed to slow and eventually halt and reverse the accumulation of GHGs. Mitigation duties include the reduction of GHG emissions, providing economic and technological resources necessary for others (e.g., poor nations) to reduce emissions, and preserving "carbon sinks" (e.g., rainforests) that absorb GHGs that otherwise would accumulate in the atmosphere. The second type of responsibility involves duties of *adaptation*, for example, modifying human behavior or the environment in order to avoid the harmful consequences produced by climate change. The focus of this chapter is on duties of mitigation because the appropriate assignment of adaptation duties depends, in part, on what steps are taken, and by whom, to avoid climate-induced harms through mitigation efforts (Jamieson 2010b).

Questions regarding the proper assignment of mitigation duties are complicated by the fact that global climate change is a problem with a peculiar, though perhaps not unique moral shape. The Earth's atmosphere has a finite, rapidly approaching limit on its capacity to store GHGs without producing dangerous climate change. Global warming and its harmful effects are caused by the total stock of emissions produced and accumulated in the atmosphere from the dawn of the industrial revolution down through the present. The harm produced by climate change therefore is due to the fact that over hundreds of years millions of individuals, firms, and governments will have made small causal contributions by generating and using electricity, building cities, driving cars, cutting trees, and so on (Jamieson 2010a; Sinnott-Armstrong 2010). It is only when the total stock of atmospheric emissions from all sources, produced across many generations, reaches some critical threshold that the harms result. Hence, the critical nature of settling on the appropriate target for the maximum atmospheric emissions concentration.

The problem of climate change represents a challenge to traditional conceptions of moral responsibility found in ordinary moral thought, leading moral theories, and the moral foundations of environmental tort law. Two examples illustrate the source of the primary difficulties in assigning moral responsibility.

First, our inherited conception of individual moral responsibility "presupposes that harms and their causes are individual, that they can be readily identified, and that they are local in time and space" (Jamieson 2010a: 83). Responsibility for remedying or compensating for oil pipeline spills and industrial pollution of rivers and streams are familiar examples. Climate change does not conform to this standard pattern. With global warming, the causally responsible parties act separately and without coordination over extended periods of time, across great geographic distances, resulting in the joint production of a still unfolding set of harms. Climate change is thus a problem that is inherently different from and more complex than the familiar environmental problems in which the assignment of moral responsibility proceeds from individually identifiable and morally accountable agents.

Second, climate change poses a challenge to conceptions of moral responsibility presupposed in some prominent political theories. Consider the twin assumptions in Article 3 of the Convention. If the world collectively should act to reduce cumulative emissions from all sources, *and* the claims of developing nations for continuing emissions necessary to meet their pressing needs for poverty alleviation merit some priority, then absent a technological "magic bullet," the highest per capita emitters, concentrated in the developed nations, must decrease their emissions, even as emissions from less developed nations continue to rise (Shue 2011: 306). The fact that the entire world shares a common, but declining pool of available future emissions necessary to prevent the triggering of dangerous climate change means that the fates of nations are bound together in ways some leading theories of justice deny. Such theories assume that the fortunes of nations are largely a function of autonomous domestic policy choices, and that the primary determinants of wellbeing are tied to local factors under state control (Rawls 2001). Duties of distributive justice are then said to be largely domestic in scope because the primary causes of distributive inequalities are domestic, and global principles of distributive justice are not needed. Climate change shows that it is no longer plausible to think of the fates of nations, and of the global poor in particular, as substantially independent from external forces that exert profound and pervasive impact on a country's citizens in ways largely beyond domestic control.

I first discuss principles that link the moral responsibility of persons and firms to their individual causal contributions and I then examine some further issues arising from the assignment of primary moral responsibility for climate change to nation-states rather than to such individuals.

Holding Individual Polluters Responsible

The main alternative to the Convention's assignment of moral responsibility to nation-states is the Polluter Pays Principle (PPP). The potential sources of PPP's attraction are various, but in each instance, there are powerful objections to the use of the principle in the context of global warming that limit its plausible scope of application.

One of the main attractions of the PPP is the fact that it figures centrally in environmental ethics and is prominent in the normative foundations of environmental tort law. It is appealing for a simple reason. It answers to the intuitive idea that all and only the causal contributors to some problem should have duties to prevent future harm, mitigate ongoing harm, or remedy or compensate for the harms created by their actions (Adler 2007; Perry 1992; Caney 2010a).

PPP is attractive for a second reason. Its application does not depend upon, or serve the ends of, any particular theory of distributive justice (Shue 2010a: 209–10; 2010b: 103; Miller 2008: 126). The PPP is a principle of corrective justice, which means that its sole purpose is to restore the injured party to his or her status prior to some injurious action, or if restoration is not possible, to compensate for irreparable injury. If climate change makes already badly off nations or peoples even more badly off, then there is a duty to restore them to their status quo position, but nothing more is required. PPP therefore does not alter the existing distribution of advantages, for example, in the way that the Convention contemplates in its proposal for giving priority in the allocation of future emissions to developing nations for poverty alleviation (Shue 2010a: 207).

A third source of PPP's enduring appeal in the climate change context is that it might seem like a useful way to pin the primary burdens of responsibility on citizens and businesses located in the nations that have gained so much in their standard of living from their historically higher use of GHG-producing fossil fuels.

However, there are numerous difficulties in applying PPP to climate change. One major problem is that the apportionment of causal responsibility among so many causal contributors, over an extended and continuing time frame, is so indefinite and speculative that it is neither feasible nor fair (Caney 2010c: 207; Posner and Sunstein 2008: 18). In particular, the worry is that the complete identification of wrongdoers is thwarted by the fact that some individuals are no longer living and some corporate entities are no longer doing business (Posner and Sunstein 2008: 18; Caney 2010a: 130; Miller 2008: 126–7). PPP then would seem both unfair and unworkable because it can hold accountable only a small fraction of the causal contributors to global warming, and even then, issues of fair apportionment of responsibility exceed the epistemic capacities of human judgment.

Moreover, if the aim of proponents of PPP is to penalize the rich or get the big emitters of the past to make amends for their large historical role thus far in causing global warming, there are numerous problems with that approach (Miller 2008: 126; Caney 2010c: 205, 212). While the biggest historical contributors to the accumulated stock of emissions thus far are based in the rich industrial nations, the composition of the biggest historical emitters will change as the threshold of dangerous climate change is approached. Because the bulk of accumulated emissions have been generated since the mid-twentieth century, it provides an important benchmark for comparison. One widely respected projection estimates that by 2050 the percentage of total emissions since 1970 attributable to the thirty economically most developed nations will be surpassed by the cumulative emissions generated during that period from within the BRIC nations—Brazil, Russia, India, and China—and the share attributable to the rest of the world is projected to lag only slightly behind the combined total for the thirty most developed nations (OECD 2008). Whatever the precise proportions turn out to be in 2050, the clear trend is one in which the historical emissions attributable to developing or less developed nations is catching up to the historical emissions attributable to developed nations. Application of PPP will result in greatly declining responsibility being assigned to developed nations because the logic of PPP is such that moral responsibility follows strictly the path of proportionate causal responsibility. It is indifferent to how much any of the causally responsible parties benefited and whether anyone who benefited did so at the expense of others.

Perhaps the main objection against PPP is a lack of a plausible theory of morally culpable action by the emitters of the distant past for which they should be held accountable. Even if we can identify with sufficient precision the main contributors and find a feasible way to hold them or their successors accountable, it is unclear what makes their actions morally wrong. Arguably very few causal contributors at any stage of history are culpable due to malign intent or because their actions were inherently unjust in the way slavery can be said to be wrong in itself (Sinnott-Armstrong 2010; Miller 2008: 129). Even the weaker notion of negligence in tort law, from which we might construct a moral analogue, is problematic. As a condition for imposing liability it requires a showing of harm from some conduct that was in violation of existing norms of due care, for which the parties being held responsible either knew or should have known they were violating (Posner and Sunstein 2008: 18–19). The problem is that, until quite recently, there was no reliable scientific information upon which such norms could have been based, and hence, no reasonable basis for second-guessing conduct of the sort that many once assumed to be either morally benign or even socially valuable (Caney 2010a: 130–1; Caney 2010c: 207–10).

Some defenders of PPP argue "that the objection of ignorance runs together punishment for an action and being held responsible for an action" (Shue 2010b: 104). Shue agrees that it would be unfair to punish someone for actions they could not have known were harmful to others, but not unfair to make them pay the costs of problems they caused. Some arguments of this sort rest on a moral analogue to legal doctrines of strict liability (Neumayer 2000: 188; Baer 2010: 250–1; Shue 2010c). Under theories of strict liability, those individuals causally responsible for harms of some types should be made to bear the associated costs without regard for their intentions or what they knew or should have known at the time.

Even if a moral analogue of legal doctrines of strict liability offers a plausible account of moral culpability for actions in the distant past, the weight of other objections to the application of PPP to climate change is significant. Problems of identity, apportioning causal responsibility, and the fact that the creation of harm is ongoing undermine its plausibility. Moreover, PPP is a conservative moral principle, at least from the perspective of those who have reservations about the current global distribution of advantages and disadvantages, and by itself it offers no prospective guide to deciding how to allocate emissions. Most of the large emitters from the past are off the hook because they are no longer available, and their proportional share of causal contribution to dangerous climate change is in steep decline. Under PPP, a greater share of the moral responsibility will fall on individual polluters from within developing nations that neither accrued massive developmental benefits nor have the resources to pay their share for mitigation without eroding recent gains in poverty reduction.

However intuitively attractive it might seem to hold all and only those individuals morally responsible for their individual causal contributions, assignment of moral responsibility for climate change to individuals through the application of PPP is unfair and unfeasible.

Holding Nation-States Responsible

A variety of justifications have been proposed for assigning primary moral responsibility for climate change to nation-states, rather than to individuals. However, critics argue that nation-states are not the right kind of entities for assignment of moral responsibility. This section surveys several lines of argument for holding nation-states responsible for addressing climate change and the main objections. The conclusion is that nation-states are plausible entities for assignment of moral responsibility, but only with some caveats, and not for the reasons most often cited.

One line of argument appears to be designed to rescue at least a part of the underlying rationale of PPP by treating the industrialized nation-states that have been home to the largest carbon emitters as proxies for the diverse and unidentifiable polluters that have been causally responsible for the harm of climate change and by treating current generations as their appropriate successors. The argument rests on the claim that the citizens of developed countries are the contemporary beneficiaries of past carbon-intensive activities that have been harmful. This principle has been called the Beneficiary Pays Principle (BPP) (Caney 2010a: 128). The essence of the argument is that the high standard of living of the developed nations has been made possible only through their ancestors' contribution to GHG accumulation to date and that these nations should be held responsible because of the benefits derived from the harmful side effects of earlier emissions (Shue 2010b: 105; Neumayer 2000: 189). In effect, this construal of BPP attempts to circumvent the main difficulties of PPP while retaining many of its intuitively attractive aspects as a principle of compensatory justice.

The first objection is that, even if current citizens of developed nations are the continuing beneficiaries of prior generations of GHG emitters, the lack of clearly articulated grounds for assigning moral culpability to those earlier emitters under PPP reappears as a problem for BPP. If the rationale for BPP is that their predecessors caused the harm from which current generations benefited, then compensation to those who have been harmed is due from those who benefited only if the actions of their predecessors can be shown to be morally culpable (Miller 2008: 129). Under BPP, if intended as a principle of compensatory justice, the current beneficiaries may be held responsible only for what amounts to ill-gotten gains. Absent a theory of moral culpability of past emitters heavily clustered in developed nations, current citizens are merely the beneficiaries of an undeserved windfall, not ill-gotten gains for which their moral claim is nullified.

Alternatively, BPP might be construed as a general principle of distributive justice, for example, on the theory that it is just, all things considered, to place the burden of responsibility on parties who benefited from some windfall and thereby are better able to bear the burdens. Similarly, it has been argued that nations that are prepared to accept the benefits of past actions should be prepared to accept the burdens as well (Neumayer 2000: 189). Indeed, human rights arguments discussed later in the chapter reach that very same conclusion. But proponents of BPP muddy the waters insofar as they tend to tout its merits as a principle that satisfies a demand for compensation for past harms, rather than a principle grounded in a general theory of distributive justice, or theory regarding the fair distribution of benefits and burdens.

Even if the moral culpability objection can be met, such that BPP *should be applied* even if the beneficiaries gain from activities of predecessors who could not have known the harmful effects of their actions, the BPP is vulnerable to a further objection. The further complaint is against the speculative character of the counterfactual arguments that are necessary to back up the crucial empirical assumption that developed nations actually benefit in the way that the principle requires and that their actions resulted in a net harm to others.

Some observers might conclude that the continuing benefit from prior emissions is patently obvious, as is the net harm, but counterfactual claims regarding benefit or harm that accrues *but for* some activity are more complex than often supposed. The simplest examples of counterfactual arguments are found in environmental tort cases. In order to establish that agricultural waste runoff from factory farms is responsible for degradation of a water well, the plaintiff's burden is to show that "but for" the negligent actions of some specific polluter there would not be dangerous toxic substances present in the drinking water. Such cases are often factually difficult to sort out, especially where the polluters are numerous, the actions are spread across a long time horizon, and other causally contributing factors may be at work. However, the difficulties in establishing "but for" arguments in ordinary water pollution cases are not nearly as great as counterfactual arguments involving sweeping historical claims (Posner and Sunstein 2008: 18–20).

An example of a grand historical counterfactual is the argument that but for the 500-year legacy of colonialism and slavery, developed nations would not enjoy the same high standard of living and lesser developed nations would not experience their current level of poverty (Pogge 2005). Critics argue that counterfactuals of such sweep pose insuperable problems (Risse 2005). In order to argue that, as a consequence of previous wrongs to earlier generations, the current residents of some nations have been made worse off than they otherwise would have been, or that current residents of some nation would not enjoy their high standard of living, it must be possible to rule out all of the intervening variables that might have altered the broad sweep of human history.

Objections to the reliance on counterfactual arguments of this sort do not dispute that slavery and the practices of colonialism were unjust in themselves. Nor do they dispute that members of past generations were harmed by those practices. However, the objection is that conclusions regarding the continuing harms, as well as the continuing benefits, that flow from those practices are speculative. While there is no dispute about the unfairness of an initial distribution of advantages and disadvantages, there is uncertainty about the enduring effects of that initial, unjustly created distribution. The same sort of objection applies to counterfactuals regarding the enduring effects of GHG consumption. Rich nations might have become rich even without as much GHG production, and poor nations might still be poor even with more GHG production.

Third, for the sake of argument, assume that defenders of BPP are justified in claiming that but for a history of carbon-intensive activities, current citizens of some nations would not enjoy their high standard of living. A further objection is that holding nation-states morally responsible is potentially unfair to particular citizens in both rich and poor nations. Because carbon-intensive lifestyles are imperfectly correlated with the wealth of states, holding nation-states responsible fails to take account of the fact that there are rich, carbon-intensive consumers in poor states and less carbon-intensive, poor consumers in rich states (Baer 2010: 247–8, 253; Socolow and English 2011: 183; Baer et al. 2010: 216–17). For any assignment of moral responsibility to nation-states, based on contribution to the problem from which citizens derived (or continue to derive) benefit, fairness requires some mechanism or formula that ensures that all high emitters are treated alike across nations and that citizens who live in affluent nations, but who have not benefited (or do not now benefit from ongoing activities), are not penalized (Socolow and English 2011: 185; Caney 2010c). The objection is not decisive against a principle of holding nation-states morally responsible for what happens within their borders. It simply alters the conditions under which holding nation-states responsible is justified and it makes large epistemic demands on the state's ability to distinguish properly among its citizens.

Fourth, some objections to holding nation-states accountable for the actions of their citizens do not depend on any of the historical claims discussed so far. Critics argue that even in the case of very recent or ongoing GHG emissions produced by their citizens, only individual persons or firms and not nation-states are the right sort of entities to be held morally responsible (Posner and Sunstein 2008: 20). The claim is that all ascriptions of moral responsibility should attach to individuals and corporate entities that are the direct causal agents of environmental problems, and not to collective governmental entities that have only indirect relationship to the harms.

The counterargument is that citizens of all countries, by virtue of membership in the state, readily accept, and claim as justified, the benefits and advantages derived from whatever harms their predecessors have produced, as well as the harms produced by co-nations who are their contemporaries, at least insofar as the nature of the harms were well understood at the time of the emissions (Neumayer 2000: 189; Miller 2008: 128).

Arguments for a blanket exclusion of nation-states from any assignment of a share of moral responsibility ignore the fact that modern states play important causal roles in climate change. Numerous forms of state involvement can be cited, including state owned or operated carbon-intensive industries. In addition, nations exert substantial influence on the carbon-intensive conduct of both industrial polluters and consumers within their borders. Such influences include direct subsidies of industries, government-backed bonds and other complex financing mechanisms for the construction of power plants and other energy facilities, fossil fuel mining and drilling operations conducted on public lands, and individual and corporate tax deductions that incentivize the purchase of large homes, automobiles, and other energy-intensive products. Nation-states have contributed, and continue to contribute to GHG accumulation by direct GHG production, fostering consumer demand, shaping both the preferences and the options of everyone within its boundaries, and implementing policies that sustain carbon-intensive modes of production and consumption. Failure to ascribe moral responsibility to nation-states ignores the fact that the carbon footprints of individuals and corporations within its territories are what they are only because of governmental fingerprints.

The real question, then, is not whether nation-states are eligible for being held responsible for mitigation. The question is whether the case for holding them responsible should be made to depend on assumptions about the benefits accrued from past activities or the wrongness of the means from which those benefits were derived. The answer, it seems, is that it is not necessary to look to the distant past to find sufficient reasons to question the fairness of current emissions, especially when those emissions support an affluent lifestyle for a minority of the world's population. Some human rights approaches explore arguments of this sort as alternatives to historical principles such as BPP.

Two Human Rights Approaches

Simon Caney (2009, 2010a) argues that the basis for climate change duties is found in Henry Shue's cosmopolitan conception of human rights. The cosmopolitan conception proceeds under the assumption that everyone has duties to everyone else to ensure circumstances necessary for the fulfillment of rights to life, health, and subsistence (Shue 2011: 305). These are rights "that persons have in virtue of their humanity, and not because of the nation or state into which they were born or any actions that they have performed" (Caney 2010a: 164). Caney surveys the list of adverse consequences expected from climate change and identifies them as harms to the very interests that these specific rights are meant to protect (Caney 2010a: 166). The harms are then shown to be very substantial and in violation of human rights insofar as human rights "represent moral thresholds," below which people should not fall. They designate the most basic moral standards to which persons are entitled" (Caney 2010a: 136, 164–5). The adverse consequences of climate change are said to be an injustice when those who have the ability to mitigate the dangerous accumulation of GHGs fail to do so and the consequence is that some people fall below the moral thresholds established by these human rights. For example, many people in the hottest regions of the world already face significant challenges in meeting their own food needs, but the impact of global warming in these regions is a much further reduction of available ground water, accelerated desertification, and the increase of pests and diseases (Samson et al. 2011). The loss of the economically most viable and most heavily populated coastal lands, and even the loss of entire island nations, are examples of the further threats to the minimum requirements of a decent life posed by global warming, resulting in the potential for massive global migration of climate refugees unable to meet their needs in their countries of origin (WDR 2010).

Central to the cosmopolitan conception of human rights is the fact that it grounds universal duties with respect to health, life, and subsistence in the vital needs of others. The basis upon which the specific moral responsibility for addressing climate change is assigned is not tied to history, or to any active harming of the interests of others, but to the ability to pay. "In principle, the Ability to Pay approach is indifferent to who caused a harm: its emphasis is on who can rectify that harm" (Caney 2010c: 213). In fact, Caney claims that the existence of duties of the affluent nations to address climate change "does not necessarily rest on the assumption that climate change is human-induced. Its insistence is that persons' preeminent interests be protected, and it is not, in itself, concerned with the causes of climate change" (Caney 2010a: 136).

Climate change duties, then, on the cosmopolitan account, do not differ in their rationale from duties that would arise if an asteroid were hurtling toward a vulnerable country. The existence of profound human need and the ability of others to meet it are jointly sufficient to trigger duties that correspond to human rights claims.

Critical readers will raise questions about what supports the cosmopolitan's conclusion. In response, Caney invokes what he takes to be the widely shared conviction that even when someone plays no part in causing the suffering of others, there are sufficient reasons to render assistance, especially when the costs of doing so are not substantial. Caney takes the central intuition as well established (Caney 2010c: 216). Shue argues in similar fashion that what is of paramount moral importance is that everyone have enough of the various goods that are necessary for a "decently human, if modest, life" (Shue 2010b: 108), and that "[i]f the aggregate of resources is enough for some parties to have more than enough, and they do in fact have more than enough, and other parties have less than enough, then it is unfair not to guarantee everyone at least an adequate minimum" (Shue 2010b: 108).

Not everyone will find such arguments persuasive. Libertarian critics, for example, argue that for such an argument to be successful it must establish a link between someone's need, however great, and the reasons for holding specific persons or entities under a moral duty to meet that need (Nozick 1974: 168; Lomasky 1987: 85–94). The critic rejects, as unsupported by clear philosophical argument, the cosmopolitan's core claim that there is universal duty of everyone—including specific nation-states—to guarantee to everyone else, regardless of nationality, and regardless of how need arose, the means to the satisfaction of their most basic human needs.

Even many of the defenders of universal duties of humanitarian assistance, or duties to relieve extreme human suffering such as famine, augment their arguments with the strategic proviso that such duties apply only when they could be performed without significant sacrifice (Singer 1972). However, it is worth noting that duties of climate change mitigation might prove difficult to square with the proviso. The IPCC (Solomon et al. 2007) estimates that a cut in the annual global per capita emissions from 2000 levels of 4 tons by 50–80 percent by 2050 would be necessary in order to keep the temperature rise in the range of 2°. Given the fact that the world's population is expected to grow by 2 billion people by then, the estimated per capita global average in 2050 has to be reduced to a level between 1.33 tons and 1.5 tons (Moellendorf 2011: 118–19; Baer 2010: 219–21). The significance of these numbers becomes clear when we observe that the per capita emissions in the U.S. in 2008 was roughly 18 tons compared with just over 5 tons for China (World Bank 2012). Without a rapid technological transition toward a radically decarbonized world, life in a country at or near the global average would be one in which "few could be described as well-off" (Socolow and English 2010: 181).

Both Caney and Shue concede that the stringent demands of their cosmopolitan conception of human rights will be resisted in various quarters. Accordingly, they offer an alternative conception of human rights designed to enlist wider support. They argue that at the very least their critics should accept a negative rights construal of their trio of human rights (Caney 2010a: 166). The core claim of the negative rights account is that we "should not do things that interfere with others' ability to maintain a decent human life for themselves" (Shue 2010b: 109). Similarly, Caney argues that what is often ignored is "a morally relevant aspect of current climate change, namely that some persons are imposing grave risks on others" (Caney 2010a: 170).

A negative rights construal fundamentally shifts the grounds of the argument. The upshot is that whatever we might think about the duties of the developed nations in the asteroid case, global warming should not be seen as morally equivalent. By focusing on the causal role played by large emitting nations, Caney and Shue strategically retreat from their much stronger compound claim that it makes no moral difference how the harms were created and that ability to pay is the only morally relevant factor in the assignment of duties to guarantee a minimum human rights standard for all. The negative rights alternative attempts to show that the real moral difference does in fact rest with how the harms are created (Caney 2010a: 169).

Moreover, the negative rights construal need not rely upon claims regarding the harms generated by activities in the distant past or upon counterfactual speculations about how the current benefits enjoyed by developed nations were caused. All that is necessary to make the case that global warming constitutes a violation of human rights, negatively construed, is to point to the current failure of affluent nations to take the available steps necessary to alter the technological and economic basis that supports their way of life, when that failure eventuates in a human-made disaster for much, if not, all of the rest of the planet.

We might, then, re-state the point of the negative rights construal in the language of moral thresholds. Instead of conceptualizing human rights as moral thresholds below which no one *should be allowed to fall*, the negative rights construal argues for a moral threshold below which no one should be *driven* by the actions of others. The negative rights construal thus challenges its critics to provide sufficient reasons for failing to curb current high levels of emissions that support a very high standard of living for some when their level of emissions contributes to the deprivation of a decent human life for others.

Systematic Disadvantage

The further consequences of a failure to mitigate the production of GHGs are dramatically portrayed in estimates of the differential impact of climate change on poorer, less developed nations, especially in the global South, the less developed regions of Asia, and island nations (Parry et al. 2007; WDR 2010; UNDP 2008). The effects are already being felt by, and will be greatest for, the nations that are the poorest, hottest, agriculturally most vulnerable to weather pattern disruption, economically most dependent on agriculture, most vulnerable to vector borne diseases that are expected to increase dramatically, and least able to adapt by virtue of both disadvantaging geography and fewer economic resources. All the while, some nations of the global North will experience far less negative impact at GHG concentration levels of around 450 ppm. In some cases, nations in the northern latitudes may even experience some economic benefits (Samson et al. 2011), and certainly they have the economic resources that will make adaptation to any negative effects much easier. The stark truth about climate change is that it is not an ordinary collective action problem in which all stand to lose in roughly comparable ways, at the same threshold of harm, unless all act to prevent it. It is a problem in which the poorest, most vulnerable will be hurt first and worst.

Moreover, the harms associated with global warming for the global poor are not confined to losses in health, subsistence, and life. As important as these are, at stake additionally is the loss of even a minimal degree of self-determination over the most fundamental matters affecting them. The populations most vulnerable to climate change experience complete powerlessness in the face of a set of global social arrangements in which developed and developing nations can decide unilaterally whether to mitigate the unfolding of a human-made disaster that imposes the greatest burdens on the global poor. Indifference of this magnitude, if that is the outcome over the years ahead, is incompatible with any plausible understanding of what is required by a commitment to the equality of moral standing among human beings. For such indifference means that the most vital human interests of wholly dependent peoples are given no moral weight in the decisions of those who hold asymmetric political and economic power over their fates.

What can be expected from business-as-usual energy policies of the more affluent nations is the perpetuation and exacerbation of a densely woven web of systematic disadvantage, characterized by deprivations of wellbeing across multiple dimensions, from which those most adversely affected groups are largely powerless to escape, and could not, on their own, have taken steps to avoid (Powers and Faden 2006).

The fact that ongoing economic and political interactions among nation-states can create or perpetuate global patterns of systematic disadvantage underscores the point that there are sources of injustice beyond those associated with policies that have the effect of driving citizens of other nations below a moral threshold for a decent human life. Many in the global South are already below that threshold due to a variety of causes other than climate change. The global poor are profoundly and pervasively affected by extra-national energy policies that make them even worse off, lock in lower long-term life prospects by making it far less likely that they can rise above the threshold for a decent human life, and ensure that they will not lead sufficiently self-determining lives or exercise significant domestic political control over their vital interests in health, life, and subsistence. These impacts of global climate change demand a global response to the issue of moral responsibility. Responsibility must be assigned somewhere to ensure that urgent action is taken to prevent great and irreparable harm being done to the poorest and most vulnerable.

Related Topics

Chapter 2, "Social Determinants of Health and Health Inequalities," Sridhar Venkatapuram and Michael Marmot

Chapter 31, "Population Growth and Decline: Issues of Justice," Margaret P. Battin

References

Adler, M. (2007) "Corrective Justice and Liability for Global Warming," *University of Pennsylvania Law Review* 155: 1859–67.

Baer, P. (2010) "Adaptation: Who Pays Whom? Fairness in Adaptation to Climate Change," in S.M. Gardiner, S. Caney, D. Jamieson and H. Shue (eds.) *Climate Ethics: Essential Readings*, Oxford and New York: Oxford University Press, pp. 247–62.

Baer, P., Athanasiou, T., Kartha, S. and Kemp-Benedict, E. (2010) "Greenhouse Development Rights: A Framework for Climate Protection that is 'More Fair' Than Equal Per Capita Emissions Rights," in S.M. Gardiner, S. Caney, D. Jamieson and H. Shue (eds.) *Climate Ethics: Essential Readings*, Oxford and New York: Oxford University Press, pp. 215–30.

Caney, S. (2009) "Human Rights, Responsibilities and Climate Change," in C. Beitz and R. Goodin (eds.) *Global Basic Rights*, Oxford: Oxford University Press, pp. 227–47.

Caney, S. (2010a) "Cosmopolitan Justice, Responsibility, and Global Climate Change," in S. M. Gardiner, S. Caney, D. Jamieson and H. Shue (eds.) *Climate Ethics: Essential Readings*, Oxford and New York: Oxford University Press, pp. 122–45.

Caney, S. (2010b) "Climate Change, Human Rights, and Moral Thresholds," in S.M. Gardiner, S. Caney, D. Jamieson and H. Shue (eds.) *Climate Ethics: Essential Readings*, Oxford and New York: Oxford University Press, pp. 163–77.

Caney, S. (2010c) "Climate Change and the Duties of the Advantaged," *Critical Review of International Social and Political Philosophy* 13 (1): 203–28.

Gardiner, S. (2011) "Is No One Responsible for Global Environmental Tragedy? Climate Change as a Challenge to Our Ethical Concepts," in D. Arnold (ed.) *The Ethics of Climate Change*, Cambridge: Cambridge University Press, pp. 38–59.

Hansen, J. (2008) "Target Atmospheric CO2: Where Should Humanity Aim?" *Open Atmospheric Science Journal* 2: 217–31.

Jamieson, D. (2010a) "Ethics, Public Policy, and Global Warming," in S.M. Gardiner, S. Caney, D. Jamieson and H. Shue (eds.) *Climate Ethics: Essential Readings*, Oxford and New York: Oxford University Press, pp. 77–86.

Jamieson, D. (2010b) "Adaptation, Mitigation, and Justice," in S.M. Gardiner, S. Caney, D. Jamieson and H. Shue (eds.) *Climate Ethics: Essential Readings*, Oxford and New York: Oxford University Press, pp. 263–83.

Lomasky, L. (1987) *Persons, Rights, and the Moral Community*, New York and Oxford: Oxford University Press.

Miller, D. (2008) "Global Justice and Climate Change: How Should Responsibilities Be Distributed? Parts I and II," in G.B. Peterson (ed.) *Tanner Lectures on Human Values 28*, Salt Lake City, UT: University of Utah Press, pp. 119–56.

Moellendorf, D. (2011) "Common Atmospheric Ownership and Equal Emissions Entitlements," in D. Arnold (ed.) *The Ethics of Global Climate Change*, Cambridge: Cambridge University Press, pp. 104–23.

Neumayer, E. (2000) "In Defence of Historical Accountability for Greenhouse Gas Emissions," *Ecological Economics* 33 (2): 185–92.

Nozick, R. (1974) *Anarchy, State, and Utopia*, New York: Basic Books.

OECD (Organization for Economic Cooperation and Development) (2008) *OECD Environmental Outlook to 2030*, Paris: OECD Publishing.

Parry, M.L., Canziani, O.F., Palutikof, J.P., van der Linden, P.J. and Hanson, C.E. (2007) *Climate Change 2007: Impacts, Adaptation and Vulnerability: Contribution of Working Group II to the Fourth Assessment Report of the Intergovernmental Panel on Climate Change*, Cambridge: Cambridge University Press.

Perry, S. (1992) "The Moral Foundations of Tort Law," *Iowa Law Review* 77: 449–514.

Pogge, T. (2005) "World Poverty and Human Rights," *Ethics and International Affairs* 19 (1): 1–7.

Posner, E. and Sunstein, C. (2008) "Global Warming and Social Justice: Do We Owe the World for Climate Change?" *Regulation* 31 (1): 14–20.

Powers, M. and Faden, R. (2006) *Social Justice: The Moral Foundations of Public Health and Health Policy*, Oxford and New York: Oxford University Press.

Rawls, J. (2001) *The Law of Peoples*, Cambridge, MA: Harvard University Press.

Risse, M. (2005) Do We Owe the Global Poor Assistance or Rectification? A Response to Pogge," *Ethics and International Affairs* 19 (1): 9–18.

Samson, J., Berteaux, D., McGill, B.J. and Humphries, M.M. (2011) "Geographic disparities and moral hazards in the predicted impacts of climate change on human populations," *Global Ecology and Biogeography* 20 (July): 532–44.

Shue, H. (2010a) "Subsistence Emissions and Luxury Emissions," in S.M. Gardiner, S. Caney, D. Jamieson and H. Shue (eds.) *Climate Ethics: Essential Readings*, Oxford and New York: Oxford University Press, pp. 200–14.

Shue, H. (2010b) "Global Environment and International Inequality," in S.M. Gardiner, S. Caney, D. Jamieson and H. Shue (eds.) *Climate Ethics: Essential Readings*, Oxford and New York: Oxford University Press, pp. 101–11.

Shue, H. (2010c) "Deadly Delays, Saving Opportunities: Creating a More Dangerous World?" in S.M. Gardiner, S. Caney, D. Jamieson and H. Shue (eds.) *Climate Ethics: Essential Readings*, Oxford and New York: Oxford University Press, pp. 146–62.

Shue, H. (2011) "Human Rights, Climate Change, and the Trillionth Ton," in D. Arnold (ed.)*The Ethics of Global Climate Change*, Cambridge: Cambridge University Press, pp. 292–314.

Singer, P. (1972) "Famine, Affluence, and Morality," *Philosophy and Public Affairs* 1 (3): 229–43.

Sinnott-Armstrong, W. (2010) "It's Not My Fault: Global Warming and Individual Moral Obligations," in S.M. Gardiner, S. Caney, D. Jamieso and H. Shue (eds.) *Climate Ethics: Essential Readings*, Oxford and New York: Oxford University Press, pp. 332–46.

Socolow, R. and English, M. (2011) "Living Ethically in a Greenhouse," in D. Arnold (ed.) *The Ethics of Global Climate Change*, Cambridge: Cambridge University Press, pp. 170–91.

Solomon, S., Qin, D., Manning, M., Chen, Z., Marquis, M., Averyt, K.B. et al. (eds.) (2007) "Technical Summary," in *Climate Change 2007: The Physical Basis. Contribution of Working Group I to the Fourth Assessment Report of the Intergovernmental Panel on Climate Change*, Cambridge: Cambridge University Press.

UNDP (United Nations Development Programme) (2008) *Human Development Report 2007/8: Fighting Climate Change: Human Solidarity in a Divided World*, New York: Palgrave Macmillan.

UNFCCC (1992) United Nations Framework Convention on Climate Change. Available at: http://unfccc.int/key_documents/the_convention/items/2853.php (accessed July 7, 2014).

WDR (2010) *World Development Report 2010: Development and Climate Change*, Washington, DC: World Bank.

World Bank (2012) "CO2 emissions (metric tons per capita)." Available at: http://data.worldbank.org/indicator/EN.ATM.CO2E.PC (accessed July 7, 2014).

Part III

INTELLECTUAL PROPERTY AND COMMODIFICATION

In June 1980, the Supreme Court handed down its decision in the landmark case of *Diamond v. Chakrabarty*. In a close 5–4 ruling, the court upheld a patent initially granted to the General Electric Company for a genetically modified organism created in its labs by Ananda Chakrabarty. Living things had previously been thought outside the realm of patentable subject matter; but in *Chakrabarty* the court ruled that the modified genome of a bacterium, *Pseudomonas putida*, was no different than any other invented "composition of matter" and thus was eligible for a patent. The decision was (and still is) a landmark; the *Chakrabarty* case opened up a whole set of items—genetically modified organisms, cell lines, and genes, among others—to patenting, and made what were previously thought to be research tools into valuable commercial properties. Biomedical scientists doing research on, for example, cell lines extracted from patients with cancer were no longer working with "merely" biological materials; they were now working with resources worth (potentially) millions of dollars.

Changes to law and policy over the last 30–40 years like the *Chakrabarty* decision have had big effects on the conduct of biomedical research. The upshot of these changes has been a steady process of commercialization of medicine, with profound consequences for research in the biomedical sciences as well as the practice of medicine. How best to understand commercialization, as well as the evaluation of its effects, are hotly contested topics. Commercialization raises a number of questions that overlap with many of the traditional concerns of bioethics: access to health care resources, exploitation in the doctor–patient relationship, the treatment of research subjects, and the use of human biological materials in research, among others. It also generates questions at the frontiers of work in research ethics and the ethics of the life sciences.

This section explores ethical questions about intellectual property and commercialization in medicine and biomedical research, focusing on the potential harms of commercialization. Biddle surveys ethical questions about the role of intellectual property in the biomedical sciences. He focuses on two problems in particular, each of which has been the subject of intense debate: the potentially negative effects of intellectual property on access to health care resources (especially medicines), and the possibility that increased patenting of upstream research tools (such as cell lines) will have a chilling effect on research activity. Biddle views these two problems as objections to the dominant (consequentialist) justification for patents, the incentives argument. The central function of intellectual property, according to this argument, is to generate incentives for investment in certain kinds of costly productive activity (such as biomedical research) that otherwise would be very difficult to profit from (due to the difficulty of excluding others from—and charging a price for access to—their products, such as medicines). In exchange for the welfare-decreasing effects of patents (due to the high prices patent holders can charge), there is (allegedly) a net benefit over the long term in the form of more and better medical innovation. But, as Biddle points out, if there is reason to doubt whether patents generate this benefit, then there is reason to doubt whether the incentives argument offers a sufficient justification for intellectual property rights in biomedical research.

Biddle explores the two problems in depth, and surveys a great deal of existing commentary on these two issues; he also discusses some of the potential solutions. Ultimately, he concludes that the potential harms patents pose are serious enough to warrant a revision of current patent criteria (at least as they pertain to biomedical research). Biddle's concern is with the impacts of the biomedical sciences: with the ways in which research and its results in these disciplines affect the health and wellbeing of consumers of medicine. Resnik, however, is concerned with the way commercialization will affect the conduct of research itself. Scientists, as Resnik points out, are bound by standards of research integrity, and adherence to those standards is required not only to ensure that research is ethically above board, but also to maintain the credibility of scientific expertise and public trust in science. Resnik makes a distinction between two sorts of threats to scientific integrity posed by interactions with commercial interests: the possibility of biasing research, and outright misconduct. Whereas bias is unintentional and largely unconscious, misconduct involves the deliberate intent to deceive through, for example, the fabrication of research results. Because of the potential harms of both of these sorts of behaviors, Resnik argues that dealing with both should be a top priority for those institutions responsible for regulating research.

Like Resnik and Biddle, Brody discusses issues in research ethics, but his contribution also deals with a topic of longstanding interest to bioethicists: the ethics of the doctor–patient relationship. Brody's subject is the influence of the pharmaceutical industry on both medical research and patient care; he explores a number of questions about the potential for interaction with the pharmaceutical industry to generate conflicts of interest for physicians and medical researchers. Brody considers the available evidence that financial and other relationships with pharmaceutical companies creates conflicts of interest, and analyzes the arguments for and against different harms associated with these. He also discusses where primary responsibility for dealing with these harms lies (for example, whether it is industry or physicians who are responsible), and what the proper response to these harms should be.

Together these entries survey a wide range of issues and work on commercialization and intellectual property in medicine and the biomedical sciences. Given the sheer amount of money, brain power, and resources—not to mention hopes and dreams—invested in the biotechnology and pharmaceutical industries, and the real potential of work in the biomedical sciences to greatly alter (for better or worse) the human condition over the coming decades, this topic area will only increase in importance, and should be one that will generate worthwhile issues for bioethicists to explore for the foreseeable future.

11
INTELLECTUAL PROPERTY IN THE BIOMEDICAL SCIENCES

Justin B. Biddle

Introduction

Since the late 1970s and early 1980s, intellectual property rights (IPRs) have become increasingly important in many areas of science, including (and perhaps especially) biomedical research. This is evidenced by a dramatic rise in patenting activity. Between 1983 and 2003, the number of patents issued to U.S. universities rose from 434 to 3,259 (Walsh et al. 2007: 1184); patenting in biotechnology has also risen significantly, from 2,000 in 1985 to over 13,000 in 2000 (Walsh et al. 2003: 293). Other countries have witnessed similar trends (American Association for the Advancement of Science (AAAS) 2007a).

While there are a number of factors that have contributed to the increase in patenting, three are particularly important. The first is the development of recombinant DNA technology by Stanley Cohen and Herbert Boyer in the early 1970s, which allowed scientists to isolate specific segments of DNA and transfer them into the DNA of other organisms. This development, which ushered in the age of biotechnology, also laid the groundwork for the patenting of living organisms, as it created the possibility of engineering living organisms that are not "naturally occurring." The second factor is a legal development concerning the patentability of living organisms. In 1972, Ananda Chakrabarty applied to the U.S. Patent and Trademark Office (USPTO) for a number of patents on a genetically engineered bacterium—including a patent on the process of engineering this organism and a patent on the organism itself. The USPTO granted the process patent but initially argued that the organism itself is not patentable because it is a product of nature, and living. Chakrabarty appealed the case to the Supreme Court, which ultimately granted the patent (*Diamond v. Chakrabarty*, 447 U.S. 303 (1980)). The Court argued that Chakrabarty had engineered a bacterium that does not occur naturally, and it claimed that the fact that the organism was living was irrelevant to the question of patentability; the relevant distinction is between products of nature and human-made inventions, not between the living and non-living. In the U.S., this decision provided legal groundwork for the patenting of life. Subsequent to this decision, the

European Patent Office reached a similar conclusion, in part to ensure that the U.S. biotech industry, which could patent living organisms, did not have a competitive advantage over its European counterpart (Brody 2007).

The third factor that contributed to the rise in patenting is a series of U.S. legislative initiatives passed in the early 1980s, especially the *Bayh–Dole Act* of 1980 (PL 96-517) and the *Stevenson–Wydler Technology Innovation Act* of 1980 (PL 96-480). Prior to these enactments, inventions resulting from privately funded research could be privately appropriated, whereas inventions resulting from publicly funded research typically remained in the public domain. The *Bayh–Dole Act* allowed universities and private corporations to patent the results of publicly funded research, while the *Stevenson–Wydler Act* allowed for the patenting of results obtained in government laboratories. The explicit intention behind these acts was to encourage patenting in order to facilitate the transfer of research results into the marketplace (Biddle 2011).

The growing importance of intellectual property (IP) in the biomedical sciences raises a number of important philosophical issues. As will be discussed in the next section, one of the most important moral justifications of IPRs, especially patents, is that they incentivize research and development (R&D) that ultimately benefits society. Patents give patent holders the right to exclude others from making, using, or selling patented entities; as such, they give patent holders a temporary monopoly over those entities. One of the most important arguments in favor of patents is that these temporary monopolies facilitate the production of knowledge, which in turn benefits society. However, there are reasons to doubt that patents in biomedical research have this effect; this essay will examine some of these reasons.

Intellectual Property and Its Justifications

There are four types of IP: patents, copyrights, trademarks, and trade secrets. The subject of this essay is IP in the biomedical sciences, and because the type of IP that is most relevant to the sciences is patents, this essay will deal exclusively with them. In the U.S., patents cover inventions and discoveries that are: statutory, novel, useful, and non-obvious. Most other patent systems, including the European Patent Office, have similar requirements. To be statutory, an invention or discovery must be the kind of thing that is patentable; while different countries interpret this requirement in different ways, all require that patentable objects be "non-natural"—e.g., not an abstract idea or law of nature. Novelty requires of an invention that it not be known publicly prior to the submission of the patent application. Usefulness requires that an object be capable of being utilized in a practical context for the attainment of specific goals. Finally, to be non-obvious, the discovery or invention cannot be obvious to a person with ordinary skill in the art. Clearly, each of these requirements is open to interpretation and has been the object of a long legal and policy debate. Excellent narrative histories of recent debates in the U.S. and in Europe have been provided by Brody (2006a, 2006b) and Brody (2007), respectively.

The recent increase in patenting activity in science raises philosophical questions about the moral and epistemological justifiability of IP. There are at least three types of justifications: labor based, personality based, and incentive based (Hughes 1988). The labor-based account begins with the premise that every human being has a property right over herself, including her labor. When an individual mixes her labor with a previously unowned object, she thereby acquires a property right over it (subject to certain restrictions).

This account, which derives from John Locke (1980 [1690]), has been defended more recently by Nozick (1974), Moore (2001), and others.

According to the personality-based account, property provides a particularly suitable means for self-actualization and personal expression (Hughes 1988: 330). The process of self-actualization requires that we maintain some degree of control over our external environment, both tangible and intangible; personality-based justifications argue that property rights are the most effective means of maintaining such control. This view, which derives from G.W.F. Hegel (1991 [1821]), is discussed in detail by Hughes (1988).

According to the third type of account, IP is justified on the basis of its incentivizing effects. This justification includes both an epistemic and a moral component. IPRs are thought to incentivize R&D that would otherwise not get done, or not get done as quickly, and thereby facilitate the development of useful knowledge (the epistemic component). In facilitating the development of useful knowledge, IPRs thus quicken the transfer of research into the marketplace, which ultimately benefits society (the moral component). This justification, which is associated with the utilitarian tradition in moral philosophy, is widely accepted in the arena of science and technology policy, and it has been used to justify initiatives aimed at increasing patenting activity in science, such as the *Bayh–Dole Act*.

While the labor-based and personality-based accounts might provide plausible justifications for some kinds of IP, they face serious obstacles as justifications of patenting in science. Scientific research is a communal enterprise. Advances in science and technology require not just teams of researchers working toward particular developments but also prior generations of researchers who provide the requisite groundwork for those advances. Cohen and Boyer's work on recombinant DNA technology, for example, would have been impossible without Watson and Crick's earlier discovery of the structure of DNA. The communal nature of research presents serious difficulties for both labor-based and personality-based accounts, as such accounts would seem to require that we be able to draw a sharp line between those who have contributed their labor or their "personality" toward an advance and those who have not. While it is easy enough to draw a line for pragmatic reasons, it is difficult if not impossible to draw it in a principled way. Personality-based accounts face the additional problem that they seem incapable of justifying property rights over objects that are useful but that have little of their developer's "personality" in them (Hughes 1988). It is perhaps plausible to argue that an individual has a property right over a poem that she wrote, on the grounds that it is an expression of her personhood; this argument is much less plausible when the object in question is a genetically modified microorganism.

The incentive-based, consequentialist justification of patenting is arguably the most plausible of the three, at least with respect to biomedical research—and, as noted, it is the most commonly maintained justification in science and technology policy. The remainder of this essay will examine two important sets of criticisms of patenting in biomedical research, both of which call into question the consequentialist justification. The first is the "tragedy of the anticommons" thesis, which concerns the effects of patenting items of basic research, while the second pertains to the effects of patenting in pharmaceutical research, especially for the developing world.

Tragedy of the Anticommons?

Many have argued that the proliferation of patenting in science—particularly in basic, or upstream, research—is obstructing the flow of information, which in turn impedes progress in science and technology (Nelson 2004). One of the most important of these arguments is the "tragedy of the anticommons," put forward by Heller and Eisenberg (1998). The tragedy of the anticommons thesis is a play on Garrett Hardin's "tragedy of the commons," according to which common ownership of scarce resources leads, by way of a series of individually rational decisions, to overexploitation (Hardin 1968). The solution to this problem, according to Hardin, is private appropriation of the commons. According to Heller and Eisenberg, however, too many property rights can lead to underutilization and impede the development of potentially beneficial technologies. A "proliferation of intellectual property rights upstream may be stifling life-saving innovations further downstream in the course of research and product development" (Heller and Eisenberg 1998: 698).

An example that Heller and Eisenberg provide in support of their thesis is patents on concurrent gene fragments. In situations in which the development of a product requires access to multiple concurrent gene fragments, patents can slow down, and even stop, the development of a product. For example, the development of DNA diagnostic tests can require access to multiple patented DNA segments; obtaining access to these segments can be either so complex or so expensive that, in many cases, researchers will cease developing these tests and turn their attention elsewhere. While Heller and Eisenberg do not explicitly defend a particular solution to this problem, I interpret them as maintaining that patents on the results of upstream scientific research—and particularly research inputs—should be prohibited.

The anticommons thesis has generated much controversy. Several studies have been conducted to test the thesis empirically, and many hold that these studies effectively falsify the thesis. One of the most commonly cited of these studies is that of American Association for the Advancement of Science's Project on Intellectual Property in the Public Interest (AAAS-SIPPI), one of the conclusions of which is that there is "very little evidence of an 'anticommons problem'" (AAAS 2007a: 12). In order to reach this conclusion, the authors surveyed over 8,000 randomly selected members of the AAAS from a variety of different fields and asked them about their experiences acquiring IP-protected materials. Many of the results provide grounds for concern. Thirty-three percent of respondents reported that they had experienced difficulties acquiring IP-protected material, including 25 percent of academic respondents and 40 percent of industry respondents (AAAS 2007b: 24). Of those who reported difficulties, 60 percent stated that licensing negotiations were "overly complex" and 38 percent reported a "breakdown of licensing negotiations" (AAAS 2007b: 24). Given these results, it is at first difficult to see why the authors would conclude that there is very little evidence of an anticommons problem; the basis for this conclusion is that only 1 percent of all respondents reported abandoning their projects (AAAS 2007b: 25, 61). The study authors have thus interpreted "anticommons problem" rather narrowly, which is how they could reach the conclusion that they did. While the results of this study do not suggest that IPRs are leading to widespread project abandonment, they do provide reason to worry that IPRs are inhibiting research in a number of ways.

Perhaps the most important of the studies cited in response to the anticommons thesis are those of J. Walsh, W. Cohen, and colleagues (e.g., Walsh et al. 2007). One of these surveyed over 1,000 researchers in genomics and proteomics—two fields with extensive patenting activity—in order to determine the effects of patenting on the choice of problems to address and the decision not to pursue a project. To determine the former, the authors listed a variety of potential reasons for choosing a project and asked respondents to rate the importance of each. While "scientific importance" and "interest" were widely reported to be "very important" or "moderately important" reasons for choosing a project (by 97 and 95 percent, respectively), only 7 percent reported that "inputs patent free" was an important reason for choosing a project, with the same percentage reporting that the patentability of results was an important reason (Walsh et al. 2007: 1188). With respect to the decision not to pursue a project, only 3 percent of respondents reported that too many patents upstream was an important reason for not pursuing a project. These results cohere well with those of the AAAS-SIPPI study in finding that IPRs—at least in some areas of research—do not seem to be leading to widespread project abandonment.

The results reached by Walsh et al. are curious: In the patent-rich fields of genomics and proteomics, patents do not appear to be doing what they are designed to do—i.e., exclude others from using patent-protected objects. Walsh et al. investigate this issue and argue that scientists have developed "working solutions" to the problem of obtaining access to IP-protected materials; perhaps the most important of these is infringement. The authors ask how often scientists believe they require access to other people's IP-protected materials, and of those who responded, 8 percent believed that they had, within the past two years, used knowledge or information covered by someone else's patent, but only 5 percent of respondents reported that they regularly check to see if the information they are using is patent protected (Walsh et al. 2007: 1189). Given the frequency of patenting activity in these fields, and given the infrequency with which scientists report checking for patents, it is hard not to conclude that infringement is widespread.

It is common to believe that these studies provide evidence against the anticommons thesis. The AAAS-SIPPI study states this explicitly, and it is often cited to this effect (e.g., Gold et al. 2010). However, a closer examination reveals that the evidence presented in the AAAS-SIPPI study and in the studies of Walsh et al. is largely irrelevant to an evaluation of the anticommons thesis (Biddle 2012; Eisenberg 2008: 1069). The anticommons thesis, recall, states that a proliferation of patenting and licensing *upstream*—i.e., in more basic research—is inhibiting *downstream* research and product development. The aforementioned studies, however, do not examine the effects of patenting and licensing in upstream research on downstream research and product development. The AAAS-SIPPI study focuses upon research scientists and did not ask which patented materials were being acquired or how these materials were being used (AAAS 2007b: 19); as a result, it is not relevant to the question of how patents upstream effect downstream research and product development. The studies of Walsh et al. examine the effects of patenting and licensing upon the sharing of information among academic researchers, the vast majority of whom are engaged in basic research (Walsh et al. 2007: 1086). The data in these studies, as a result, are also irrelevant to the anticommons thesis. In this regard, it is worth noting that, despite the fact that the studies of Walsh et al. are sometimes taken to disconfirm the anticommons thesis, the authors themselves never make this claim. Rather, they claim that, at the present time, access to patents "rarely imposes a significant burden for academic biomedical researchers" who are engaged in basic research (Walsh et al. 2007: 1191).

There are other empirical studies that do provide data that are relevant to the anticommons thesis, and these studies support the thesis—though the data they provide are limited to a small number of fields. DNA diagnostics is one area in which we do seem to be witnessing anticommons problems. Mildred Cho et al. surveyed 132 directors of diagnostic laboratories; 75 percent of respondents held patent licenses, 65 percent had been contacted by a patent or license holder regarding potential infringement, *25 percent had stopped performing a clinical genetic test as a result of a patent or license, and 53 percent had decided not to develop a new clinical genetic test as a result of a patent or license* (Cho et al. 2003: 5, emphasis added). This is exactly the sort of problem anticipated by Heller and Eisenberg.

While it is not clear why we are witnessing problems in this area and not in the areas of more basic research examined by Walsh et al., one can hypothesize a plausible explanation in terms of a simple cost–benefit analysis (Walsh and Cohen 2008). The burden of enforcing IPRs falls on the patent holder, and in many areas of basic research, there is little incentive to enforce these rights, as the development of a marketable product is typically a long way away. In these areas, the expected benefits of enforcement are typically negligible. The situation is different, however, in areas of research that straddle the line between basic research and product development—areas such as DNA diagnostics. In DNA diagnostics, a significant part of the research is isolating genes and determining their functions in disease processes; but once this is done, one is not far from having a marketable product—namely, a test for the gene(s) in question. In areas such as this, the benefits of enforcement can be great.

These empirical investigations have important implications for the questions of the moral and epistemic justifiability of patenting in the biomedical sciences. Patents increase the cost and complexity of research, and while they do not seem to be leading to widespread project abandonment in academic research, this is in large part due to the prevalence of patent infringement. And while there are relatively few data concerning the effects of patents over items of basic research on downstream research and product development, the data that we do have provide reason to believe that patents are having an inhibiting, rather than an incentivizing, effect. More specifically, patents in areas such as DNA diagnostics appear to be inhibiting the development of certain kinds of knowledge and certain technological capabilities that have the potential to save lives. Thus, with respect to patents on items of basic biomedical research, the consequentialist justification of IPRs is on shaky ground.

Intellectual Property and Pharmaceutical Innovation

The pharmaceutical industry is ostensibly an area in which IPRs play a crucial role in incentivizing research and development. Putting a new drug on the market is a long and expensive process; some have estimated the cost at $800 million per drug (DiMasi et al. 2003), though others argue that this figure is highly inflated (Angell 2004). Nonetheless, it is clear that commercial enterprises will be reluctant to invest in drugs unless they have reason to believe that they can recoup their investments—and patents provide a mechanism for doing so. For many commentators, cases like this—in which the outcomes of research are uncertain and the costs of developing a product prohibitive—are paradigm examples of why patents are necessary.

The claim that patents incentivize *innovative* pharmaceutical research is, however, questionable. Much of what the pharmaceutical industry produces are duplicative drugs—or “me-too” drugs—that are sufficiently different from already-existing medicines to obtain a separate patent, but that have therapeutic effects that are the same as, or very similar to, drugs already on the market. For example, between 1990 and 2004, 77 percent of drugs approved by the U.S. Food and Drug Administration were duplicative in this sense (Angell 2004: 75). Developing "me-too" drugs is profitable for industry; it can charge monopoly prices because the drugs are patent protected, and the risk involved in R&D is much lower than in the case of truly innovative drugs. All of this suggests that while IPRs might be necessary for innovation, they are not sufficient, and that at present, they are not adequately incentivizing the development of innovative pharmaceuticals. The consequentialist justification of patenting requires that patents incentivize not just any research, but research that benefits society. In this respect, the consequentialist justification of patenting is again on shaky ground.

While the innovativeness of the pharmaceutical industry in the developed world is debatable, it is unquestionable that IPRs are failing to incentivize the development of innovative medicines for the developing world. Nearly 2 billion people, or almost 30 percent of the world population, do not have access to potentially life-saving medicines; as a result, roughly 10 million people die needlessly every year, most of whom live in the developing world (Grover 2009: 7). This situation represents one of the greatest collective moral failures of our time, and IP is at the center of it. Discussions of this tragedy focus upon two problems. The first is the problem of gaining access to medicines that already exist (the "problem of access"); the second is the problem of developing new drugs to treat diseases that afflict primarily or exclusively the developing world (the "problem of availability").

There are a myriad of factors that contribute to the problem of access to essential medicines; one of them is the high cost of medicines that are patent protected. By granting legal rights to exclude others from making, using, or selling patent-protected materials, patents provide temporary monopolies; this gives patent holders and licensees the ability to sell their products at whatever price the market will bear. The vast majority of inhabitants of developing countries cannot afford to purchase life-saving medicines at these prices (or their impoverished health systems cannot afford to buy them on their behalf). Other factors that contribute to the problem of access include inadequate infrastructure in developing countries, which makes storing and distributing medicines difficult, and extreme poverty, which prohibits some people from affording *any* drugs, even those that are no longer patent protected.

The problem of access has been exacerbated by the Agreement on Trade-Related Aspects of Intellectual Property Rights (TRIPS). This agreement, which was negotiated in 1994 at the Uruguay Round of the General Agreement on Tariffs and Trade (GATT), set minimum standards for IP policies for all World Trade Organization (WTO) members. One of these standards requires all WTO members to grant product patents. Prior to this agreement, some developing countries (such as India) granted patents on processes but not products. This allowed generic drug makers to reverse engineer new drugs that were still patent protected in other countries, allowing them to be sold in the developing world for prices much lower than their patented equivalents. Once the TRIPS agreement took effect, WTO countries could no longer produce generics for many medicines.

While IPRs represent only one contributing factor among many to the problem of access, they are by far the most important contributing factor to the problem of availability. Pharmaceutical R&D, as noted, is expensive, and it is conducted almost exclusively by industry; because for-profit corporations must be profitable in order to survive, and because inhabitants of the developing world cannot afford medicines at monopoly prices, there is little incentive for firms to invest in medicines that treat diseases that afflict primarily or exclusively the developing world (or type II or type III diseases, respectively). Thus, for example, of the 1,393 drugs approved for sale between 1975 and 1999, only 13 specifically treated tropical diseases (Trouiller et al. 2002). Between 2000 and 2004, an additional 163 new chemical entities were marketed, and only five were for neglected diseases (Chirac and Torreele 2006).

Potential Solutions

While the problems discussed thus far (the anticommons problem and the problems of access and availability) are recognized to varying degrees—the anticommons problem is still much debated, and the problems of access and availability are widely acknowledged—there is little consensus about how best to solve them. Potential solutions can be placed into one of three mutually exclusive categories:

1. Maintain the current system of IPRs (perhaps supplemented with additional rewards).
2. Eliminate IPRs.
3. Revise the current system of IPRs.

The vast majority of proposals for solving the problems of access and availability fall within (1). One proposal that has already been implemented is governmental and non-governmental donations and bulk buying, which involves governments, sometimes in combination with one another, targeting particular diseases and donating drugs that treat these diseases, or negotiating with pharmaceutical companies to sell drugs for particular diseases at lower prices. These programs address the problem of access by ensuring that (at least some) medicines are sold at either a lower cost or at no cost at all, and they address the problem of availability by providing a market for drugs for (at least some) neglected diseases. The overall effect of these programs, however, is modest, due to the fact that they tend to target diseases that have well-organized lobbying groups. Thus, they have had some success with regard to HIV/AIDS medications but are unlikely to have much of an effect in the treatment of type III diseases such as African sleeping sickness (Ravvin 2008). There are a number of other proposals that work entirely within the current system of IPRs—including differential pricing and compulsory licensing—but none is likely to serve as a general solution to either the problem of access or the problem of availability (Ravvin 2008), and none addresses the anticommons problem.

Others have proposed supplementing the current system of IPRs by offering additional financial incentives to firms that develop vaccines or medicines that treat neglected diseases. One such proposal, which is already in effect, is Advanced Market Commitments (AMCs). On this proposal, sponsors (e.g., governments, non-governmental organizations) incentivize the development of new vaccines by guaranteeing that they will purchase vaccines that meet predetermined technical specifications. The purchase price is predetermined, and once the vaccine is purchased, they are sold at predetermined, affordable prices. AMCs thus have the potential to alleviate both the problems of availability and access; but while they have had some successes, there are a number of drawbacks, which make them unlikely to serve as a general solution to either problem. Perhaps most significantly, AMCs require of innovators that they create vaccines that meet technical specifications that are predetermined by a committee. Medical research, by its very nature, is uncertain, and it is difficult to know ahead of time whether a particular intervention will meet predetermined specifications; the demand to meet such specifications thus places significant limits on the incentivizing effect of AMCs (Ravvin 2008).

Arguably the most promising of the proposals to supplement the current system of IPRs is the Health Impact Fund (HIF), developed by Aidan Hollis and Thomas Pogge (Hollis 2008; Pogge 2005). Under this proposal, innovators would have the choice of selling a drug or vaccine under the current IP system or registering it with the HIF. If the latter option were chosen, the innovator would be rewarded on the basis of the extent to which the innovation actually reduced the global burden of disease (GBD). This proposal has a number of advantages. Depending upon the size of the prize (Hollis (2008) suggests somewhere between $2 and 20 billion per year), it could provide a significant incentive to develop treatments for neglected diseases. Moreover, because the innovator would be rewarded on the basis of the extent to which the treatment *actually* reduced the GBD, the HIF provides incentive not just to develop treatments, but also to ensure that the treatments are affordable, that they reach targeted populations, and that they are taken properly. The proposal also has the benefit of being acceptable to the pharmaceutical industry; it leaves the current IP system completely intact. Perhaps the most significant problem with the proposal is the technical one of determining the extent to which an intervention actually reduces the GBD. Determining the causal effect of an intervention upon the GBD is difficult for both theoretical and practical reasons; this is especially so when multiple interventions are introduced simultaneously (Selgelid 2008). Neither the HIF nor AMCs is intended to address the anticommons problem.

The second class of proposals recommends eliminating IPRs in medical research. Brown (2008) defends a version of this, which he calls "scientific socialism." Under this proposal, patents in medical research should be eliminated, and public funding for research should be adjusted to appropriate levels. Brown argues that patents are not necessary for incentivizing medical innovation; recognition within the scientific community has been a sufficient incentive to innovate for most of the history of science, and it still can be (cf. Hollis 2008; Reiss 2010). Moreover, taking research out of the hands of private corporations would allow scientists the freedom to investigate treatments for all diseases—not just those that afflict the wealthy—and the lack of monopoly pricing would help to solve the problem of access. Furthermore, while Brown does not emphasize this consequence, the proposal would solve the anticommons problem.

The proposal to eliminate IPRs in medical research is a radical one, which would have profound repercussions not just for the entire complex of biomedical research, but for the global economy as well. The radical nature of the proposal brings with it a practical problem of political feasibility: Even if it were advisable in the ideal to eliminate IPRs in medical research, it is unlikely that this proposal would garner much political support. The radical nature of the proposal also, however, brings an epistemological problem of knowing precisely how such a change would affect our systems of knowledge production. Given this, it is perhaps wiser—both practically and epistemically—to proceed in a piecemeal and iterative fashion, by examining the current system of IPRs, predicting the effects of adjusting components of this system, making adjustments, examining the actual effects of these adjustments, and beginning the iterative process anew. This strategy of "adaptive management" has been defended by Mitchell (2009) in the context of policy-relevant research and by Reiss (2010) in the context of biomedical research.

In the remainder of this section, I will analyze the current system into five different components, for the purpose of illustrating the variety of ways in which the current system could be revised, and I will discuss briefly a few possibilities for revising the current system.[1] The focus is on the U.S.; the European system is very similar, with one exception, which I will highlight below.

The first component of the current system of IPRs is the permissibility of patents on products as well as processes. In other words, it is not only possible to patent something for use in a particular specified process; it is also possible to patent something for any usage whatsoever. This has not always been the case; as I noted earlier, some countries have refused to allow patents on products (e.g., India prior to the TRIPS agreement).

The second component is that patents are granted to the first to file a patent application, as opposed to the first to invent. Most countries operate under a first-to-file system; the U.S. previously operated under a first-to-invent system, but changed to first-to-file with the *America Invents Act* of 2011.

The third component is extensive rights of exclusion. Patents, again, provide legal rights to patent holders to exclude others from making, using, and selling patented inventions—but these rights can be weaker or stronger, and they can apply to different ranges of activities. The term "use," for example, is open to different interpretations. The U.S. legal system has traditionally allowed that non-commercial research falls outside the range of activities that patent holders can exclude; however, in the important Federal Court of Appeals decision, *Madey v. Duke University* (2002), the concept of a non-commercial activity was interpreted so narrowly that almost no activity falls within it. Another issue that is open to interpretation is the limits to the demands that patent holders can place to grant access to patent-protected materials. At present, there are no limits upon the demands that can be placed—even in cases where inventions were made through the use of public funds. Finally, there is the issue of the duration of rights to exclude, which is currently placed at 20 years.

The fourth component is the full sufficiency of meeting the USPTO requirements for obtaining a patent. (A discovery or invention, again, must be statutory, novel, useful, and non-obvious in order to be patentable.) There are other patent systems—for example, that of the European Union—in which these four requirements are not sufficient; according to Article 53(a) of the European Patent Convention, discoveries or inventions that are "contrary to the 'ordre public' or morality" are not patentable. The full sufficiency of these requirements in the U.S. does not allow any exceptions, such as for items of basic research or research tools. It also does not allow for exceptions for living organisms. There are some patent systems that place restrictions upon the types of living organisms that can be patented; Canada, for example, does not grant patents on "higher life forms" (such as plants and animals)—though it does allow for patents on single-celled organisms.

The fifth component is the liberality of USPTO requirements. As noted, the notions of novelty, usefulness, and non-obviousness are open to interpretation, as is the question of whether or not an invention or discovery is statutory. There is a long history of decisions by the USPTO and cases within the U.S. legal system that have dealt with these issues of interpretation, and most of these, especially since 1980, have sided on behalf of those seeking stronger IP protection (Brody 2006a, 2006b). For example, the question of whether isolated and purified DNA segments are statutory is one that is currently making its way through the U.S. legal system; the outcome could have significant implications for the extent to which upstream biomedical research can be shared openly (e.g., *Association for Molecular Pathology et al. v. USPTO* (2010)).

Given this analysis, what kinds of revisions to the current system might alleviate the anticommons problem and the problems of access and availability? I will briefly highlight a couple of different possibilities. One would be to revise the first component by allowing patents on processes but not on products. This would have the effect of weakening IP protection, which in turn would facilitate the free flow of information, so much so that the anticommons problem would be greatly alleviated, if not solved completely. It would also reduce the problem of access to essential medicines, as it would allow firms to reverse engineer new drugs and create generics. However, in a pharmaceutical system dominated by industry, this reduction might come at the cost of exacerbating the problem of availability, as it would decrease the financial incentives of firms to develop new drugs (Schroeder and Singer 2011).

A different possibility would be to continue to allow product patents but to restrict the rights that patent holders have over these products (the third component). Creating a more robust research exemption by interpreting "non-commercial use" more broadly could have the effect of alleviating the anticommons problem. Placing limits on prices that patent holders can charge for access, especially in cases in which inventions were made through the use of public funds, could help to reduce the problem of access. Shortening the duration of patent rights from 20 years would also help to reduce the problem of access, while arguably still providing sufficient incentive to develop new medicines (Reiss and Kitcher 2009).

Revising the third component in the ways just suggested could be supplemented by a revision of the fourth component, by granting exceptions to the full sufficiency of the four requirements for obtaining a patent. One such potential exception could be for research inputs, which could help to alleviate the anticommons problem. Finally, supplementing the revisions of the third and/or fourth components with targeted, market-based proposals such as AMCs and the HIF could further incentivize the development of new, low-cost drugs that target type II and III diseases, thereby increasing both access and availability.

Conclusion

According to the consequentialist justification, IPRs are both epistemically and morally justifiable, because they incentivize innovative research that leads to social benefits. The preceding discussion has highlighted a number of respects in which IPRs in biomedical research are not adequately incentivizing R&D. The tragedy of the anticommons thesis holds that the proliferation of patenting and licensing in upstream biomedical research is actually *impeding* downstream research and product development. In the area of pharmaceuticals, IPRs might be incentivizing innovation in the developing world (though this is questionable), but they do not incentivize the types of innovations that, on the global scale, are most necessary from a moral perspective. The fact that the current system of IPRs is not adequately incentivizing innovative research, and in some cases is inhibiting the ability of the poor to obtain access to life-saving medicines, poses a serious problem for the consequentialist justification of IPRs in biomedical research.

I have argued that the best strategy for solving these problems is to revise the current system of IPRs. I have provided a framework for examining the ways in which this might be done and have discussed the following possibilities: prohibiting product patents; placing greater restrictions on the rights of patent holders, and allowing exceptions to the full sufficiency of the four requirements for obtaining a patent. The second and third of these revisions could be supplemented by market-based proposals such as AMCs and the HIF in order to increase the incentive to innovate, as well as lower costs further. Determining which, if any, of these revisions and supplements would be most successful is a project for further investigation.

Related Topics

Chapter 13, "Influence of the Pharmaceutical Industry on Research and Clinical Care," Howard Brody

Note

1 This analysis is a slightly modified version of Brody's (2006a, 2006b).

Bibliography

AAAS (American Association for the Advancement of Science) (2007a) *International Intellectual Property Experiences: A Report of Four Countries*, Washington, DC: Project on Science and Intellectual Property in the Public Interest. Available at: http://sippi.aaas.org/Pubs/SIPPI_Four_Country_Report.pdf (accessed July 19, 2012).

AAAS (American Association for the Advancement of Science) (2007b) *Intellectual Property Experiences in the United States Scientific Community*, Washington, DC: Project on Science and Intellectual Property in the Public Interest. Available at: http://sippi.aaas.org/Pubs/SIPPI_US_IP_Survey.pdf (accessed July 21, 2012).

Angell, M. (2004) *The Truth about the Drug Companies: How They Deceive Us and What to Do About It*, New York: Random House.

Biddle, J. (2011) "Bringing the Marketplace into Science: On the Neoliberal Defense of the Commercialization of Scientific Research," in M. Carrier and A. Nordmann (eds.) *Science in the Context of Application*, Dordrecht: Springer, pp. 245–69.

Biddle, J. (2012) "Tragedy of the Anticommons? Intellectual Property and the Sharing of Scientific Information," *Philosophy of Science* 79: 821–32.

Brody, B. (2006a) "Intellectual Property and Biotechnology: The U.S. Internal Experience—Part I," *Kennedy Institute of Ethics Journal* 16: 1–37.

Brody, B. (2006b) "Intellectual Property and Biotechnology: The U.S. Internal Experience—Part II," *Kennedy Institute of Ethics Journal* 16: 105–28.

Brody, B. (2007) "Intellectual Property and Biotechnology: The European Debate," *Kennedy Institute of Ethics Journal* 17: 69–110.

Brown, J.R. (2008) "The Community of Science®," in M. Carrier, D.A. Howard and J. Kourany (eds.) *The Challenge of the Social and the Pressure of Practice*, Pittsburgh: University of Pittsburgh Press, pp. 189–216.

Chirac, P. and Torreele, E (2006) "Global Framework on Essential Health R&D," *The Lancet* 367: 1560–1.

Cho, M., Illangasekare, S., Weaver, M., Leonard, D. and Merz, J. (2003) "Effects of Patents and Licenses on the Provision of Clinical Genetic Testing Services," *Journal of Molecular Diagnostics* 5: 3–8.

DiMasi, J., Hansen, R. and Grabowski, H. (2003) "The Price of Innovation: New Estimates of Drug Development Costs," *Journal of Health Economics* 22: 151–85.

Eisenberg, R. (2008) "Noncompliance, Nonenforcement, Nonproblem? Rethinking the Anticommons in Biomedical Research," *Houston Law Review* 45: 1060–99.

Gold, E.R., Kaplan, W., Orbinski, J., Harland-Logan, S. and N-Marandi, S. (2010) "Are Patents Impeding Medical Care and Innovation?" *PLoS Med* 7 (1): e1000208.

Grover, A. (2009) *Promotion and Protection of All Human Rights, Civil, Political, Economic, Social and Cultural Rights, Including the Right to Development, a Report of the Special Rapporteur on the Right of Everyone to the Enjoyment of the Highest Attainable Standard of Physical and Mental Health*, United Nations, A/HRC/11/12. Available at: http://www2.ohchr.org/english/bodies/hrcouncil/docs/11session/A.HRC.11.12_en.pdf (accessed July 21, 2012).

Hardin, G. (1968) "The Tragedy of the Commons," *Science* 162: 1243–8.

Hegel, G.W.F. (1991 [1821]) *Elements of the Philosophy of Right*, A.W. Wood and H.B. Nisbet (eds.), Cambridge: Cambridge University Press.

Heller, M. and Eisenberg, R. (1998) "Can Patents Deter Innovation? The Anticommons in Biomedical Research?" *Science* 280: 698–701.
Hollis, A. (2008) "The Health Impact Fund: A Useful Supplement to the Patent System?" *Public Health Ethics* 1: 124–33.
Hughes, J. (1988) "The Philosophy of Intellectual Property," *Georgetown Law Journal* 77: 287–366.
Locke, J. (1980 [1690]) *Second Treatise of Government*, C.B. Macpherson (ed.), Indianapolis: Hackett.
Mitchell, S. (2009) *Unsimple Truths: Science, Complexity, and Policy*, Chicago: University of Chicago Press.
Moore, A. (2001) *Intellectual Property and Information Control*, New Brunswick, NJ: Transaction Publishing.
Moore, A. (2008) "Personality-Based, Rule-Utilitarian, and Lockean Justifications of Intellectual Property," in H. Tavani and K. Himma (eds.) *Information and Computer Ethics*, Hoboken, NJ: John Wiley & Sons, pp. 105–30.
Nelson, R. (2004) "The Market Economy, and the Scientific Commons," *Research Policy* 33: 455–71.
Nozick, R. (1974) *Anarchy, State, and Utopia*, Oxford: Blackwell.
Pogge, T. (2005) "Human Rights and Global Health: A Research Program," *Metaphilosophy* 36: 182–209.
Ravvin, M. (2008) "Incentivizing Access and Innovation for Essential Medicines: A Survey of the Problem and Potential Solutions," *Public Health Ethics* 2: 110–23.
Reiss, J. (2010) "In Favor of a Millian Proposal to Reform Biomedical Research," *Synthese* 177: 427–47.
Reiss, J. and Kitcher, P. (2009) "Biomedical Research, Neglected Diseases, and Well-Ordered Science," *Theoria* 24: 263–82.
Schroeder, D. and Singer, P. (2011) "Access to Life-Saving Medicines and Intellectual Property Rights: An Ethical Assessment," *Cambridge Quarterly of Healthcare Assessment* 20: 279–89.
Selgelid, M. (2008) "A Full-Pull Program for the Provision of Pharmaceuticals: Practical Issues," *Public Health Ethics* 1: 134–45.
Trouiller, P., Olliaro, P., Torreele, E., Orbinski, J., Laing, R. and Ford, N. (2002) "Drug Development for Neglected Diseases: A Deficient Market and a Public-Health Policy Failure," *The Lancet* 359: 2188–94.
Walsh, J. and Cohen, W. (2008) "Real Impediments to Biomedical Research," *Innovation Policy and the Economy* 8: 1–30.
Walsh, J., Cohen, W. and Arora, A. (2003) "Patenting and Licensing of Research Tools and Biomedical Innovation," in W.M. Cohen and S. Merrill (eds.) *Patents in the Knowledge Based Economy*, Washington, DC: NAP, pp. 285–340.
Walsh, J., Cohen, W. and Cho, C. (2007) "Where Excludability Matters," *Research Policy* 36: 1184–203.
World Trade Organization (WTO) (2001) *Declaration on the TRIPS Agreement and Public Health*, Ministerial Conference. Available at: http://www.wto.org/english/thewto_e/minist_e/min01_e/mindecl_trips_e.pdf (accessed July 21, 2012).

12

BIAS, MISCONDUCT, AND INTEGRITY IN SCIENTIFIC RESEARCH

David B. Resnik

Introduction

Integrity in science involves adherence to ethical norms for the conduct of research. Integrity is essential to good scientific research, as it plays a key role in collaboration, peer review, publication, confirmation, mentoring and education, and data acquisition, analysis, and management. Integrity helps scientists to secure the public's trust and support, and is important in interactions with the public, such as communicating with the media and providing expert testimony in legal proceedings on government advisory committees. Integrity is also indispensable in research involving human subjects or animals. Some of science's ethical norms include honesty, openness, carefulness, objectivity, fair sharing of credit, social responsibility, and respect for students, peers, and research subjects (Shamoo and Resnik 2009).

One reason why integrity is essential in research is that scientists build on each other's work and share information, materials, methods, and ideas. As Isaac Newton once said, "If I have seen further, it is by standing on the shoulders of giants" (Newton 1676). Scientists must be able to trust that the data and results reported in publications are truthful, accurate, and reliable, and that collaborators, editors, and reviewers will honor their obligations and commitments.

Two different types of ethical problems in science can undermine trust: bias and misconduct. The difference between bias and misconduct is that bias may be unintended, whereas misconduct is intentional. Although both bias and misconduct can compromise the integrity of research, misconduct is regarded as a worse ethical transgression because it involves deliberate deception. The person who publishes biased research may be regarded as negligent or incompetent, whereas the person who publishes fraudulent research may be viewed as morally corrupt (Shamoo and Resnik 2009).

Bias

One of the overarching goals of scientific research is to develop knowledge that is free from personal, financial, political, religious, or other biases. Scientific hypotheses and theories should be based on empirical evidence and sound argumentation, not on subjective opinions or beliefs, erroneous assumptions, careless mistakes, political ideologies, or religious dogma. Because scientific knowledge is based on human observations, concepts, and theories, it is impossible to eliminate all types of bias, but scientific methods can help reduce or control for bias. Objectivity is worth pursuing as a goal even it is not completely attainable (Haack 2003; Resnik 2007).

Clinical trials, for example, include several different methods to control for bias. Randomization helps to reduce biases that might arise if investigators or subjects decide which treatment to take. In a clinical trial that compares an experimental drug and one that is already approved (the control), subjects are randomly assigned to receive either the experimental drug or the control. If investigators determine the assignment, they might decide that the healthiest patients should receive the new drug, which could bias the results. Double-blinding helps to control biases related to the placebo effect, a phenomenon in which a person's belief that they are receiving an effective therapy influences their response to treatment. Preventing investigators and subjects from knowing who is receiving the experimental drug or the control helps to counteract biases due to the placebo effect (Gallin 2007).

Science's peer review system also helps to reduce and control bias. When scientists submit a paper to journal, the editors ask independent experts to review the work to determine whether it meets appropriate standards of research and scholarship. In their critical assessment of the paper, reviewers will typically address the following questions: Is the research original and important? Does the evidence support the conclusions? Are the methods well described and appropriate for the research? Have the authors reviewed and cited the appropriate literature? Is the paper well written and organized? Have the authors made any unjustified assumptions? Though the peer review system is not perfect—editors and reviewers sometimes fail to catch obvious errors and other flaws and have their own biases—it is by far the best way of ensuring that published research is accurate, reliable, and significant (Shamoo and Resnik 2009).

Different types of bias can still impact the publication process, despite peer review. One of these is the tendency to publish positive results rather than negative ones. A positive result is evidence showing support for a particular hypothesis, while a negative (or null) result is evidence showing no support for the hypothesis. In clinical research, a positive result could be evidence that an experimental drug is more effective than placebo or that an approved drug is more effective than competing drugs (Easterbrook et al. 1991). Negative results are still published in science, especially when they challenge well known and accepted hypotheses or theories, but they are published less often than positive ones.

The underreporting of negative results can skew the publication record. For example, in meta-analysis scientists use statistical techniques to synthesize data from many different studies. If an investigator performs a meta-analysis of different studies of a particular drug, the analysis may be biased in favor of the drug if it does not include unpublished, negative data, or results. A similar type of bias may arise when a scientist writes a review article that does not include unpublished data or results (Resnik 2007).

There are several reasons for a bias in favor of publishing positive results. First, editors and reviewers may be more interested in positive results rather than negative ones. A study that reports new and exciting positive results is more likely to pique the interest of editors and reviewers than a study that reports negative ones (Olson et al. 2002). Second, investigators may decide not to submit negative results to journals, because they believe there is little chance of publication or they don't regard the results as interesting

(Easterbrook et al. 1991). Third, negative results sometimes have less statistical significance than positive results, and statistical significance is an important factor in editorial decision-making (Dickersin et al. 2002). Fourth, private companies may decide not to publish results that are unfavorable to their products. For example, a pharmaceutical company that sponsors several different studies of its drug might publish only the studies that show its drug is effective (Resnik 2007).

Problems with pharmaceutical company Merck's drug Vioxx illustrate the hazards of repressing negative results. The U.S. Food and Drug Administration (FDA) approved Vioxx in 1999 as a treatment for arthritis and chronic pain. In 2001, Merck scientists possessed data showing that Vioxx increases cardiovascular risks, but the company did not publish these data. Merck sponsored a study, known as the VIGOR trial, which compared Vioxx with other pain medicines. The study showed that patients receiving Vioxx had five times the risk of heart attack or stroke compared with those taking naproxen. The VIGOR study did not include all the cardiovascular risk data. Merck did not publish these data, although it submitted them to the FDA, which treated the data as confidential business information. In 2001, the FDA warned Merck that it had misrepresented Vioxx's safety profile, and in 2002 it issued a black box warning. A subsequent trial, known as the APPROVE study, showed that Vioxx had twice the cardiovascular risks compared with placebo. The study was stopped prematurely in 2002 to protect patients taking Vioxx from risks. On September 30, 2004, Merck withdrew Vioxx due to patient safety and legal liability concerns. Since then, thousands of lawsuits have been filed against the company (Resnik 2007).

Repression of negative results conflicts with the normative ideal of openness. Openness—the sharing of data, methods, materials, and tools—helps advance scientific knowledge by enabling scientists to build on each other's work, thereby saving time, effort, and resources. Openness is also crucial for the exchange of information and ideas that stimulates creativity, innovation, dialogue, criticism, and debate in science. Although some secrecy is justifiable in science for legitimate reasons, such as to protect preliminary work and the confidentiality of research participants or the peer review process, openness that leads to biased results or harms the public is not justifiable (Resnik 2007).

In response to suppression of data by Merck and other pharmaceutical companies, biomedical journals now require clinical trial registration as a condition for publication of research reporting the results of clinical trials. Clinical trial registration involves submitting key information about a study to a public database, such as ClinicalTrials.gov, which is run by the National Library of Medicine. Submitted information includes the treatments under investigation, study design and objectives, methods and procedures, research sites, related publications, and contact information. The FDA also requires registration of most clinical trials, except phase I studies in which drugs or biologics are tested for the first time in human beings to assess their safety (Laine et al. 2007).

Although clinical trial registration can make it more difficult for companies to suppress data, it does not guarantee that all clinical trial data will be published or made otherwise available to investigators or clinicians, because registrants are not required to submit original data. However, there are good reasons for not making all data immediately available to the public, because data must be validated, analyzed, and interpreted prior to publication to deal with errors, inconsistencies, and other problems. Publishing raw clinical trial data on a public website could be misleading. Even though clinical trial registration does not eliminate the problem of data suppression, it makes investigators and clinicians aware of the studies that are being conducted and whom to contact if they want more information (Resnik 2007).

Another way of dealing with the problem of unpublished data is to provide a forum for the publication of negative and non-significant results. Some journals have been established that focus specifically on negative results, such as the *Journal of Negative Results* and the *Journal of Negative Results in Biomedicine* (O'Hara 2011). Others have suggested that computer databases be established to provide open access to unpublished data (Schooler 2011). However, the idea of publishing negative and non-significant results, which has been discussed for two decades, has failed to catch on. One reason why scientists have not made much progress in this direction is that they are not adequately rewarded for publishing negative and non-significant results, since tenure and promotion committees are interested in publications that report positive, significant results. An ethical concern with publishing insignificant results is that they might be misleading due to small sample sizes. Scientists who use these results should be aware of their limitations.

Conflicts of interest (COIs) can also bias research and skew the publication record. Many scientists today have relationships with research sponsors, such as stock or equity, consulting arrangements, and intellectual property, which can bias their judgment and undermine the integrity of research. For example, 11 out of the 12 investigators conducting the VIGOR study had financial ties to Merck (Resnik 2007). There is considerable evidence that financial interests can influence the outcome of a study. A review of the literature on financial interests found that industry-funded clinical trials are more likely to report results that favor a company's product than publicly funded studies (Ridker and Torres 2006). Most journals today have policies that require authors to disclose their financial interests related to the research. Disclosure may not prevent bias, but it at least helps readers to understand the financial relationships that may impact a study, which may be useful in evaluating the research (Resnik and Elliott 2013). A critical examination of the ethics of COIs in science would take us well beyond the main focus of this article, so this topic will not be explored in depth here. For further discussion, see Krimsky (2004), Resnik (2007), and Elliott (2011).

Misconduct

As mentioned earlier, misconduct involves the deliberate violation of science's ethical norms. The U.S. government defines misconduct as fabrication, falsification, or plagiarism (FFP). Fabrication is making up data or results; falsification is changing, omitting, or manipulating data or materials in a way that misrepresents the research; and plagiarism is claiming someone else's words, ideas, methods, data, or images as one's own (Office of Science and Technology Policy 2000). Most organizations include FFP in the definition of misconduct, and some include other misbehaviors, such as interference with a misconduct investigation or egregious violations of rules for conducting research with human or animal subjects (Resnik 2003).

Misconduct is not just unethical; it is also usually illegal. In the U.S., federal regulations prohibit misconduct in research supported by government funds. An individual who is found to have committed misconduct may be barred from receiving federal funds for research. He or she may also receive sanctions from his or her institution, such as loss of employment. In some cases, researchers who have committed misconduct may be prosecuted for criminal fraud. For example, University of Vermont clinical researcher Eric Poehlman was sentenced to serve one year and one day in a federal prison in 2006 for defrauding the government. An investigation by the university found that Poehlman fabricated or falsified data on 17 grant applications (worth $2.9 million) and 10 papers from 1992 to 2001. Seoul National University stem cell scientist Woo Suk Wang, who was found by a university investigation to have fabricated data in two papers on human therapeutic cloning published in the journal *Science* in 2004 and 2005, was sentenced to serve two years in prison in 2009 for embezzlement and bioethics law violations, though his sentence was suspended (Shamoo and Resnik 2009).

It is difficult to get an accurate estimate of the incidence of misconduct, due to limitations of surveys methods. In one survey of 2,000 university faculty and students, 6–9 percent said they had direct knowledge of faculty falsifying data or plagiarizing research (Swazey et al. 1993). Other surveys with similar designs found similar results (Titus et al. 2008). In a more recent survey of over 3,000 federally funded researchers, 0.3 percent admitted that they falsified or cooked data in the last three years (Martinson et al. 2005). Fanelli (2009) examined 21 surveys and 18 meta-analyses of misconduct and found that, on average, about 2 percent of scientists admitted to fabricating or falsifying at least once in their careers and 14 percent said they had observed colleagues falsifying data.

Surveys have potential shortcomings. Surveys in which participants are asked whether they have observed misconduct tend to overestimate the incidence of misconduct because some of the behaviors the participants have observed may appear to be misconduct, but are, in fact, not. The participants may not have sufficient knowledge to determine whether misconduct has occurred. Surveys in which participants report their own misconduct tend to underestimate the incidence of misconduct, because people may not be willing to admit to unethical or illegal behavior, even on an anonymous survey (Shamoo and Resnik 2009).

Steneck (2000) estimated the incidence of misconduct to be 1 event per 100,000 researchers, based on 200 confirmed cases of misconduct in 20 years of National Institutes of Health funded research. This methodology probably grossly underestimates the rate of misconduct, because it only includes data from confirmed cases. Probably many more people commit misconduct than are caught doing it (Titus et al. 2008).

Misconduct has adverse impacts on those directly affected by it (such as individuals who collaborate or study with someone who commits misconduct), the institution, and the research community. A misconduct investigation is burdensome for all involved parties, from the defendant to the witnesses to investigators. It can take several years to completely resolve a misconduct allegation. An investigation can be stressful not only for the defendant but for others as well. Misconduct investigations usually involve major disruptions of scientific work, because records may be seized and research may be suspended, pending the outcome of the investigation. A student who is working with a researcher who is found to have committed misconduct may lose funding and may need to transfer to another university. An innocent researcher who is wrongly accused of misconduct may still have to endure a lengthy investigation, and the researcher's reputation may be damaged. The research community can also be negatively impacted because misconduct can tarnish the integrity of science and erode the public's trust in research (Shamoo and Resnik 2009). And last, but certainly not least, misconduct leads to the publication of fraudulent and erroneous results that undermine the search for knowledge. Scientists who rely, unknowingly, on fabricated or falsified data may be led astray.

There are two different explanations of why misconduct occurs. According to the "bad apples" theory, misconduct is committed by people who are morally corrupt or psychologically unstable. Some cases seem to fit this pattern. For example, in 1974, Sloan Kettering immunology researcher William Summerlin admitted to fabricating data in skin transplant experiments. He was attempting to develop a technique to make white-haired mice accept skin transplants from black-haired mice. His deception was discovered when a laboratory assistant who was cleaning the mice noticed that the black patches on the white mice could be washed off with alcohol. Summerlin admitted that he used a black felt-tip pen to draw the black patches on the white-haired mice. A committee that investigated the incident determined that Summerlin was suffering from mental health problems (Shamoo and Resnik 2009).

In 2002, Bell Laboratories physicist Jan Hendrik Schön was found to have fabricated data in at least 17 publications. Schön was a rising star who had been publishing at an unbelievable rate of a paper every eight days. His papers had appeared in *Science*, *Nature*, *Physical Review Letters*, and other prestigious journals. An investigation by the University of Konstanz, which had awarded Schön his PhD, found that he had also fabricated data in his dissertation. The university revoked his degree (Shamoo and Resnik 2009).

The Summerlin and Schön cases seem to fit the bad apples theory. Summerlin had mental health problems. Indeed, a person who was mentally well would probably not attempt to get away with such an obvious scam. Even if no one detected the initial data fabrication, problems would arise when other investigators attempted to replicate his results. In Schön's case, it seems likely that he was incredibly arrogant to think that he could get away with such a tremendous amount of deception throughout his career. At some point someone would question his unprecedented rise to stardom, and his fraud would be detected.

The other explanation of misconduct is that it is produced by a research environment that encourages unethical behavior. Scientists face tremendous pressures to produce results, publish, and obtain funding. Competition for government grant dollars has grown even more intense as the budgets of funding organizations have shrunk in the recent economic downturn. In defending his actions, Poehlman said that he falsified data because he felt immense pressure to keep grant dollars flowing into his laboratory to support students and staff. The pressure to produce can be overwhelming for post-doctoral fellows, graduate students, and other researchers who depend on grants for their employment (Shamoo and Resnik 2009). In some countries, such as China, the government provides economic incentives for publishing research in top-tier journals and requires graduate students to have a specific number of first-author publications before they can receive their doctorate (Zeng and Resnik 2010). In the United States, hiring, tenure, and promotion decisions are usually based, in large part, on the number of publications one has (Shamoo and Resnik 2009).

Inadequate supervision of students and subordinates can also encourage or at least fail to prevent misbehavior. Many scientists are in charge of large laboratories staffed by students, post-doctoral fellows, and research staff. They sometimes do not take time to explain to their students and subordinates how to design experiments, keep adequate records, analyze data, produce figures and tables, cite articles, and so on. Lab directors (and other supervisory scientists) may fail to communicate properly and inform students and subordinates about research expectations. Additionally, cross-cultural variations in practices related to authorship, plagiarism, data management, and other aspects of scientific behavior may lead to misunderstandings and differences of opinion concerning the ethical conduct of research (Resnik and Shamoo 2009).

Industry ties may also encourage misbehavior. As noted earlier, many scientists today own stock in companies that sponsor their research or have paid positions with industry. Scientists also pursue patents and other forms of intellectual property. These conflicts of interest may encourage not only bias but also misconduct. A scientist who has an economic stake in the outcome of a study may be tempted to cut corners or manipulate data in order to produce results. Since COIs are a risk factor for misconduct, it is important to manage them properly (Shamoo and Resnik 2009).

Additional evidence for the research environment theory is that ethically questionable behaviors, such as inappropriate authorship assignment, republishing data or results without proper citation, violating animal or human research rules, unauthorized use of confidential information, failing to disclose conflicts of interest, and poor record-keeping, are much more common than misconduct (Swazey et al. 1993; Martinson et al. 2005). Researchers who commit minor infractions may be more willing to engage in major transgressions, such as misconduct.

Both of these explanations of misconduct probably contain part of the truth. Psychological factors, such as mental illness and moral depravity, probably play an important role, but so do social and economic factors, such as the pressure to produce results, poor supervision, and financial interests. Efforts to prevent misconduct via education, mentoring, policy development, and enforcement should therefore take all of these different factors into account. Though education and mentoring may have little impact on researchers who are "bad apples," they may help guide ordinary researchers who are tempted to bend or break the rules or who do not understand what is expected of them.

Preventing misconduct needs to be a top priority for research institutions. Some strategies for prevention include education and mentoring on the responsible conduct of research, policy development, institutional leadership involving a commitment to ethics, mechanisms for reporting misconduct and other ethical concerns, and enforcement of ethics policies. Additionally, institutions should consider reforming their hiring and promotion practices so that there is less emphasis on the quantity of publications (Titus et al. 2008; Shamoo and Resnik 2009; Koocher and Keith-Spiegel 2010).

Deciding whether to report misconduct can be a difficult dilemma for would-be whistle-blowers because fulfilling the ethical duty to report suspected misconduct can come at considerable personal expense. Witnesses must be available to testify, which can take time and effort and cause stress. If the defendant is the accuser's supervisor, the accuser may lose his job or need to transfer to another institution if the defendant is fired. In some cases, the accuser may fear retribution from the defendant or others. Although federal and state laws protect whistle-blowers from direct retaliation, such as loss of employment or demotion, other repercussions may still happen. A whistle-blower may be shunned or branded as a trouble-maker, for example. Of course, in some situations the whistle-blower may be implicated in misconduct if he does not report it. For example, if the whistle-blower is a co-author on a paper in which he believes one of his collaborators has faked data, then he may face a misconduct allegation if he does nothing and someone else discovers the impropriety. Whistle-blowers must therefore consider their options carefully when deciding whether to report misconduct. They should make sure that they have not misinterpreted the defendant's behavior and that they have sufficient evidence to make an accusation (Shamoo and Resnik 2009; Malek 2010).

A recent example of whistle-blowing occurred when research assistants and a graduate student working in Harvard psychology professor Marc Hauser's laboratory in 2007 suspected that he had fabricated data concerning pattern recognition experiments in monkeys. In these experiments, an animal listens to a sound pattern played repeatedly through a speaker, and then the pattern is changed. If the animal looks at the speaker when the pattern changes researchers infer that the animal can recognize sound patterns. In the experiment, two independent observers, Hauser and an assistant, coded videotaped monkey responses. To reduce bias, both observers were not allowed to hear the sound. A second assistant analyzed the results and found that while Hauser's coding indicated that the monkeys recognized sound patterns, the assistant's did not. The second assistant and a graduate student asked Hauser if they could recode his data to make sure they were correct, but Hauser refused. The assistant and the student then recoded Hauser's data without his permission, and they found that the videotaped behavior bore little relation to what Hauser claimed that he observed. The assistants and the student consulted other people in Hauser's laboratory and found that they had similar concerns about his work for several years. The whistle-blowers made an official allegation to the university ombudsman, which led to an informal inquiry and then a misconduct investigation. In August 2010, a Harvard committee determined that Hauser committed eight counts of research misconduct. In August 2011, Hauser resigned his position at Harvard. He has not admitted to misconduct, though he does claim to regret some mistakes he made (Gross 2011). In 2012, the Office of Research Integrity (ORI) reviewed Hauser's case and determined that he had fabricated and falsified data in several publications. Under the terms of the agreement reached with ORI, Hauser's research must be supervised for three years. Hauser did not admit that he committed misconduct as part of the agreement, though he did admit that ORI had evidence that he did (Office of Research Integrity 2012).

The Hauser case illustrates several important points about bias and misconduct. First, the methods used in cognitive ethology are designed to reduce bias, so that researchers will not inappropriately infer that animals display human-like behaviors. Assigning two people to independently code data concerning the animal's behavior without knowledge of whether the sound pattern has been changed provides a way of producing results that are reliable and replicable. It also minimizes the chance that the coders will draw conclusions based on what they expect or hope to observe. One of the main problems with Hauser's research, according to the investigatory committee, is that he did not follow these methods properly (Gross 2011). Second, Hauser's research has misled the scientific community, because he published results that cannot be verified or replicated. He made bold claims about pattern recognition in monkeys, some of which do not stand up to further scrutiny. Third, the entire incident has caused considerable harm to Hauser, Harvard University, and the field of animal cognition. Hauser's reputation and career prospects have been damaged permanently. These and other adverse consequences underscore the importance of preventing bias and misconduct in research.

Conclusion

Bias and misconduct are unethical because they undermine the integrity of research and erode the public's support for science. It is crucial for scientists to avoid them, and to teach their students and staff how to avoid them. Institutions, government agencies, and journals can help promote the responsible conduct of research by developing policies that prohibit misconduct and promote the objective reporting of data and results. Institutions and government agencies can also support education and mentoring in the responsible conduct of research by providing scientists with teaching resources and requiring that students, trainees, and others receive instruction in research ethics.

Acknowledgments

This article is the work product of an employee or group of employees of the National Institute of Environmental Health Sciences (NIEHS), National Institutes of Health (NIH). The statements, opinions, and conclusions contained herein do not necessarily represent the statements, opinions, or conclusions of NIEHS, NIH, or the U.S. government.

Related Topics

Chapter 11, "Intellectual Property in the Biomedical Sciences," Justin B. Biddle
Chapter 19, "The Ethics of Incentives for Participation in Research: What's the Problem?" Alan Wertheimer

References

Dickersin, K., Olson, C.M., Rennie, D., Cook, D., Flanagin, A., Zhu, Q., Reiling, J. and Pace, B. (2002) "Association Between Time Interval to Publication and Statistical Significance," *Journal of the American Medical Association* 287: 2829–31.

Easterbrook, P.J., Berlin, J.A., Gopalan, R. and Matthews, D.R. (1991) "Publication Bias in Clinical Research," *Lancet* 337: 867–72.

Elliott, K.C. (2011) *Is a Little Pollution Good for You? Incorporating Societal Values in Environmental Research*, New York: Oxford University Press.

Fanelli, D. (2009) "How Many Scientists Fabricate and Falsify Research? A Systematic Review and Meta-analysis of Survey Data," *PLoS One* 4 (5): e5738.

Gallin, J. (2007) *Principles and Practice of Clinical Research* (2nd edition), Burlington, MA: Academic Press.

Gross, C. (2011) "Disgrace: on Marc Hauser," *The Nation* December 21, 2011. Available at: http://www.thenation.com/article/165313/disgrace-marc-hauser (accessed December 29, 2011).

Haack, S. (2003) *Defending Science within Reason*, New York: Prometheus Books.

Koocher, G.P. and Keith-Spiegel, P. (2010) "Peers Nip Misconduct in the Bud," *Nature* 466: 438–40.

Krimsky, S. (2004) *Science in the Private Interest: Has the Lure of Profits Corrupted Biomedical Research?* Lanham, MD: Rowman and Littlefield.

Laine, C., De Angelis, C., Delamothe, T., Drazen, J.M., Frizelle, F.A., Haug, C., Hébert, P.C., Horton, R., Kotzin, S., Marusic, A., Sahni, P., Schroeder, T.V., Sox, H.C., Van der Weyden, M.B. and Verheugt, F.W. (2007) "Clinical Trial Registration: Looking Back and Moving Ahead," *Annals of Internal Medicine* 147: 275–7.

Malek, J. (2010) "To Tell or Not To Tell? The Ethical Dilemma of the Would-Be Whistleblower," *Accountability in Research* 17: 115–29.

Martinson, B., Anderson, M. and De Vries, R. (2005) "Scientists Behaving Badly," *Nature* 435: 737–8.

Newton, I. (1676) Letter to Robert Hooke. February 5, 1676.

Office of Research Integrity (2012) "Case Summary: Hauser, Marc." Available at: http://ori.dhhs.gov/content/case-summary-hauser-marc (accessed June 24, 2013).

Office of Science and Technology Policy (2000) "Federal Research Misconduct Policy," *Federal Register* 65 (235): 76262.

O'Hara, B. (2011) "Negative Results Are Published," *Nature* 471: 448–9.

Olson, C.M., Rennie, D., Cook, D., Dickersin, K., Flanagin, A., Hogan, J.W., Zhu, Q., Reiling, J. and Pace, B. (2002) "Publication Bias in Editorial Decision Making," *Journal of the American Medical Association* 287: 2825–8.

Resnik, D.B. (2003) "From Baltimore to Bell Labs: Reflections on Two Decades of Debate about Scientific Misconduct," *Accountability in Research* 10: 123–5.

Resnik, D.B. (2007) *The Price of Truth: How Money Affects the Norms of Science*, New York: Oxford University Press.

Resnik, D.B. and Elliott, K.C. (2013) "Taking Financial Relationships into Account When Assessing Research," *Accountability in Research* 20: 184–205.

Ridker, P. and Torres, J. (2006) "Reported Outcomes in Major Cardiovascular Clinical Trials Funded by For-Profit and Not-for-Profit Organizations: 2000–2005," *Journal of the American Medical Association* 295: 2270–4.

Schooler, J. (2011) "Unpublished Results Hide the Decline Effect," *Nature* 470: 437.

Shamoo, A.S. and Resnik, D.B. (2009) *Responsible Conduct of Research*, 2nd edition. New York: Oxford University Press.

Steneck N. (2000) "Assessing the Integrity of Publicly Funded Research," in *Proceedings from the ORI Conference on Research Integrity*, Washington, DC: Office of Research Integrity.

Swazey, J.P., Anderson, M. and Louis, K. (1993) "Ethical Problems in Academic Research," *American Scientist* 81: 542–53.

Titus, S.L., Wells, J.A. and Rhoades, L.J. (2008) "Repairing Research Integrity," *Nature* 453: 980–2.

Zeng, W. and Resnik, D.B. (2010) "Research Integrity in China: Problems and Prospects," *Developing World Bioethics* 10: 164–71.

13

INFLUENCE OF THE PHARMACEUTICAL INDUSTRY ON RESEARCH AND CLINICAL CARE

Howard Brody

Since the beginning of the twenty-first century, bioethicists have begun to pay serious attention to the influence that the pharmaceutical and medical-device industries exert over both medical research and patient care. Most authorities agree that the main ethical concern, if there is one, is conflict of interest. According to one viewpoint, the main goal of research is discovery of scientific truths for the benefit of the health of future patients, and the main goal of clinical care is the health benefit of the patient receiving attention. While it is possible that the drug and device industries can maximize their profits while also serving these goals, in too many cases there is a conflict between the goal of patient benefit and the goal of profit maximization. In such cases, influence exerted by industry may be deleterious to patients. To the extent that health care professionalism is defined as giving highest priority to the interests of patients, then industry influence becomes a threat to professionalism.

Alternative points of view dispute this portrayal. One such view is that the entrepreneurialism of industry provides a net patient benefit, through continued innovation in health care, so that any interference with the current system of relationships of physicians and medical scientists with industry would result in significant patient harm. Another related view is that the very idea of "conflict of interest," in this context, is vague and incoherent, and amounts to an *ad hominem* attack rather than a tool of ethical analysis.

Accordingly, a discussion of the bioethical significance of industry influence ought to answer these questions:

1. What are the available facts regarding the influence of industry over medical research and clinical care?
2. How is "conflict of interest" defined by those who believe that it serves a useful function in bioethical analysis?
3. What arguments are raised against the above view of "conflict of interest"?
4. If industry influence is detrimental to patient interests, with whom does the major responsibility lie?

Factual Concerns

Since about 2004, a number of book-length treatments expressing concern about the consequences of industry influence over medicine have appeared (Abramson 2004; Angell 2004; Kassirer 2005; Avorn 2004; Brody 2007; Weber 2006) though some books raising similar concerns were published much earlier (Silverman and Lee 1974; Braithwaite 1984). These works amass a considerable body of data showing that deleterious consequences arise from industry influence.

The degree of industry influence is substantial. One analysis claimed that in 2004 the total expenditures for marketing drugs to physicians and patients in the U.S. totaled $57 billion, many times the total budget for all medical schools and residency training programs (Gagnon and Lexchin 2008). Surveys showed that 94 percent of American practitioners reported some sort of contact with pharmaceutical marketers in 2004; by 2009 the number had dropped slightly, to 84 percent (Campbell et al. 2007, 2010).

Regarding clinical practice, a recent review systematically analyzed 58 published studies of the results of industry influence. The authors concluded that the majority of the studies showed that industry influence over practitioners was associated with a higher number of prescriptions, higher costs of prescriptions, and less rational prescribing. Virtually no studies found the opposite effects (Spurling et al. 2010).

A repeated finding in studies of physician attitudes is that while industry marketing appears to influence physician behavior, physicians themselves routinely deny that they are influenced in this manner (Orlowski and Wateska 1992). Physicians routinely report that they personally remain uninfluenced by industry marketing strategies, while admitting that their peers are readily swayed by the same types of marketing (Steinman et al. 2001).

Currently, a large majority of clinical studies related to pharmaceuticals are funded by industry. Numerous studies comparing commercially sponsored medical research with research funded by government agencies or non-profit foundations demonstrate a systematically greater likelihood that industry-funded research will favor the drug under study, by up to a four-fold difference (Lexchin et al. 2003). A particularly worrisome aspect of industry marketing is the practice of ghostwriting, in which medical writers hired by firms paid by a drug company write articles favorable to the company's drug, which are then submitted to widely read journals under the name of a respected academic physician, with no admission of the role of the hired writer (Leo et al. 2011). Ghostwriting assures that the commercial firm will exercise the maximum control over the content of the article, while creating the impression that the true author is an academic expert who is presumably unbiased. In the more extreme cases, what are actually infomercials touting a drug are disguised as scientific publications.

Influencing individual physicians to prescribe drugs for patients that may be inferior to alternative drugs, or to non-drug therapies such as diet and exercise, causes harm to individual patients. Exerting marketing control over the content of the medical literature, by contrast, potentially harms a much larger number of patients, because even physicians who conscientiously avoid industry marketing will be unable to tell the difference between scientifically valid results and industry-biased reporting. Increasingly, physicians rely on clinical practice guidelines written by expert panels to summarize scientific data in usable form. Studies have shown that many physicians sitting on these panels, as well as the organizations that produce the guidelines, receive substantial sums of money from the industry and so may be biased (Choudhry et al. 2002; Rose 2008).

One telling illustration of the degree to which the medical literature can be skewed through commercial influence is provided by a study of 12 different antidepressant drugs. The authors compared the published literature with the data supplied to the U.S. Food and Drug Administration (FDA) by the firms seeking approval to market their drugs (the latter obtained through the *Freedom of Information Act* as the FDA usually protects proprietary industry information from public release) (Turner et al. 2008). The authors found that about half of the clinical trials of these antidepressants failed to show that the drug was superior to placebo. The vast majority of these negative studies either were never published in medical journals, or were published with "spin" to represent the results as being positive. If a physician were to consult only the published literature, it would appear that scientific evidence strongly supported the efficacy of these medications. If the same physician had access to the complete and unbiased body of clinical trial data, it would seem a toss-up as to whether these drugs were effective or not.

An "Inverse Benefit Law" has been proposed to describe the relationship between pharmaceutical marketing and patient benefit (Brody and Light 2011). The "Law" (a heuristic device) claims that the ratio between benefit and harm of a drug turns more unfavorable the more vigorously the drug is marketed. To market a drug, a company must persuade physicians to lower the threshold at which the drug is prescribed, so that a larger percentage of the total patient population become candidates. As a rule, a drug is most beneficial when used among patients with the severest symptoms or the most severe physiological abnormality. An antihypertensive drug, for instance, will usually benefit someone whose baseline blood pressure is 180/110 much more than someone whose pressure is 150/95. Adverse reactions to drugs, by contrast, are randomly spread throughout the entire patient population. Therefore, lowering the prescribing threshold and exposing more patients with milder disease to the drug reduces population benefit and increases population harm.

In summary, the pharmaceutical industry spends considerable resources to influence both medical practice and medical science. The available evidence suggests that this influence has the potential to harm patient interests. Patients may be harmed when individual practitioners are influenced by contacts with drug sales representatives, for example, and prescribe less effective or less safe products. A more basic level of harm arises when the scientific evidence base is distorted by commercial influence over scientific research and publication. We assume that most of what is true of the pharmaceutical industry is also true of the medical device industry, but the latter industry has been less thoroughly studied.

Understanding Conflict of Interest

An often-quoted definition of "conflict of interest" in medicine is: "a set of conditions in which professional judgment concerning a primary interest (such as the patient's welfare or the validity of research) tends to be unduly influenced by a secondary interest (such as financial gain)" (Thompson 1993: 573). Arthur Schafer (2004) has objected to this definition, noting that it trivializes the problem to see it as a conflict between competing *interests*. Physicians have an *interest* in receiving such gifts and emoluments from industry as free dinners, consulting and speaking fees, and research grants. By contrast, physicians have a *duty* to protect the patient's welfare and the integrity of research.

Ed Erde (1996) provides a more in-depth discussion of the definition of "conflict of interest." He notes first that the basic notion that conflict of interest addresses is *trust in a social role*. This means that the often-cited distinction between "conflict of interest" and "apparent conflict of interest" is frequently spurious. The appearance of a conflict of interest can be just as destructive of trust as actual bad behavior.

Erde proceeds to suggest that two further distinctions *are* pertinent to describing a conflict. First, a physician may have a motive to act in a way that violates a professional duty; or she may merely have entered into certain social arrangements that increase a tendency or temptation to neglect that professional duty. The available evidence strongly suggests that an actual motive to neglect or violate professional duty is rare, and most conflicts in practice consist of entering into social arrangements that constitute serious temptations to neglect duties (such as relying on drug salespeople or detailers for information about new drugs rather than taking the time to consult less biased, evidence-based information sources).

A second distinction is between entering into the wrong sorts of arrangements without violating one's duty, and actually succumbing to the temptation and violating a duty. For example, one physician-scientist might accept company grants and consulting and speaker's fees while still remaining rigorous in conducting unbiased research. A different scientist might accept those fees and, as a result, allow his name to be attached to a ghostwritten article that inappropriately recommends a less beneficial or even harmful drug. The appropriate moral response in the first case is a warning, while in the second case it is moral condemnation. Again, the record suggests that the need for warning is a much more common occurrence in today's practice than outright bad moral behavior.

While Erde tries to describe a topology of conflict of interest rather than providing a single definition, it seems possible to employ his insights and to construct the following definition: *A conflict of interest exists in medicine when the following conditions have all been met:*

1. The physician has a duty to advocate for the interests of the patient (or public).
2. The physician is also subject to other interests—her own, or those of a third party.
3. The physician becomes a party to certain social arrangements.
4. Those arrangements, as viewed by a reasonable onlooker, would tempt a person of normal human psychology to neglect the patient's/public's interests in favor of the physician's (or third party's).

(Brody 2011)

This definition makes it clear that to allege a conflict of interest is not to accuse a physician of actually violating duties to patients. Rather, such an allegation points out a situation in which public trust in medicine could be weakened, through the reasonable interpretation that the physician would be strongly tempted to neglect duties to patients in that situation.

The next ethical question is whether a conflict of interest, having been identified, can best be handled by management or avoidance. Many recent guidelines promulgated by medical institutions speak predominantly of "managing" conflicts of interest, assuming that they cannot be eliminated or else that it would be undesirable to do so. A case example where management seems the appropriate strategy might be a research trial involving a novel device that shows great therapeutic promise. One particular surgeon has invented this device and has invested in a biotechnology firm that has agreed to develop the device. No other physician currently has enough experience with this device to design and administer a clinical trial. To allow this physician to serve as the principal investigator in a clinical trial of this device, while appointing a special oversight committee to review all aspects of the trial design and conduct to be sure that the physician's financial interests in the device do not affect scientific integrity, might be the best way to handle this particular situation.

In other situations, however, the better approach might be to prohibit conflicts of interest and to demand that academic physicians divest themselves of conflicted financial ties to industry. Many commentators have characterized the "management" strategy as a too-facile acceptance of the status quo, and have called for a divestment strategy as superior in most cases (Schafer 2004; Kassirer 2005; Brody 2007). While a physician cannot be accused of violating duties to patients merely because a conflict of interest exists, a physician can be held ethically accountable for entering into social arrangements of the sort where neglect of patient duties becomes much more likely. This is especially so when the arrangements are not necessary for the conduct of clinical care or scientific research. No physician *needs* to visit regularly with drug detailers or accept free dinners from them in order to provide quality patient care. No investigator *needs* to accept speaker or consulting fees from a drug or device company in order to do research.

For many years such arrangements were accepted as part of the medical landscape and shielded from criticism. More recently, ethical concern has mounted over these practices and calls have increased for their prohibition (Brennan et al. 2006; Lo and Field 2009). One sign of the effectiveness of this ethical criticism is a step taken by the Pharmaceutical Research and Manufacturers of America (PhRMA), the national organization representing brand-name drug firms. In January 2009, PhRMA voluntarily inaugurated a new set of guidelines that eliminated many common marketing practices—perhaps most notably, pens and other "reminder items" emblazoned with the names of drugs. These guidelines were voluntary for industry and skeptical questions were raised as to their actual impact (PhRMA 2008). The point, however, is that the climate of public perception had changed sufficiently so that PhRMA apparently felt that previous marketing practices were unsustainable, and it was necessary to create at least the appearance of reform.

Conflict of Interest: Objections

The increased scrutiny of pharmaceutical marketing practices appears to represent a widely held ethical view, but a small but vocal group has raised some objections. This group of critics includes members of the Association of Clinical Researchers and Investigators, who appear especially concerned to advocate for free-market solutions in health care. One objection focuses especially on the concept of "conflict of interest."

Philosopher Lance Stell objects to current usage of "conflict of interest" as an epithet that amounts to an illogical *ad hominem* attack rather than a substantive mode of ethical inquiry (Stell 2009). He argues, first, that conflicts of interest are ubiquitous in medicine, as evidenced by the long history of fee-for-service payment (in which physicians are tempted to do extra, unnecessary procedures in order to maximize income). Fiduciaries, he states, are generally conflicted in multiple ways; it is simply unrealistic to imagine that one set of conflicts, financial ties to drug manufacturers, are uniquely incapacitating of one's ability to adhere to one's duties to patients.

Stell next notes the subjective elements of definitions like Erde's, "reasonable onlooker," "tempt a person of normal human psychology," etc. For a term to be of use in ethical inquiry, he suggests, there ought to be a reasonably agreed-upon, objective threshold for its application. There is no such agreed-upon standard for conflict of interest.

Hence this term can serve only as a kind of name-calling. Conflict-of-interest guidelines, Stell asserts, violate the industry's rights to free commercial speech, and potentially deny physicians useful information and resources that can benefit patients.

Stell's objections are open to several rebuttals. If, as Erde claims, the basic concept underlying conflict of interest is trust in a social role, then it is not surprising that the concept includes an irreducible element of subjectivity, since it is a subjective judgment when trust has been violated and how severely. Stell also appears to dispute the evidence summarized in an earlier section, and tends to assume that financial relationships will probably lead only to beneficial exchanges of information between medicine and industry. Finally, he lumps financial conflicts of interest with all other sources of bias that afflict medical science and practice. While it is indeed unrealistic to imagine one could eliminate all those sources of bias, financial conflicts of interest are generally unnecessary for medical practice and research and could in theory at least be eliminated. In addition, many other sources of bias, such as the desire of scientists to confirm their favored hypotheses, are obvious to the scientific reader. By contrast, financial conflicts of interest would remain hidden unless specific disclosure policies are adopted. Sander Greenland, an epidemiologist, has looked at different sources of investigator bias from a biostatistician's standpoint and argues that the rational reader, concerned to know the likelihood that the conclusions of a given study are true, would wish to be informed about financial conflicts of interest as a distinct, important category (Greenland 2009).

Law professor Richard Epstein (2007) agrees with Stell that conflicts of interest are ubiquitous, so that it is arbitrary to single out financial or gift ties between physicians and drug/device companies as particularly problematic. He adds the further concern that the cost of regulating or policing conflicts of interest would be greater than the cost of a laissez-faire approach. Citing the adage, "Who guards the guardians?" he argues that any oversight system would do little more than introduce an additional layer of further conflicts of interest, leading to an infinite regress. Epstein ignores two logical implications of his position, however: First, that all attempted regulation of commercial transactions is vain; and second, that there is no effective possibility of professional self-regulation (an odd position for a law professor to adopt). The most effective rebuttal to Epstein's claims would be a reasonable set of proposals for regulating financial conflicts of interest in medicine. I will discuss some such proposals briefly below.

Harmful Effects of Influence: Objections

Presumably, the whole reason to try to identify and deal with conflicts of interest in this area is because of the dangers of harm to patient interests. While a great many works have documented a large number of examples of possible harms, a few have objected that these harms are in fact illusory.

Stell has joined forces with physician-investigator Thomas Stossel to argue that patients are best served by a robust system of financial ties between physicians and medical scientists with industry (Stell and Stossel 2011). As in other areas of life, financial incentives work to stimulate the maximum effort toward innovation, leading to improved cures. If "professional" efforts to rein in conflicts of interest were successful, innovation would be severely curtailed, leading to significant harm to patients in the future. Stossel argues further that the examples cited by critics of the deleterious consequences of industry influence over science and practice are unrepresentative and constitute unreliable anecdotal evidence. Presumably, critics of the drug industry object to the publication of biased research reports because these make it difficult for physicians to practice evidence-based medicine. If the critics were consistent, then they would require the same high evidence-based standards before accusing the industry of exerting a deleterious influence over medical practice and research. This evidentiary standard, argues Stossel, is one from which critics have fallen short (Stossel 2007).

It is worth asking what would count as evidence for a deleterious influence that would meet the high standards Stossel recommends. Focus for now on medical practice only. It is often held that the gold standard for evidence of a causal connection is a randomized controlled trial. Meeting Stossel's standards of evidence would require that medical students, on matriculation, be randomly assigned to two groups. One group would be encouraged to have maximum contact with drug industry representatives and marketing, while the other would be strictly forbidden to have such contact. After perhaps 10 years, the health of the patients cared for by the two groups of physicians would be measured and compared. Only if the health of the patients of the second group of physicians was significantly better than that of the first group would the conclusion be allowed that industry marketing exerted a negative influence over medical practice.

The point about this hypothetical randomized trial is its utter impracticality. Since no such definitive trial is ever going to be conducted, a better question is the degree to which the partial, incomplete evidence assembled to date is sufficiently suggestive to yield policy recommendations. As noted, the review by Spurling and colleagues (2010) suggests a substantial unanimity in the direction of findings among the available research studies, all tending in the direction that the influence of industry contact among practitioners yields potentially deleterious effects. Since Stell and Stossel apparently remain unpersuaded by the evidence amassed by investigators such as Spurling et al., one has to question whether, by demanding "better quality" evidence, they are deliberately setting the bar so high as to be practically unreachable.

Defenders of close financial relationships between medicine and the pharmaceutical industry commonly cite a series of research studies by the economist Frank Lichtenberg (2001). Lichtenberg has searched large databases and concluded that there is a close association between greater life expectancy and higher expenditures for newer, brand-name drugs. The implication is that physicians who have closer contacts with industry marketers are more likely to prescribe such drugs (a finding with which Spurling et al. (2010) would concur). Since the result of prescribing more of these drugs is patients who live longer, whatever influence the industry exerts over physicians is beneficial. There are, however, several problems with the methods used by Lichtenberg (Law and Grepin 2010). To mention just two concerns related to biological implausibility, Lichtenberg's methodology appears to assume that a new brand-name antihistamine for allergies is as likely to extend patients' lives as a drug to prevent heart attacks, and that a drug that is preventive in nature, and so might at best reduce mortality after a 5–10-year lag period, can demonstrate reduced mortality in the first year after it is prescribed. Moreover, considerable evidence exists to show that a number of widely prescribed, newer, brand-name drugs are no better than older generics, or else have little beneficial effect on health outcomes (Leucht et al. 2009; Gale 2001; Roberts 2012).

Assigning Ethical Responsibility

Even if some of the objections defending closer ties between medicine and industry appear to be plausible if not conclusive, one might accept for purposes of argument that the case has been made that conflicts of interest at the interface between medicine and the drug and device industries threaten patients' health. Assuming this to be the case, the final question is where ethical responsibility lies for taking effective remedial action.

I will address three arguments:

1. Fault lies primarily with the industry, and the correct action is tighter government regulation.
2. Fault lies at least in part with industry, and a part of the solution lies in more ethical business practices.
3. Fault lies to a large degree within the medical profession, and solutions require a heightened sense of and dedication to high professional standards of behavior.

Assigning primary responsibility to industry may seem warranted in light of the frequency with which industry behavior crosses the line from the ethically questionable to the illegal. Sociologist John Braithwaite alleged as long ago as 1984 that the global pharmaceutical industry was disproportionately engaged in corporate crime (Braithwaite 1984). More recently, drug firms have prominently led the list of U.S. corporations settling with the Federal government over allegations of illegal acts, in some cases paying fines in excess of $1 billion (Feeley and Fisk 2012). The fact that several of these companies are repeat offenders suggests that skating as close as possible to legal limits is seen by industry as a routine business practice. Sen. Charles Grassley (R-IA) has been a consistent critic of the industry and has led investigations into its misdeeds (Wadman 2009). The *Federal Sunshine Act*, which became law as a part of the *Affordable Care Act* of 2010, is a significant legislative step to require public access to information about payments made by drug firms to physicians (Anonymous 2012).

Leonard Weber suggested a somewhat different approach in his study of the business ethics of the pharmaceutical industry (Weber 2006). Weber argued that the current behavior of the industry, which threatens medical professionalism through promoting deleterious conflicts of interest, falls distinctly short of the ethical responsibility of these firms as good corporate citizens. On the assumption that ethical business behavior is, in the long run, in the interests of the industry as well as society generally, Weber proceeds to argue for reforms that can be brought about within the drug industry.

These two approaches are not necessarily in competition. In the present climate, a single drug or device firm that chooses to act more ethically might lose market share when competitors are not similarly constrained. Appropriate government regulation might level the playing field and thereby encourage enhanced attention to ethics among the firms.

Other authors have focused more on the responsibility of the medical profession itself to police the interface with the pharmaceutical and device industries (Kassirer 2005; Brody 2007). On this line of argument, when companies ignore ethics, patient well-being, and sound science in order to maximize profit, they are simply doing what they are expected to do in a capitalist society. On completion of their business degrees, corporate executives swore no oath to protect patients and adhere to the integrity of medical practice, but physicians did. The primary obligation, therefore, lies with physicians and scientists to refuse to collaborate with industry in ways that create serious conflicts of interest. It is important to note, for example, that all drug detailers would be out of a job tomorrow if all physicians refused to see them; and drug company speakers' bureaus would largely cease to exist if all physicians declined to participate. That physicians and medical scientists so frequently accept the gifts and payments offered by industry reflects much more on their own professionalism than on industry ethics.

The marketing of medical drugs and devices is a complex activity. Kalman Applbaum, an anthropologist, analyzes industry behavior in terms of "controlling the channels," by which he means that the company seeks to manage every aspect of a drug from discovery through manufacture through its eventual prescription to patients (Applbaum 2009). It would seem to follow that a program to achieve ethically optimal discovery and use of drugs and devices would need to be similarly complex and multi-faceted. Appropriate government regulations, an enhanced sense of business ethics, and greater attention to professional responsibilities would all seem to be vital parts of an overall program of reform (Brody 2007).

Those like Stell (2009) and Epstein (2007) who dismiss concerns about conflicts of interest allege that any set of regulations addressing this pseudo-problem would simply add unnecessary and ineffective layers of bureaucracy. Indeed this argument might have merit if close financial ties between medical scientists and the pharmaceutical industry were absolutely essential for desired innovation to occur; intrusive efforts to police the financial ties might well then detract from an environment fully conducive to innovation and discovery. But as Schafer (2004) pointed out, all arguments in favor of close connections between the drug industry and the medical profession call for the ready exchange *of information* so as to facilitate innovation. There is, Schafer notes, no reason besides habit and greed to imagine that this exchange of information need be accompanied in all cases by an exchange of *money*. The ideal direction for reforms, both intraprofessional and governmentally imposed, would therefore be to assure that information flows freely but without the corrupting influence of gifts of value. In the realm of medical practice, for example, there already exist a number of sources of commercially unbiased information about pharmaceuticals; the question is whether practitioners will develop the professional integrity to seek out those sources and refuse to see industry sales representatives as their preferred source of information (and free lunches and dinners) (Evans et al. 2013). By contrast, removing inappropriate financial incentives in research will probably require more than professional action alone; many believe that ultimately, the financing of clinical trials needs to be removed from industry and placed in the hands of a neutral government agency such as the National Institutes of Health (Avorn 2004; Brody 2007).

If intraprofessional reforms have an important role to play in governing conflicts of interest, then the education of future physicians and other professionals becomes paramount. It is encouraging in this regard that some of the earliest calls for substantial reforms came from leaders of academic medical centers, and many such centers have made great progress in removing sources of industry influence (Brennan et al. 2006).

While I have assumed that medical devices raise most of the same ethical issues as drugs, and require many of the same measures to address conflicts of interest, there are a few important differences. One is the greater importance of hands-on contact with the sales representative in the case of devices. Devices often require practical demonstration before physicians can use them properly and many device representatives are highly trained biomedical engineers. While the need for this hands-on contact can easily be exploited by device companies, it cannot be easily eliminated. Regulations for device marketing will of necessity be different from those for drugs.

Related Topics

Chapter 11, "Intellectual Property in the Biomedical Sciences," Justin B. Biddle
Chapter 12, "Bias, Misconduct, and Integrity in Scientific Research," David B. Resnik

References

Abramson, J. (2004) *Overdo$ed America: The Broken Promise of American Medicine*, New York: HarperCollins.

Angell, M. (2004) *The Truth about the Drug Companies: How They Deceive Us and What to Do about It*, New York: Random House.

Anonymous (2012) "Of Doctors and Drug Makers [editorial]," *Los Angeles Times*, January 27.

Applbaum, K. (2009) "Getting to Yes: Corporate Power and the Creation of a Psychopharmaceutical Blockbuster," *Culture, Medicine and Psychiatry* 33: 185–215.

Avorn, J. (2004) *Powerful Medicines: The Benefits, Risks and Costs of Prescription Drugs*, New York: Knopf.

Braithwaite, J. (1984) *Corporate Crime in the Pharmaceutical Industry*, Boston: Routledge & Kegan Paul.

Brennan, T.A., Rothman, D.J., Blank, L., et al. (2006) "Health Industry Practices that Create Conflicts of Interest: A Policy Proposal for Academic Medical Centers," *JAMA* 295: 429–33.

Brody, H. (2007) *Hooked: Ethics, the Medical Profession, and the Pharmaceutical Industry*, Lanham, MD: Rowman and Littlefield.

Brody, H. (2011) "Clarifying Conflicts of Interest," *American Journal of Bioethics* 11 (1): 23–8.

Brody, H. and Light, D.W. (2011) "The Inverse Benefit Law: How Drug Marketing Undermines Patient Safety and Public Health," *American Journal of Public Health* 101: 399–404.

Campbell, E.G., Gruen, R.L., Mountford, J., Miller, L.G., Cleary, P.D. and Blumenthal, D. (2007) "A National Survey of Physician–Industry Relationships," *New England Journal of Medicine* 356: 1742–50.

Campbell, E.G., Rao, S.R., Desroches, C.M., Iezzoni, L.I., Vogeli, C., Bolcic-Jankovic, D. and Miralles, P.D. (2010) "Physician Professionalism and Changes in Physician–Industry Relationships from 2004 to 2009," *Archives of Internal Medicine* 170: 1820–6.

Choudhry, N.K., Stelfox, H.T. and Detsky, A.S. (2002). "Relationships between Authors of Clinical Practice Guidelines and the Pharmaceutical Industry," *JAMA* 287: 612–17.

Epstein, R.A. (2007) "Conflicts of Interest in Health Care: Who Guards the Guardians?" *Perspectives in Biology and Medicine* 50: 72–88.

Erde, E.L. (1996) "Conflicts of Interest in Medicine: A Philosophical and Ethical Morphology," in R.G. Speece, D.S. Shimm and A.E. Buchanan (eds.) *Conflicts of Interest in Clinical Practice and Research*, New York: Oxford University Press.

Evans, D., Hartung, D.M., Beasley, D. and Fagnan, L.J. (2013). "Breaking Up Is Hard to Do: Lessons Learned from a Pharm-Free Practice Transformation," *Journal of the American Board of Family Medicine* 26: 332–8.

Feeley, J. and Fisk, M.C. (2012) "Abbott to Pay $1.6 Billion to Settle Depakote Drug Allegations," *Business Week/Bloomberg News*, May 8.

Gagnon, M.A. and Lexchin, J. (2008) "The Cost of Pushing Pills: A New Estimate of Pharmaceutical Promotion Expenditures in the United States," *PLoS Medicine* 5 (1): e1.

Gale, E.A. (2001) "Lessons from the Glitazones: A Story of Drug Development," *Lancet* 357: 1870–5.

Greenland, S. (2009) "Accounting for Uncertainty about Investigator Bias: Disclosure Is Informative," *Journal of Epidemiology and Community Health* 63: 593–8.

Kassirer, J.P. (2005) *On the Take: How Medicine's Complicity with Big Business Can Endanger Your Health*, New York: Oxford University Press.

Law, M.R. and Grepin, K.A. (2010) "Is Newer Always Better? Re-evaluating the Benefits of Newer Pharmaceuticals," *Journal of Health Economics* 29: 743–50.

Leo, J., Lacasse, J.R. and Cimino, A.N. (2011) "Why Does Academic Medicine Allow Ghostwriting? A Prescription for Reform," *Society* 48: 371–5.

Leucht, S., Corves, C., Arbter, D., Engel, R.R. and Davis, J.M. (2009) "Second-Generation vs. First-Generation Antipsychotic Drugs for Schizophrenia: A Meta-Analysis," *Lancet* 373: 31–41.

Lexchin, J., Bero, L.A., Djulbegovic, B. and Clark, O. (2003) "Pharmaceutical Industry Sponsorship and Research Outcome and Quality: Systematic Review," *BMJ* 326: 1167–70.

Lichtenberg, F.R. (2001) "Are the Benefits of Newer Drugs Worth Their Costs? Evidence from the 1996 MEPS," *Health Affairs* 20: 241–51.

Lo, B. and Field, M.J. (2009) *Conflict of Interest in Medical Research, Education, and Practice*, Washington, DC: National Academies Press.

Orlowski, J.P. and Wateska, L. (1992) "The Effects of Pharmaceutical Firm Enticements on Physician Prescribing Patterns. There's No Such Thing as a Free Lunch," *Chest* 102: 270–3.
PhRMA (2008) *Code on Interactions with Health Professionals*, Washington DC: Pharmaceutical Research and Manufacturers of America.
Roberts, B. (2012) *The Truth about Statins: Risks and Alternatives to Cholesterol-Lowering Drugs*, New York: Pocket Books.
Rose, J. (2008) "Industry Influence in the Creation of Pay-for-Performance Quality Measures," *Quality Management in Health Care* 17: 27–34.
Schafer, A. (2004) "Biomedical Conflicts of Interest: A Defence of the Sequestration Thesis—Learning from the Cases of Nancy Olivieri and David Healy," *Journal of Medical Ethics* 30: 8–24.
Silverman, M. and Lee, P.R. (1974) *Pills, Profits, and Politics*, Berkeley, CA: University of California Press.
Spurling, G.K., Mansfield, P.R., Montgomery, B.D., Lexchin, J., Doust, J., Othman, N. and Vitry, A.I. (2010) "Information from Pharmaceutical Companies and the Quality, Quantity, and Cost of Physicians' Prescribing: A Systematic Review," *PLoS Medicine* 7 (10): e1000352.
Steinman, M.A., Shlipak, M.G. and McPhee, S.J. (2001) "Of Principles and Pens: Attitudes and Practices of Medicine Housestaff toward Pharmaceutical Industry Promotions," *American Journal of Medicine* 110: 551–7.
Stell, L.K. (2009) "Drug Reps Off Campus! Promoting Professional Purity by Suppressing Commercial Speech," *Journal of Law, Medicine and Ethics* 37: 431–43.
Stell, L.K. and Stossel, T.P. (2011) "Another Dip into the Muddy Waters of COI," *American Journal of Bioethics* 11 (1): 49–50.
Stossel, T.P. (2007) "Regulation of Financial Conflicts of Interest in Medical Practice and Medical Research: A Damaging Solution in Search of a Problem," *Perspectives in Biology and Medicine* 50: 54–71.
Thompson, D.F. (1993) "Understanding Financial Conflicts of Interest," *New England Journal of Medicine* 329: 573–6.
Turner, E.H., Matthews, A.M., Linardatos, E., Tell, R.A. and Rosenthal, R. (2008) "Selective Publication of Antidepressant Trials and Its Influence on Apparent Efficacy," *New England Journal of Medicine* 358: 252–60.
Wadman, M. (2009) "The Senator's Sleuth," *Nature* 461: 330–4.
Weber, L. (2006) *Profits before People? Ethical Standards and the Marketing of Prescription Drugs*, Bloomington, IN: Indiana University Press.

Part IV

RESEARCH

The ethics of biomedical research pits the personhood, the moral inviolability of the individual against the goal of scientific progress. Research is required not only to develop new cures for dread diseases but also to teach us which existing treatments and diagnostics are beneficial and which are useless or even positively harmful. Are good ethics and good science compatible?

At the beginning of the era of contemporary bioethics, this question focused on the moral necessity of obtaining research subjects' informed consent. The traditional view in medicine had been that physician-researchers should enjoy nearly complete discretion in determining how much information should be shared with prospective subjects and even whether subjects should be asked for their consent. As Jonathan Moreno and Dominic Sisti demonstrate, this longstanding professional prerogative was challenged and eventually overturned by a series of scandalous revelations of research abuses at Nuremberg, Tuskegee, and leading U.S. universities. These authors also show us how what began as a quite narrowly focused and straightforward question—namely, is informed consent a moral requirement of ethical research?—has exploded into a highly variegated set of complex and morally contentious questions: e.g., is the randomized clinical trial (RCT), the current "gold standard" of evidence in biomedicine, compatible with good ethics? Who should be asked to participate? Should monetary incentives be offered to increase enrollment, or would this be "coercive"? Should certain categories of "vulnerable" subjects—e.g., prisoners, children, pregnant women, the poor—be afforded special protections? Are such protections compatible with equitable access to participation in research? Moreno and Sisti also note that biomedical research, formerly a kind of localized cottage industry, has gone global in recent decades, making possible important advances in our knowledge of genetics and pharmaceuticals but also posing serious problems for the ethical conduct and oversight of research in the developing world.

The compatibility of rigorous research design and good ethics is a central concern for the conduct of biomedical research today. How can the key structural ingredients of the RCT, such as randomization, the blinding of subjects and researchers, and placebo controls—i.e., features of the RCT designed to eliminate or reduce biases that can degrade the results of research—be squared with the physician-researcher's fiduciary duties of loyalty to the health and welfare of the individual patient-subject? Charles Weijer, Paul Miller, and Mackenzie Graham argue that good science is indeed compatible with a rigorous, non-utilitarian ethic of patient protection.

Although obtaining research participants' informed consent is now universally regarded as a requirement of ethical research, it is less clear whether informed consent, as currently practiced, actually succeeds in meeting its original goals of precluding abusive research and enabling participants to make informed decisions. Indeed, many empirical studies have shown that increasingly lengthy consent forms can impede genuine understanding of the goals and most salient risks of research protocols. Moreover, the current practice of consent does little to alleviate the so-called "therapeutic misconception"—i.e., tendency of potential research subjects to assume that the goals and methods of RCTs exist for their own individualized benefit. This confusion is problematic because it means that potential research participants often agree to join studies without a genuine understanding of what they are doing. Paul Appelbaum contributes a helpful history of informed consent in the research context as well as an alternative model of consent that might solve the problems of information overload and the therapeutic misconception.

Issues of informed consent also loom large in particular areas of biomedical research, such as genetics and genome studies, that hold great promise for our understanding of many diseases. Such research is based on tissue samples that can be stored indefinitely, shared with other researchers, and reexamined in future research projects having little, if any, connection to the study for which the tissues were originally obtained. Thus, in addition to the usual problems of informed consent, genetic research poses novel problems relating to unanticipated future uses of stored samples. When we sign onto any given genetics research project, are we consenting to the use of our tissues exclusively within this particular study, to any and all uses of our tissues in a vast array of unrelated studies in the near and distant future, or perhaps only for certain kinds of research on certain kinds of problems, excluding uses that we might find morally objectionable? Such questions, as well as the threats of genetic research to personal privacy, are addressed in Dena Davis's chapter.

The field of research ethics was "born in scandal, and raised in protectionism." The dominant ethos at the birth of contemporary bioethics was one of protecting vulnerable parties—e.g., prisoners, children with mental retardation, pregnant women—from the risks of research participation. This ethos was challenged during the 1980s by advocates for people with HIV/AIDS, women, and children who began to view participation in research as a benefit, and categorical exclusion from research as a violation of justice. Toby Schonfeld surveys the history of this problem and offers a useful analytical framework for more nuanced and respectful approaches to worries about vulnerability.

A related question in research ethics concerns the use of various incentives, including money and medical care, to facilitate greater participation in studies. One proposed remedy for this situation is to make participation more attractive by paying participants extra money or offering access to medical treatments unavailable to them off trial. Such an approach has been resisted by many in the bioethics community as being either coercive, an undue inducement, or exploitative of poor and sick populations. Alan Wertheimer argues that many, if not most, of such criticisms are either mistaken or misapplied.

Finally in this section, Tom Beauchamp tackles the controversial issue of the use of animals in biomedical research. Key questions here focus on the moral status of different species of animals, gauging their most important interests, and discerning how best to protect those interests in research. The most important question, however, is exactly how research on animals might be ethically justified. How much pain and suffering do various kinds of studies inflict? What are the realistic prospects of human benefit, and is research on animals strictly necessary to achieve such benefits?

14
BIOMEDICAL RESEARCH ETHICS
Landmark Cases, Scandals, and Conceptual Shifts

Jonathan D. Moreno and Dominic Sisti

Introduction

Charting the history of biomedical research ethics is as much an exercise in reporting a litany of past scandals as it is an examination of shifts in scientific, political, and broader cultural mores. In this chapter, we provide a brief accounting of both by describing landmark cases and how reactions to these cases gave purchase to significant conceptual shifts in the ethics of human subjects research.

To do this, we first present a typology for these cases, which, we should note, is neither strictly chronological nor exhaustive. We begin by describing several infamous scandals in the history of research ethics, such as the experiments conducted on prisoner-victims by the Nazis, the examples inventoried in Henry Beecher's seminal paper, "Ethics and Clinical Research" (Beecher 1966), and the Tuskegee Syphilis study.

From there we present three groups of cases. The first group is culled from findings related to the research conducted by the U.S. and British military from the 1940s through the 1970s. We highlight the work of the Advisory Committee on Human Radiation Experiments, a commission created by President Clinton and charged with the investigation of experiments conducted by half a dozen government agencies on unsuspecting persons.

The second group of cases features examples from psychiatric, psychological, and social science research. These include the well known Milgram Obedience Study and the Stanford Prison Experiment, illustrating the ethically fraught practice of deception in social science research as well as investigator–participant role conflicts.

In the third set of cases, we describe more recent incidents, including the death of Jesse Gelsinger in a 1999 gene therapy experiment. Issues here related to lapses in informed consent, protocol adherence, subject selection, and concerns about financial conflicts of interest. Again highlighting the role of federal ethics committees, we discuss recent revelations concerning the sexually transmissible disease (STD) experiments conducted in Guatemala in the late 1940s in this section as well.

We chose these cases to bring into conceptual relief several key developments in biomedical research ethics. First, as a result of the early scandals, a moment of clarity occurred revealing voluntariness as a necessary but not sufficient condition for ethical research. This now-seemingly common sense notion was not universally apparent to the practitioners of biomedical science prior to 1960. Second and more fundamentally, as we will see, the principle of respect for persons was precipitated by legal issues and, in reaction, theoretical discussions among philosophers as the early bioethicists applied it to bio-behavioral research.

Third, we also find that the scientific enterprise, in general, and human subjects research, specifically, have been transformed from protected activities shielded by the elite status of medicine into a more transparent and publically accountable activity. The advent of human subjects protection rules and committees provided unprecedented power to both the government and the lay public to check the ambitions of scientists.

Finally, the historical arc presented here reveals that the ideals of informed consent and respect for persons—arguably the most fundamental touchstones of American biomedical ethics—are pockmarked with both conceptual ambiguity and practical challenges that make their full realization difficult, if not impossible. These conceptual and theoretical lacunae set the stage for ongoing and future challenges in human subjects research. We conclude by prognosticating about issues on the horizon of research ethics.

Early Scandals

Holocaust-Related Experiments

The atrocities perpetrated by Nazi physicians and scientists are extensively documented (Annas and Grodin 1992; Caplan 1993; Lifton 2000 [1986]). Although these atrocities represent the coalescence of political, social, and scientific ideologies, distinct research programs were designed and executed to support particular military goals, to reinforce claims of Nazi superiority, and to investigate particular "scientific" interests of SS researchers (*U.S. v. Karl Brandt et al.* 1947).

From 1940 to 1945, thousands of victims were culled from concentration and work camps. They included Jews, Roma, Poles, and others who were deemed "scientifically" appropriate subjects or—in the parlance of the efficiently orchestrated Nazi "euthanasia" program— "lives not worthy of life."

On the military research track, victims were forced into cold water and extreme barometric exposure trials. Led by Sigmund Rascher, the researchers at Dachau presided over experiments aimed to better understand the physiology of hypothermia in support of the Luftwaffe, as German pilots were being increasingly shot down or shipwrecked in frigid waters (Berger 1990). In a related episode, 100 victims were forced to drink seawater to observe the impact of extreme dehydration and test new desalination methods (Katz 1992b).

As Lifton describes, experiments were also conducted that were "a direct expression of racial theory and policy" (Lifton 2000 [1986]: 267). For example, at Auschwitz's notorious Block 10, Carl Clauberg conducted mass sterilization experiments of racially "inferior" female prisoners, which involved the injection of caustic compounds into the cervix to block the fallopian tubes (Proctor 1992). Similarly, Horst Schumann implemented X-ray and surgical castration protocols. Of the approximately 1000 victims, all were left severally maimed or shuttled to the gas chambers and killed (*U.S. v. Karl Brandt et al.* 1946).

Josef Mengele perpetrated the most infamous Holocaust-related experiments. Mengele's studies of identical twins at Auschwitz were an extension of his previous heredity and morphology evaluations conducted under the direction of Baron Otmar von Vertschuer, with whom he worked in the racial courts established by the Nuremberg race laws (Seidelman 1988). At Auschwitz, Mengele was the medical gatekeeper. He selected research subjects for any number of experimental protocols, determining who would be sentenced to the brutality of the Nazi scientific enterprise, to slave labor, or sent to die in the gas chambers.

The curiosities of Nazi doctors were satisfied in a number of horribly strange experimental programs that seemed to be motivated as much by pseudoscientific ambition and a distorted notion of public hygiene as by military strategy or Nazi ideology. Certainly, many of Mengele's twin studies fit within this rubric. These included injecting colored dyes into the eyes of twins to see if eye color would permanently change and the sewing together of twins in an attempt to conjoin them. Mengele was never tried for his crimes. He spent his post-war life in hiding in South America, evading justice.

In the end, as Annas and Grodin (1992) point out, the horrors of Nazi medical research represented several recurrent perverse motivations: The dehumanization of particular members of society, the medicalization of social and political problems, the political indoctrination of physicians, and lack of concern for human rights. Nazi doctors saw their role as physicians not of individual patients but of the Reich, which was existentially threatened by Total War (Caplan 2007). This belief led the Nazi doctors to justify their actions by appealing to both the doctrine of "superior orders" (that they were obliged to those above them in the chain of command) and to a crude utilitarianism that in war some must be sacrificed for the good of the state.

The Nuremberg Trial and Code

"The voluntary consent of the human subject is absolutely essential" (*U.S. v. Karl Brandt et al.* 1947). So reads the first sentence of ten provisions of what posterity has come to know as the Nuremberg Code, promulgated by the three-judge panel in their ruling at the Nazi Doctors trial, delivered in August 1947. The Nuremberg Code represented the embodiment of principles that were thought by the judges to be implicitly accepted by medical researchers.

Of the twenty-three defendants on trial, sixteen were found guilty, and seven of those were executed. In a surprising reversal, the defense argued that the Allies had conducted similar human experiments with prison populations. The claims were accurate (and in fact certain other Allied experiments were not discovered until decades later), but ultimately the court found that the Nazi experiments were uniquely barbaric (Moreno 2000). Ultimately, the defendants were found guilty of murder, not for the violation of research ethics.

Moreover, the prosecution struggled to cite any formal research ethics code with jurisdiction over the conduct of Nazi researchers, with the exception—perhaps ironically—of those previously promulgated in Germany (Katz 1996; Sass 1997). This void prompted Dr Andrew Ivy, the prosecution's primary medical expert witness, to urge the American Medical Association to adopt his proposed principles of research ethics, which were ratified by the AMA shortly after the trial began and to which Ivy pointed as evidence of prevailing ethics conventions in his testimony (Shuster 1997).

The legacy and impact of the Nuremberg Code on research ethics in the United States continues to be debated. On the one hand, some have argued that, as a matter of historical fact, the Code exerted little practical influence on American researchers, who initially considered "it a good code for barbarians but an unnecessary code for ordinary physicians" (Katz 1992a). In fact, Henry Beecher, himself an icon of research ethics, as we shall see below, expressed reservations about the usefulness and appropriateness of the Code in American research universities (Beecher 1959).

On the other hand, as Faden et al. (1996) state, "the Nuremberg Code stands alone as the most eloquent and principled statement of the significance of human rights in the conduct of research involving human subjects." As such, the Code laid the conceptual foundations for a half-century of research ethics innovations both directly and as a result of reaction to it. For example, physician researchers of the World Medical Association, who were skeptical of the usefulness of the Nuremberg Code—and who perhaps wished to preserve the prerogatives of physicians in framing medical ethics—developed and adopted the Declaration of Helsinki in 1964 and amended it six times. The Declaration is a highly influential set of global standards, but to its detractors it serves as "recommendations by physicians for physicians" (Annas 1992).

Beecher's Inventory

Neither international conventions nor codes of ethics—whether from Nuremberg, Geneva, or Helsinki—proved sufficient to prevent abuses perpetuated throughout the next half century. Harvard anesthesiologist, Henry Knowles Beecher, provided the first inventory of such abuses in his seminal paper, "Ethics and Clinical Research" (Beecher 1966).

In this brief article, Beecher first reiterates his concerns about the applicability of codes of ethics that naively demand full consent, as if it is "readily available for the asking." He instead espouses a model of virtue ethics for biomedical researchers, according to which a "*responsible* investigator" is a "far more dependable safeguard" than consent guidelines (Beecher 1966: 1355; italics in original). But because consent information was not normally reported in published accounts, Beecher's list of 22 ethically compromised experiments focused on those that were scientifically questionable in design, carried a high ratio of risk to benefit, employed bizarre methods, and, most importantly, placed vulnerable subjects at extreme risk for no justifiable therapeutic purpose (Levine 1986).

Beecher referred to one study that did in fact involve questionable consent. Example 16 involved the inoculation of cognitively disabled children with hepatitis who lived in an institution where the disease was endemic. Beecher questioned the validity of the parents' consent, a concern that would be vindicated, as the details of this study were uncovered over the course of the next decade that we now know as the Willowbrook Hepatitis Study.

Willowbrook

In 1954, Dr Saul Krugman, an infectious disease researcher from New York University, began to study hepatitis within the population of children living at the Willowbrook

State School for children who were mentally disabled on Staten Island, New York. The study involved exposing subjects to hepatitis, ostensibly in order to devise preventative measures for the disease, which was endemic in the institution particularly due to its squalid condition.

Critics of the study reiterated Beecher's concern about the means by which the study was conducted—that children who were mentally disabled were intentionally and unjustly harmed for the sake of science—and they argued the consent procedures were coercive. There was a long waiting list for admission to the school and parents who agreed to enroll their children in the study were granted admission. This inducement was viewed as undue and extreme and invalidated the consent process (Rothman and Rothman 1984).

Krugman (1986) contended that his research was ethically justifiable since the study risks were equal to the inevitability of children contracting hepatitis. Moreover, he claimed that carefully controlled inoculation of the virus increased the likelihood of a subclinical manifestation of symptoms, which could bestow immunity later in life. Krugman also insisted that the consent procedures were carefully designed and vetted by all appropriate regulatory entities and endorsed by subjects' parents (Emanuel et al. 2003). Indeed, Krugman found support not only among his professional and scientific boosters and funding agencies, but also the Benevolent Society of Retarded Children—a parents' advocacy group that lauded Krugman's "distinguished, pioneering, humanitarian research in the prevention of infectious disease and their resultant complication in children, born and unborn" (Krugman 1986: 162).

The controversy generated by the Willowbrook Hepatitis Study points to fundamental disagreements over the essential elements of surrogate consent for vulnerable and incapacitated persons. While most would agree that voluntariness is an essential element, ascertaining the limits of subjects' or surrogates' free choice within the context of real world pressures is often exceedingly difficult. Nonetheless, there is a broad if not universal consensus that the Willowbrook Hepatitis Study was patently unethical because of the duress under which the parents agreed to their children's participation.

Jewish Chronic Disease Hospital

Example 17 of Beecher's inventory was the soon-to-be infamous case involving two physicians who injected cancer cells into terminally ill patients at the Jewish Chronic Disease Hospital in Brooklyn, New York. The aim of the study was to examine patients' immune response to foreign cells. Twenty-two patients were never told that they were research subjects and that they were being injected with "live cancer cells." Dr Chester Southam, the study's primary investigator, recounted that a full explanation had been given to patients in the early years of the research, but that,

> . . . as our body of knowledge has increased and the course of reaction to the injections became more predictable, we have simply explained that the procedure was a test which had nothing to do with treatment, that it involved the injection of foreign material, described the expected course of reaction, and that its purpose was to determine the rate at which the expected nodules would develop and then regress.
>
> (Arras in Emanuel et al. 2003)

Southam articulated an unequivocal position in favor of *therapeutic privilege*—the withholding of medical information from patients by physicians (or researchers) because they believe that such disclosure would somehow harm the patient:

> Unless the patient inquired, we refrained from describing the precise nature of the human cells for the reason that in my own professional judgment as well as that of my professional colleagues . . . the precise nature of the foreign cells was irrelevant to the bodily reactions which could be expected to occur . . . Furthermore, in my own clinical judgment . . . to use the dreaded word "cancer" in connection with any clinical procedure on an ill person is potentially deleterious to the patient's well-being because it may suggest to him (rightly or wrongly) that his diagnosis is cancer or that his prognosis is poor . . . I believe such revelation is generally contraindicated in the best consideration of the patient's welfare and therefore to withhold such emotionally disturbing but medically nonpertinent details (unless requested by the patient) is in the best tradition of responsible clinical practice.
> (Emanuel et al. 2003)

We also find here the commingling of the therapeutic and research roles by clinicians—a role conflict that is ethically problematic precisely because the duties each role entails are at times directly opposed. For example, physicians, when acting as researchers, are appropriately concerned with the advancement of biomedical science and the treatment of future patients; but when acting in their capacity as clinicians, physicians have a strict duty to advance the best interests of their particular patients. We will see similar role conflicts and their ethical consequences in future cases.

U.S. Public Health Service Syphilis Study

Starting in 1932, the U.S. Public Health Service Syphilis Study (better known as the Tuskegee Syphilis Study) spanned the entire period of the above episodes in research ethics. In fact, the study went on for four decades, and although it was conducted openly and generated several publications, it ended in 1972 only when it was exposed by the popular press.

Dr Taliaferro Clark, Chief of the U.S. Public Health Service, devised the study as a way to learn about the life history of untreated syphilis among black men. He decided that Macon County in rural Alabama would be the ideal location to conduct the study because of the high incidence of untreated syphilis there. As Brandt (1978) argues, the belief held by researchers that black men suffering from syphilis would not avail themselves of treatment, even if available, was a self-fulfilling prophesy steeped in racist ideology. Note that arguments that appeal to the "inevitability" of disease are similar to those made by Krugman in his "natural history" study of hepatitis (Rothman 1982).

The study conscripted 399 black men who had syphilis and, to serve as the control group, 200 who were not infected. Throughout the research, subjects were subjected to spinal taps and physical examinations under the ruse that they were being treated. In the early part of the study, a treatment regime involving heavy metal injections was available but denied to participants of the study. Macon County served as the observatory for untreated syphilis even after penicillin was discovered to cure the disease. Throughout the study, local African American physicians continued to conspire with researchers in denying subjects penicillin.

In the end, 128 men had died of syphilis or complications, 40 wives were infected with syphilis and 19 children were born with the disease. Uproar was sparked by a story in the *Washington Star*, which stimulated political investigations and action that led eventually to the Belmont Report, Common Rule and, much later, an apology and reparations from President Bill Clinton.

It is widely thought that Tuskegee continues to foment and reinforce deep mistrust of medicine and biomedical research among black Americans, but data on the scope of this phenomenon are equivocal (Katz et al. 2006; Wendler et al. 2005). However, it is indisputable that the Tuskegee Syphilis Study represents one of the worst ethical lapses in the history of American biomedical research and stands out as the case that has had the most influence in the reform of ethics standards. The fact that it spanned such a long period and so clearly violated basic principles of medical and research ethics—even while they were being formulated at Nuremberg—illustrates that the American biomedical enterprise was largely shielded from ethical scrutiny. This would change in coming years as Presidential commissions were formed to examine not just Tuskegee but also military experimentation, the topic of our next section.

Military Research

Imperial Japanese Experiments

While the Nazi atrocities of World War II received substantial attention in the West, little attention was paid to the lethal wartime human experimentation conducted by the Imperial Japanese army. Officially the Water Purification Bureau, the construction of the Ping Fan prison complex was completed in 1939 and housed in excess of 1,000 human experimental subjects. Later known infamously as Unit 731, this complex was the site of substantial biological and chemical warfare research. The experimental subjects, predominantly Han Chinese and Soviets, were often prisoners or civilians and included both men and women. From 1939 to 1942 they were subjected to horrendous biological and chemical weaponry testing.

Prior to experimentation the subjects were fed well and generally kept in good health; they also received medical treatment following the completion of successful experimentation. However, the health of the subjects was important to the Imperial Army only insofar as healthy subjects yield superior results. Cyclic experimentation of subjects was therefore continued until the subject was too weak to yield reliable data. Many subjects died during the course of experimentation, while survivors were subsequently killed by poison injection. Subjects were inoculated with any number of diseases, often including anthrax, plague, and/or cholera. Similarly, experiments reminiscent of those conducted in Nazi Germany—for example frostbite studies—were undertaken.

Impressing his superiors in the Imperial Japanese military with preliminary biological warfare experimentation, General Shiro Ishii, chief medical officer, received authorization for the initial construction of Unit 731 and the undertaking of the human experimentation trials. The trials resulted in the subsequent death or intentional extermination of at least 400–600 Ping Fan prisoners a year; the uneven accuracy of the records kept makes precise estimates beyond these figures impossible. Additionally, it is believed that at least 1,485 British, American, Australian, and New Zealand Prisoners of War (POWs) were forced to drink liquids containing a number a pathogens for further human experimentation.

Despite the atrocious level of violence towards human prisoners exercised by Ishii, the U.S. was initially consciously inattentive. Decisions were made by American officials to avoid a war crimes investigation or a compromise of their own biological weapons experimentation. However, following the occupation of Japan and the accumulation of a growing body of evidence, American officials finally prepared charges against Ishii and fellow Unit 731 researchers and conducted a series of interrogations.

As international relations between the U.S. and the Soviet Union began to deteriorate, military intelligence ultimately granted Ishii immunity in exchange for the information previously obtained from Unit 731 warfare experimentation. Despite the insistence that Unit 731 bore information crucial for U.S. intelligence, and the eagerness of American officials to be privy to this information, it became apparent that Unit 731 was unable to discover little more than what had already been learned in the U.S. Subsequently, American officials were concerned less with ethical ramifications than with potential embarrassment if the deal were publicized.

The Plutonium Injections

The bombings of Hiroshima and Nagaski in 1945 during the final days of World War II were the result of significant military funding, known as The Manhattan Project. Manhattan Project scientists were directed by the White House to manufacture nuclear weaponry by January of 1945. It was unlikely that sufficient uranium-235 could be obtained and used to create any more than one atomic bomb by that date, so the managers of the project explored alternative sources of fissionable energy. In 1941 a solution was obtained through the creation of plutonium from uranium. Plutonium could both sufficiently power an atomic bomb and be generated in substantial quantities—with production likely to meet the required deadline.

In light of this discovery, concerns were raised about the risks faced by plutonium workers, given that they were exposed to high levels of plutonium dust and that nothing was known about this newly created and potentially poisonous substance. Following six accidents involving exposure of researchers to plutonium during animal experiments, and only a year until the urgent Manhattan Project deadline, it appears that Manhattan Project director J. Robert Oppenheimer endorsed human experimentation.

The first human trial did not occur until April 1945. Ebb Cade, a 43-year-old cement worker, was brought into the Manhattan Army Project Hospital in March 1945, suffering broken bones in three limbs following a car accident. Requiring several surgeries to set the bones and a number of weeks in hospital, Cade became "Human Product 1." Without his knowledge or consent Cade was injected with 4.7 micrograms of plutonium. Acting physicians were instructed not to divulge the names of the institutions from which they received the plutonium; indeed, the very word *plutonium* was classified until the bombings of Japan in August 1945.

The second and third subjects selected were both patients with carcinoma at the University of California's hospital; like Cade, they were long-stay patients. San Francisco researchers have since claimed that their interest in these patients extended beyond the Manhattan Project, and that they believed plutonium may confer help in the treatment of cancer. Later investigation by the University of California revealed that these subjects could not have benefitted from the injections, nor were they expected to. Fourteen additional patients were subjected to plutonium injections at the Universities of

California and Rochester during wartime, along with one additional patient at the University of California following its cessation.

In October 1995 Clinton's Advisory Committee on Human Radiation Experiments concluded that all but the final subjects were not aware that they were part of experimental procedures relating to the development of the atomic bomb. The plutonium trials raised significant issues of consent, with experiments failing to meet even the most modest ethical expectations for human subjects research. Similarly, when no longer overshadowed by the necessity of wartime—as in the case of subject eighteen—the plutonium trials raised concern regarding the limitations of human experimentation in the U.S.

The Maddison Case

In some instances decades are required for information about unethical human experiments to become available to scholars, especially when the activities take place under the cover of national security. For legal and political reasons, the U.S. has been the site of most of the cases uncovered since World War II. One exception is the series of sarin gas experiments undertaken at Porton Down in the U.K. during the 1950s (Schmidt 2006).

In 1953 a 20-year-old Royal Air Force engineer named Ronald Maddison was one of the servicemen exposed to the lethal gas. He was the only one out of hundreds of test subjects to die in the experiment, a death that was covered up by the Ministry of Defense (MoD). Responding to repeated allegations and rumors in the decades following chemical weapons experiments in the U.K., especially from veterans and their families, a British judge quashed the MoD's original inquest finding in 1953 as "death by misadventure."

Following a new inquest fifty-one years after Maddison's death, in February 2006, the MoD and Maddison's family settled on the charge of "gross negligence." After this ruling, Porton Down veterans filed claims relating to Cold War experiments. The House of Commons agreed to a compensation package worth about $5 billion and an apology in 2008 (Schmidt 2006).

Behavioral and Social Science Research

National Commission Reports

Several of the reports promulgated by the National Commission for the Protection of Human Subjects of Biomedical and Behavioral Research focused on research involving mentally ill persons.

In its 1975 report, *Psychosurgery*, the Commission investigated the use of surgical procedures aimed at "controlling, changing, or affecting any behavioral or emotional disturbance of such individual[s]." Public concern about the misuse of psychosurgery intensified in the late 1960s, as both researchers and the lay press began to publish accounts of the haphazard use of psychosurgery. Popular worries were stoked by books and films centering around the use of psychosurgery for social control, such as Stanley Kubrick's *A Clockwork Orange*, Ken Kesey's *One Flew Over the Cuckoo's Nest*, and Michael Crichton's *The Terminal Man*.

The key ethical issue considered in *Psychosurgery* was the scientific merit of the surgical procedures in increasingly common use. Although surgeons considered psychosurgery to be a therapeutic device, the Commission argued it ought to be "considered experimental and should be conducted within the context of research, subject to all review provisions and procedures for the protection of human subjects which that implies" (page 10). Indeed, most research had been performed in the context of clinical practice—there were no protocols, ethics reviews, or systematic evaluation of outcomes—using questionably competent research subjects.

In *Research Involving Those Institutionalized as Mentally Ill* (1978) the Commission explicated a set of five comprehensive recommendations for guiding the conduct of research on mentally ill subjects. These recommendations included several criteria to guide IRB review, including clear directives about research involving more than minimal risk to subjects, and recommendations for elevating review to a national board in very specific circumstances. Many of the theoretical underpinnings and practical applications outlined in these reports would be embodied in the *Belmont Report* (1979).

Deception and Forbidden Knowledge

As scrutiny of research involving mentally ill persons increased, ethically fraught psychological research on healthy volunteers continued to attract attention and criticism. These studies involved deception or unauthorized surveillance—methods that continue to be used and are considered permissible in very specific contexts (American Psychological Association 2010). Studies that employ deception involve a basic conflict—or balancing—between utilitarian aims and the deontological duty of veracity (Pittenger 2008).

For example, the Yale psychologist Stanley Milgram conducted an experiment in which subjects were misled to think they were enrolling in a study on the effect of punishment on memory and learning (Milgram 1963). In an elegantly designed protocol, naïve subjects were told they were "teachers" whose job it was to punish "learners" with increasingly high voltages of electricity whenever learners made mistakes in a memory test. The learners were experimental accomplices and actors, who expressed pain and suffering as subjects (i.e., the "teachers") inflicted fake electric shocks. Experimenters prodded the subjects to increase the strength of the electrical shocks despite learners' faux cries and pleas to stop the experiment. A majority of subjects, although visibly disturbed, deeply conflicted, and seriously stressed, obeyed the orders of the experimenter and increased the voltage to what would have been extremely high and possibly lethal levels (450 volts).

According to Milgram, the experiment pointed to conflicting tendencies of human nature—the intrinsic tendency to avoid harming others was in conflict with the disposition to respect and obey persons of authority. In this case, the latter tendency won out. The findings of the Milgram Obedience study, along with video footage of the experiment, raised issues about the ethical permissibility of deception of psychological research subjects, particularly in experiments that may reveal disturbing facts or behavioral dispositions. Although the point of the study was to assess the extent to which "ordinary" people might be induced to engage in sadistic acts, it seemed to many that the experimenters themselves were behaving in a sadistic manner by implementing an experimental design that could traumatize the subjects if they came to see themselves as easily manifesting cruelty.

Similarly, the Stanford Prison experiment, conducted by Philip Zimbardo in 1971, revealed a disturbing tendency of individuals to abuse authority, while others submitted helplessly to their abuse. Zimbardo randomly assigned research subjects to one of two roles—prison guard or prisoner—and then allowed each group to act out their roles in a mock prison. The experiment lasted only six days, as it became clear that the study had taken on a life of its own, with guards verbally abusing and humiliating prisoners. Even Zimbardo—acting in a conflicted role as prison superintendent—allowed abuse of prisoners to continue. Christina Maslach, a graduate student who would later marry Zimbardo, urged him to stop the experiment after she witnessed the guards abusing prisoners (O'Toole 1997).

The paradigmatic example of behavioral research involving not only deception but also unauthorized surveillance was Laud Humphreys' ethnography of anonymous homosexual encounters that transpired in public restrooms between men. To study this sexual practice—the so-called "Tearoom Trade"—Humphreys impersonated the "watchqueen" who was the third man meant to be a lookout for the other two men engaging in sex. In this role, Humphreys was able to observe and document their behavior, collect their license plate numbers, and identify them in the community. Humphreys then interviewed them under the guise of a health service researcher. He reported his results in his book *Tearoom Trade: A Study of Homosexual Encounters in Public Places* (1970).

The results of Humphreys' study were significant in raising awareness about the nature of sexuality and public versus private personas. Serious ethical concerns were raised about Humphreys' study on the grounds that he had never received consent from his unknowing subjects, that he invaded their privacy by identifying them, and that he lied to subjects about his role and the intent of his interviews. Deception is still viewed as an indispensable tool of much social science research. The deontological concerns raised by critics—e.g., that deception was incompatible with treating subjects as autonomous agents—do not seem to have resonated with social psychologists, many of whose research agendas are based on deceptive practices.

Recent Cases and the Future of Research Ethics

The Case of Jesse Gelsinger

On September 17, 1999, Jesse Gelsinger, an 18-year-old participant in a gene therapy trial at the University of Pennsylvania, died after receiving an experimental adenovirus vector designed to deliver genetic material to treat a metabolic condition. Gelsinger's death triggered a new round of political, scientific, and ethical investigation into deficiencies in subject protections practices across the entire American biomedical research enterprise (Walters 2000). At least three important ethical issues emerged from the Gelsinger affair. The first issue related to the selection of subjects for the experiment. Debate ensued about placing relatively healthy adults such as Gelsinger at unnecessary risk in this phase I trial to test safety. While some argued that newborns with the lethal form of the disorder would have been more appropriate research subjects, others contended that parents of such severely ill newborns could not adequately provide consent without erroneously expecting a therapeutic benefit (Sisti and Caplan 2003).

The second issue concerned the investigators' informed consent procedures, their adherence to the approved protocol, and general problems in study management and oversight. Gelsinger had not been told about problems related to the adenovirus vector found in pre-clinical animal trials and with other research subjects. Animal data are not typically part of informed consent procedures, but it is beyond dispute that issues with other subjects should be addressed. At the time of the experiment, Gelsinger's liver was functioning below the inclusion criteria stipulated on the protocol and he should not have received the infusion. This turned out to be one of several changes the investigators made to the protocol about which they had failed to inform the proper authorities (Steinbrook 2008).

Third, the Gelsinger case highlighted the complexities of individual and institutional financial conflicts of interest. James Wilson, the lead investigator and director of the research institute at Penn, held a 30 percent equity stake as the founder of Genovo, Inc., which held the rights to market gene therapies discovered at Penn. Likewise, the University and others affiliated with the University held minor equity shares in Genovo.

These relationships raised ethical concerns about the conflicted role of Wilson and others, and sparked a broader conversation about the ethical perils of commingling financial and scientific goals. The number of academic–industry relationships vastly increased in the 1980s and 1990s in part as a result of the *Bayh–Dole Act*, which allowed private institutions or individuals to patent and profit from biomedical innovations made with federal funding. By 2009 academic–industrial relationships had become the norm, with more than half of academic scientists engaged in some form of industrial relationship (Zinner et al. 2009).

Historiography and Human Research Ethics

Historiography refers to the methodology of historical studies. How can valid conclusions be drawn about events in the past? What counts as validity in historical judgment? How can people appreciate the circumstances of those who lived before them, and is "appreciation of prior circumstances" even necessary for doing history? The historiography of ethics is perhaps still more puzzling. Considering that moral judgments are often hard to understand and justify with regard to current or very recent events, valid *moral* judgments about the past as it recedes from living memory seem to add still another layer of complexity. These are not abstract problems. Because so much of the modern regulatory apparatus and the field of research ethics rely on the sorts of crucial cases we have described, "getting the history right" is anything but a trivial pursuit.

Consider, for example, the plutonium injection experiment. In 1945 the boundaries between research and practice were not carefully drawn. Patients were not generally considered to be partners in the research enterprise (although it was not uncommon for scientific articles to express gratitude for their sacrifice). Further, a wartime ethos prevailed under conditions of total mobilization and pervasive government controls that have not been experienced since. Subjects seem to have been selected based on a diagnosis of bone cancer, suggesting that there was a secondary therapeutic intent that might have helped justify the experiment in the minds of the scientists. Can later persons confidently conclude that the experiment was ethically unacceptable?

Here, as in other cases we have described in this chapter, we are confronted with the problem of retrospective moral judgment, a form of anachronistic ethical assessment. Averting this criticism requires a detailed knowledge of the historical facts—a pursuit that is not always evident in casual recitations of landmark cases. For instance, we would need to know that there had been discussions of research ethics in other contexts prior to 1945, including experiments with prisoners, in order for the general ethical principle of subject voluntariness to have been available to persons at the time. Interestingly, just two years after the last plutonium injection, the newly formed Atomic Energy Commission determined that the experiment should be kept secret in order to avoid government embarrassment, a sure indication that the relevant ethical norm was appreciable at the time.

Yet that experiment took place under the auspices of the atomic bomb project, a scientific endeavor that was then and now widely accepted as a matter of military necessity, even national emergency. More than most treatments of the history of human research ethics, we have emphasized the role of national security needs and military sponsorship in a number of the cited cases. As military and intelligence technologies are increasingly reliant on basic science or its products, including the life sciences, we may expect increasing pressures to reconcile the aims of ethical research and national security imperatives.

Research Ethics on the Horizon

Those who believe in moral progress and those who are skeptical about the improvement of regard for the rights and interests of vulnerable human beings may both find support in the history of research involving human subjects. While there is no question that far more systematic attention is paid to the welfare of human subjects of biomedical and behavioral research than was the case prior to World War II, it is also true that abuses continue to be alleged, especially in developing countries where the regulatory environment is lax.

Whether the reporting of current ethical lapses is a result of greater scrutiny or intractable features of scientific research, like professional ambition or simple ethical obtuseness, is hard to know. What is certain is that the increasingly global nature of scientific research has cast a new and brighter light on international research standards. For example, in the wake of the revelations of the Guatemala STD studies of the late 1940s, a Presidential commission published both an historical reconstruction of the incident and a study of the extent to which a similar transgression could occur in the contemporary practice of human experiments in underdeveloped countries (Presidential Commission for the Study of Bioethical Issues 2011).

A debate about whether research standards should in any sense be made more flexible in light of local conditions has long bedeviled the World Health Organization's revisions of the Declaration of Helsinki. There are valid scientific, humanitarian, and business reasons to engage in research in sites beyond the borders of the most highly developed societies, especially in the fields of genetics and public health. In recent years there has also been a discernible shift away from a "protectionist" priority and toward making access to research more available to potential subjects. A variety of groups—including women, patients with HIV, and children's advocates—have argued convincingly that an overemphasis on the "vulnerability" of such groups has precluded them from access to important studies that could potentially improve their health. Taken together, these and other factors suggest that international research ethics will continue to be a site of ethical transgressions and an important field of further inquiry for bioethics.

Acknowledgments

The authors thank Skye Kinder and Katherine Buckley for their assistance.

Related Topics

Chapter 18, "Research Involving "Vulnerable Populations": A Critical Analysis," Toby Schonfeld
Chapter 20, "The Ethics of Biomedical Research Involving Animals," Tom L. Beauchamp

References

American Psychological Association (2010) "Ethical Principles of Psychologists and Code of Conduct," Standard 8.07, Deception in Research. Available at: http://www.apa.org/ethics/code/index.aspx?item=11#807 (accessed July 8, 2014).

Annas, G. (1992) "The Changing Landscape of Human Experimentation: Nuremberg, Helsinki, and Beyond," *Health Matrix* 2: 119–40.

Annas, G. and Grodin, M. (1992) *The Nazi Doctors and the Nuremberg Code*, New York, NY: Oxford University Press.

Beecher, H. (1959) "Experimentation in Man," *Journal of the American Medical Association* 169 (5): 461–78.

Beecher, H. (1966) "Ethics and Clinical Research," *New England Journal of Medicine* 274 (24): 1354–60.

Berger, R. (1990) "Nazi Science: The Dachau Hypothermia Experiments," *New England Journal of Medicine* 322 (20): 1435–40.

Brandt, A. (1978) "Racism and Research: The Case of the Tuskegee Syphilis Study," *Hastings Center Report* 8 (6): 21–9.

Caplan, A. (1993) *When Medicine Went Mad: Bioethics and the Holocaust*, Totowa, NJ: Humana Press.

Caplan, A. (2007) "The Ethics of Evil: The Challenge and the Lessons of Nazi Medical Experiments," in W. Lafleur, G. Böhme and S. Shimazono (eds.) *Dark Medicine: Rationalizing Unethical Medical Research*, Bloomington, IN: Indiana University Press.

Emanuel, E., Crouch, R., Arras, J., Moreno, J. and Grady, C. (2003) *Ethical and Regulatory Aspects of Clinical Research: Readings and Commentaries*, Baltimore, MD: The Johns Hopkins University Press.

Faden, R., Lederer, S. and Moreno, J. (1996) "US Medical Researchers, the Nuremberg Doctors Trial, and the Nuremberg Code: A Review of Findings of the Advisory Committee on Human Radiation Experiments," *Journal of the American Medical Association* 276 (20): 1667–71.

Humphreys, L. (1970) *Tearoom Trade: Impersonal Sex in Public Places*, Chicago: Aldine.

Katz, J. (1992a) "The Consent Principle in the Nuremberg Code," in G. Annas and M. Grodin (eds.) *The Nazi Doctors and the Nuremberg Code*, New York, NY: Oxford University Press, pp. 227–39.

Katz, J. (1992b) "Abuse of Human Beings for the Sake of Science," in A. Caplan (ed.) *When Medicine Went Mad*, Totowa, NJ: The Humana Press, pp. 233–70.

Katz, J. (1996) "The Nuremberg Code and the Nuremberg Trial: A Reappraisal," *Journal of the American Medical Association* 276 (20): 1662–6.

Katz, R., Russell, S., Kressin, N., Green, B.L., Wang, M.Q., James, S. and Claudio, C. (2006) "The Tuskegee Legacy Project: Willingness of Minorities to Participate in Biomedical Research," *Journal of Health Care for the Poor and Underserved* 17 (4): 698–715.

Krugman, S. (1986) "The Willowbrook Hepatitis Studies Revisited: Ethical Aspects," *Reviews of Infectious Diseases* 8 (1): 157–62.

Levine, R. (1986) *Ethics and Regulation of Clinical Research*, 2nd edition, New Haven, CT: Yale University Press.

Lifton, R.J. (2000) [1986] *The Nazi Doctors: Medical Killing and the Psychology of Genocide*, New York: Basic Books.

Milgram, S. (1963). "Behavioral Study of Obedience," *Journal of Abnormal and Social Psychology* 67 (4): 371–8.

Moreno, J. (2000) *Undue Risk: Secret State Experiments on Humans*, New York: Routledge.

Myser, C. (ed.) (2011) *Bioethics Around the Globe*, New York: Oxford University Press.

National Commission for the Protection of Human Subjects of Biomedical and Behavioral Research (1977) *Psychosurgery: Report and Recommendations*, DHEW Publication No. (OS) 77-0001.

National Commission for the Protection of Human Subjects of Biomedical and Behavioral Research (1978) *Research Involving Those Institutionalized as Mentally Infirm*, DHEW Publication No. (OS) 78-0006.

National Commission for the Protection of Human Subjects of Biomedical and Behavioral Research (1979) *The Belmont Report: Ethical Principles and Guidelines for the Protection of Human Subjects of Research*, DHEW Publication No. (OS) 78-0012.

O'Toole, K. (1997) "The Stanford Prison Experiment: Still Powerful After All These Years," *Stanford University News Service*, January 8.

Pittenger, D. (2008) "Deception in Research: Distinctions and Solutions from the Perspective of Utilitarianism," in D. Bersoff (ed.) *Ethical Conflicts in Psychology*, 4th edition, Washington, DC: American Psychological Association.

Presidential Commission for the Study of Bioethical Issues (2011) "'Ethically Impossible' STD Research in Guatemala from 1946 to 1948." Available at: http://bioethics.gov/cms/node/654 (accessed July 8, 2014).

Proctor, R. (1992) "Nazi Doctors, Racial Medicine and Human Experimentation," in G. Annas and M. Grodin (eds.) *The Nazi Doctors and the Nuremberg Code: Human Rights in Human Experimentation*, New York, NY: Oxford University Press.

Rothman, D. (1982) "Were Tuskegee & Willowbrook 'Studies in Nature'?" *The Hastings Center Report* 12 (2): 5–7.

Rothman, D. and Rothman, S. (1984) *The Willowbrook Wars*, New York, NY: Harper & Row.

Sass, H.M. (1997) "Letter: The Nuremberg Code, German Laws and Prominent Physician-Thinkers," *Journal of the American Medical Association* 277 (9): 709.

Schmidt, U. (2006) "Cold War at Porton Down: Informed Consent in Britain's Biological and Chemical Warfare Experiments," *Cambridge Quarterly of Ethics* 15 (4): 366–80.

Seidelman, W. (1988) "Megele Medicus: Medicine's Nazi Heritage," *The Milbank Quarterly* 66 (2): 221–39.

Shuster, E. (1997) "Fifty Years Later: The Significance of the Nuremberg Code," *New England Journal of Medicine* 337: 1436–40.

Sisti, D. and Caplan, A. (2003) "Back to Basics: Research Ethics and Oversight in the Post-Gelsinger Era," in C. Rehmann-Sutter and H. Müller (eds.) *Ethik und Gentherapie: Zum praktischen Diskurs um die Molekulare Medizin*, Stuttgart and Basel: Francke Verlag, 2. Auflage.

Steinbrook, R. (2008) "The Gelsinger Case," in E. Emanuel, C. Grady, R. Crouch, R. Lie, F. Miller and D. Wendler (eds.) *The Oxford Textbook of Clinical Research Ethics*, New York: Oxford University Press.

Walters, L. (2000) "The Oversight of Human Gene Transfer Research," *Kennedy Institute of Ethics Journal* 10: 171–4.

Wendler, D., Kington, R., Madans, J., Van Wye, G., Christ-Schmidt, H., Pratt, L.A., Brawley, O.W., Gross, C.P. and Emanuel, E. (2005) "Are Racial and Ethnic Minorities Less Willing to Participate in Health Research?" *PLoS Med* 3 (2): e19.

U.S. v. Karl Brandt et al. (1947) Nuremberg Military Tribunal, The Nuremberg Code.

Zinner, D., Bolcic-Jankovic, D., Clarridge, B., Blumenthal, D. and Campbell, E. (2009) "Participation of Academic Scientists in Relationships with Industry," *Health Affairs* 28 (6): 1814–25.

15
THE DUTY OF CARE AND EQUIPOISE IN RANDOMIZED CONTROLLED TRIALS

Charles Weijer, Paul B. Miller, and Mackenzie Graham

The Ethical Challenge of Randomization

The randomized controlled trial (RCT) is widely regarded as a key approach to assessing the efficacy and safety of new medical treatments. RCTs are near the top of the evidence-based medicine hierarchy, and the results of well designed and carefully conducted RCTs influence physicians, drugs regulators, and health policy-makers (Sackett et al. 1996). In an RCT, patients with a medical illness are allocated by chance to one of two or more study arms or "conditions." Patients allocated to the experimental condition receive the new treatment under investigation, while patients allocated to the control condition receive a standard treatment to which the new treatment is being compared. All patients are followed for a defined period of time, and information on prespecified outcome measures is collected. Physician-researchers conclude that the new treatment is effective if patients in the experimental condition outperform those in the control condition in the primary outcome measure according to statistical tests of significance.

Randomization is an important methodological strength of the RCT: It helps ensure the comparability of patients in the experimental and control conditions; it enables both patient and physician-researcher to remain ignorant as to assignment of conditions; and it guarantees the validity of statistical tests of significance (Friedman et al. 1998). Despite the advantages, randomization is the source of one of the most difficult and persistent challenges in the ethics of research. Until recently, most patients were offered enrollment in an RCT by their own physician; in many cases, the physician-researcher conducting the RCT was the patient's physician. Physicians are widely regarded as having special ethical obligations to their patients. These include the obligation to ensure that the patient receives competent treatment. The problem is how can the physician, consistent with this ethical obligation, offer the patient enrollment in an RCT? As we have seen, in an RCT the patient will be randomly allocated to the experimental or control condition. On the face of it at least, tossing a coin to determine which treatment a patient will receive seems inconsistent with the physician's obligation. Can the physician ever ethically offer RCT enrollment to his or her patient? If so, under what circumstances?

In order to address these questions, we require a clearer picture of the physician's ethical obligations to his patient. The physician–patient relationship is a trust relationship. Trust relationships play a very important role in our lives. These relationships have been described as having a tri-partite, purposive structure: A trusts B *to do* C (Baier 1986). In this three-part relationship, the truster (in this case, the patient) trusts the trustee (the physician) to protect and promote a significant practical interest (the patient's health). The truster cedes control of the significant practical interest, and as a result, the trustee has discretionary power over the interest at stake (Miller and Weijer 2006b). Trust relationships are, as a result, not relationships between equals; rather, they are relationships of structural inequality in which the truster is dependent on the loyalty, judgment, and competence of the trustee. To mitigate the vulnerability of the truster, moral obligations accrue to the trustee, including a duty to act and advise the truster so as to protect and promote the significant practical interests at stake. Socially important trust relationships, including those between doctor and patient, lawyer and client, and chief executive officer and shareholder, are closely mirrored in a legal context by the law of fiduciary relationships (Miller and Weijer 2006a).

Thus, we argue that it is the trust relationship between physician and patient that grounds the physician's ethical duties to the patient. Prominent among these duties is the ethical duty of care: The physician must act and advise the patient so as to protect and promote the patient's health. And it is the duty of care that comes into conflict with randomization. Given the randomized nature of treatment allocation in an RCT, physicians cannot ensure that their patient will receive one treatment as opposed to another. How can physicians fulfill their duty of care to the patient if they cannot be sure which treatment their patient will receive? Finding a way to answer this question is a matter of considerable importance. If physicians cannot ethically offer their patients enrollment in RCTs, important medical research will be impeded and the development of new treatments will slow. The ethical challenge of randomization has troubled many bioethicists for decades. In this chapter, we will consider a few of the most prominent arguments that have been offered to address the problem, examine closely their underlying ethical foundations, and situate the debate as a part of a larger question regarding the origins of ethical norms. At stake is a foundational question in the ethics of research: To what degree, if any, may the medical interests of a patient be put at risk for the potential benefit of future patients and society?

Fried and Freedman's Solutions

In his 1974 book *Medical Experimentation: Personal Integrity and Social Policy*, Charles Fried argued that the physician–patient relationship is a trust relationship, and concluded that the physician's duty of personal care to his patient requires "unqualified fidelity to that patient's health" (Fried 1974: 50). The physician must exercise his judgment in a manner that considers both the specific health interests and particular circumstances of the patient. Fried believed that personal care is a right that a physician "may not compromise in the general pursuit of the common good" (Fried 1974: 92). When a physician sacrifices the interests of the patient in receiving competent care in favor of the welfare of others, he violates the integrity of the relationship and thus his obligations to the patient. Fried argued that participation in an RCT is consistent with a patient's right to personal care only when a state of "equipoise" obtains, that is, when the physician is genuinely uncertain as to the preferred treatment for the patient (hereafter,

"Fried's equipoise"). Importantly, Fried's equipoise is specific to a particular patient, taking into account the patient's symptoms, diagnosis, and personal preferences. So long as Fried's equipoise exists, the physician does not know which treatment is best for the patient and, accordingly, the duty of personal care is indifferent to the patient being allocated to one condition or another in an RCT—both treatments are consistent with the considered judgment of the physician.

Fried's equipoise has been interpreted as an absolute standard in which physicians' uncertainty is balanced on a knife's edge; that is, their preference for one treatment compared with another is precisely 50:50 across a whole range of criteria (Schafer 1982; Marquis 1983). On this reading, Fried's equipoise sets a nearly impossible standard, one that is both too rigid and too fragile. Promising results from preparatory research required to motivate an RCT seem likely to disrupt Fried's equipoise. Even if Fried's equipoise exists at the start of an RCT, accumulating data on patients in the RCT would surely disrupt it long before the study is completed. Because of the difficulties, commentators have been skeptical of Fried's equipoise as a solution to the ethics of randomization (Joffe and Truog 2011).

In an effort to resolve this impasse, Benjamin Freedman proposed a more robust version of equipoise, which he called "clinical equipoise" (Freedman 1987). Clinical equipoise relocates the site of uncertainty regarding the preferred treatment from the individual physician to the expert medical community as a whole. Thus, when there exists "an honest, professional disagreement among expert clinicians about the preferred treatment . . . a state of clinical equipoise exists" (Freedman 1987: 144). For Freedman, the purpose of an RCT is to disrupt clinical equipoise and change clinical practice. When the accumulated evidence in favor of one treatment is such that no open-minded physician informed of the results would favor the other treatment, clinical equipoise is disturbed and the RCT must stop. Because preliminary research data or interim RCT results would be unlikely to resolve disagreement within the medical community, RCTs will generally need to continue to the planned point of completion in order to provide data sufficiently robust and reliable to change medical practice.

Clinical equipoise, with its emphasis on collective norms rather than individual opinion, can be understood as a reflection of a larger shift within the medical community towards evidence-based medicine (Sackett et al. 1996). For Freedman, standards of care are determined by consensus within the medical community. Clinical equipoise promotes consistent standards of care across groups of expert physicians, and diminishes the import of the (potentially idiosyncratic) judgment of individual physicians. As Freedman points out:

> competent (hence, ethical) medicine is social in nature. Progress in medicine relies on progressive consensus within the medical and research communities . . . Normative judgments of behavior rely on a comparison with what is done by the community of medical practitioners.
>
> (Freedman 1987: 144)

Accordingly, the physician's duty of care consists less of the individualized judgment advocated by Fried, and more of the provision of competent care consistent with broad communal practices among expert physicians. Indeed, such is the emphasis on communal norms that, consistent with clinical equipoise, an individual physician with a strong treatment preference may nonetheless ethically offer his patient trial enrolment, provided the less-favored treatment is preferred by responsible and competent colleagues.

Clinical equipoise is an important deontological constraint upon science. It requires that the experimental and control conditions in an RCT be consistent with competent care. It thereby prohibits exposing patients to the risks of an experimental or control condition that is known to involve substandard care. While placebo-controlled trials may offer certain advantages, including being cheaper and arguably easier to interpret, clinical equipoise restricts the use of placebos in RCTs (Freedman 1990). A placebo control may only be used when no proven and effective treatment exists, the trial selectively enrolls patients who have not responded to standard treatment, the medical condition is minor and non-treatment is consistent with competent practice, or all study participants receive standard medical care (as in an RCT in which the addition of a new drug to a standard regimen is compared with the standard regimen plus placebo) (Weijer and Miller 2004).

At the time that Fried and Freedman were writing, most patients were offered enrollment in an RCT by their own physician, and sometimes the physician-researcher conducting the RCT was that same physician. As a result, Fried and Freedman understood norms governing RCTs in terms of the physician–patient relationship. They both acknowledged that physicians owe a duty of care to their patients, and they both saw the duty of care as a key point of conflict with random allocation of patients to study conditions in an RCT. However, Fried and Freedman understood the demands of the duty of care somewhat differently. Fried understood the duty of personal care to require that physicians exercise individualized judgment on behalf of patients. This understanding of the duty of care in turn shaped Fried's equipoise: Only when the physician is uncertain as to the preferred treatment for his or her patient (considering the patient's history, diagnosis, and preferences) would an offer of RCT enrollment be ethically permissible. For Freedman, the norms of practice derive from the community of physicians and not the opinions of individual physicians; accordingly, the duty of care necessitates consistency with accepted communal practices. This understanding of the duty of care in turn shaped Freedman's concept of clinical equipoise: Only when there is disagreement in the relevant community of expert physicians as to the preferred treatment may the patient be approached for enrollment in an RCT.

Critics

Freedman's concept of clinical equipoise was—for a period of time at least—regarded by many as the definitive solution to the ethics of randomization. Clinical equipoise is widely used (and cited) by those who design and conduct RCTs to justify the choice of study conditions and the decision whether to continue a trial in light of interim data. Its role as an ethical constraint upon the practice of science has been particularly important. Clinical equipoise has been cited prominently in criticism of placebo-controlled trials and trials in developing countries (Rothman and Michels 1994; Angell 1997). Finally, it is a key concept in a systematic approach to the ethical analysis by research ethics committees of benefits and harms in clinical research called "component analysis" (Weijer and Miller 2004).

However, the years since 2002 have witnessed a vigorous debate in the bioethics literature about clinical equipoise and the duty of care as solutions to the ethical problem of randomization (Joffe and Truog 2011). Critics can be divided into at least three groups: Those who endorse the duty of care but deny clinical equipoise; those who endorse clinical equipoise but deny the duty of care as its moral foundation; and those who deny both clinical equipoise and the duty of care. The first group of critics believes that clinical equipoise ignores the pivotal importance of clinical judgment in protecting the medical interests of patients in RCTs. Like Fried, they understand the duty of care as requiring that physicians exercise individual judgment on behalf of their patients, and the appeal of clinical equipoise to communal norms does not satisfy the duty of care so understood. For instance, Deborah Hellman points out that "what matters ethically is not whether the medical community is in equipoise about the merits of the standard versus the experimental therapy, but rather whether the individual physician enrolling patients in the study himself favors one treatment or another" (Hellman 2002: 375). As a result, she rejects clinical equipoise and argues that the ethical problem of randomization is "real and fairly intractable" (Hellman 2002: 379).

The second group of critics acknowledge the importance of clinical equipoise as an ethical constraint upon science, but questions whether it can be grounded in the role of the physician-researcher and his attendant duty of care to the patient. At least two reasons are given. First, as argued above, clinical equipoise seems inconsistent with Fried's view of the duty of care and its requirement of individual clinical judgment. As a result, Alex London concludes that clinical equipoise must be "revised or rejected because it is . . .. insufficiently responsive to the physician's fiduciary obligations to the individual patient" (London 2007: 106). Second, critics point out—correctly—that RCTs in health services and public health research may not involve physician-researchers, and thus clinical equipoise seems not to apply. Rebecca Kukla sees this as a troubling result: "To the extent that one grounds research ethics on the ethics of therapeutic clinical medicine, these other kinds of research will be left in an unconstrained ethical vacuum" (Kukla 2007: 172). Both London and Kukla go on to propose alternative moral foundations for clinical equipoise (or cognates), appealing to egalitarian political theory and the researcher's moral obligations to persons, respectively (London 2007; Kukla 2007).

The third group of critics rejects altogether the role of the duty of care and clinical equipoise in the ethics of randomization. Franklin Miller and colleagues have argued that invoking an ethical duty of care and the moral rule of clinical equipoise in RCTs conflates the ethics of research with the ethics of medical practice (Miller and Brody 2003a; Miller 2004). The differing roles of researchers and physicians are incompatible, according to Miller and colleagues, because the ends of the activities in which they are engaged are different. Medical practice aims *solely* to protect and promote the health of the patient, while medical research aims *solely* to produce generalizable knowledge. When a physician-researcher recruits a patient in an RCT, she is no longer acting as a physician, but rather as a researcher. As such, different ethical obligations apply. In particular, the physician-researcher does not have a duty of care to the patient in an RCT because the purpose of research is not to provide medical care. As a result, Miller and colleagues claim that clinical equipoise is "neither necessary nor sufficient for ethically justifiable RCTs" (Miller and Brody 2003a: 25). Since the ethical problem of randomization is generated by the special moral duties that physicians have to patients, they deny that there is an ethical problem in need of resolution.

To understand the force of Miller and colleagues' position, it is important to take account of recent changes in clinical research. Currently, although some patients may be approached for RCT enrollment by their physician, many—if not most—learn of RCTs through other sources, including the Internet. Typically, the patient has had no prior relationship with the physician-researcher conducting the RCT. Thus, the norms of the physician–patient relationship may *not* be immediately relevant. Given that the ends of research are separable from those of medical practice, it would be hasty to assume that the ethical obligations of one domain *automatically* apply to the other. An argument is needed as to why the relationship between physician-researcher and patient in an RCT ought to be understood as one of trust.

Skeptical of the existence of a trust relationship, Miller and colleagues believe that it is the "the basic goal and nature of the activity [which] determines the ethical standards that ought to apply" (Miller and Brody 2003a: 22). In their view, the differing purposes of research and medical practice entail separate ethical standards. The ethical obligations of the physician-researcher are defined by the norms internal to the practice of good science. These scientific norms require that physician-researchers ensure that the RCT asks an important question, the methodology is sound, the risks to the patient are outweighed by the benefits to future patients, patients provide informed consent, and are not exploited.[1] Physician-researchers do not, in their view, have a duty to protect and promote the medical interests of patients in an RCT. According to Miller and colleagues, "clinical research is dedicated primarily to promoting the medical good of future patients by means of scientific knowledge derived from experimentation with current research participants—a frankly utilitarian purpose" (Miller and Brody 2003a: 21).

Central to Miller and colleagues' rejection of the duty of care in clinical research is their resistance to the role of clinical equipoise as an ethical constraint upon science. As we have noted, clinical equipoise prohibits exposing patients to experimental or control conditions that are known to involve substandard care, and this limits the ethical use of placebo controls when proven, effective treatment exists for a medical condition. Miller and colleagues have argued that placebo-controlled trials have important scientific advantages, particularly in illnesses such as schizophrenia or depression, in which deterioration or improvement is difficult to measure accurately (Miller and Brody 2002). The importance of generating reliable scientific data from RCTs, they believe, outweighs the medical interests of patients. Thus, they claim that patients with schizophrenia and depression—conditions for which proven, effective treatment exists—can ethically be enrolled in an RCT with placebo as the control condition (Miller and Brody 2002, 2003a).

But can an appeal to the internal norms of science alone successfully ground the ethical obligations that Miller and colleagues would substitute for those that underlie clinical equipoise? For some requirements, the answer seems to be yes. The requirement of a well formulated scientific question and the use of an appropriate study method are scientific norms. In other cases, though, the answer is less clear. What norm internal to science grounds obligations to ensure that study benefits exceed harms, to obtain informed consent, or to ensure that participants are not exploited? These claims might be justified by appeal to broader ethical principles (e.g., Mill's Harm Principle) or utilitarianism, but doing so seems to violate the assumption that the "goal and nature of the activity determines the ethical standards" (Miller and Brody 2003a; Miller and Weijer 2007). Further, even if clinical research has a "frankly utilitarian purpose," deontological constraints, such as clinical equipoise, may have an important role to play. Consider the analogy with criminal punishment, which may be viewed as a utilitarian project limited by deontological constraints not grounded in utility, including "don't punish the innocent" (Hart 1968). Finally, their argument ignores the possibility that the moral obligations inherent in medical practice and research arise because of the nature of the relationships involved, and not simply the goals of the activities. We return to these issues in the final section of this chapter.

Revisions

We believe that a successful resolution to the ethical challenge of randomization must take account of these criticisms. First, the justification of clinical equipoise cannot rest solely on the trust relationship between physician-researcher and patient. Research ethics committees review RCTs prior to enrollment of any patients in the study (and hence prior to any physician-researcher and patient relationship) and some health research, including public health research, does not even involve physician-researchers. Second, there must be a defined role for clinical judgment in the enrollment and continuation of patients in RCTs. Third, if it is the case that a physician-researcher owes the patient in an RCT a duty of care, an argument must be given as to why the duty applies in research without appeal to the norms of medical practice. In this section we provide a revised account of equipoise and the duty of care responding to the first two points; in the next section we give an account of the trust relationship between the physician-researcher and patient.

There is something deeply appealing about both Fried's and Freedman's solutions to the conflict between randomization and the duty of care. Fried identifies an essential feature of medical practice, namely, the personalized judgment exercised by a physician on behalf of his patient; Freedman recognizes the role of the professional community as a whole in setting standards for medical care. However, we have argued that neither concept presents a sufficient moral condition for the conduct of RCTs (Miller and Weijer 2003). The lengthy history of abuses in research makes clear the shortcomings of relying solely on the character and judgment of physician-researchers, and highlights the importance of having research ethics committees in place to judge the ethical acceptability of RCTs. Indeed, it is difficult to see how Fried's equipoise provides research ethics committees with any guidance. While clinical equipoise seems well suited to guiding research ethics committees, it does not account for the protective judgment of individual physician-researchers. Given this, we argue that the two concepts may be productively viewed as having differing roles in the ethical justification of randomization.

While Freedman understood the physician–patient relationship as the sole foundation for clinical equipoise, we believe another trust relationship, namely that between the state and research participant, plays an important role in grounding the concept (Miller and Weijer 2006b). RCTs are key to the rigorous assessment of the safety and effectiveness of novel medical treatments, and the resulting evidence base for medicine is a public good. Without the voluntary participation of patients in RCTs, this evidence could not be generated and the public would be deprived of an important good. Patients enroll in RCTs trusting that the state will protect their interests in exchange for their contribution to the scientific enterprise. The interests of patients in RCTs are several, and include interests in receiving competent medical care and not being exposed to undue risk for the benefit of others. As a result of the public good of RCTs and the trust shown by patients who agree to participate in them, the state is obligated to protect the interests of patients in RCTs. The state fulfills its trust-based obligations in promulgating guidelines for the ethical conduct of research and ensuring that they are enforced. On this view, the research ethics committee may be viewed as an arm of the state that ensures the protection of the liberty and welfare interests of research participants (Miller and Weijer 2006b).

Clinical equipoise is a specification of the state's trust-based obligation to protect the patient's interest in receiving competent medical care (Miller and Weijer 2006b). It guides research ethics committees in their review of RCTs by directing their attention to the relative merits of study treatments (or therapeutic procedures) in light of available evidence and current medical practices. The research ethics committee must ensure that sufficient evidence exists to support the experimental condition; they must also ensure that the control condition does not involve treatment known to be substandard. Study conditions are permissible if the research ethics committee concludes that honest, professional disagreement in the community of expert practitioners exists (or would exist, were the evidence widely known) as to the preferred treatment. Research ethics committee approval signifies that study conditions conform to broad professional standards for the treatment of a defined population of patients. As such, clinical equipoise is a key concept in a systematic and comprehensive approach to the ethical analysis of study benefits and harms we call "component analysis" (Weijer and Miller 2004).

It is important, however, to recognize the limits of research ethics committee approval. Conformity with clinical equipoise does not entail the moral acceptability of either enrolling or retaining *particular* patients in an RCT. For instance, patients may satisfy all of an RCT's eligibility criteria, but their medical history may suggest that study participation will be unduly harmful or burdensome. Physician-researchers meet their duty of care in enrolling and retaining patients in an RCT by making an expert judgment that takes into account the evidence on treatment alternatives *and* the particular circumstances of the patient. Knowing that a research ethics committee has determined that clinical equipoise is fulfilled, the physician-researcher may enroll or retain a patient in an RCT unless the physician-researcher believes it would be medically irresponsible to do so, and this belief is supported by evidence that would be convincing to colleagues. We refer to this ethical requirement as the "clinical judgment principle," a more robust variant of Fried's equipoise. Protecting the medical interests of patients in RCTs requires that both clinical equipoise *and* the clinical judgment principle are satisfied in the design, review, and conduct of an RCT (Miller and Weijer 2006b).

A Moral Foundation for the Physician-Researcher and Patient Relationship

The explanation in the previous section both grounds clinical equipoise in the trust relationship between the state and research participant and articulates a clear role for the expert judgment of the physician-researcher in enrolling or continuing patients in RCTs. Here we address the third concern: Why should we think that physician-researchers owe a duty of care to patients in RCTs similar to that which physicians owe their patients? Both of these are fiduciary relationships characterized by trust (Miller and Weijer 2006a, 2006b). As discussed in the first section of this chapter, a trust relationship is defined by several important features. First, it involves a relationship characterized by structural inequality. Second, it typically involves the transfer of discretionary power over certain interests from the truster to the trustee. Third, because the trustee has been entrusted with these powers, he incurs an obligation to use them in a way that protects and promotes the interests of the truster. Because the duty of care is rooted in the nature of the trust relationship, this duty applies whether the physician's goal is to improve the health of a patient in a care context, or to produce generalizable knowledge in a research context. The ends of the activities are immaterial to the moral obligations of the parties involved; it is the structure of the relationship between the parties that is morally salient.

The physician-researcher and patient relationship in an RCT bears all of the hallmarks of a trust relationship. First, given that therapeutic modalities are administered in RCTs, the patient necessarily relies on the expertise of the physician-researcher in improving his or her health. Only the physician-researcher is socially authorized to provide the patient with the treatments prescribed by the study protocol. Further, the physician-researcher possesses specialized knowledge that the patient does not have. Thus the relationship between physician-researcher and patient is structurally unequal.

Second, the patient grants the physician-researcher discretionary powers over the former's health interests, and by ceding these powers the patient is exposed to the risk of having these interests compromised. Among other things, physician-researchers are authorized to:

- collect and use confidential information about patients;
- determine eligibility for RCT participation;
- administer and withdraw therapeutic interventions (standard and experimental drugs and procedures);
- administer and withdraw non-therapeutic procedures;
- order alternative therapy (or the resumption of standard therapy) in the event the study must be terminated or the patient removed from the RCT.

Exercise of these powers entails considerable discretion. Physician-researchers must exercise judgment regarding patient eligibility, as well as in the development and execution of study protocols. It is up to the discretion of the physician-researcher to determine whether protocol adherence is appropriate for a particular patient. Whether the patient receives competent care and is protected from undue harm will thus depend on the decisions made by the physician-researcher.

Third, because the physician-researcher has been entrusted with these powers, he incurs a duty to protect and promote the health interests of the patient. That is, in the context of an RCT, the physician-researcher owes the patient a duty of care.

The trust-based nature of the physician-researcher and patient relationship is underscored by the fact that it fits the legal definition of a fiduciary relationship as well. We have argued that a fiduciary relationship is established where, "One party entrusts another with discretionary power over the legal, economic or other practical interests of a beneficiary, and the other party undertakes, expressly or impliedly, to exercise that power" (Miller and Weijer 2006a: 427–8).

In contrast to most private law relationships, in which parties are presumed to have an equal and independent capacity to pursue their respective interests, the transfer of discretionary power that characterizes the fiduciary relationship results in structural inequality and dependence. Haavi Morreim has argued that the relationship between physician-researchers and patients cannot be fiduciary because RCT protocols constrain the exercise of discretion by physician-researchers (Morreim 2005). However, she misapprehends the nature of fiduciary discretion. Fiduciaries are not expected to enjoy—and rarely do enjoy—unfettered discretion to advance the interests of their beneficiaries. Rather, they have a contextual kind of discretion, that is, discretion within the ambit of constraints peculiar to the activity in which they and their beneficiaries are involved. These constraints may be owing to the nature of the activities, the environment within which they are undertaken, or overarching legal or regulatory requirements. As we explain above (and elsewhere in a detailed response to Morreim), physician-researchers have discretion in determining whether to enroll or to continue the enrolment of patient-subjects in RCTs, notwithstanding that their fiduciary discretion differs in certain particulars from the kind of discretion enjoyed by physicians in clinical settings (Miller and Weijer 2006a).

What obligations arise from the relationship between the physician-researcher and patient, understood in terms of the discretionary power that the former enjoys over the latter? As noted above, the vulnerability inherent in the trust relationship determines the obligations of the physician-researcher. Perhaps the most obvious vulnerability of the patient is to exploitation by the physician-researcher when discretionary power is misused to promote the interests or goals of the latter at the expense of the former. Exercise of power in this way is exploitative because it involves treating the patient as a mere means to an end; that is, the patient's interests are actively subordinated in service of the interests of others. Vulnerability to exploitation grounds a duty of loyalty, which requires the physician-researcher to avoid or properly manage conflicts of interest and duty.

Additionally, the patient is vulnerable to neglect by the physician-researcher. Because exercise of discretionary power requires judgment, the patient is vulnerable to failure by the physician-researcher to make responsible judgments. Accordingly, the physician-researcher owes the patient a "duty of discretion," which requires the former to exercise discretion or judgment when making decisions on behalf of the latter.

Finally, the patient is vulnerable to carelessness. Accordingly, the physician-researcher owes the patient a "duty of care." One way in which the physician-researcher can fulfill this obligation is by appealing to the "clinical judgment principle," which permits the enrollment of patients in an RCT by physician-researchers (provided the study has been reviewed by a research ethics committee and found to be consistent with clinical equipoise) unless "they believe that it would be medically irresponsible to do so and this belief is supported by evidence that ought to be convincing to colleagues" (Miller and Weijer 2006b: 546). This principle emphasizes the role of expert judgment in fulfilling the duty of care. If the physician-researcher has good reason to believe that one of the treatments being tested in an RCT would expose a patient to undue harm, enrollment would be medically irresponsible and ethically impermissible.

We have seen that although the goals of clinical research and medical practice are different, the relationship between the physician-researcher and patient is similar to that between physician and patient; both are trust relationships. It is because both are trust relationships—and *not* because they are similar in other respects—that the duties of loyalty, discretion, and care apply equally to both physicians and physician-researchers. Denying the relevance of the duty of care is not an acceptable answer to the ethical challenge of randomization. Physician-researchers must abide by some form of equipoise (as exemplified by clinical equipoise and the clinical judgment principle) when enrolling and continuing patients in RCTs.

Normative Externalism and Internalism

In the final section of this chapter, we situate the debate about the ethics of randomization as a part of a larger question regarding the origins of ethical norms. As we have seen, at stake is whether and, if so, to what degree the medical interests of a patient in an RCT may be put at risk for the potential benefit of future patients and society. We argue that both the state and the physician-researcher have a trust-based duty of care to the patient that grounds clinical equipoise and the clinical judgment principle. These moral rules are important deontological constraints on science; they prohibit knowingly providing patients with substandard care and require physician-researchers to exercise expert judgment on their behalf. Franklin Miller and colleagues reject this approach. They deny the existence of a duty of care and reject related deontological constraints upon science. In their place, they offer an essentially utilitarian apparatus in which the medical interests of patients may be put at risk provided that the potential benefits to future patients and society are sufficiently significant. They endorse as ethical placebo-controlled trials involving patients with conditions such as schizophrenia and depression, for which proven effective treatment exists. Finally, they deny that physician-researchers have a duty to exercise judgment to protect the medical interests of patients.

A key feature of the debate is disagreement as to the source of norms in clinical research, one that we might productively characterize as a debate between ethical externalism and internalism. For the externalist, norms governing an activity are imposed from without, either by broad ethical or legal norms that apply to society as a whole, or the more fundamental ethical principles upon which these norms are based. For the internalist, the norms governing an activity are generated by the nature of the activity itself. So long as the nature of the activity or practice can be adequately specified, choosing among competing ethical norms will not raise intractable problems.

Charles Fried, Benjamin Freedman, Rebecca Kukla, Alex London, Paul Miller, and Charles Weijer adopt an externalist view of ethical norms. For Fried, Freedman, Miller, and Weijer, physician-researchers owe an ethical duty of care to patients in RCTs because of the asymmetry, dependence, and vulnerability of the trust relationship. Miller and Weijer argue further that the state also owes a trust-based duty of care to patients in RCTs. Importantly, all trust relationships possess these characteristics, and thus, the ethical obligations of the actors in RCTs are imposed from outside of the activity. While the norms of science, including the importance of a valuable study question and appropriate methodology, are a part of the ethics of RCTs, the ends of science are constrained by ethical duties that trustees owe trusters broadly within society. For instance, even if the use of a placebo control would be scientifically desirable in some cases, clinical equipoise (and the duty of care) prohibit its use when proven, effective treatment exists and is available in a sustainable manner.

Franklin Miller and colleagues' critique of the duty of care and equipoise may be viewed as a rejection of externalism. Defenders of the duty of care err, according to them, in "drawing the line" in the wrong place because they fail to give sufficient weight to the ends of science (Miller and Brody 2003a). In their internalist approach, Franklin Miller and colleagues argue that physician-researchers must see themselves as "scientists only and not as doctors," and should thus derive their ethical obligations from the goals of science (Joffe and Miller 2008). This explains why they argue that norms cannot be imported from one activity into another (i.e., from clinical practice to research); the differing ends of each activity generate different ethical norms. In their view, the duty of care does not apply within the research context because it is the ends of medical practice, and *only* these ends, that generate such obligations (Miller and Brody 2003b).

Franklin Miller and Steven Joffe, in the most detailed exposition of this internalist view, point out that "biomedical research constitutes a spectrum of activities," with in vitro experimentation at one end, and clinical research on patients at the other (Joffe and Miller 2008: 32). They claim that it is a necessary condition of biomedical research that its goal be the production of generalizable knowledge, and that it respect "the internal norms of science," which requires the use of the scientific method as well as respect for scientific integrity (Joffe and Miller 2008: 33). Biomedical research is also subject to ethical constraints, which accumulate incrementally.

Research involving inanimate or nonsentient materials, such as molecules, DNA, and cell lines, must "minimize external risks," and "proceed under the good-faith assumption that the societal benefits of the research are likely to outweigh any potential harms" (Joffe and Miller 2008: 35). When research involves laboratory animals, including mice, cats, dogs, pigs, and primates, these same ethical constraints apply, with the additional requirement that the risks and burdens to the animals be minimized. Research on healthy human volunteers imposes additional constraints, including avoiding unacceptable risks, respecting participants, ensuring fairness in subject selection, and satisfying ancillary care obligations. When research involves patients, further ethical constraints must be observed, including "maximizing direct benefits, consistent with achieving the scientific aims of the study," honesty regarding the nature of the research, and the adoption of a "caring attitude" which acknowledges the patient's illness or limitation (Joffe and Miller 2008: 35). Due respect for the variable moral status of the experimental materials coupled with regard for the internal norms of science is thought sufficient to ensure that patients are protected.

The internalist view is not without difficulties. If the internalist seeks to ground specific moral constraints in the ends of an activity, she must first determine what precisely constitute the "ends of research." Numerous stakeholders may be involved in a particular research study (patients, families, research ethics committees, academic institutions, public funding bodies, and private sector funders), and research can take many different forms (e.g., market surveys, ethnographies, gene sequencing, and RCTs). Many social scientists would deny that their research is designed to produce generalizable knowledge. Even if we take the core end of science to be production of generalizable knowledge, this goal needs to be refined further for it to be useful: Who or what is the knowledge for? Is it knowledge purely for its own sake? How generalizable must it be?

Moreover, research is a complex activity, and it is not entirely clear just what is meant by the term "research context." Rather than playing a single role at any given time, researchers often perform many different roles. For example, if a physician-researcher undertakes a routine examination of a patient, performs an extra blood draw to monitor the experimental drug the patient is taking for hypertension, and then prescribes a medication for an ear infection, all in the span of 15 minutes, what role is the physician-researcher actually playing? In a theoretical sense, one might say that he starts out in the role of the physician, and then takes on the role of the researcher, before returning to his previous role. In practice, however, this exchange of roles is not obvious to either the patient or the physician-researcher.

The internalist might respond that an externalist view offers no clearer a picture of what the "ends of research" are or ought to be. But this is less of a problem for the externalist, as she doesn't seek to ground ethical constraints upon science in the ends of research. Moreover, the internalist might agree that research is a complex activity, yet insist that it is incumbent upon researchers that they do their utmost for their own sake to maintain a clear separation between roles (Miller and Rosenstein 2003).

The difficulty of justifying moral constraints becomes more pronounced when the internalist considers research on human participants. Miller and Joffe claim that researchers are required to fulfill familiar moral obligations (non-maleficence, respect for persons, justice) in the conduct of their research on healthy human participants, with additional requirements for patients who are in need of care. In order to remain consistent with the view that researchers are acting as scientists, the internalist must reject constraints on study design (such as equipoise requirements) which are not entailed by good scientific practice. Miller and Joffe argue that such constraints result from physicians "graft[ing] the pursuit of research objectives onto [their] primary therapeutic commitments," and that these are external to the practice of good science (Joffe and Miller 2008).

What sort of argument can the internalist employ to justify appropriate moral constraints on research, without resorting to moral principles that go beyond the practice of "good science"? Miller and Joffe claim that, in all instances, researchers must minimize the external risks associated with their research, and proceed under the good-faith assumption that the social benefits of their work will outweigh any potential individual or societal harms. When research requires testing on laboratory animals, researchers must ensure that the number of animals used is minimal, and that the pains or burdens to which these animals are subjected are minimized. One could envision this constraint emerging from a scientific requirement to maximize the use of limited scientific materials; subjecting animals to unnecessary testing would simply be wasting a valuable resource. Perhaps this same justification could be applied to minimizing harm to human subjects, although this would seem somewhat morally obtuse.

Miller and Joffe also state that there must be some limit on the acceptable level of risk to which research participants can be exposed (though it is not clear what that limit is), and assert that researchers must maximize direct benefit to participants, provided doing so is consistent with answering the relevant scientific questions (Joffe and Miller 2008). They also suggest that researchers adopt a "caring attitude" towards participants in recognition that they are "human beings rather than data points" (Joffe and Miller 2008: 38). But these harm–benefit requirements rest on a utilitarian foundation. Any plausible view of utilitarianism requires a principle of utility and a theory of welfare and, thus, their view of acceptable harms and benefits appeals to norms external to the practice of good science (Miller and Weijer 2007). The same can be said for adopting a "caring attitude." Why is adopting a "caring attitude" an inherent norm of scientific activity, and not a moral constraint that is grounded in more general moral principles? Imagine a physician-researcher who has the same attitude to patients as Dr Harry Harlow, the author of the now notorious monkey maternal separation experiments, had to his experimental subjects. (Harlow once remarked: "The only thing I care about is whether the monkeys will turn out a property I can publish. I don't have any love for them. Never have. I don't really like animals. I despise cats. I hate dogs. How could you like monkeys?") (Blum 1994: 92). Such an attitude would surely be unethical, but it seems tenuous to call it unscientific. Finally, if the ethical norms that govern activities do not in fact overlap, then it is difficult to see how Miller and colleagues could argue that physician-researchers have an obligation to obtain informed consent when this is clearly an obligation for physicians.

We conclude that internalists encounter several obstacles in their attempt to justify an acceptable level of protection for research participants, and are forced to import supplemental moral constraints that are externally derived. Miller and colleagues repeatedly invoke utilitarian moral philosophy and general ethical principles in explaining their position (Miller and Weijer 2007). Unsurprisingly, many proponents of the internalist position have come to recognize the deficiencies of their account, and have moved towards more open and sophisticated externalist orientations (Dickert and Wendler

2009; Rid and Wendler 2011). An externalist orientation provides principled constraints on what we can do to patients in the service of producing generalizable knowledge. It asserts that patient-subjects' right to competent care limits the design and conduct of RCTs, such that patients may not be randomly assigned to therapeutic modalities when existing evidence suggests this would entail substandard treatment. The account given here locates these constraints in the trust relationships that bind the state and physician-researchers with patients in RCTs.

Related Topics

Chapter 12, "Bias, Misconduct, and Integrity in Scientific Research," David B. Resnik
Chapter 14, "Biomedical Research Ethics: Landmark Cases, Scandals, and Conceptual Shifts," Jonathan D. Moreno and Dominic Sisti

Note

1 Exploitation is a contested concept in the bioethics literature. For further discussion, see: Wertheimer (1996); Resnik (2003).

References

Angell, M. (1997) "The Ethics of Clinical Research in the Third World," *New England Journal of Medicine* 337: 847–9.
Baier, A. (1986) "Trust and Antitrust," *Ethics* 96: 231–60.
Blum, D. (1994) *The Monkey Wars*, New York: Oxford University Press.
Dickert, N. and Wendler, D. (2009) "Ancillary Care Obligations of Medical Researchers,"' *JAMA* 302: 424–8.
Freedman, B. (1987) "Equipoise and the Ethics of Clinical Research," *New England Journal of Medicine* 317: 141–5.
Freedman, B. (1990) "Placebo-Controlled Trials and the Logic of Clinical Purpose," *IRB* 12 (6): 1–6.
Fried, C. (1974) *Medical Experimentation: Personal Integrity and Social Policy*, Amsterdam: North Holland Publishing Company.
Friedman, L.M., Furberg, C.D. and DeMets, D.L. (1998) *Fundamentals of Clinical Trials*, New York: Springer.
Hart, H.L.A. (1968) *Punishment and Responsibility: Essays in the Philosophy of Law*, New York: Oxford University Press.
Hellman, D. (2002) "Evidence, Belief, and Action: The Failure of Equipoise to Resolve the Ethical Tension in the Randomized Clinical Trial," *Journal of Law, Medicine, and Ethics* 30: 375–80.
Joffe, S. and Miller, F. (2008) "From Bench to Bedside: Mapping the Moral Terrain of Clinical Research," *Hastings Center Report* 38: 30–42.
Joffe, S. and Truog, R.D. (2011) "Equipoise and Randomization," in E.J. Emanuel, C. Grady, R.A. Crouch, R.K. Lie, F.G. Miller and D. Wendler, *The Oxford Textbook of Clinical Research Ethics*, New York: Oxford University Press, 245–60.
Kukla, R. (2007) "Resituating the Principle of Equipoise: Justice and Access to Care in Non-ideal Conditions," *Kennedy Institute of Ethics Journal* 17: 171–202.
London, A.J. (2007) "Two Dogmas of Research Ethics and the Integrative Approach to Human-Subjects Research," *Journal of Medicine and Philosophy* 32: 99–116.
Marquis, D. (1983) "Leaving Therapy to Chance," *Hastings Center Report* 13: 40–7.
Miller, F. (2004) "Research Ethics and Misguided Moral Intuition," *Journal of Law, Medicine, and Ethics* 32: 111–17.
Miller, F.G. and Brody, H. (2002) "What Makes Placebo-Controlled Trials Unethical?" *American Journal of Bioethics* 2 (2): 3–9.
Miller, F.G. and Brody, H. (2003a) "A Critique of Clinical Equipoise: Therapeutic Misconception in the Ethics of Clinical Trials," *Hastings Center Report* 33: 19–28.
Miller, F.G. and Brody, H. (2003b) "The Clinician-Investigator: Unavoidable but Manageable Tension," *Kennedy Institute of Ethics Journal* 13: 329–46.

Miller, F.G. and Rosenstein, D. (2003) "The Therapeutic Orientation to Clinical Trials," *New England Journal of Medicine* 348: 1383–6

Miller, P.B. and Weijer, C. (2003) "Rehabilitating Equipoise," *Kennedy Institute of Ethics Journal* 13: 93–118.

Miller, P.B. and Weijer, C. (2006a) "Fiduciary Obligation in Clinical Research," *Journal of Law, Medicine and Ethics* 34: 424–40.

Miller, P.B. and Weijer, C. (2006b) "Trust Based Obligations of the State and Physician-Researchers to Patient-Subjects," *Journal of Medical Ethics* 32: 542–7.

Miller, P.B. and Weijer, C. (2007) Equipoise and the Duty of Care in Clinical Research: A Philosophical Response to Our Critics," *Journal of Medicine and Philosophy* 32 (2): 117–33.

Morreim, E.H. (2005) "The Clinical Investigator as Fiduciary: Discarding a Misguided Idea," *Journal of Law, Medicine and Ethics* 33 (3): 586–98.

Resnik, D. (2003) "Exploitation in Biomedical Research," *Theoretical Medicine* 24: 233–59.

Rid, A. and Wendler, D. (2011) "A Framework for Risk–Benefit Evaluations in Biomedical Research," *Kennedy Institute of Ethics Journal* 21: 141–79.

Rothman, K.J. and Michels, K.B. (1994) "The Continuing Unethical Use of Placebo Controls," *New England Journal of Medicine* 331: 394–8.

Sackett, D.L., Rosenberg, W.M., Gray, J.A., Haynes, R.B. and Richardson W.S. (1996) "Evidence Based Medicine: What It Is and What It Isn't," *British Medical Journal* 312: 71–2.

Schafer, A. (1982) "The Ethics of the Randomized Clinical Trial," *New England Journal of Medicine* 307: 719–24.

Weijer, C. and Miller, P.B. (2004) "When Are Research Risks Reasonable in Relation to Anticipated Benefits?" *Nature Medicine* 10 (6): 570–3.

Wertheimer, A. (1996) *Exploitation*, Princeton: Princeton University Press.

16

THE FUTURE OF INFORMED CONSENT TO RESEARCH

Reconceptualizing the Process

Paul S. Appelbaum

Informed consent has become a *sine qua non* for the ethical conduct of human subjects research, with few exceptions. Indeed, so taken for granted is the notion that investigators must obtain subjects' consent before proceeding with research that it is difficult for most investigators and research staff to imagine that human subjects research was ever conducted in any other way. An examination of the history of informed consent to research, however, reveals that it is largely a creation of the second half of the twentieth century and has never been without controversy. Moreover, a careful examination of informed consent as actually applied in research settings reveals a highly imperfect process, much in need of adjustment. Thus, the future of informed consent to research is by no means clear.

In this chapter, I present a brief history of informed consent to research, distinguishing it from the very different evolution of consent in the treatment setting, consider the lessons of research that has been conducted on the consent process itself, and suggest a conceptual reorientation of consent to participate in research that holds the promise of more meaningfully engaging participants in the decisional process.

The History and Current Status of Consent to Research

Medical research—at least in the modern sense of a systematic investigation—is a relatively recent innovation in the long history of medicine. Lind's controlled trial of treatments for scurvy in the British navy in 1747 may well have been the first clinical trial ever performed, followed late in the century by additional studies of scurvy in sailors (Lind 1753). Despite the practical impact of the scurvy studies, which led to plummeting death rates among British sailors, and of Pierre-Charles-Alexandre Louis' publication in France of his conclusions regarding the inefficacy of bloodletting as a therapy for fevers (Louis 1836), systematic clinical investigation remained the rare exception in medicine. Most new treatments continued to be introduced and promoted on the basis of hypothesis and anecdote rather than firm supportive data. However, in the late nineteenth century the pace of experimentation accelerated, with the nutritional origins of beriberi (Hawk 2006) and pellagra (National Institutes of Health no date) discovered in studies with human subjects, and the origins of and treatments for a variety of infectious diseases pursued (Lederer 1995).

During these early years of systematic medical investigation, attention to consent-related issues appears to have been sporadic. Statements can be found from some leading physicians endorsing disclosure of information about the risks and benefits of experimental treatment (though not necessarily in the context of systematic research) (Lederer 1995: 1–2). Information as to whether subjects were even informed that they were part of a research study does not appear in most reports of the era, and the strong inference from the circumstances presented suggests that they were not (e.g., the Japanese beriberi studies, undertaken by feeding distinct diets to the crews of two battleships). A scandal in Prussia in the 1890s over experimental inoculation of unknowing patients with the syphilis spirochete led the Prussian government to establish the first governmental requirement for consent of human subjects prior to the conduct of research (Moreno 2000: 20). The earliest extant consent form derives from the studies of yellow fever, conducted with American soldiers in Cuba by Col. Walter Reed. Its resemblance to contemporary consent forms is striking, although its length—a single page—sets it clearly apart (Lederer 1995: 21). Pre-Nazi Germany, in 1931, adopted regulations requiring clear explanations of the experimental or innovative nature of proffered treatments (Howard-Jones 1982). However, accounts of the years before the Second World War make clear that obtaining consent was not routine in research settings in any part of the world (Lederer 1995; Parson 1984).

The turning point came with the revelations of the horrors committed by Nazi doctors in the concentration camps and death camps of the Third Reich. Among the experiments they conducted were exposure of prisoners to frigid seawater and low oxygen pressure to the point of death; mass sterilization by means of gonadal irradiation; and deliberate induction of gangrene in artificially created wounds (Proctor 1992). The Doctors' Trial in Nuremberg culminated in 1947 with the promulgation of what came to be called the Nuremberg Code, encompassing 10 principles of the conduct of research rooted in the notion that "[t]he voluntary consent of the human subject is absolutely essential," and requiring that:

> before the acceptance of an affirmative decision by the experimental subject there should be made known to him the nature, duration, and purpose of the experiment; the method and means by which it is to be conducted; all inconveniences and hazards reasonably to be expected; and the effects upon his health or person which may possibly come from his participation in the experiment.
>
> (*Trials of War Criminals* 1949)

The controversies regarding the derivation of the Nuremberg principles—i.e., whether they represented actual practice at the time or were constructed on an *ad hoc* basis to justify punishment for the horrific behaviors of the Nazi doctors—have been discussed extensively (Schmidt 2004). Suffice it to say that it is likely that little medical research in Allied countries was being carried out in conformance with the dictates of the Code, although it is also true that Allied researchers were generally not engaged in the deliberate infliction of suffering and death that characterized much of the Nazi work.

Perhaps because the circumstances in the concentration camps seemed so alien to medical researchers in other countries, it was easy for them to conclude that the Nuremberg principles—including the requirement for consent—were not meant to apply to them. They were not, after all, coercing prisoners into participating in research certain to induce harm. Most, though certainly not all, medical research was performed to test new treatment approaches that presented some prospect of benefit. The seeming inapplicability of Nuremberg to civil settings around the world was one of the motivators for the development of the Declaration of Helsinki by the World Medical Association in 1964, a much-revised version of which continues in effect today (World Medical Association 2008). Unlike the Nuremberg Code, the original Declaration held that "clinical research combined with patient care"—unlike "non-therapeutic clinical research"—could proceed without consent, if physicians concluded that obtaining consent would not be in the best interests of patients. As late as 1964, therefore, world medicine had still not accepted the idea that consent played a critical role in legitimizing experimental interventions and the deviations entailed from the usual approach to treatment.

Two forces converged in the 1970s to change that stance, exemplified by developments in the United States. A decade of scandals revealed that experiments had been conducted without subjects' consent, and sometimes with considerable risk of harm. This culminated in the expose of the Tuskegee syphilis study in 1971. Approximately 400 African-American men in Alabama who had contracted syphilis were followed for 40 years by the U.S. Public Health Service to observe the natural history of syphilis in blacks (Jones 1981). Their diagnosis was not revealed to them—indeed extraordinary efforts were taken to prevent discovery—and even after effective treatment for the disease became available, therapy was not provided. In response, the *National Research Act* of 1974 was passed, establishing a commission to make recommendations for preventing such abuses in the future. Although some federal subject protections existed as early as 1966 (Stewart 1972), the first comprehensive set of regulations was adopted by the Department of Health and Human Services in 1981. Current regulations, often referred to as the "Common Rule," were promulgated in 1991 and have been modified in only minor ways since (Department of Health and Human Services 2009).

The shape of those regulations, at least with regard to the requirements for consent, was influenced as well by developments in American courts beginning in the 1950s. Although it long had been a common law expectation that physicians would obtain patients' consent prior to intrusive (especially surgical) interventions, this "simple consent" required little in the way of disclosure to patients beyond the nature of the intervention proposed (Berg et al. 2001: 41–4). But U.S. courts in the mid and late 1950s began to formulate a more expansive doctrine of "informed consent" (the term first being used in this context in a 1957 decision (*Salgo v. Stanford* 1957)), which was widely accepted by the courts in the early 1970s (*Canterbury v. Spence* 1972; *Cobbs v. Grant* 1972). Physicians were now obligated to reveal information regarding the risks and benefits of the proposed treatment, along with alternative treatments—including the option of no treatment—and their risks and benefits. Many jurisdictions declared the standard of disclosure to be the amount of information on these topics that a reasonable patient would want to know before making a treatment decision. It was clear that patients were expected to play a major role in selecting their preferred treatments, and were to be given sufficient information to make meaningful choices (Berg et al. 2001: 46–65).

Combining the imperative to protect research subjects from abuse with the developments in informed consent law in the clinical setting, the drafters of the federal regulations elaborated a complex set of procedures and substantive requirements for investigators, which if anything have only become more intricate over time. Informed consent of subjects is required except when an Institutional Review Board (IRB) waives consent or when subjects are incompetent, in which case the consent of a legally authorized representative might be acceptable. In general, consent is to be obtained on a printed consent form, containing the relevant information and the subject's signature. Eight essential elements of information have to be disclosed to all subjects, along with six optional elements (Department of Health and Human Services 2009: 46.116b), and some studies require additional disclosures. Although these rules are specific to the U.S., the regulatory regime is roughly similar in most other developed areas of the world.

Informed Consent to Research: How Well Does It Work?

Almost from the inception of consent to research as a systematic policy, there have been studies of how well the process functions. The body of literature that has accumulated cannot be reviewed comprehensively here, but it is possible to summarize the findings and to provide illustrative examples.

The initial focus must be on written consent forms, given their salience to investigators and IRBs. In the years since the adoption of the federal regulations, consent forms have become more comprehensive in their coverage and grown steadily in length (Albala et al. 2010). A 2004 study of 107 consent forms for oncology clinical trials found an average length of eleven pages and 2700 words (Sharp 2004). Today, single-spaced forms exceeding twenty or even thirty pages in length are not uncommon. Among the drivers of increased content has been the tendency for regulatory agencies to add required boilerplate (e.g., most recently that U.S. clinical trials will be registered with a government agency (Department of Health and Human Services, Food and Drug Administration 2009)). Sponsors and investigators also have begun to include information about what will happen at each visit in longitudinal studies. Medical procedures and tests are described in increasing detail, among them procedures of negligible risk such as neuropsychological test batteries. It is often said that the impetus for ever-more-inclusive forms derives from concern about lawsuits alleging lack of informed consent if relevant information is missing, but it seems clear that by now investigators and IRBs have internalized the notion that more detail is better, quite apart from any realistic legal threats.

Remarkably, this stunning growth in the length of consent forms has come in the face of data indicating an inverse relationship between length and comprehension of the information provided (i.e., the longer the form, the less information subjects take from the process) (Mann 1994). Sharp has pointed to data suggesting that consent forms longer than 1,000 words (four double-spaced pages) are unlikely to be read, perhaps in part because of the time involved. He recommends that length be limited to no more than 1,250 words, which would take an average high-school graduate five to seven minutes to read (Sharp 2004). In addition, forms typically are written at a level of complexity that makes it unlikely that most research subjects will comprehend their contents (Paasche-Orlow et al. 2003; Williams et al. 2003). For example, a study of consent forms intended for use with patients with chronic mental illnesses showed that they had overall mean readability scores well above the educational level of most potential participants; the forms were even more complex in higher-risk studies (Christopher et al. 2007). Readability levels, moreover, may not tell the whole story about the challenges facing potential subjects in interpreting consent forms. Hochhauser noted a consent form reviewed by his IRB that was twenty-three single-spaced pages, contained 10,100 words, and "was so complicated that the risk section for the three drugs [being studied] included 160 possible side effects . . ." He asks, quite reasonably, "Is it possible for prospective subjects to remember and make informed decisions based on so many risks?" (Hochhauser 2008).

The length and complexity of consent forms might be of less concern if they did not play such a key role in informing potential research subjects. Few observational studies exist of how consent is routinely obtained, but there seems to be general agreement that primary reliance on the forms is widespread, especially when the disclosure process is delegated to research staff other than the investigator (Appelbaum and Roth 1983). Thus, the information in the form becomes the prime, and in some cases the only, disclosure that subjects receive about the study. Although it is routine for subjects to be asked whether they have any questions about the study, their limited comprehension often means that little additional information is requested or conveyed.

The answer to the question posed by Hochhauser—whether subjects are likely to grasp the extensive, complicated information with which they are presented—is evident from the large number of studies examining subjects' comprehension and appreciation of informed consent disclosures. Although there is some diversity in the literature, in general the studies suggest that research subjects are unable to recall much—in many cases most—of the information that has been conveyed to them (Verheggen and van Wijmen 1996). Subjects typically fail to grasp the purpose of research studies, the likelihood of benefit, and the range of risks (e.g., Daugherty et al. 2000). This has been found to be true for a broad array of research subjects with a wide range of disorders.

In addition to purely factual information about the study, which presents challenges of its own, subjects seem to have a particularly difficult time grasping some of the ways in which participation in a clinical trial differs from engaging in ordinary treatment. Joffe and colleagues' interviews of 207 oncology subjects, for example, revealed that 48 percent of subjects were willing to endorse the statement that "All the treatments and procedures in my clinical trial are standard for my type of cancer," when the purpose of the studies was precisely to test non-standard treatments (Joffe et al. 2001). Similarly, 29 percent agreed that "The treatment being researched in my clinical trial has been proven to be the best treatment for my type of cancer"; had that been correct, of course, the studies would not have been conducted. My colleagues and I have characterized this failure to appreciate the nature of a clinical trial as a "therapeutic misconception" (Appelbaum et al. 1987). The problem seems to manifest itself along two dimensions: Failure to understand the absence of individualization of treatment in clinical trials, and mistaken beliefs about the likely benefits of participation based on a misunderstanding of the study's methods. When so defined, we found that 61% of research subjects from a diverse array of studies at two academic medical centers manifested some degree of therapeutic misconception (Appelbaum et al. 2004).

To be sure, studies of subjects' comprehension of consent disclosures can be subject to a variety of methodologic criticisms (Hochhauser 2008; Verheggen and van Wijmen 1996). Definitions of comprehension are often vague and inconsistent, and the instruments used in many studies are unvalidated. Moreover, demonstrating a lack of understanding about one or more aspects of a study is different than showing a causal link between defective understanding or appreciation and potential subjects' decisions to enter (or to avoid) clinical trials. Acknowledging the limitations in the current data, there are strong reasons to accept the validity of the conclusion that subjects are frequently clueless about important aspects of clinical studies. The reasons to credit these findings include their consistency, the degree to which they comport with the impressions of clinical investigators and researchers studying informed consent, and the confirmation provided by more methodologically precise efforts. Indeed, the field as a whole has embraced the idea that our current approaches to informed consent often—perhaps usually—do not result in subjects having a sufficient grasp of the study to make meaningfully informed decisions.

As a consequence, a growing literature documents the attempts of researchers to do a better job of conveying information to their subjects. Flory and Emanuel published a review of this work in 2004, the findings of which have largely been confirmed by subsequent analyses (Cohn and Larson 2007). Among the efforts they catalogued to improve the consent process were videotaped disclosures and computer-based multimedia interventions; more user-friendly consent forms, with simplified language and streamlined content; extended or repetitive informational sessions with subjects; post-disclosure testing with feedback and correction; and some combinations of these various approaches. Their analysis suggested a lack of consistent improvement with video and computer technology (confirmed by a later Cochrane review (Ryan et al. 2008))—although some recent studies have been more promising (Jeste et al. 2009)—or with improved or simplified consent forms, although there was some evidence that simplifying forms might be helpful. However, extended discussions with potential subjects and testing with feedback both seemed more promising, perhaps because of the human interaction involved. An interactive process, Flory and Emanuel noted, encourages responsiveness of the information provider to the individual needs of each participant, in contrast to the fixed content of even the best consent forms or multimedia presentations. (It is of interest that consent to treatment appears to be more amenable to improvement with a wide variety of interventions (Schenker et al. 2011), perhaps because information concerning research is more difficult to comprehend or because information is so much more poorly presented in treatment settings.)

Two examples of a more interactive approach exemplify the rather small literature on this means of improving subjects' understanding. The earliest such study detailed the use of a "neutral educator"—a person unaffiliated with the team conducting the primary study but knowledgeable about the research—to instruct subjects on the elements of the research project (Benson et al. 1988). Although the study was underpowered to demonstrate statistically significant effects, the results showed a clear trend in the direction of improved understanding compared with standard procedures, even when the latter were augmented by the use of videotape. Given the time-intensive nature of individual sessions with subjects, the results of a subsequent study that used a group approach are of particular interest. Working with subjects with schizophrenia who had poorly understood the original disclosure, Carpenter and colleagues (2000) provided two thirty-minute group teaching sessions, along with the opportunity to review a computerized program about research in general and a flip-chart on the details of the study in question. Of the twenty subjects who went through this procedure, eleven subsequently scored above the *a priori* cut-off for adequate understanding and the group's mean understanding scores did not differ from that of a normal control group exposed to the usual consent process.

To sum up what is known about the quality of informed consent in the research setting, it seems fair to conclude that: (1) The process is conducted in a less-than-optimal fashion, with heavy reliance on written consent forms that subjects are unlikely to comprehend; and (2) the result is that research subjects display significant impairments in their understanding of the factual elements of their studies and of the ways in which they differ from ordinary treatment. Although a variety of interventions have been attempted to improve this situation, their use still appears to be the exception rather than the rule, and the most effective intervention—direct human interaction with potential subjects—is the most expensive to implement and thus may be least likely to be adopted.

Rethinking the Future of Informed Consent to Research

The promise of informed consent was that prospective research subjects would be sufficiently knowledgeable that they would make meaningful choices regarding their participation. Although by no means a complete remedy for the abuses in human subjects research, informed consent has been seen as a crucial component of that effort. The data reviewed above, however, suggest that the hopes for informed consent have not been realized: Many potential subjects still make relatively uninformed decisions. Efforts to improve the situation, although commendable, have generally tinkered at the edges of the consent process without getting to the heart of the problem. A more radical fix would appear to be in order if we are serious about actualizing the potential of informed consent.

Part of the problem lies in the conceptualization of the informed consent process itself, as evidenced by the language used to describe it. Borrowing from judicial decisions establishing a requirement for treating physicians to obtain patients' informed consent, the researcher's obligation is often described as a duty to *disclose* specific types of information (Berg et al. 2001: 46–65). The federal regulations on protection of human subjects specify "in seeking informed consent the following information shall be *provided* to each subject . . ." (Department of Health and Human Services 2009: 46.116, emphasis added). In the Nuremberg Code, researchers are told that part of their obligation to potential subjects can be discharged when certain information is "*made known* to . . ." them (*Trials of War Criminals* 1949, emphasis added). These terms have in common the notion that mere exposure of subjects to the relevant information will be sufficient to permit an informed decision. This model implicitly envisions subjects who knowingly receive information, grasp its meaning and implications, and use it in an informed way to make a decision whether to enter a research study.

As we have seen, however, this model does not reflect the reality of most human subjects research today. The information that is *disclosed*, *provided* or *made known* to potential subjects is often poorly understood and appreciated. This situation is due in varying parts to the inherent complexity of the information revealed, the difficulty that investigators have in presenting it clearly (notwithstanding the statement in the federal rules that the information provided "shall be in language understandable to the subject," Department of Health and Human Services 2009: 46.116), the educational, literacy, and numeracy limitations of subjects themselves, and the unfamiliar and counterintuitive aspects of the research setting (e.g., the fact that the physician supervising a subject's care will not be selecting a treatment based on that person's individualized needs). Simple revelation of information turns out to be inadequate to insure that prospective research subjects can make meaningful decisions.

What more might we ask of investigators? One aspect of the Nuremberg Code's formulation is helpful here. A research subject, the Code indicates, "should have sufficient knowledge and comprehension of the elements of the subject matter involved as to enable him to make an understanding and enlightened decision." Moreover, "[t]he duty and responsibility for ascertaining the quality of the consent rests upon each individual who initiates, directs or engages in the experiment." The term "quality of consent" is ambiguous, to be sure, but combined with the suggestion that subjects should comprehend the information made known to them, it could be taken to indicate the investigator's responsibility to determine that disclosure has actually resulted in a knowledgeable subject, able to make a meaningful choice. The Declaration of Helsinki, though also problematic in some ways, is more direct, indicating that researchers should "ensur[e] that the potential subject has understood the information" about which they have been informed. Taken seriously, these formulations would suggest that mere disclosure is inadequate unless the effectiveness of the informational process is ascertained.

Why, then, are these exhortations to assess subjects' comprehension so often honored only in the breach? The answer is undoubtedly multidimensional and includes the absence of clear language to this effect in many of the regulatory codes, such as the one in the U.S. But the influence of the doctrine of informed consent as it has developed in the clinical realm may be relevant here, too. Many of the foundational court decisions elaborating the doctrine deliberately adopted the language of "disclosure" and were decidedly ambiguous as to whether physicians must insure that patients in fact comprehended the information (Berg et al. 2001: 65–7). Judicial aversion to a more rigorous requirement of patient understanding may have derived from concern that some patients would be deprived of highly beneficial medical treatment because of their inabilities to grasp sufficient information. Although this may be sensible policy in a clinical context, where it can usually be assumed that physicians are recommending treatment believed to be in a patient's best interests, it makes less sense in the research environment in which other ends—namely the advancement of knowledge—often take precedence (Miller and Brody 2003). However, in the minds of clinical researchers, who often alternate between treatment and research duties, the idea may be firmly embedded that disclosure *to* the person rather than comprehension *by* the person is the goal of the consent process.

In addition, many researchers (and others, including some bioethicists) continue to doubt whether subjects can comprehend the information necessary for genuinely informed consent (Glannon 2006; Sreenivasan 2003). These doubts relate to the volume of information associated with modern clinical studies, the difficult methodologic concepts that may be involved, and the differences—which many people find counterintuitive—between research procedures and the ordinary provision of treatment. As a result, commentators have proposed reconceptualizing the goals of informed consent in a variety of ways. For example, Manson and O'Neill (2007) suggested that the informed consent process should be understood as a mechanism for waiving rights to which subjects would otherwise be entitled (e.g., privacy of medical information). A practical consequence of this conceptual difference, they argue, is that it would lead to a more manageable consent process, one focused on effective communication of a limited range of critical information, as opposed to the current tendency toward massive—and often incomprehensible—disclosure. Similarly disturbed by the failures of many research subjects to absorb consent disclosures, Miller and Wertheimer (2011) argue for a "fair transaction model" of informed consent, whereby investigators would disclose the information necessary for fair consideration of participation in a study, but without an expectation that subjects would necessary grasp the disclosure in its entirety. They, too, believe that it is unrealistic to expect informed consent to result in fully autonomous decision-making, but more explicitly rely on the vetting of research studies by research ethics committees to ensure that potential subjects are not being asked to participate unreasonably. Sreenivasan (2003) urges us not to mistake the "aspirational" goal of subject comprehension of the standard disclosure for a "minimum ethical standard," and argues that consent is the core ethical requirement, whether or not the subjects who offer their consent do so knowledgeably.

Although it is not possible here to do full justice to the arguments urged in favor of altering current notions of the purpose of informed consent, and the differences among them, two responses can be offered. From a normative perspective, substantial dilution of the informed consent requirement—whether by limiting disclosure to some subset of concerns or by discounting subjects' failures to grasp the information disclosed—diminishes subjects' abilities to make meaningful (i.e., informed) choices about participation. Whether viewed as limiting subjects' autonomous choice or failing to respect them as persons, this constricted view of the consent process is particularly problematic in research, as opposed to clinical care, since subjects cannot assume that offers of participation in research studies are intended to advance their interests. Defending those interests requires something more—at a minimum some clear notion of what would be involved in research participation and how it differs from ordinary clinical care.

Insofar as many of the leading critiques of informed consent have at their core certain empirical presumptions, their validity is worth considering. Data showing that many research subjects have a poor grasp of the nature of the research process and the specifics of their own studies are sometimes recruited to support the conclusion that striving for genuine comprehension would be futile. Of course, these arguments are circular. Given that information today is provided poorly, often with reliance on consent forms that are well beyond most people's capacity to understand, researchers are correct in their judgment that subjects' decisions are less than fully informed. However, as suggested by some of the studies reviewed above, when consent processes are better designed, subjects generally prove capable of grasping essential information about the studies and of making more meaningful decisions.

Overcoming nihilism regarding the possibility of an effective consent process will require nothing less than reconceptualizing what we are asking researchers to do. The model of mere disclosure is clearly inadequate. Whether conducted verbally or in writing, simply laying out information—in ever-increasing aliquots—guarantees only more of the situation we have today. Researchers will continue to view informed consent as a charade, and subjects will be inclined to see it as something researchers are doing to protect themselves from administrative sanctions or liability. Instead, I would suggest, we should view the consent process as one centered on the *education* of the subject. Mathematics teachers in our secondary schools, after all, are not expected merely to *disclose* algebraic equations to their students, accepting that most will be mystified but some small number may know intuitively what they mean. We ask teachers to educate their students about the nature and use of those equations, including their practical implications. This is precisely what we should be demanding of those people (more about their identity later) who obtain consent from research subjects: To teach, to instruct, to educate. Their success should not be judged by the number of subjects who consent to participate in their studies, as it often is today, but by the degree of comprehension manifested by potential subjects regardless of the decisions they reach.

A reorientation of the consent process from disclosure to education would have implications for who should be interacting with prospective subjects, how that exchange takes place, and what information should be taught. With regard to the identity of the subject educator—precisely the role envisioned under this approach—we may need to rethink who should carry out this task. Admittedly, there are advantages to having investigators themselves conduct the informational process. They know their studies best, and will usually be optimally situated to answer subjects' questions. But there are disadvantages as well. The time of senior personnel is expensive and often limited. They frequently have strong vested interests in maximizing enrollment—indeed their careers may depend on it—and thus they may be less than forthcoming about negative aspects of participation. And, though they may be wonderful researchers, they may lack the "people skills" of the best educators.

Thus, we might consider turning this instructional endeavor over to a group of people trained specifically for the purpose. Candidates for this role might have research backgrounds, perhaps having served as research coordinators or nurses. Large research groups might develop cadres of their own subject educators, whereas other studies could draw from a central pool of educators maintained by large research organizations. By way of qualifying for this job, subject educators would be trained and certified in effective instructional techniques, along with the nuances of research methods and the particular concerns of research subjects. For settings in which it would be impractical to maintain staff members dedicated to this role, certified members of the research team—in some cases investigators themselves—could serve instead. Requirements for training in the ethics of human subjects research are becoming routine in the U.S.; it would not be unimaginable to add a component to the training regarding effective communication with subjects. Whatever the details of implementation, it will be critical to set aside sufficient time for an effective teaching interaction with subjects. May and colleagues (2007) suggested a model of "translational informed consent" that shares some of these characteristics, and at least one institution has begun to implement a program involving trained personnel whose role is to educate potential subjects (Foglia et al. 2009).

The methods used for teaching, of necessity, will differ from those typical of the current disclosure process. Central to the education of prospective subjects will be interactions with the subject educator. However, for studies with a sufficient flow of referrals, these sessions need not be carried out one-on-one, but could be conducted in groups. Most schooling, after all, occurs in classes rather than individual tutorials. Group presentations not only maximize efficiency, an obvious advantage, but also permit subjects to discuss issues with each other and to pose relevant questions that some participants might not have considered. In contrast to the hospital and clinic, the classroom will be a familiar setting for most potential subjects, perhaps making it easier for them to absorb information and ask questions.

Although existing studies suggest that direct human interaction is crucial for subject comprehension—it is unlikely that any preprogrammed teaching device, for example, could answer the full range of queries subjects may have about their own medical and personal situations—innovative educational technologies can supplement person-to-person interactions. Data on computer-aided approaches have been variable, but some efforts have shown success. Moreover, advantage can be taken of newer technologies that would allow instruction to be individualized. Interactive DVDs or hyperlinked webpages, for example, would permit viewers to select particular components that might be important to some potential subjects (e.g., an explanation of randomization) but might be well known to others. Subjects could review matters that they found confusing. Video images of research procedures would give prospective participants a better feel for what would be involved if they enroll in the study. Periodic quizzes might be embedded in the DVD or webpage, with subjects required to attain a passing score before proceeding to the next module, a common procedure in online learning today. Technological approaches such as these might supplement, but would not supplant, direct interaction with a subject educator.

A reoriented process of subject education would require changes in the kind of information that is provided to would-be subjects as well. The welter of detail included in the current disclosure-oriented process overwhelms subjects and distracts them from the very information that is likely to be material to their decisions. When the risks of the study are buried on page 11 of a 21-page consent form, or when minor risks (like the ubiquitously disclosed "risk" of bruising from a blood draw) proliferate, providing perhaps inadvertent camouflage for the substantial adverse effects on which subjects should be focused, it is no wonder that consent forms provide relatively little usable information. As noted above, it has been known for decades that when it comes to informed consent less is more, i.e., patients and subjects take more information away from briefer presentations (Epstein and Lasagna 1969). Thus, the new subject educators would be encouraged to prune the content of their disclosures to potential subjects. Every subject could get a booklet with extensive information that they could consult if they so choose. I would guess most will not, but for those in the minority that values comprehensive information, they would have it in hand. Teaching sessions, however, would focus on major procedures in the study, the key benefits, the most salient risks, and a small number of other items.

Along with this slimming of the information taught to subjects, some additional refocusing is needed. Multiple studies have demonstrated the prevalence of therapeutic misconception among research subjects, manifested by the difficulty that they have distinguishing between the nature and procedures of research and the ordinary treatment setting. Some commentators have despaired of ever breaking through this misconception, but their anguish is premature. Almost no systematic efforts have been made to diminish therapeutic misconception, yet a new educationally focused informed consent process would seem ideal for the task. Subject educators could provide background information on how the purposes of research differ from the goals of treatment, the unique methods of research (e.g., double blinds), why they are used, and how they are likely to affect subjects in this particular study. We may finally have an opportunity to assess the extent to which therapeutic misconception is remediable, and to identify successful techniques for addressing the problem.

Needless to say, it would be a mistake to rush into a full-scale reorientation of consent to research participation without testing these approaches to ensure that they are practical and effective. However appealing this model might be, unless it yields significantly better-educated research subjects who can make more meaningful choices about participation, there is little reason to adopt it. We do not need additional studies of how poorly informed subjects currently are; the point has been made. It is to the testing of educational approaches such as those suggested here that our efforts should be directed. We need to acknowledge as well that it will not always be possible to engage in an idealized consent process. Some studies, such as those carried out in emergency settings, will not offer an opportunity for extended interactions with potential subjects. In other cases, only the investigator, rather than a trained educator, will be in a position to provide instruction about the study. However, recognition that this approach may not always be feasible does not detract from it as an ideal towards which we can aspire.

Conclusion

Informed consent to participate in research evolved from two sources: Basic notions of fairness towards people whose participation in research was sought, and a strong desire to avoid the abuses of the past, in which unknowing and unwilling participants found themselves placed at risk for the supposed advancement of medical science. The peculiarities of the development and application of informed consent to research, however, have resulted in a process that meets none of its original goals and that imposes substantial costs. Investigators find it time-consuming and irrelevant to subjects' decision-making; potential subjects—though they often report themselves satisfied with the information they have received—frequently lack basic knowledge about the studies they have entered; and regulators ostensibly charged with protecting human subjects and facilitating their choices find themselves caught up instead in the minutia of an ever-growing body of rules and procedures. To extricate all of us from this situation, we need to reconceptualize the aims of the consent process: It should be targeted at yielding an educated, not merely an informed, subject. If that is not the future of informed consent to research participation, the unappetizing alternative is simply more of the same.

Related Topics

Chapter 19, "The Ethics of Incentives for Participation in Research: What's the Problem?" Alan Wertheimer
Chapter 22, "Capacity and Competence," Jessica Berg and Katherine Shaw Makielski

References

Albala, I., Doyle, M. and Appelbaum, P.S. (2010) "The Evolution of Informed Consent Forms for Research: An Evaluation of Changes Over a Quarter Century," *IRB: Ethics and Human Research* 32 (3): 7–11.

Appelbaum, P.S. and Roth, L.H. (1983) "The Structure of Informed Consent in Psychiatric Research," *Behavioral Sciences and the Law* 1 (4): 9–19.

Appelbaum, P.S., Roth, L.H., Lidz, C.W., Benson, P. and Winslade, W. (1987) "False Hopes and Best Data: Consent to Research and the Therapeutic Misconception," *Hastings Center Report* 17 (2): 20–4.

Appelbaum, P.S., Lidz, C.W. and Grisso, T. (2004) "Therapeutic Misconception in Clinical Research: Frequency and Risk Factors," *IRB: Ethics and Human Research* 26 (2): 1–8; "Correction and Clarification," 26 (5): 18.

Benson, P.R., Roth, L.H., Appelbaum, P.S., Lidz, C.W. and Winslade, W.J. (1988) "Information Disclosure, Subject Understanding, and Informed Consent in Psychiatric Research," *Law & Human Behavior* 12: 455–75.

Berg, J.W., Appelbaum, P.S., Lidz, C.W. and Parker, L. (2001) *Informed Consent: Legal Theory and Clinical Practice*, 2nd edition, New York: Oxford University Press.

Canterbury v. Spence, 464 F.2d 772 (D.C. Cir. 1972).

Carpenter, W.T., Gold, J.M., Lahti, A.C., Queern, C.A., Conley, R.R., Bartko, J.J., Kovnick, J. and Appelbaum, P.S. (2000) "Decisional Capacity for Informed Consent in Schizophrenia Research," *Archives of General Psychiatry* 57: 533–8.

Christopher, P.P., Foti, M.E., Roy-Bujnowski, K. and Appelbaum, P.S. (2007) "Consent Form Readability and Educational Levels of Potential Participants in Mental Health Research," *Psychiatric Services* 58 (2): 227–32.

Cobbs v. Grant, 502 P.2d 1 (Cal. 1972).

Cohn, E. and Larson, E. (2007) "Improving Participant Comprehension in the Informed Consent Process," *Journal of Nursing Scholarship* 39: 273–80.

Daugherty, C.K., Banik, D.M., Janish, L. and Ratain, M.J. (2000) "Quantitative Analysis of Ethical Issues in Phase I Trials: A Survey Interview of 144 Advanced Cancer Patients," *IRB: Ethics and Human Research* 22 (3): 6–14.

Department of Health and Human Services (2009) "Protection of Human Subjects," 45 Code of Federal Regulations Part 46, January 15. Available at: http://www.hhs.gov/ohrp/humansubjects/guidance/45cfr46.html (accessed July 11, 2014).

Department of Health and Human Services, Food and Drug Administration (2009) "Informed Consent Elements (21 CFR Part 50)," December 29, *Federal Register* 74 (248): 68750–6.

Department of Health and Human Services, Office of the Secretary (1981) "Final Regulations Amending Basic HHS Policy for the Protection of Human Research Subjects," 45 CFR Part 46, January 26, *Federal Register* 46 (16): 8366–92.

Epstein, L.C. and Lasagna, L. (1969) "Obtaining Informed Consent: Form or Substance?" *Archives of Internal Medicine* 123: 682–8.

Flory, J. and Emanuel, E. (2004) "Interventions to Improve Research Participants' Understanding in Informed Consent for Research: A Systematic Review," *JAMA* 292 (13): 1593–601.

Foglia, M.B., Salas, H.S. and Dieckema, D.S. (2009) "A Quality Improvement Approach to Improving Informed Consent Practices in Pediatric Research," *Journal of Clinical Ethics* 20: 343–52.

Glannon, W. (2006) "Phase I Oncology Trials: Why the Therapeutic Misconception Will Not Go Away," *Journal of Medical Ethics* 32: 252–5.

Hawk, A. (2006) "The Great Disease Enemy, Kak'ke (beriberi) and the Imperial Japanese Army," *Military Medicine* 171: 333–9.

Hochhauser, M. (2008) "Consent Comprehension in the 21st Century: What Is Missing?" *Drug Information Journal* 42: 375–84.

Howard-Jones, N. (1982) "Human Experimentation in Historical and Ethical Perspectives," *Social Science and Medicine* 16: 1429–48.

Jeste, D.V., Palmer, B.W., Golshan, S., Eyler, L.T., Dunn, L.B. Meeks, T. et al. (2009) "Multimedia Consent for Research in People with Schizophrenia and Normal Subjects: A Randomized Controlled Trial," *Schizophrenia Bulletin* 35: 719–29.

Joffe, S., Cook, E.F., Cleary, P.D., Clark, J.W. and Weeks, J.C. (2001) "Quality of Informed Consent in Cancer Clinical Trials: A Cross-Sectional Survey," *Lancet* 358: 1772–7.

Jones, J. (1981) *Bad Blood: The Tuskegee Syphilis Experiment*, New York: Free Press.

Lederer, S.E. (1995) *Subjected to Science: Human Experimentation in America Before the Second World War*, Baltimore, MD: Johns Hopkins University Press.

Lind, J. (1753) *A Treatise of the Scurvy. In Three Parts Containing An Inquiry into the Nature, Causes and Cure, of that Disease. Together with a Critical and Chronological View of What Has Been Published on the Subject*, Edinburgh: Sands, Murray and Cochran for A. Kincaid and A. Donaldson.

Louis, P.C.A. (1836) *Researches on the Effects of Bloodletting in Some Inflammatory Diseases*, Boston: Hilliard, Gray.

Mann, T. (1994) "Informed Consent for Psychological Research: Do Subjects Comprehend Consent Forms and Understand Their Legal Rights?" *Psychological Science* 5 (3): 140–3.

Manson, N.C. and O'Neill, O. (2007) *Rethinking Informed Consent in Bioethics*, New York: Cambridge University Press.

May, T., Craig, J.M. and Spellecy, R. (2007) "IRBs, Hospital Ethics Committees, and the Need for Translational Informed Consent," *Academic Medicine* 82: 670–4.

Miller, F.G. and Brody, H. (2003) "A Critique of Clinical Equipoise: Therapeutic Misconception in the Ethics of Clinical Trials," *Hastings Center Report* 33 (3): 19–28.

Miller, F.G. and Wertheimer, A. (2011) "The Fair Transaction Model of Informed Consent: An Alternative to Autonomous Authorization," *Kennedy Institute of Ethics Journal* 21: 201–18.

Moreno, J.D. (2000) *Undue Risk: Secret State Experiments on Humans*, New York: W.H. Freeman.

National Institutes of Health (no date) "Dr. Joseph Goldberger and the War on Pellagra." Available at: http://history.nih.gov/exhibits/goldberger/index.html (accessed July 11, 2014).

Paasche-Orlow, M.K., Taylor, H.A. and Brancati, F.L. (2003) "Readability Standards for Informed Consent Forms as Compared with Actual Readability," *New England Journal of Medicine* 348 (8): 721–6.

Parson, W. (1984) "Uninformed Consent in 1942," *New England Journal of Medicine* 310: 1397.

Proctor, R.N. (1992) "Nazi Doctors, Racial Medicine, and Human Experimentation," in G.J. Annas and M.A. Grodin (eds.) *The Nazi Doctors and the Nuremberg Code: Human Rights in Human Experimentation*, New York: Oxford University Press.

Ryan, R.E., Prictor, M.J., McLaughlin, K.H. and Hill, S.J. (2008) "Audio-visual Presentation of Information for Informed Consent for Participation in Clinical Trials," *Cochrane Database of Systematic Reviews* CD003717. DOI:10.1002/14651858.CD003717.pub2.

Salgo v. Leland Stanford Jr. University Board of Trustees, 154 Cal. App. 2d 560 (Cal.Ct. App. 1957).

Schenker, Y., Fernandez, A., Sudore, R. and Schillinger, D. (2011) "Interventions to Improve Patient Comprehension in Informed Consent for Medical and Surgical Procedures: A Systematic Review," *Medical Decision Making* 31: 151–73.

Schmidt, U. (2004) *Justice at Nuremberg: Leo Alexander and the Nazi Doctors' Trial*, Hampshire: Palgrave MacMillan.

Sharp, S.M. (2004) "Consent Documents for Oncology Trials: Does Anybody Read These Things?" *American Journal of Clinical Oncology* 27 (6): 570–5.

Sreenivasan, G. (2003) "Does Informed Consent to Research Require Comprehension?" *Lancet* 362: 2016–18.

Stewart, W.H. (1972) "Memorandum of Surgeon General William H. Stewart to the Heads of Institutions Conducting Research with Public Health Grants (Febraury 8, 1966)," in J. Katz, A. Capron and E.S. Glass (eds.) *Experimentation with Human Beings: The Authority of the Investigator, Subject, Professions and State in the Human Experimentation Process*, New York: Russell Sage Foundation.

Trials of War Criminals before the Nuremberg Military Tribunals under Control Council Law No. 10, Vol. 2. (1949) Washington, DC: U.S. Government Printing Office. Available at: http://www.hhs.gov/ohrp/archive/nurember.html (accessed July 18, 2014).

Verheggen, F.W.S.M. and van Wijmen, F.C.B. (1996) "Informed Consent in Clinical Trials," *Health Policy* 36: 131–53.

Williams, B.F., French, J.K., White, H.D., HERO-2 Consent Substudy Investigators (2003) "Informed Consent During the Clinical Emergency of Acute Myocardial Infarction (HERO-2 Consent Substudy): A Prospective Observational Study," *Lancet* 361: 918–22.

World Medical Association (1964) "Declaration of Helsinki: Ethical Principles for Medical Research Involving Human Subjects." *New England Journal of Medicine* 271: 473–4.

World Medical Association (2008) "Declaration of Helsinki: Ethical Principles for Medical Research Involving Human Subjects." Available at: http://www.wma.net/en/30publications/10policies/b3/index.html (accessed July 11, 2014).

17
ETHICAL ISSUES IN GENETIC RESEARCH

Dena S. Davis

Introduction

Last week I gave a blood sample as part of research in which I am a volunteer. VITAL is a large study that seeks to learn about the effects of certain dietary supplements. VITAL often asks its subjects to consider "extra" participation, including this blood sample. The blood draw had its own informed consent for the actual procedure and for the use of the information. Interestingly, there is a separate box for me to check to indicate whether I am willing to have the sample used for genetic research.

Why this degree of concern? Why do I give specific consent to genetic analysis of my blood, but not to the possibility that my blood will yield evidence of tuberculosis or gonorrhea? Why is genetic information considered special?

In fact, the question of whether genetic information carries special potential for harm and is thus in need of special protections continues to be controversial. Thomas Murray coined the term *genetic exceptionalism* to describe the belief that "genetic information is sufficiently different from other types of health-related information that it deserves special protection," a view with which he vigorously disagrees (1997: 61).

The claims for genetic exceptionalism include its predictive quality for one's future health, a kind of "probabilistic future diary" (Murray 1997: 62); the relevance of genetic information for one's relatives as well as for oneself; the history of stigma and discrimination associated with claims about genetic traits, leading to everything from forced sterilization to genocide and the Nazis' Final Solution. Other "special" qualities include the way in which research on a small segment of an identified group can confer risk on all members of the group, without their prior knowledge or consent, and the ability to track population migration through genetic research.

Murray's point, however, is that there are very few traits that are entirely genetic (or entirely environmental), and that most of the factors associated with genetic information and genetic research have non-genetic analogs that deserve the same level of protection. Knowing about my cholesterol level and my sky-diving hobby, for example, provides as much of a "future diary" as most genetic information. Murray concludes that genetic exceptionalism is an "overly dramatic" (Murray 1997: 71) view of the significance of genetic information, born of genetic reductionism and genetic determinism. Further, he warns of a "vicious circularity" (Murray 1997: 71): The more we treat genetic information as fundamentally different, the more support we provide for genetic determinism, that is, "the notion that genetics exerts special power over our lives" (Murray 1997: 71).

A common concern regarding genetic research with identifiable populations (such as Ashkenazi Jews or specific Native American tribes) is that information published about the group subjects all members to possible stigma, whereas only a few members actually gave consent and agreed to participate. However, one could raise equal concerns about other forms of research on groups. A sociological study of the sex habits of long-distance truck drivers, for example, potentially stigmatizes all members of that profession, most of whom never gave consent.

One signpost that genetic exceptionalism has won the day is the passage of the *Genetic Information Non-Discrimination Act* (GINA) of 2008, which was strongly supported by research scientists because they hoped it would reassure potential volunteers about participation in genetic research studies. While people may not agree with Dorothy Nelkin and Susan Lindee that the gene has "become the secular equivalent of the human soul" (Murray 1997: 70), we often act as if genetic information is uniquely perilous if it gets into the wrong hands.

History

For millennia philosophers and scientists have been fascinated by the contributions of heredity to human characteristics. Belief in the strength of heredity as opposed to environment (the "nature/nurture" debate) has waxed and waned over the years, but folk idioms such as "chip off the old block" and "the apple doesn't fall far from the tree" all attest to the importance of heredity in the human imagination. Before the Human Genome Project was launched in 1990, it was not possible to look directly at a person's genetic blueprint. Nor can we treat humans like peas or fruitflies, breeding them with mathematical precision in the hope of scientifically useful outcomes. Instead, research on human genetics was, and often still is, a matter of attempting to impose scientific sense on existing family histories. The genetic contribution to alcoholism, for example, was originally quantified through research involving twin, adoption, and family studies. If identical twins had a higher degree of concordance for alcoholism than non-identical twins, or if children whose biological parents were alcoholics had a higher than average likelihood of alcoholism even when adopted by non-alcoholic parents, this was evidence of a genetic contribution to the risk of alcoholism (Foroud et al. 2010).

Most genes are not 100 percent penetrant; most phenotypes are not engendered by only one gene; many genes are pleiotropic, influencing more than one characteristic; most human characteristics result from a confluence of genetics and environment. For example, we now believe that genetic factors account for 50–60 percent of the probable risk of developing alcoholism (Foroud et al. 2010), with the remainder attributable to "environment." Cystic fibrosis, however, is believed to be entirely genetic, with a classic recessive pattern, but with more than 1,800 mutations of the gene, different mutations may account for more or less severe variations of the disease. As these examples attest, genetic research on humans is a complicated business. Research can range from a narrowly focused study of one unique family, to worldwide studies involving thousands of subjects. Genome wide association studies (the search of the genomes of individuals with disease compared with those without the disease) requires thousands of participants in order to arrive at statistically significant results (Rotimi and Marshall 2010).

Because few health states are completely lacking in a genetic component (even a broken leg may reflect an inborn tendency to clumsiness or to risk-taking), genetic research holds out great promise for understanding disease and ameliorating human suffering. More controversial goals include understanding population migration and the narrative of human ancestry, and prenatal or preconception testing for traits future parents may prefer to avoid. One ethically complex field of study involves behavioral genetics, which seeks to explain human behavior through genetics and genetic–environmental interaction. Claims of genetic components to intelligence, violence, sexual orientation, and so on carry complex societal implications. A society that believed that intelligence was largely due to genetics, for example, would perhaps be more likely to engage in eugenic activities and to spend less on education for "below average" children.

Genetic Research on Stored Tissue Samples

Genetic research is also unusual, although not unique, because it can be carried out without the participation, cooperation, or even knowledge of the research subjects (Clayton et al. 1995). Genetic research can use tissue samples such as blood, saliva, and solid tissue, including samples originally obtained and stored for other uses and from sources long deceased, and also samples shared with researchers pursuing different projects in different institutions.

When scholars in the 1970s were scrutinizing the ethics of research with human subjects and writing the original documents and regulations, the typical research experience involved a time-limited intervention designed to answer a small number of questions. Perhaps the volunteer was asked to take an antibiotic for 10 days, to compare with a comparable drug for efficacy in responding to a specific health problem. Even long-term projects followed participants only until their deaths. The best example is the Framingham Heart Study, which began in 1948 and follows thousands of men and women from Framingham, Massachusetts, looking at factors contributing to cardiovascular disease. The study is now looking at the grandchildren of the original cohort. Although the Framingham questions have changed and expanded over time, participants can stop participating if they no longer want to be part of it. In the traditional research context, participation is active: Subjects typically take a pill or fill out a questionnaire, and if they become disaffected by the research they can end their involvement. However, research using stored biospecimens, while "critical" to understanding genetic variation and its health implications, "challenge[s] the established norms of informed consent" (McGuire and Beskow 2010: 361). Specimens can be stored and used indefinitely, and traded and shared with other researchers working on different questions in different institutions. When specimens are "anonymized," by being stripped of all identifying information, the work is no longer considered to be research with human subjects and falls outside of regulatory protections (Clayton et al. 1995). Thus, research never ends; autonomy rights are limited; future use is unspecified; privacy risks are "uncertain" and persist throughout the subject's lifetime and perhaps beyond; consent is "forever" (McGuire and Beskow 2010).

Privacy is a primary concern for many commentators, and risks to privacy are taken seriously in the practice and regulation of research with human subjects (at least when those subjects are alive). Specimens and research results that cannot be connected to their sources are usually thought to pose little risk. To some people, however, the lack of identifiers is irrelevant, because it is the specimen itself, and not the information obtained from it, that needs to be considered. Many Native Americans would refuse to participate in research if they suspected that their blood specimens would be stored too close to that of a specimen from a taboo clan, breaking the rules against comingling.

Among the Navajo, illness is commonly attributed to the mishandling of specimens separate from the body (Bowekaty and Davis 2003).

Genetic research on stored tissue samples is unusual in that research use can persist long after the source of the tissue is dead. Thus, research on stored tissue has highlighted an old philosophical debate on whether deceased persons can have interests and whether those interests can be harmed.

It is not uncommon for members of minority groups or their advocates to oppose genetic research that they view as threatening the continued existence of their community, e.g., by giving prospective parents the tools to avoid having children with those characteristics. Deaf Pride activists, autistic persons who support "neurodiversity," sexual minorities, and advocates for people with Down syndrome, have all expressed these fears; their interests would be harmed even after their deaths were their specimens to be used in research that threatened to lessen their numbers. Should these beliefs be respected even after these persons are dead?

Federal regulations do not require consent for the use of specimens for research if the specimen is not identifiable or if the subject is dead, although some commentators believe that institutional review board (IRB) review is still worthwhile (Clayton et al. 1995). And yet, I would argue that even dead people can be wronged, and even anonymous specimens can pose risks to the interests of sources both dead and alive. Philosophers such as Joel Feinberg (1984) argue that some interests (for example, in reputation) persist even after death, as do interests in the welfare of one's descendants, and in certain hopes for the future. Feinberg writes "we can think of some of a person's interests as surviving his death, just as some of the debts and claims of his estate do, and that in virtue of the defeat of these interests, either by death itself or by subsequent events, we can think of the person who was, as harmed" (1984: 176). Just as I would be wronged if money that I willed to the Anti-Defamation League were somehow diverted after my death to the Ku Klux Klan (or the other way around!), I would arguably be wronged if genetic researchers discovered and published information about me or my relatives that destroyed my reputation, and to which I would never have consented while alive.

Persons can be wronged if their specimens are used in ways that harm what they perceived to be their interests and values, even if they are not aware of that use. We understand that it would be wrong to use someone's estate to pursue goals inimical to their values. Feinberg (1984) argues that a person would be harmed if some enemy started a whispering campaign that ruined his reputation and humiliated his family, even if his loved ones were somehow able to keep this reality from him, perhaps because he was in a coma. Thus, it can be wrong to use the specimen of someone to pursue research he or she would have opposed when alive, even though, being dead, he or she cannot suffer from that knowledge.

Another way of arguing for this same point is to say that those of us who are now alive and conscious want our own wishes to be honored once we are dead or permanently unaware, and therefore have an interest in protecting the interests of the dead and unaware. Imagine a government with a policy to take organs from all brain dead persons, even those with strong convictions against organ donation. Persons now alive who shared those convictions would oppose the policy, even though it could be argued that they cannot be harmed by what happens to them when they are dead. If I had strong convictions against certain types of genetic research, I would work now to protect myself against contributing involuntarily to that research after my death.

Tomlinson (2013: 42) mounts a strong critique of a research ethics framework that is "all about risk." To protect subjects against risk of harm, we ask their consent for the risk associated with the actual blood draw or biopsy, and the risk to the confidentiality of information garnered from the sample.

> But once a donor to a research biobank has willingly parted with his tissue, and both it and any accompanying medical information have been de-identified, then the donor's welfare is no longer at risk—and she no longer needs any ethical protection. Subject to no risk, she's no longer a human "subject." As for her tissue? It's like her trash. Once left by the curb it's no longer "hers."
>
> (Tomlinson 2013: 42)

Tomlinson believes that respect for donors requires researchers to be transparent about possible future uses of donor tissue, to protect donors against "*nonwelfare* interests in preserving the moral significance of their donation" (Tomlinson 2013: 42). He identifies a number of concerns donors could have about the uses of their gift, including research into prenatal diagnostic testing; research that may stigmatize minority groups; research whose benefits will likely not be justly distributed.

To address similar issues to those Tomlinson raises, Mello and Wolf (2010) support a system of tiered consent. Tiered consent gives donors, at the time of donation, a choice to narrow their gift to this one project, to have their samples used in the future for other health-related projects, to be used only on research on a specific disease, only with additional consent, and so on. Thus, the relatively small percentage of people who want to limit the use of their tissue can do so.

Privacy and Confidentiality

As mentioned above, loss of privacy, or being publicly identified with a genetic trait associated with stigma or discrimination, is a major focus of policy and regulation. Potential research subjects are regularly reassured that their privacy will be protected, and much energy goes into "de-identifying" information. Researchers are required to explain to IRBs and recruits alike, how privacy will be guarded. However, there are a number of ways in which genetic information may elude the protective efforts of even the most conscientious researchers.

Pedigree charts (genetic "family trees") are an efficient and perhaps even an indispensable vehicle for reporting on certain types of genetic research, but the uniqueness of family constellations makes it difficult to protect privacy and confidentiality when pedigrees are published. One can protect privacy by changing details such as birth order and gender, but this is controversial, as it may erode the usefulness of the information. To make matters more complex, a pedigree may threaten the privacy of many family members, but usually only a few people have actually given their consent to be part of the study and to incur that risk. U.S. regulations call for specific written consent of the study subjects when pedigrees are published, but Botkin et al. found that "current practices . . . do not conform with established recommendations and risk the privacy and confidentiality of subjects, often without informed consent" (Botkin et al. 1998: 1808).

Confidentiality can also be threatened by publishing findings about an identifiable group, even though the identities of individuals are adequately protected. Identifying a specific Native American tribe with a high rate of diabetes, or Ashkenazi Jews with a high rate of a mutation that confers an added risk of certain cancers, may cause at least some members to feel threatened or that their privacy has been invaded (Davis 2000). Of course, opponents of genetic exceptionalism could well point out that high rates of diabetes or cancer in specific groups are public knowledge with or without a genetic narrative.

Finally, the very uniqueness of individual genetic blueprints may render privacy impossible, so that "de-identified DNA" becomes an oxymoron. Although research with de-identified specimens does not currently fall under the umbrella of the Common Rule, McGuire and Gibbs (2006) argue that it ought to do so, given the risk of individual identification from publicly available databases. McGuire and Gibbs recommend required informed consent, with a three-tiered, "stratified" consent process in which participants elect the degree of risk to their privacy with which they are comfortable. However, the authors acknowledge that stratifying consent in this way may create deleterious subject bias.

Community Consent

As we have seen, genetic research may hold out special risks to "socially identifiable populations." These populations might include ethnic groups, indigenous groups, and geographically identified groups. Genetic researchers often focus on small, cohesive groups because genetic traits can be concentrated in groups of people who descended from a small number of common ancestors, the "founder effect." Researchers are especially attracted to groups who have been socially or physically isolated, or who rarely marry outside the group. Even when a group has no higher incidence of a particular trait than the general population, a relatively homogenous population cuts down on background "noise" and can foreground genes of interest. Thus, Ashkenazi Jews, the Amish, Icelanders, and Native American tribes are common foci of genetic interest.

Special risks of genetic research might include undermining the group's creation narrative, challenging the prevailing power structure, or publicizing the results in ways that create stigma or engender discrimination. For example, genetic research that was widely interpreted by lay people to validate the Jewish descent of the Lemba, a South African tribe, resulted in an onslaught of attention from Western Jewish groups, and a shift in tribal culture that challenged the power of existing leaders (Davis 2004). A news headline that drew attention to the high number of "mutant genes" among Ashkenazi Jews, did not sit well with that group of people. Genetics has captured the public imagination, and researchers have no control over how their results are expressed in the popular press.

Because the risks and benefits of genetic research devolve upon the entire "community," while only a relatively few members actively participate and give their consent, some commentators have argued for a type of *community consent* which in its strongest form would give the community a veto over research it deemed unacceptable. A softer form of this argument would require *community consultation* with "recognized cultural authorities" (Weijer and Emanuel 2000). However, even supporters of this view admit that it works well only with indigenous groups, who already have a political structure and relatively clear membership criteria. Critics argue that people who share a genetic heritage are not necessarily a "community" in any social or political sense, and that where communities do exist, they often enshrine the values of subgroups (Davis 2000). (The Lemba, Amish, and Hutterites are examples of groups that are often the subject of genetic research, and whose political leaders are exclusively male. Thus, a "community consent" from "recognized cultural authorities" would risk ignoring the perspectives of women in the community and would violate the principles of "respect for persons" and "justice" that are two key values of ethical research with human subjects.)

The Havasupai: A Perfect Storm

The long, complicated, and ultimately bitter relationship between genetic researchers at Arizona State University (ASU) and the Havasupai tribe highlights some of the many ways in which genetic research can fall afoul of ethics and the law. The Havasupai are a federally recognized Native American tribe, living in an isolated and stunningly beautiful reservation just west of Grand Canyon National Park. In 2012, the tribe numbered 639 people.

Native tribes have good reason to be wary of genetic research, and a number have described themselves as "just a hairsbreadth away" from shutting it down in their jurisdictions (Bowekaty and Davis 2003: 12). For centuries, white people have dug up the bones and sacred possessions of native people and used them for sale and display. Thus when researchers ask for blood, hair, cheek swabs, or other bodily substances, their requests are framed by this history.

Indigenous peoples are also concerned about "ownership" of their creation stories and communal narratives. Research into tribal origins, such as migration over the Bering Strait, are often met with hostility. Migration studies that can call into question treaty rights or exacerbate tensions with neighboring tribes may pose serious risks to native communities.

Non-Indians who interact with Native American and Alaskan Native people quickly notice the importance of two concepts: Theft and respect (Bowekaty and Davis 2003). Theft has been the primary experience of native people in North America: Theft of land, sovereignty, natural resources, religious and cultural artifacts, children sold into slavery, and so on. In response, respect is a term often voiced by native peoples: Respect for their culture, religion, and values, for their sovereignty, for their sacred artifacts.

There is also a long history of researchers from many disciplines using native peoples as objects of study with little concern for benefiting the people themselves. Genetic research is vulnerable to this criticism, because it can appear to be looking for solutions where the money is, rather than seeking to make the biggest impact on tribal health. Although many tribes struggle with crippling rates of type 2 diabetes, they notice that cheap and proven interventions such as nutrition and exercise programs are often ignored in favor of expensive and highly speculative genetic research.

It is against this background that the Havasupai agreed in 1990 to participate in a genetic study to attempt to tease out some of the causes of the tribe's high rate of type 2 diabetes. In fact, a member of the tribe initiated the collaboration, approaching John Martin, an ASU anthropologist who had a long and mutually respectful relationship with the tribe (Harmon 2010). It is impossible to recount here all the details of this long and sorry story. There was a serious discrepancy between the understanding of tribal members, based on their discussions with the researchers, that the work would be limited to diabetes, and the actual consent form, in which members gave their signed consent to "study the causes of behavioral/medical disorders" (Drybiak-Syed 2010). Martin's colleague, Therese Markow, had initially indicated her interest in studying schizophrenia as well as diabetes, but had been told by Martin that the tribe would not accept that. Confusingly, ASU's IRB gave its approval to a proposal by Markow to study schizophrenia, not diabetes;

in addition, Markow had begun taking blood samples the summer before she received IRB approval. Between 1991 and 1993, recruitment of participants devolved onto Daniel Benyshek, who switched to oral consent only and told participants, apparently in good faith, that the study would focus solely on diabetes. Finally, Markow did not abide by the provisions in the consent form about conducting the research at ASU and keeping "all information" private. Samples were sent to other researchers, other universities, and other countries. Researchers other than Markow had access to codebooks allowing for the reidentification of samples, thus enabling them to look for documentation of schizophrenia among tribal members (Drybiak-Syed 2010).

The Havasupai became aware of what was going on only in 2003, when a member of the tribe (who had herself volunteered for the study) happened to attend a presentation by a doctoral student who had done his work on the tribal samples. When she questioned him about permission to use the samples, the problems began to unfold. Martin asked ASU to remedy the situation by returning the samples to the tribe, but the university refused. Later investigation discovered more than two dozen articles published using the Havasupai samples, on topics including schizophrenia and migration history. In 2004, the Havasupai issued a banishment order, forbidding ASU employees to step onto the reservation; lawsuits were filed against ASU, alleging wrongdoing that had resulted in harm to the tribe as a whole and to individual study subjects. ASU spent in excess of a million dollars in legal fees (Drybiak-Syed 2010).

In 2010, the Havasupai and ASU entered into a settlement, involving return of the specimens; compensation of $700,000; and return of all documents relating to research with the specimens (Harmon 2010). In the wake of this scandal, ASU had an uphill struggle to rebuild trust with its tribal neighbors, and other researchers who were engaged in studies on genetics with southwest tribes had their projects halted. The Havasupai themselves never learned if any of this research held out any hope for their battle with diabetes (Harmon 2010).

Commenting on this case, Mello and Wolf (2010: 206) echo Tomlinson's perspective on "risk," by arguing that "at least some participants consider factors other than individual risk when evaluating future uses of their specimens." But Markow insists that she was merely doing good science, and that her detractors did not understand the peculiarities of genetic research (Harmon 2010).

Conclusion

For every risk of genetic research we can find an analogous risk in some "non-genetic" sphere. In addition, the more we learn about genetics, the more we realize how few conditions are exclusively genetic or environmental. However, genetic research presents a phalanx of ethical issues, often layered within a single piece of research. For that reason alone, genetic research with human subjects deserves the highest level of ethical scrutiny.

Related Topics

Chapter 16, "The Future of Informed Consent to Research: Reconceptualizing the Process," Paul Appelbaum
Chapter 24, "Privacy, Surveillance, and Autonomy," Alan Rubel
Chapter 32, "Reproductive Testing for Disability," Adrienne Asch and David Wasserman

References

Botkin, J.R., McMahon, W.M., Smith, K.R. and Nash, J.E. (1998) "Privacy and Confidentiality in the Publication of Pedigrees: A Survey of Investigators and Biomedical Journals," *JAMA* 279 (22): 1808–12.
Bowekaty, M. and Davis, D.S. (2003) "Cultural Issues in Genetic Research with American Indian and Alaskan Native People," *IRB: Ethics & Human Research* July–August.
Clayton, E.W., Steinberg, K.K., Khoury, M.J., Thomson, E., Andrews, L., Kahn, M.J. et al. (1995) "Informed Consent for Genetic Research on Stored Tissue Samples," *JAMA* 274: 1786–92.
Davis, D.S. (2000) "Groups, Communities, and Contested Identities in Genetic Research," *Hastings Center Report* 30: 38–45.
Davis, D.S. (2004) "Genetic Research and Communal Narratives," *Hastings Center Report* 34: 40–9.
Drybiak-Syed, K. (2010) "Lessons from Havasupai Tribe v. Arizona State University Board of Regents: Recognizing Group, Cultural, and Dignitary Harms as Legitimate Risks Warranting Integration into Research Practice," *Journal of Health and Biomedical Law* 6: 175–225.
Feinberg, J. (1984) "Death and Posthumous Harms," in *Harm to Others*, Oxford: Oxford University Press, 74–95.
Foroud, T., Edenberg, H. and Crabbe, J. (2010) "Genetic Research: Who Is at Risk for Alcoholism?" *Alcohol Research & Health* 33: 64–75.
Harmon, A. (2010) "Indian Tribe Wins Fight to Limit Research of Its DNA," *New York Times*, April 21.
McGuire, A.L. and Beskow, L.M. (2010) "Informed Consent in Genomics and Genetics Research," *Annual Review of Genomics and Human Genetics* 11: 361–81.
McGuire, A.L. and Gibbs, R.A. (2006) "No Longer De-identified," *Science* 312: 370–1.
Mello, M.M. and Wolf, L.E. (2010) "The Havasupai Indian Tribe Case—Lessons for Research Involving Stored Biologic Samples," *New England Journal of Medicine* 363: 204–7.
Murray, T.J. (1997) "Genetic Exceptionalism and 'Future Diaries': Is Genetic Information Different from Other Medical Information?" in M.A. Rothstein (ed.) *Genetic Secrets: Protecting Privacy and Confidentiality in the Genetic Era*, New Haven, CT: Yale, pp. 60–73.
Rotimi, C.N. and Marshall, P.A. (2010) "Tailoring the Process of Informed Consent in Genetic and Genomic Research," *Genome Medicine* 2: 20. Available at: http://genomemedicine.com/content/2/3/20 (accessed July 11, 2014).
Tomlinson, T (2013) "Respecting Donors to Biobank Research," *Hastings Center Report* 43/1: 41–7.
Weijer, C. and Emanuel, J. (2000) "Protecting Communities in Biomedical Research," *Science* 289: 1142–4.

18

RESEARCH INVOLVING "VULNERABLE POPULATIONS"

A Critical Analysis

Toby Schonfeld

Much of the contemporary context of research ethics can be understood as a response to the United States Public Health Service Syphilis Study becoming public knowledge. In this study, 400 black men with untreated syphilis from rural Alabama were recruited to participate in a research study that would last 40 years (Jones 1993). The public outcry about this study was substantial, but some of the most scathing criticism centered around the notion that these research participants were particularly vulnerable: They were economically depressed and therefore had strong motivation to participate in order to garner additional income (and later, burial money for their families), they were uneducated and therefore had difficulty understanding the study, and they had little access to healthcare and therefore were likely to agree to participate simply to have access to healthcare professionals (Jones 1993; Reverby 2009).

In addition to arguing for the scientific merit of the study, investigators (from the U.S. government) argued that there were no formal research guidelines to dictate the "proper" conduct of research involving human participants, nor was there any formal designation of populations as "vulnerable" (Reverby 2009). In fact, it was not until much later that considerations about research ethics were codified into U.S. law (Porter and Koski 2008), which can now be found in part 46 of title 45 of the Code of Federal Regulations (CFR). In addition to detailing for investigators and reviewers what constitutes ethical study design and participant recruitment, Subpart A (known as the "Common Rule") also includes guidance for conducting research with groups identified as requiring "additional protections." These groups are referred to as "vulnerable populations": "When some or all of the subjects are likely to be vulnerable to coercion or undue influence, such as children, prisoners, pregnant women, mentally disabled persons, or economically or educationally disadvantaged persons, additional safeguards have been included in the study to protect the rights and welfare of these subjects" (45 CFR 46.111b). However, the regulations only include special sections for three specific populations: Pregnant Women, Human Fetuses, and Neonates involved in Research (Subpart B), Prisoners (Subpart C), and Children (Subpart D).

There are at least three problems with these regulations as they stand. (1) It is unclear what defining characteristics make an individual or a subpopulation "vulnerable" and therefore deserving of additional protections. (2) It is unclear whether or not the additional safeguards written into the regulations do in fact protect these subpopulations from their vulnerability. (3) There are other groups of individuals that scholars have argued deserve special protections, including the terminally ill, the politically exiled, and the elderly, among others. It is not clear why federal regulations only apply to the three subpopulations listed above and not others that may in fact be more at risk depending upon the context of the research, regardless of historic instances of abuse. For example, it is difficult to see how a prisoner is at relatively increased risk from participating in a brief anonymous survey (DuBois et al. 2012: 2222), whereas a series of interviews with members of a politically oppressed group are likely to pose substantial risk to participants from the oppressive regime.

In this chapter, I will explore the concept of vulnerability in research, using the situation of pregnant women as our paradigm case. The regulations regarding research conducted with pregnant participants are both problematic and misleading, and therefore focusing on this particular excluded group will demonstrate how the critical analysis of regulations can provide insight into the ethical issues associated with conducting research involving historically excluded participants.

Concepts of Vulnerability in Research

Given that our concern is how regulations influence the notion of vulnerability, it makes sense to begin an analysis of the concept by investigating what a variety of regulatory documents seem to mean by the term "vulnerability." In the United States, that means we begin with the CFR, in which vulnerability is not defined except by pointing to examples of populations that need additional protections (Coleman 2009). For example, the CFR requires institutional review boards (IRBs) to have individuals "knowledgeable about and experienced working with" members of vulnerable groups (45 CFR 46.107a), and to be "particularly cognizant of the special problems of research involving vulnerable populations" (45 CFR 46.111a3). The closest the CFR comes to outlining essential characteristics of these groups is in the section detailing criteria for IRB approval of research. In this section, the regulations include language that says "when some or all of the subjects are *likely to be vulnerable to coercion or undue influence* . . . additional safeguards have been included in the study to protect the rights and welfare of these subjects" (45 CFR 46.111b, emphasis added).

Other international guidelines fail to be more specific or helpful when it comes to definitions. The newly revised Declaration of Helsinki (World Medical Association 2013) includes a section on "Vulnerable Groups and Individuals," but it simply states that "[s]ome groups and individuals are particularly vulnerable and may have an increased likelihood of being wronged or incurring additional harm," and as a result deserve "specifically considered protection." One safeguard included in the Declaration is that the investigators must assure the regulatory body that the proposed research could not be conducted adequately with a non-vulnerable population.

The most helpful regulatory framework comes in the form of the International Ethical Guidelines for Biomedical Research Involving Human Subjects from the Council for International Organizations of Medical Sciences (CIOMS). Here, there is some attempt at definition. Guide 13 states the following: "Vulnerable persons are those who are relatively (or absolutely) incapable of protecting their own interests. More formally, they may have insufficient power, intelligence, education, resources, strength, or other needed attributes to protect their own interests" (Council for International Organizations of Medical Sciences 2002). Subsequent information links the inability to protect their own interests to the process of informed consent, and identifies particular groups as vulnerable to different parts of the consent process. (For example, students may be vulnerable in the context where an instructor with control over their future asks them to agree to participate in a study, whereas these same students would not be vulnerable in a different context.)

The conclusion one can draw, then, is that there is no clear definition of vulnerability to which everyone refers. Scholars' attempts to define vulnerability or vulnerable populations in research include: Susceptibility to exploitation (Macklin 2003), those at an increased likelihood to incur "additional or greater wrong" (Hurst 2008), and those facing "a significant probability of incurring an identifiable harm while substantially lacking ability and/or means to protect oneself" (Schroeder and Gefenas 2009). Others link vulnerability to the precise notions of that to which human subjects are especially vulnerable: Issues with informed consent, the risk/benefit ratio in research, and the distribution of benefits and burdens are commonly cited (Coleman 2009).

Linking the concept of vulnerability to specific protections is another strategy. The Consortium to Examine Clinical Research Ethics suggests that the concept of vulnerability be replaced with the notion of "special scrutiny," and identifies three criteria that should trigger careful attention to a protocol and certain relevant features (Levine et al. 2004). Florencia Luna and Sheryl Vanderpoel (2013) are also concerned with identifying the appropriate safeguard and worry that the traditional ascription of vulnerability to groups of people (the "categorical model") overlooks the notion that an individual can be vulnerable in a number of different respects—and therefore protections must address these multiple "layers" of vulnerability. Additionally, it is clear that individuals who do not fall into traditionally vulnerable subgroups may also need additional safeguards in some circumstances (Luna and Vanderpoel consider the case of middle-class pregnant women who are considering umbilical cord bank storage), and the categorical model offers no way to provide such protections. Instead, they advocate a "layered account" of vulnerability, where researchers and policy-makers are encouraged to attend to the multiple ways in which individuals or groups can be vulnerable, and to develop policies and processes that facilitate the creation of appropriate safeguard for these complex situations.

Lange et al. (2013) take the approach one step further and create a "typology of sources of vulnerability and attendant duties." In their view, vulnerabilities can be inherent (those that are unavoidable features of the human condition), situational (those that pertain to the particular context of the participant), or pathogenic (related to dysfunctional social or personal relationships). Each of these vulnerabilities can be experienced either acutely (what they term "occurrent") or chronically ("dispositional—latent or background"). It is important, they claim, to identify the type of vulnerability in order to properly identify our responsibilities related to the vulnerability-making feature, and in this way it is similar to Luna's layering theory of vulnerabilities. Without the proper identification of the vulnerability, we are likely to make sweeping regulations that are over-inclusive, under-inclusive, or both. In any case, the regulations will miss their mark.

Many scholars who have deep interest in the concept of vulnerability have turned to Ken Kipnis' analysis (Kipnis 2001, 2003). Kipnis expressly challenges what he terms the "subpopulation view" of the concept of vulnerability in research and instead replaces it with analytical categories. Combining two different works, Kipnis identifies seven exhaustive categories that are meant to identify the morally relevant features of vulnerability: Cognitive, juridic, deferential, medical, allocational, structural, and social. He argues that this analysis serves three purposes: (1) To provide a "checklist of circumstances that, along with other conditions, can invalidate the permissibility of research"; (2) to identify the necessary features of vulnerability and determine the "supplementary measures" required to address these vulnerabilities; and (3) to serve as grounds for adjudicating an investigator's culpability in taking unfair advantage of a particular population (Kipnis 2001: G-6). A group is considered "vulnerable" if there is a positive response to any of the questions pertaining to a particular analytic category. Kipnis' analysis will be useful for our considerations here.

Application of Vulnerability

Before proceeding, it is useful to describe a few representative studies that may be helpful to keep in the back of one's mind when assessing the forthcoming analysis. Essentially, why does it matter if vulnerable populations are included as research participants? Consider an experimental dermatological ointment that is not thought to be systemically absorbed. Even if a pregnant woman suffers from an uncomfortable or embarrassing skin condition, some IRBs may interpret the regulations in such a way as to prevent pregnant women from participating in this research, despite the low probability of harm from this topical medication (for either the woman or the fetus) and potential for benefit. Or consider a case from the world of pediatrics: Suppose researchers are proposing a trial of medical countermeasures (or vaccines, etc.) to combat (or as prophylaxis against) a biological attack. Surely, in the event of such an event we want to have effective methods of treating children who might have been exposed to the agent. Yet to have compelling evidence about therapeutic options, we will have to expose children to the risks of the treatment (and perhaps even the agent, should intentional exposure studies be warranted) without the possibility of direct benefit to the child (Presidential Commission for the Study of Bioethical Issues 2013).

In either case, there may be good reasons for proceeding with the research—carefully, respectfully, and with sufficient safeguards to minimize risks. Yet the regulations often serve as an impediment to research by limiting meaningful conversations about research with pregnant women. In this way, the regulations can in fact create harms—or vulnerabilities—rather than mitigate them. In what follows, I will briefly describe how Kipnis' analysis of vulnerability (originally applied to pediatric research) supports the argument that regulations can create or exacerbate vulnerabilities by demonstrating the harms obtaining to vulnerable populations (predominantly pregnant women and fetuses here) from the so-called "additional protections" of the federal requirements. (For a full treatment of this topic, see Schonfeld 2013.)

First, consider cognitive vulnerability, which Kipnis claims is obtained when potential participants have some intellectual barrier to participating fully in an informed consent process. Certainly this does not apply to pregnant women (or if it does apply to a particular pregnant woman, it is not by virtue of the pregnancy that it does so). And while it may be true that the fetus is cognitively vulnerable in that it cannot make decisions for itself, there is no reason to think that having a woman make a decision for the fetus is any more inappropriate than it is once the child is born and the parent is required to make decisions for him/her. That is, it is not clear that the regulations offer any additional protections greater than those that would normally be the case of the appropriate proxy decision-maker.

Cognitive vulnerability is also interesting in the context of prisoners. While some prisoners may be cognitively vulnerable, this vulnerability is not due to the incarceration itself. In fact, it is a common stereotype that prisoners have some cognitive vulnerability (because surely someone whose rationality was intact would not commit a crime!). So in one sense, ascribing vulnerability of this kind to prisoners may in fact *increase* their vulnerability as it makes them more susceptible to the biases and prejudices of others.

Medical vulnerability is commonly cited as a reason to offer additional safeguards to research participants; the idea is that because of their medical situation, research participants with medical vulnerabilities may be more likely to consent to participate in a study regardless of the attendant risks. Consider here the pregnant woman who is willing to do *anything* to preserve the health of her fetus, or the parent who is willing to do *anything* to improve the health of his/her (acutely or chronically) ill child.

While it is true that pregnant women may be selected for inclusion in research specifically because of their condition, it is not clear that such selection makes them medically vulnerable to the extent that they would be willing to take risks they would otherwise deem unreasonable (Kipnis 2003: 115). There may be occasions, however, when the fact of pregnancy *coupled* with another medical problem confers medical vulnerability on the pregnant woman. The classic example would be a pregnant woman with a newly diagnosed cancer, where treatment for the cancer may require a woman to consider therapies that put her fetus at heightened risk. If there is an experimental therapy that purports to shrink her tumors without exposing the fetus to radiation, for example, she might be inclined to choose that option over a regimen that has a higher probability of success at curing her cancer but also a higher probability of fetal harm. In this way, she is in a situation of medical vulnerability, when she chooses a research option that she might otherwise not consider. Yet one could plausibly argue that the cancer is responsible for the medical vulnerability here, not the pregnancy, even though treatment decisions about one will invariably affect decisions about the other. Such a situation might require a particularly nuanced consent process in order to separate these issues, but it is not clear whether additional regulatory protections are required for this above and beyond the standard guidance for adequate informed consent.

Ironically, the most plausible account of ways in which pregnant women are medically vulnerable is as a direct result of their *lack* of inclusion in research. We know that women are consistently prescribed medication during pregnancy, and many of those prescriptions involve a drug of either unknown teratogenicity or drugs that had demonstrated teratogenic effects (Daw et al. 2012; Yang et al. 2008; Andrade et al. 2004). Women who have a chronic health problem are four times as likely to be exposed to risk to themselves and their offspring via pharmaceuticals during their pregnancy as are women without chronic illness (Yang et al. 2008: 272). This is a pressing concern, since, as Françoise Baylis notes, "pregnant women get sick and sick women get pregnant" (Baylis 2010). Additionally, since approximately half of all pregnancies in the United States are unplanned (Guttmacher Institute 2012), fetuses are exposed to medications when their mothers unexpectedly become pregnant (Lyerly et al. 2009).

What this means is that any of the medications used to treat women during pregnancy are used "off label," that is, without specific guidance from the U.S. Food and Drug Administration or the manufacturer, or data on their likely outcomes. We know that pregnancy changes the way women's bodies respond to medications, and it is often difficult to predict the specific changes that a woman may experience (Lyerly et al. 2009). Therefore, clinicians cannot rely on standard evidence-based practice in order to prescribe medications for pregnant women, since the data available from clinical trials that included only non-pregnant women may be inaccurate or misleading in this context (Lyerly et al. 2009; Baylis 2010; Lyerly et al. 2008; Chambers et al. 2008).

This does more than create a situation of uncertainty; rather, it is a failure to respect the principle of justice. Pregnant women deserve to have effective treatment during pregnancy, and this goal can only be fostered by responsibly including pregnant women in clinical research (Baylis 2010). As Lyerly et al. argue, " . . . a pregnant woman is not just a woman with a bigger belly . . . if we are to treat pregnant women's illnesses effectively—something crucial to the health of *both* pregnant women and that of the children they may bear—we must study medications in pregnant women" (Lyerly et al. 2009: 4).

Finally, consider the case of juridic vulnerability. Juridic vulnerability is obtained in situations when others have legal authority over the decisional processes of others. This is certainly the standard case in the parent–child relationship until the child reaches the "legal age" of decision-making. The pediatric context is the easiest in which to see the justification for protections related to jurdic vulnerability: Given that cognitive development is such that children are often willing to forego long-term risks in favor of short-term rewards, it is important that others who have developed the skills to evaluate a risk/benefit ratio appropriately do so on behalf of the child. The idea is to ensure that children are safe and healthy in order to enable them to develop the appropriate cognitive skills that will enable them to make well-informed decisions later in life.

It is difficult to see how any of this could apply, however, to pregnant adult women (leaving aside, of course, the situation of pregnant children).[1] Assuming typical cognition, pregnant women are not under the juridic control of others. Some argue, however, that it is the fetus that is juridicially vulnerable, in some ways no different from children: Others have to make decisions on their behalf. The difficulty lies in how the regulations have addressed this vulnerability. The federal regulations confer juridic authority to *both* the biological mother and biological father in certain instances of research: Namely, when the research holds out the prospect of direct benefit solely to the fetus (provided that the father is not unavailable, incompetent, or temporarily incapacitated or that the pregnancy resulted from incest or rape) (45 CFR 46.204e). The parallel to this situation in the regulations is for research involving children that is greater than minimal risk to the child (45 CFR 46.406–407). In those cases, consent from both parents is required (with similar exceptions as those listed above).

The "protections" offered for the juridically vulnerable fetus, then, are the same as for children being considered for research that is greater than minimal risk. The justification for two-parent consent in the latter case is that the increased level of risk requires an increased level of protection; ostensibly, the child's welfare is better safeguarded with both parents providing permission for research participation than simply one parent doing so (recognizing, of course, that there are exceptions to this situation). The implication with fetuses, therefore, is that all research involving the potential for direct benefit to the fetus alone must be considered of a sufficient risk to require what is known as "two parent consent." Yet recall that the fetus exists dependently with the woman; as a result, many things that confer risk to a fetus also confer risk to a woman. A particularly vivid example of this are the rare instances of fetal surgery that confer significant risk (but the possibility of benefit) on the fetus, but also involve surgical procedures on the woman herself. But there are other examples as well: Interventions to reduce preterm labor, placental insufficiency, or other issues of necessity affect the woman (either because they are ingested by her or bodily affect her in some way, such as cervical cerclage or stitching) despite the potential for fetal benefit. And while there may not be significant risk to the woman with these agents, they are still actions being taken within her body. The implication of conferring juridic authority on the father, then, is that it gives him the power to consent to research that will happen to someone *who does not lack decisional authority*. This is odd, to say the least. The regulations remain silent on what happens if the mother and the father disagree about research participation in these instances, although presumably refusal by one would fail to meet the criterion that consent is obtained by both parties. Regardless, the purported juridic vulnerability of the fetus has the paradoxical effect of *making* the pregnant woman juridically vulnerable, which gives others authority over choices affecting her own body—a situation we would judge unethical in any other population retaining cognitive decisional capacity (Cantor 2012). Therefore, as it stands, the regulations do *not* protect the rights and welfare of pregnant women who are research participants; rather, they serve to *create* additional vulnerability for them.

Consequences of Additional Protections

This creation of vulnerabilities is not restricted to pregnant women. In the creation of their typology of vulnerability, Lange et al. (2013) worry that failing to connect protections precisely to the type of vulnerability a participant is experiencing may result in those extra protections exacerbating or creating vulnerability. In 2011, the National Institute of Mental Health (NIMH) convened an interdisciplinary panel to investigate the concept of vulnerability in research and to suggest approaches to reduce such vulnerabilities or protect the vulnerable in the research context (DuBois et al. 2012). Interestingly, one of the first findings by this panel was that efforts to protect groups from harm may in fact create new harms for that same population—in this case, those with mental illness. Indeed, they identified five problems with the "status quo" approach to research protections for vulnerable populations: (1) Saddling groups with the label of "vulnerable" can reinforce, rather than reduce, stigmas associated with that group; (2) labeling groups as vulnerable may discourage researchers from including particular individuals in research when they in fact retain decisional capacity; (3) current policies regarding vulnerable subjects may create artificial barriers to research, and as a result create harms or injustice to those populations; (4) "vulnerability" becomes an easy scapegoat for reasons to exclude particular populations when system or other problems are the actual causal factors in a potential participant's inability, for example, to understand a proposed study; (5) denying individuals the ability to choose to participate in research when they are capable of making such choices, even if they are members of a traditionally "vulnerable" group, unjustifiably impedes the exercise of their autonomy (DuBois et al. 2012).

It seems, then, that some of our "additional protections" may in fact be backfiring: Rather than safeguarding subpopulations from abuse, these protections are actually creating the vulnerabilities they purport to resolve. Yet this is not the only harm possible from the improper use of additional protections. Many research protocols also offer the prospect of benefit to the participants; to the extent that particular subpopulations are excluded without justification from participation, they are denied this benefit, which violates the principle of justice (Koffman et al. 2009). But even more than this, if members of certain subpopulations are denied the ability to participate in research, then the results of any studies will not apply to them; and as in the case of medical vulnerabilities, this denies pregnant women the benefits of medical advances relevant to their needs or situation" (Koffman et al. 2009: 440). Similar results have been described regarding patients requiring palliative care (Koffman et al. 2009), older people (deKlerk 2012), indigenous native populations (Clough et al. 2013), and mental health research among internationally displaced people (Siriwardhana et al. 2013), among others.

Possible Remedies for Exclusion

To address the barriers to the protection of vulnerable groups in research, the NIMH panel recommends a series of six guidelines designed for researchers and ethics review boards. The hope is that by attending carefully to these guidelines, those who are truly vulnerable will be identified and additional measures can be established to protect them; and others who have the ability and desire to participate in research will not be unjustly barred from doing so. Interestingly, the authors claim that their guidelines are consistent with current federal regulations, which makes them even more appealing. The overall approach is to design a system of considerations that demonstrates "genuine respect" for research participants while at the same time attending to broader considerations of vulnerabilities. Their recommendations are as follows (DuBois et al. 2012):

1. Risk: Rather than starting with the additional protections, the panel recommends investigators start by evaluating carefully the risk involved in the research. This will ensure that any safeguards deployed are appropriate and proportionate to the risk itself.
2. Protections: The additional measures should be proportionate to the risk, that is, offer the minimum additional safeguards necessary in relation to the actual risk. This recommendation ensures that individuals will not be unjustly prevented from participating in research because of procedures that do not relate to the risks in the study.
3. Consent Assessments: Attending carefully to the actual level of risk of a study, require universal consent assessments. That is, whenever we are significantly concerned about potential participants understanding the risks involved in a study, screen all of the potential participants for capacity rather than just those who might fall into a category of vulnerability. This policy will ensure that all potential participants have a sufficient understanding of the risks of participation, regardless of one's inclusion in a vulnerable group or not. Singling out members of particular populations disregards both individual variation and respect for persons who will be the ones to assume the risk once enrolling on the protocol.
4. Evidence: Just as medicine should be evidence based, so too should the development of additional protections in research be related to evidence about the actual risk in a particular study. Relying on high-quality evidence minimizes the impact of false assumptions based on (sometimes unconscious) bias or stereotypes and ensures that the suggested protections will actually safeguard against the identified risks.
5. Labels: Given that assessments in research are really designed to test the potential participant's understanding of the particulars of the research study in which the person may participate, the panel suggests that attending to the "subjective outcome of the

assessment process" is more appropriate than making global pronouncements about a subject's decisional capacity in general (DuBois et al. 2012: 2223). What is, or should be, relevant for investigators is whether or not the potential participant is able to adequately understand the trial and consider his or her options from among other alternatives. Individuals may be able to demonstrate this capacity without demonstrating capacity for larger issues, and that should be sufficient for the conduct of research. In this way, cognitive or other deficits that impair the broader concept of decisional capacity may not prove to be a barrier for research participation in particular contexts.

6. Additional Safeguards: Policies and procedures regarding additional safeguards should be considered in context: Community attitudes and priorities are relevant to the development and implementation of protection measures. Two examples offered by the panel are how payment for research participation can be viewed as respectful or manipulative in different contexts, or how the inclusion of patient advocates can be seen as either beneficial or as an invasion of privacy. In this way, investigators can ensure that the measures they propose to mitigate risk do not in fact confer additional vulnerabilities on participants because of external factors.

Scholars have also been working on the issue of how to include pregnant women in research responsibly. As a beginning, researchers are encouraged to take advantage of "low hanging fruit"—observational studies that incur no risk of harm to the mother or the fetus. Prospective studies including pregnant women and fetuses will require some sort of regulatory reform—a necessary step in order to make true progress. Already, researchers have initiated preliminary investigations by asking women themselves how they would feel about participating in research relative to reproductive risk (Schonfeld et al. 2009; Lyerly et al. 2012). This information may serve as the basis for regulation revision, as well as give insight into new procedural recommendations regarding informed consent. In addition, careful analyses of the risks appropriate for children to bear in the context of research, as well as the appropriateness of the consent process, may also yield fruitful directions for revised policies (Wendler et al. 2005; Nelson et al. 2013). Efforts are also underway regarding the reconsideration of issues in pediatric research. This includes justifying pediatric research without the possibility of direct benefit (Wendler 2012), reconsidering the concept of "minimal risk" (Glass and Binik 2008; Wendler 2009), and meaningfully involving children in decisions about research participation (Joffe et al. 2006; Wilfond and Diekema 2012).

What is clear from the analysis of vulnerability and its attendant protections is that one size clearly does not fit all. Investigators ought to consider carefully the appropriate population for research apart from any labeling of "vulnerability," rather than rely exclusively on regulatory frameworks to dictate when an individual participant may be "vulnerable," and how that vulnerability should be addressed. Attending carefully to contextual features will enable researchers to create a study design and process of participant recruitment that conform to ethical norms that not only cohere with regulation, but also meaningfully respect the participation of the individuals who make the study possible.

Related Topics

Chapter 14, "Biomedical Research Ethics: Landmark Cases, Scandals, and Conceptual Shifts," Jonathan D. Moreno and Dominic Sisti

Chapter 16, "The Future of Informed Consent to Research: Reconceptualizing the Process," Paul Appelbaum

Note

1 The section on juridic vulnerability comes verbatim from Schonfeld (2013: 194–5).

References

Andrade S.E., Gurwitz, J.H., Davis, R.L., Chan, K.A., Finkelstein, J.A., Fortman, K. et al. (2004) "Prescription drug use in pregnancy," *American Journal of Obstetrics and Gynecology* 191: 398–407.

Baylis, F. (2010) "Pregnant women deserve better," *Nature* 465: 689–90.

Cantor, J.D. (2012) "Court-Ordered Care: A Complication of Pregnancy to Avoid," *New England Journal of Medicine* 366: 2237–40.

Chambers, C.D., Polifka, J.E. and Friedman, J.M. (2008) "Drug safety in pregnant women and their babies: Ignorance not bliss," *Clinical Pharmacology and Therapeutics* 83: 181–3.

Clough, B.A., Campbell, M.M., Aliyeva, T.A., Mateo, N.J., Zarean, M. and O'Donovan, A. (2013) "Protocols for Protection of Human Participants: A Comparison of Five Countries," *Journal of Empirical Research on Human Research Ethics* 8: 2–11.

Coleman, C. (2009) "Vulnerability as a regulatory category in human subject research," *Journal of Law, Medicine, and Ethics* 37: 12–18.

Council for International Organizations of Medical Sciences (2002) "International Ethical Guidelines for Biomedical Research Involving Human Subjects." Available at: http://www.recerca.uab.es/ceeah/docs/CIOMS.pdf (accessed January 14, 2014).

Daw, J.R., Mintzes, B., Law, M.R., Hanley, G.E. and Morgan, S.G. (2012) "Prescription drug use in pregnancy: A retrospective, population-based study in British Columbia, Canada (2001–2006)," *Clinical Therapeutics* 34: 239–249.e2.

deClerk, C.M. (2012) "Protection of Incapacitated Elderly in Medical Research," *European Journal of Health Law* 19: 367–78.

DuBois, J.M., Beskow, L., Cambell, J., Dugosh, K., Festinger, D., Hartz, S., James, R. and Lidz, C. (2012) "Restoring Balance: A Consensus Statement on the Protection of Vulnerable Research Participants," *American Journal of Public Health* 102: 2220–5.

Glass, K.C. and Binik, A. (2008) "Rethinking Risk in Pediatric Research," *Journal of Law, Medicine and Ethics* 36: 567–76.

Guttmacher Institute (2012) "Facts on Unintended Pregnancy in the United States. In Brief: Fact Sheet." Available at: http://www.guttmacher.org/pubs/FB-Unintended-Pregnancy-US.pdf (accessed December 26, 2012).

Hurst, S.A. (2008) "Vulnerability in Research and Health Care: Describing the Elephant in the Room?" *Bioethics* 22: 191–202.

Joffe, S., Fernandez, C.V., Pentz, R.D., Ungar, D.R., Mathew, N.A., Turner, C.W., Alessandri, A.J., Woodman, C.L., Singer, D.A. and Kodish, E. (2006) "Involving Children with Cancer in Decision-Making About Research Participation," *Pediatrics* 149: 862–8.

Jones, J. (1993) *Bad Blood: The Tuskegee Syphilis Experiment*, new and expanded edition, New York: The Free Press.

Kipnis, K. (2001) "Vulnerability in Research Subjects: A Bioethical Taxonomy," in National Bioethics Advisory Commission (ed.) *Ethical and Policy Issues in Research Involving Human Participants*, volume 2, pp. G1–13.

Kipnis, K. (2003) "Seven Vulnerabilities in the Pediatric Research Subject," *Theoretical Medicine and Bioethics* 24: 107–20.

Koffman, J., Morgan, M., Edmonds, P., Speck, P. and Higginson, I.J. (2009) "Vulnerability in Palliative Care Research: Findings from a Qualitative Study of Black Caribbean and White British Patients with Advanced Cancer," *Journal of Medical Ethics* 35: 440–4.

Lange, M.M., Rogers, W. and Dodds, S. (2013) "Vulnerability in Research Ethics: A Way Forward," *Bioethics* 27: 333–40.

Levine, C., Faden, R., Grady, C., Hammerschmidt, D., Eckenwiler, L., Sugarman, J. et al. (2004) "The Limitations of 'Vulnerability' as a Protection for Human Research Participants," *American Journal of Bioethics* 4: 44–9.

Luna, F. and Vanderpoel, S. (2013) "Not the Usual Suspects: Addressing Layers of Vulnerability," *Bioethics* 27: 325–32.

Lyerly, A.D., Little, M.O. and Faden, R. (2008) "The Second Wave: Toward Responsible Inclusion of Pregnant Women in Research," *International Journal of Feminist Approaches to Bioethics* 1: 5.

Lyerly, A.D., Mitchell, L.M., Armstrong, E.M., Harris, L.H., Kukla, R., Kuppermann, M. et al. (2009) "Risk and the Pregnant Body," *Hastings Center Report* 39: 34–42.

Lyerly, A.D., Namey, E.E., Gray, B., Swamy, G. and Faden, R.R. (2012) "Women's Views About Participating in Research While Pregnant," *IRB: Ethics and Human Research* 34: 1–8.

Macklin, R. (2003) "Bioethics, Vulnerability, and Protection," *Bioethics* 17: 472–86.

Nelson, D.K., Skinner, D., Guarda, S., Choudhury, S., Sideris, J., Barnum, L. et al. (2013) "Obtaining Consent from Both Parents for Pediatric Research: What Does 'Reasonably Available' Mean?" *Pediatrics* 131: e223–9.

Porter, J.P. and Koski, G. (2008) "Regulations for the Protection of Humans in Research in the United States: The Common Rule," in E.J. Emanuel, C. Grady, R.A. Crouch, R.K. Lie, F.G. Miller and D. Wendler (eds.) *The Oxford Textbook of Clinical Research Ethics*, New York: Oxford University Press.

Presidential Commission for the Study of Bioethical Issues (2013) *Safeguarding Children: Pediatric Medical Countermeasure Research*. Available at: http://bioethics.gov/node/833 (accessed February 24, 2014).

Reverby, S.M. (2009) *Examining Tuskegee: The Infamous Syphilis Study and its Legacy*, Chapel Hill: The University of North Carolina Press.

Schroeder, D. and Gefenas, E. (2009) "Vulnerability: Too Vague and Too Broad?" *Cambridge Quarterly of Healthcare Ethics* 18: 113–21.

Schonfeld, T. (2013) "The Perils of Protection: Vulnerability and Women in Research," *Theoretical Medicine and Bioethics* 34: 189–206.

Schonfeld, T.L., Amoura, N.J., Stoner, J.A. and Gordon, B.G. (2009) "Women and Contraception in Research: A Pilot Study," *Journal of Women's Health* 18: 507–12.

Siriwardhana, C., Adikari, A., Jayaweera, K. and Sumathipala, A. (2013) "Ethical Challenges in Mental Health Research among Internationally Displaced People: Ethical Theory and Research Implementation," *BMC Medical Ethics* 14: 1–8.

Wendler, D. (2009) "Minimal Risk in Pediatric Research as a Function of Age," *Archives of Pediatric and Adolescent Medicine* 163: 115–18.

Wendler, D. (2012) "A New Justification for Pediatric Research Without the Potential for Clinical Benefit," *American Journal of Bioethics* 12: 23–31.

Wendler, D., Belsky, L., Thompson, K.M. and Emanuel, E.J. (2005) "Quantifying the Federal Minimal Risk Standard: Implications for Pediatric Research Without a Prospect of Direct Benefit," *Journal of the American Medical Association* 294: 826–32.

Wilfond, B.S. and Diekema, D.S. (2012) "Engaging Children in Genomics Research: Decoding the Meaning of Assent in Research," *Genetic Medicine* 14: 437–43.

World Medical Association (2013) "Declaration of Helsinki: Ethical Principles for Medical Research Involving Human Subjects." Available at: http://www.wma.net/en/30publications/10policies/b3/ (accessed 14 January, 2014).

Yang, T., Walker, M.C., Krewski, D., Yang, Q., Nimrod, C., Garner, P. et al. (2008) "Maternal Characteristics Associated with Pregnancy Exposure to FDA Category C, D, and X Drugs in a Canadian Population," *Pharmacoepidemiology and Drug Safety* 17: 270–7.

Further Reading

For extended reflections on women and vulnerability, see Mackenzie, C., Rogers, W. and Dodds, S. (eds.) (2013) *Vulnerability: New Essays in Ethics and Feminist Philosophy*, New York: Oxford University Press. Three texts deal importantly and differently with the involvement of children in research: Wendler, D. (2010) *The Ethics of Pediatric Research*, New York: Oxford; Ross, L.F. (2006) *Children in Medical Research*, New York: Oxford University Press; Kodish, E. (ed.) (2005) *Ethics and Research with Children*, New York: Oxford University Press; for a regulatory perspective on including prisoners in research, see Institute of Medicine (2007) *Ethical Considerations for Research involving Prisoners*, Washington: National Academies Press; for a case study involving prisoners in research, see Hornbulm, A.M. (1998) *Acres of Skin*, New York: Routledge.

19

THE ETHICS OF INCENTIVES FOR PARTICIPATION IN RESEARCH

What's the Problem?

Alan Wertheimer

The purpose of this chapter is to ask whether it is ethical to provide financial or medical incentives to people to motivate them to participate in research. It is best to put this issue in a wider context.

The ethics of medical research with human subjects raises genuine moral worries not to be found in the ethics of medical care. At the most general level, the core problem of medical (therapeutic) ethics is to determine what we can ethically do to people *for their benefit*. By contrast, the core problem of research ethics with human subjects is to determine what we can ethically do to people by using them as means to produce generalizable knowledge (Wertheimer 2011: ch. 1).

And clinical research really uses people as means. No Kantian abstractions necessary here. Researchers inject substances, draw blood, perform lumbar punctures, intubate trachea, withdraw medication for schizophrenia, perform sham arthroscopic surgery, extract and store tissue, and expose healthy volunteers to malaria-infected mosquitos. Although subjects may occasionally or even often receive medical or collateral benefits from participating in research, they emphatically do not benefit from many component procedures (for example, blood draws and lumbar punctures) that are designed to test study hypotheses.

The difficulties involved in recruiting subjects into clinical trials illustrate this problem. More than one trial in five sponsored by the National Cancer Institute failed to enroll a single subject, and only half reached the minimum needed for a meaningful result (Ramsey and Scoggins 2008). Among adults diagnosed with cancer, fewer than 5 percent participate in trials. It seems reasonable to assume that more and faster completed studies would yield greater progress in the treatment of cancer, and similar things could be said about other diseases or improvements in people's quality of life.

Although it would be desirable to facilitate recruitment of subjects into clinical trials, it is generally thought that it is unethical to enlist people in research without their valid consent. As the Nuremberg Code (1949) puts it, "The voluntary consent of the human subject is absolutely essential" (Emanuel et al. 2003). On analysis, this simple view is false. For example, most think it is ethical to conduct observational social and behavioral research without any sort of consent as when psychologists sought to determine whether wealthy drivers (as indicated by their cars) behaved more unethically than less wealthy drivers (Piff et al. 2012). It is also thought that it is ethical to conduct minimal risk social and behavioral research without informed consent when subjects must be deceived if research is to produce scientifically valid data. Indeed, Federal Regulations explicitly allow for waivers of informed consent under these very sorts of conditions (45 CFR § 46.116(d)).

Consent is more likely to be required in biomedical research, but there are exceptions there as well. Even if we set aside cases in which surrogates consent for the subject (for example, children), there are special circumstances, such as emergency research in which research may be justified even though no sort of consent is possible. Research without consent may also be justifiable when it involves public health surveillance, collection of data from health records, or cluster randomized trials when it is impractical or impossible to seek everyone's consent.

These exceptions to the Nuremberg principle deserve more attention than they receive. If much research can be ethically permissible without valid consent, it is a puzzle why informed consent is typically regarded as a *sine qua non* of ethical biomedical research. And this is especially so when we consider the general problem of recruiting research subjects (Wertheimer 2011: ch. 2).

Although it is rarely discussed in these terms, participation in research often constitutes a classic collective action problem. It is in the *ex ante* interest of most people that research be conducted, but participation in actual research can be contrary to the interests of each individual. *Ex ante*, we may all be better off if all of us do our fair share of participation in research. But the knowledge generated by research is a *public good*, i.e., it is a good that is available to all whether or not one contributed to it. And to the extent that people are self-interested, they will seek to reap the benefits of research without paying the costs. Precisely for that reason, we often rely on the use of coercion to solve collective action problems in many contexts. We tax citizens to pay for public goods, including funding research that generates knowledge that is available to all. We require that cars come equipped with catalytic converters. We can at least ask: Why not require people to participate in biomedical research in much the same way?

For present purposes, I set such concerns aside. The question remains as to how we can ethically recruit people to participate in socially valuable biomedical research that is consistent with our commitment to requiring consent. There seem to be at least four alternatives. First, we could simply accept a slower pace of medical research as the price we pay for accepting the values secured by consent. Hans Jonas famously argued that avoidable illness and death are regrettable but not of overarching moral significance because "progress is an optional goal" (Jonas 1969: 224). Second, we could do more to encourage altruistic participation or to educate people about the benefits of receiving medical care in a research context. Third, investigators can give people financial incentives to participate such that the value of the payment exceeds the disvalue of the risk and burdens of participation. Fourth, investigators can take advantage of the fact that participation may be in a person's medical interest, as when participation is the only means of gaining access to an experimental intervention or, more problematically, when subjects do not have access to or cannot afford medical care. This explains one reason why pharmaceutical corporations have increasingly conducted their research in less developed countries in Eastern Europe, South America, Asia, and Africa.

Bioethicists have viewed some of these strategies for recruiting subjects with considerable suspicion. Carl Elliott (2008: 40) maintains, "Ethicists generally prefer that subjects take part in studies for altruistic reasons." As John Harris (2005: 246) puts it, "Most research ethics protocols and guidelines are antipathetic to inducements." Australian policy states that "volunteers may be paid for inconvenience and time spent, but such payment should not be so large as to be an inducement to participate" (Wilkinson and Moore 1997: 373). With respect to research in developing countries, many have claimed that this practice is grossly exploitative—"Residents of impoverished, postcolonial countries, the majority of whom are people of color, must be protected from potential exploitation in research. Otherwise, the abominable state of health care in these countries can be used to justify studies that could never pass ethical muster in the sponsoring country" (Lurie and Wolfe 1997: 855).

So is it ethical to provide financial or medical incentives to people to motivate them to participate in research? In particular, does the use of financial or medical incentives constitute coercion or undue influence and thereby compromise the validity of consent? I will argue that offering incentives does not compromise the validity of consent. But even if people can give voluntary informed consent when participation is in their financial or medical interests, it may be wrong to exploit their financial or medical needs. And so I shall consider whether the use of incentives can constitute exploitation and whether that is a good reason to prohibit the use of such incentives.

Coercion

David Rothman has remarked that when investigators recruit lower-income patients who either need the money or cannot afford conventional treatment, it is "coercion through lack of income" (Rosen 2012: 40). Although one can legitimately use the word coercion in different ways and for different purposes, we must be careful when we claim that the use of financial incentives is coercive. Words have consequences. In a recent study of institutional review board (IRB) members' views of coercion, one of the respondents noted that "Coercion has come to mean something more along the lines of simple influence in the IRBs I have worked with—not the meaning it has in other contexts" (Largent et al. 2012: 4). This statement suggests that this respondent's IRB has adopted an excessively expansive account of coercion that may be used inappropriately to limit the activities of researchers and prospective subjects.

So what constitutes the sort of coercion that invalidates consent? *The Belmont Report*, upon which many rely for authoritative guidance, gets it basically right: "Coercion occurs when an overt threat of harm is intentionally presented by one person to another in order to obtain compliance" (The National Commission for the Protection of Human Subjects of Biomedical and Behavioral Research 1978). It is worth emphasizing that this definition states that coercion requires a *threat* of harm. I have argued elsewhere for a minor modification of Belmont's suggestion. Putting aside some minor complications, A coerces B to consent to do X only if A proposes to violate B's rights or not fulfill an obligation to B if B chooses not do X (Wertheimer and Miller 2008).

On this view, A does not coerce B to do X if A offers to give a benefit to B if B consents to do X. Threats are coercive but genuine offers are not. Threats reduce the options available to the target, whereas offers expand them, and one does not coerce another when one's proposal expands the options available to her. Ruth Macklin has said that the question as to how large a payment constitutes a coercive offer is one for "which no clear answer is forthcoming" (Macklin 1989: 3). I disagree. A clear answer is forthcoming: Genuine offers do not coerce.

Those who think that offers can coerce sometimes appeal to the well-known phrase from *The Godfather*—"My father made him an offer he couldn't refuse." But Don Corleone's proposal was coercive not because it was an exceptionally attractive offer, but because it was a paradigmatically coercive threat—"Either your signature or your brains will be on the contract."

Now to say that offers do not coerce is not to deny that offers can be seriously immoral:

> *Bribe*. A, a police officer, stops B for speeding. B offers to give A $100 if B does not write a ticket. A accepts.

It is immoral for B to offer a bribe to A and it is immoral for A to accept a bribe, but B's offer hardly coerces A in a way that negates or reduces A's responsibility for accepting it. Similarly, if A offers to pay B $10,000 to kill C, B could hardly claim that A coerced him into killing C by offering a financial incentive.

In a recent study we found that many IRB members were in the grips of serious misconceptions about the concepts of coercion and undue influence. For example, some respondents thought that offers of payment were coercive or unduly influential when they motivated people to agree to participate when they would otherwise not do so, a view that is incorporated in the Australian policy noted above (Largent et al. 2012). This view is dubious. There are numerous ways of motivating people to do things that they would otherwise not do, and most of them do not involve coercion or anything morally problematic. If A persuades B to give blood or go to a movie or invest in a mutual fund when B would otherwise not do so, it is clear that B has not been coerced. The same is true for offers. If A offers the teenager next-door $20 to mow his lawn, we would not say that the teenager has been coerced.

Another popular view claims that A coerces B to do X when A's proposal leaves B with "no reasonable alternative" but to accept A's proposal. This is a natural but deeply mistaken view. It is a natural view because one generally has no reasonable alternative but to succumb to a coercive proposal. Consider the paradigmatic case in which A (a gunman) says to B, "hand over your wallet or I'll shoot you." Although A has been coerced to hand over his wallet and although B has no reasonable alternative but to do so, it does *not* follow that B has been coerced *because* he has no reasonable alternative.

To see this, simply note that there are many situations in which people choose options because they lack reasonable alternatives without being coerced. Arthur Caplan accepts the "no reasonable alternative" view when he claims that illness is coercive. But we do not say that a patient who agrees to surgery or chemotherapy because the only alternative is death has been coerced to consent or that her consent to treatment is involuntary or invalid. Nor do we describe people as coerced if they take an unpleasant job in order to provide for their families if their only alternative is to remain unemployed.

Now consider the person who consents to participate in research in exchange for payment because her background conditions are very poor. David Rothman (2000) writes, "abject poverty is harsh enough without people having to bear the additional burdens of serving as research subjects." If research participants are *benefiting* from participation all things considered, we might just as well say that abject poverty is harsh enough without denying people the opportunity to make their lives somewhat less miserable by participating in biomedical research and receiving financial payments or medical care that they would not otherwise receive. We can grant that people "do not have enough options and that society has been unjust to them in not extending more options, while nonetheless respecting and honoring the choices they actually make in reduced circumstances" (Nussbaum 1998: 721).

I suspect that many concerned with the protection of research subjects accept a form of "research exceptionalism" whereby factors that would not compromise the validity of consent in other contexts are thought to be worrisome in the context of research. After all, we allow people to assume high-risk jobs such as police work, military, fire-fighting, timber cutting, lobster fishing, structural steel work, coal mining, and professional football. We do not think that people are coerced by the offer of payment into accepting such risks, and, similarly, we should not think that prospective subjects are coerced by the offer of payment.

What would constitute coercion to participate in research? If a doctor were to implicitly or explicitly threaten to abandon a patient if he does not agree to participate in research, then the patient's decision is coerced and involuntary. If a patient were to mistakenly *fear* that he would be abandoned if he did not agree, then we might say that his decision to participate is involuntary although he has not actually been coerced. But those sorts of situations aside, we should probably simply abandon the concern that offers of payment or medical care are coercive.

Undue Influence

Even if offers of payment or medical care do not coerce, they could constitute undue influence and thereby invalidate consent. But what sort of influence is undue in that way? *The Belmont Report* states that "Undue influence, by contrast [with coercion], occurs through an offer of an excessive, unwarranted, inappropriate or improper reward or other overture in order to obtain compliance" (The National Commission for the Protection of Human Subjects of Biomedical and Behavioral Research 1978). Unfortunately, this account is not helpful. It does not specify when or for what reasons an offer should be considered excessive, unwanted, inappropriate or improper, or indicate why such offers compromise the validity of consent.

I think that A's offer of payment is best understood as undue influence if and only if it is so attractive that it distorts subjects' evaluation of the risks and benefits of participation. The Office for Human Research Protections (OHRP 2011) guidebook for IRBs implicitly endorses this view when it says "Offers that are too attractive may blind prospective subjects to the risks or impair their ability to exercise proper judgment." For reasons noted above, it hardly makes sense to say that an incentive is unduly influential just because it gets people to consent when they would otherwise not do so. Once again, on this view an inducement is *not* morally problematic if it is *genuinely* too good to refuse. It is problematic if it would be refused if the agent's judgment were not blinded or clouded or impaired.

In principle, an agent's decision-making could be distorted by the offer of inducements in at least two ways. An agent may experience *tunnel vision* when the lure of the payment causes the agent to ignore or give inadequate consideration to other relevant interests. An agent may experience *decisional myopia* when the lure of the inducement causes her to overweight the short-term benefits and underestimate or underweight the long-term costs of participation. Distortion of judgment is the key (Wertheimer 2011: ch. 4).

The Council for the International Organization of Medical Sciences worries that the offer of monetary payments may "induce prospective subjects to consent to participate in the research *against their better judgment*" (CIOMS 2002). But what does that mean? The phrase "against one's better judgment" sometimes conveys that we do something reluctantly. For example, a professor might say to a student, "It's against my better judgment but I'll grant your request for an extension on your paper." The professor does not think that he acts involuntarily or that he is not responsible for his decision. A's offer of money (or medical benefits) may motivate B to do something that *would* have been against her better judgment in the absence of the value of the offer, but that does not show that acceptance of the offer is against her better judgment *given* the value of the offer to her.

It is sometimes argued that an offer constitutes undue influence or compromises voluntariness if it is so large or in excess that it is irresistible in this context. Once again, we must be careful. We cannot say that an offer is irresistible just because one finds it hard to reject it, for that is true of all choices for which we have strong desires. We might say that a proposal is irresistible just in case no reasonable person (in that person's situation) would reject the proposal, as when a person of modest means is offered $1,000 to mow a lawn. On that view, however, there would be nothing wrong with making an irresistible offer and no reason to question the validity of the consent.

Grant and Sugarman (2004: 728) argue that while incentives are always designed to motivate "someone to do what they otherwise might not," there is something ethically suspect about using an incentive to get "someone to do something to which they are *averse* . . . And the ethical problem is multiplied where the aversion is a principled one or a matter of moral scruple."

I'm not sure I understand the distinction between (1) getting someone to do something they would otherwise not do in the absence of an incentive, and (2) getting someone to do something to which they are averse. If I would not work unless I were paid for doing so, does it not mean that I am averse to working without being paid? Grant and Sugarman might say that I'm not averse to teaching college students but I might be averse, say, to teaching middle school students or mowing lawns. I don't think this reply will work. For whatever sum of money that would be sufficient to motivate me to teach college students (to which I would be averse in the absence of being paid that sum), there is a greater sum that would be sufficient to motivate me to teach middle school or mow lawns.

Grant and Sugarman (2004: 728) might claim that things are different if the aversion is "a principled one or a matter of moral scruple," as for example, if one tried "to induce religious people to work on the Sabbath by offering large incentives." This is tricky. It does seem perverse to offer Mormons (whose religion prohibits consumption of caffeine) a large cash incentive to participate in a study of the effects of caffeine on the brain (the research may require people who have never consumed caffeine), even if there is nothing intrinsically wrong with the consumption of caffeine. But I am not sure to what extent this intuition is defensible.

First, people do not all place the same weight on their moral commitments as contrasted with their non-moral interests. Second, and more importantly, even if an offer may motivate B to violate *one* of her moral values, people have multiple values and commitments. Consider this case:

> *Family*. A wants to hire B. The job would require that B spend much of her time traveling. B tells A that she is reluctant to accept because she thinks she has an obligation to her spouse and children to work close to home. A raises the offer. B accepts.

Grant and Sugarman might argue that A is acting wrongly because he is seeking to get B to do something to which she was averse on moral grounds (her obligation to her family). I disagree. First, it might be objectionably paternalistic for A to not offer B a payment on this ground. Unless A has reason to think that his offer will distort B's judgment, A shows respect for B's autonomy by allowing B to make her own decisions in the light of her own value structure and not by preemptively short-circuiting B's decision process or opportunities. Second, people have multiple aims, projects, and obligations. B may believe that she has an obligation to spend time with her family, but she may also believe that she has a greater obligation to provide for them financially.

That is precisely why some people choose to participate in research. Consider the story of Rambha Gajre, a woman in India:

> She and her family faced eviction from their cramped, tin-roof hut if she didn't soon repay loans she used to cover life-saving medical treatment for her son . . . "Many people commit suicide and I didn't want to become one of those and I didn't want people to think I did it to avoid repaying. I have two young kids, 10 and 12 years old. What would become of them?" So Rambha did what thousands of other desperate women and men from India's slums, and across the world, now do to survive—she signed up to be a human guinea pig in drug trials for foreign pharmaceutical companies." In explaining her decision, Rambha said "I am helpless, I have to do this . . . They don't really force us, but I don't have a choice."
>
> (NBC News 2012)

This is a sad story, but it seems that Rambha knew what she was doing. She was participating in research in order to provide for her family. I am reluctant to say that her judgment was distorted or that it would have been better to deny her that opportunity.

Absent showing that participants are making irrational judgments in response to offers of financial payment, there is no reason to reject them on this ground. Moreover, although the evidence on this is limited, several empirical studies suggest that financial incentives do *not* cause subjects to be insensitive to the risks of participation (Halpern et al. 2004). Given the difficulty of recruiting subjects into socially valuable research, we should be reluctant to reject the use or even increased use of incentives as a means of facilitating recruitment when it is compatible with the principle of informed consent.

Exploitation

The concept of exploitation has also come to play an important role in discourse about the ethics of clinical research. Indeed, some bioethicists have argued that the principle of non-exploitation is the underlying rationale for many of the oft-mentioned principles of ethical research such as social value, scientific validity, informed consent, fair participant selection, and favorable risk–benefit ratio (Emanuel et al. 2000).

Accusations of wrongful exploitation in research are most frequently invoked with respect to research with vulnerable populations, such as prisoners, people on low income, and the desperately ill. The charge seems particularly poignant in the international context when poor citizens in less developed countries (LDCs) are used as subjects in research that is primarily designed to benefit those in developed countries: "the specter of exploitation is the most serious ethical issue in multinational clinical research" (Emanuel 2007: 189). Accusations of exploitation are especially applied to the growing practice in which pharmaceutical corporations "outsource" medical research to contract research organizations that, in turn, conduct many of their studies in *LDCs*—"A huge population with a diversity of diseases that are untreated—yes, that is the 'India Advantage'" (India Resource Center).

Accusations of exploitation reached fever pitch when investigators conducted placebo-controlled trials in LDCs when proven effective treatment was available in developed countries (Angell 1997). Consider *The Short-Course ART Trial*. Placebo-controlled trials had unequivocally established the efficacy of a "long course" use of the antiretroviral drug zidovudine for reducing maternal–fetal transmission of HIV (Connor et al. 1994; Lurie and Wolfe 1997). The protocol involved administering the drug orally to women who were HIV positive during pregnancy, administering the drug intravenously during labor, and subsequently administering the drug to the newborn infant. Unfortunately, the efficacy and use of the long course regime could not be confidently extrapolated to LDCs. First, the drug might not be as efficacious in LDCs due to differences in immune status and breastfeeding practices. Second, even if the long course regime proved to be efficacious in LDCs, many thought that its use was not administratively or economically feasible. It would prove too expensive, compliance with the regime would prove virtually impossible for many women, and many LDCs lacked the medical infrastructure, such as refrigeration, to support its administration. Given these facts on the ground, investigators wanted to determine whether a cheaper and simpler "short course" use of zidovudine would be reasonably effective in reducing maternal–fetal transmission of HIV even if it would not be *as* effective as the long course regimen.

It would have been ethically impossible to conduct a placebo-controlled trial (PCT) of the short course regimen in a developed nation where the local standard of care would have included the long course regimen. It would not be approved by an IRB and even if it were approved, women would not consent to participate if the long course were available. By contrast, it was ethically feasible, many argued, to recruit subjects to a PCT of the short course treatment in an LDC where the local standard of care was to receive no treatment at all. In effect, the investigators offered subjects a 50 percent chance of getting treatment where the subjects would otherwise have received nothing. The placebo-controlled trials were conducted but were widely condemned as unethical and exploitative because the investigators deliberately withheld a proven effective intervention from those in the control group.

Exploitation in clinical research is a large topic with many dimensions. The question I want to focus on here is this: Is there reason to prohibit research just because it is exploitative? To begin, it is crucial to distinguish between types of exploitation on two axes. First, we can distinguish between *harmful exploitation* and *mutually advantageous exploitation*. By harmful exploitation, I refer to those cases in which the exploiter gains by harming the exploitee. By mutually advantageous exploitation, I refer to those cases in which both parties—including the exploitee—reasonably expect to gain from the transaction as contrasted with the pre-transaction position (Wertheimer 1996, 2011: ch. 5).

We can similarly distinguish between *non-consensual exploitation* and *consensual exploitation*. By consensual exploitation, I refer to cases in which the exploitee gives valid consent in the sense that she is competent, has adequate information, and is not coerced.

These two distinctions overlap but are not equivalent. There can be cases of mutually advantageous but non-consensual exploitation. There can also be cases of harmful but consensual exploitation, as when a self-loathing B allows A to benefit by harming her. Nonetheless, because these distinctions tend to converge, I shall rely on the distinction between harmful non-consensual exploitation and mutually advantageous and consensual exploitation.

Now it is not easy to explain how and when a mutually advantageous and consensual transaction is exploitative. When does A take unfair advantage of B? Consider *Umbrella*.

> *Umbrella*. A, a storeowner, normally charges $10 for an umbrella. B, who is wearing an expensive suede jacket, wants to buy an umbrella from A. A sees that it is pouring and tells B that the umbrella will cost $50.

The transaction is mutually advantageous because it is better for B to buy the umbrella for $50 than not to do so. It is arguably consensual because B understands that to which she is consenting, because it is rational for B to consent, and because A's proposal is not coercive, i.e., A does not threaten to violate B's rights if she declines. Nonetheless, it seems that A is taking unfair advantage of B. But what is the criterion of unfairness? Some say that a transaction is exploitative when the exploiter gains much more than the exploitee. But contrary to what is often supposed, the exploited person usually gains *more* utility from a transaction than the exploiter. For example, the utility gain to B (who preserves an expensive jacket worth $1000) is probably much greater than the utility gain to A (who gets, say, $40 more than usual). Indeed, it is precisely because the exploiter stands to gain relatively little that he can threaten to walk away from the transaction.

Let us assume for the sake of argument that the terms of *Umbrella* are exploitative. The important question for our purposes is whether we should endorse the principle that A should not be able to sell the umbrella to B for $50 or that B should not be able to buy it. In the present context, we must determine whether investigators should not be permitted to exploit research subjects by offering inadequate benefits to them *if* the subjects benefit from participating in research because they receive medical care or financial payment and if they are giving valid consent to participate.

What could justify not allowing the parties to enter into a mutually advantageous consensual transaction? This issue is too complicated to be answered here. In general, I think that we should be very reluctant to interfere with transactions between investigators and subjects if participation is beneficial to the subjects and they give valid informed consent. And that includes participation in placebo-controlled trials in which subjects consent to participate in order to get a 50 percent chance at receiving at medical care. Although I am not convinced that the short course trial actually did exploit the subjects, we can concede for the sake of argument that the subjects were treated unfairly and still maintain that it is best to allow the research to take place. We may object to and work to change the circumstances that render it reasonable for people to consent to participate in exchange for medical care or what strikes us as inadequate financial compensation, but, as a general principle, we do the people of LDCs no favor if we deny them the opportunity to participate in research when they are better off if they do so.

To put the previous point slightly differently, it is sometimes right to allow people to do an act that is wrong. It may be right to allow people to engage in wrongful or hateful speech. And it may be right to allow one person to exploit another if the exploitee benefits from the exploitation and consents to it.

It might be thought that it is one thing to employ people in LDCs to produce running shoes for low wages if the workers benefit from doing so and quite another to employ them as subjects in a trial of a new drug for type 2 diabetes, whether they do it for money or for access to medical treatment that they would otherwise not receive. Shamoo and Resnik (2006: w8) say "it is especially important to prevent pharmaceutical companies from using people in developing countries as cheap labor to test drugs that will only be used in the developed world, because this would constitute an egregious form of exploitation." Although they do not say what it is that makes this practice exploitative, it is not clear why we should want to prevent it. Would they seek to prevent running shoe manufacturers from using people in developing countries as cheap labor to manufacture shoes that will only be used in the developed world if what is cheap labor to us are among the better jobs available in such societies?

I have argued elsewhere that we would be justified in prohibiting exploitative transactions *if* doing so would result in transactions that are fairer (Wertheimer 2011: ch. 5). So we prohibit people from working for sub-minimum wages in the hope that employers will not refuse to employ people but will, instead, employ them at a fairer wage. If prohibiting investigators from exploiting subjects will result in fairer terms for the subjects, then we can justify prohibiting mutually advantageous and consensual transactions. But if prohibiting such transactions causes the research not to be done with those subjects to their detriment, then it is actually difficult to justify not allowing such exploitation to occur.

Conclusion

The recruitment of subjects into socially valuable biomedical research presents us with a difficult problem. Given that people's willingness to incur the burdens and risks of participation is rather limited, the progress of research is held back to the detriment of all of us. We should therefore support strategies that give people incentives to participate when they would otherwise not do so. At the same time, those strategies must be compatible with respect for the interests and autonomy of prospective subjects. In particular, we should not recruit people into research without their valid informed consent. Adhering to this principle is not without cost. Baruch Brody (2011) describes a placebo-controlled study of the benefits of arthroscopic surgery in which subjects were required to write by hand that they understood that they might be receiving "sham surgery." Although this procedure generated a "significant refusal rate," Brody maintains that this is "the price you may have to pay if you increase potential subjects' understanding." No one said that ethics comes cheap.

But the price need not and should not be more expensive than it needs to be. Many people object to the use of financial or medical incentives for participation on the grounds that they are or can be coercive or unduly influential or exploitative. I have argued that genuine incentives do not coerce and that incentives are unduly influential only if they distort the prospective subject's ability to make a reasonable determination as to whether the benefits of participation outweigh the burdens and risks of participation. Prospective subjects need protection when they are not capable of understanding the risks and burdens of participation (Wertheimer 2011: ch. 2). But they also need respect, and we do not respect people when we deny them the opportunity to participate when it is in their interest to do so.

Given that there is a tradition of research ethics that claims that participation should always be altruistic and, at its best, that participants should adopt the goals of the research as their own goals, it is not surprising that some IRB members will find it unseemly to introduce payment into the research equation (Jonas 1969). But such justifiable caution about payment does not warrant misconceiving and misapplying the concepts of coercion and undue influence. If, as in other contexts of life, people can reasonably regard the value of payment or other incentives as greater than the risks of engaging in some activity, be it ordinary employment or participation in research, then we do not protect subjects when we preclude their activity on grounds of coercion or undue influence or exploitation.

Related Topics

Chapter 16, "The Future of Informed Consent to Research: Reconceptualizing the Process," Paul Appelbaum
Chapter 23, "Incentives in Health: Ethical Considerations," Richard Ashcroft

Bibliography

Angell, M. (1997) "The Ethics of Clinical Research in the Third World," *New England Journal of Medicine* 337: 847–9.

Brody, B. (2001) "Making Informed Consent Meaningful," *IRB* 23 (5): 1–5.

CIOMS (2002) "International Ethical Guidelines for Biomedical Research Involving Human Subjects," The Council for International Organization of Medical Sciences, guideline 7. Available at: http://www.cioms.ch/publications/layout_guide2002.pdf (accessed July 18, 2014).

Common Rule (2009) 45 CFR Part 46.

Connor, E.M., Sperling, R.S., Gelber, R., Kiselev, P., Scott, G., O'Sullivan, M.J. et al. (1994) "Reduction of Maternal–Infant Transmission of Human Immunodeficiency Virus Type 1 with Zidovudine Treatment" [electronic version]. *New England Journal of Medicine* 331: 1173–80.

Elliott, C. (2008) "Guinea Pigging," *The New Yorker* January 7, 36–41.

Emanuel, E. (2007) "The Paradox of Exploitation," in J. Lavery, C. Grady, E.R. Wahl and E.J. Emanuel (eds.) *Issues in International Biomedical Research: A Casebook*, New York: Oxford University Press.

Emanuel, E., Wendler, D. and Grady, C. (2000) "What Makes Clinical Research Ethical?" *JAMA* 283: 2701–11.

Emanuel, E. et al. (eds.) (2003) *Ethical and Regulatory Aspects of Human Subjects Research*, Baltimore, MD: Johns Hopkins University Press.

Grant, R. and Sugarman, R. (2004) "Ethics in Human Subjects Research: Do Incentives Matter?" *Journal of Medicine and Philosophy* 29: 717–38.

Halpern, S.D., Karlawish, J.H., Casarett, D., Berlin, J.A. and Asch, D.A. (2004) "Empirical Assessment of Whether Moderate Payments are Undue or Unjust Inducements for Participation in Clinical Trials," *Archives of Internal Medicine* 164: 801–3.

Harris, J. (2005) "Scientific Research Is a Moral Duty," *Journal of Medical Ethics* 31: 242–7.

India Resource Center (2004) http://www.indiaresource.org/issues/globalization/2004/indianguineapigs.html (accessed July 11, 2014).

Jonas, H. (1969) "Philosophical Reflections on Experimenting with Human Subjects," *Daedalus* 98: 219–47.

Largent, E., Grady, C., Miller, F.G. and Wertheimer, A. (2012) "Misconceptions About Coercion and Undue Influence: Reflections on the Views of IRB Members," *Bioethics* 27: 500–7.

Lurie, P. and Wolfe, S. (1997) "Unethical trials of interventions to reduce perinatal transmission of the human immunodeficiency virus in developing countries," *New England Journal of Medicine* 33: 853–6.

Macklin, R. (1989) "The Paradoxical Case of Payment as Benefit to Research Subjects," *IRB* 11: 1–3.

Nussbaum, M. (1998) "Taking Money for Bodily Services," *Journal of Legal Studies* 27: 693–724.

NBC News (2012) http://investigations.nbcnews.com/_news/2012/03/04/10562883-in-india-oversight-lacking-in-outsourced-drug-trials (accessed July 11, 2014).

Office for Human Research Protections (OHRP) (2011) *IRB Guidebook*. Available at: http://www.hhs.gov/ohrp/archive/irb/irb_guidebook.htm (accessed July 11, 2014).

Piff, P., Stancato, D.M., Côté, S., Mendoza-Denton, R. and Keltner, D. (2012) "Higher Social Class Predicts Increased Unethical Behavior," *PNAS* 109: 4086–91.

Ramsey, S. and Scoggins, J. (2008) "Commentary: Practicing on the Tip of an Information Iceberg? Evidence of Underpublication of Registered Clinical Trials in Oncology," *The Oncologist* 13: 925–9.

Rosen, G. (2012) "Studying Drugs in All the Wrong People," *Scientific American Mind* September–October: 32–41.

Rothman, D. (2000) "The Shame of Medical Research," *The New York Review of Books*, November 30.
Shamoo A. and Resnik, D. (2006) "Strategies to Minimize Risks and Exploitation in Phase One Trials on Healthy Subjects," *American Journal of Bioethics* 6 (3): W1–13, w8.
The National Commission for the Protection of Human Subjects of Biomedical and Behavioral Research (1978) *The Belmont Report: Ethical Principles and Guidelines for the Protection of Human Subjects of Research* (DHEW Publication OS 78-0012). Washington, DC: Department of Health, Education, and Welfare. Available at: http://www.hhs.gov/ohrp/humansubjects/guidance/belmont.html (accessed July 23, 2014).
Wertheimer, A. (1987) *Coercion*, Princeton: Princeton University Press.
Wertheimer, A. (1996) *Exploitation*, Princeton: Princeton University Press.
Wertheimer, A. (2011) *Rethinking the Ethics of Clinical Research*, New York: Oxford University Press.
Wertheimer, A. and Miller, F. (2008) "Payment for Research Participation: A Coercive Offer?" *J Med Ethics* 34: 389–92.
Wilkinson, M. and Moore, A. (1997) "Inducements in Research," *Bioethics* 11: 373–89.

20

THE ETHICS OF BIOMEDICAL RESEARCH INVOLVING ANIMALS

Tom L. Beauchamp

Approximately 50–100 million vertebrate animals[1] are used, worldwide, in biomedical and behavioral experiments each year (House of Lords 2002; Taylor et al. 2008). The research occurs in universities, hospitals, laboratories, government facilities, and corporations. Animals are used to study disease and injury and to assess the risks posed by drugs, chemicals, pesticides, cosmetics, and the like. Some of the research produces useful generalizable knowledge for the treatment of human disease, injury, and discomfort, but much of it fails to yield medical applications and presents moral problems about scientific uses of animals.

Claims of human preeminence and just dominion over animals have been at work for centuries (Sorabji 1993). In the first book of the Bible, God is reported to have given humans such dominion (*Genesis* 1: 26; Regan 1986). Guided by such views, animals have often been treated as without moral or legal *status*, but many writers in ethics, scientists involved in animal research, and members of the public find themselves unsatisfied by these views about our uses of animals. When it comes to scientific research, many people are perplexed and undecided.

In some cases, though, people are not perplexed. We all tend to be angry in the face of abuses of companion animals in biomedical research. In 1965 an article appeared in *Sports Illustrated* about a dog stolen from a Pennsylvania home, later to die in a laboratory in a New York hospital (Phinizy 1965), and in 1966 a story in *Life* magazine (Silva and Wayman 1966) showed some seriously mistreated and dead dogs at a breeding facility for research animals. The ensuing public outcry from these stories galvanized the American public against such uses of "pets" in biomedical research, which eventuated in the 1966 *Laboratory Animal Welfare Act*. However, this legislation itself would show how confused and scattered our thoughts and actions have been, and no doubt remain, on problems of animal research. For at least 20 years after passage of the 1966 law, the U.S. Congress did virtually nothing to protect animals in research laboratories. The law functioned only to protect companion animals from being rounded up for or sold to research laboratories. It failed to affect how the animals were used once they were in the laboratories.

Our sympathies extend deeply to companion animals, but when we read almost identical reports about research animals who have never been companion animals, especially if they are of a despised species such as rats, these creatures are commonly framed as merely "animals." Companion animals are typically accorded more moral significance than are research animals, but can that view be morally justified? In the end, do we have a set of coherent views about research animals, or do most of us live in an incoherent world in which some animals are admired and adored friends; others are merely pests; and some just dumb beasts—but all of which may be research subjects?

I start this chapter with a short sketch of the history of human thought about animals and then turn to a recent case that has had an extraordinary impact on public policy in the United States and has reversed that country's public policy in one area.

Two Histories of Conceptions of Animals and Their Welfare

There are several largely independent histories of *animal research ethics*, a recently coined term. Various strands of history have focused on animal minds and animal welfare, and two such strands will be discussed here: (1) Moral and psychological theories, and (2) government codes, guidelines, and regulations.

The History of Moral and Psychological Theories

Many writers have been interested in questions about animal minds and animal ethics since ancient times. Cultural and philosophical diversity was extensive in the ancient world, and there was no one canonical view. The two most influential, which is not to say justified, perspectives on the use of animals descending from the ancient world to the modern were that (1) plants are for animals and animals are for use by humans, and (2) animals have minds driven by motives, but lack the rational souls possessed by humans (Sorabji 1993). These theories have had remarkable persistence.

Early modern philosophy saw some impressive work on the nature of animals, produced by, among others, René Descartes, Pierre Bayle, Francis Hutcheson, David Hume, and Immanuel Kant. They disagreed among themselves about the nature of non-human animal minds and about the moral importance of our treatment of animals, but here, for the first time, we find major philosophers thinking at a deep level about animal minds and, to a lesser extent, animal ethics.

Jeremy Bentham would become the most influential of these early modern philosophers on subsequent animal ethics literature. Bentham focused on the capacity of animals to experience pleasure, pain, and suffering—a capacity itself sufficient, he thought, to make animals morally important beings—just as these capacities make humans morally considerable. Bentham asked, "Is there any reason why we should be suffered to torment them [e.g., research animals]? Not any that I can see. Are there any why we should *not* be suffered to torment them? Yes, several." This reasoning underlies Bentham's famous rhetorical questions, "The question is not, Can they [nonhuman animals] *reason*? nor, Can they *talk*? but, Can they *suffer*?" (Bentham 1996: ch. 17, sec. 1).

Finally, Charles Darwin's theory of evolution and philosophical reflections on animal minds and their moral significance have been more influential in intellectual history than any figure before or since. In *The Descent of Man*, Darwin catalogued many similarities in mental ability between humans and apes, observing that "it is a significant fact, that the more the habits of any particular animal are studied by a naturalist, the more he ascribes to *reason* and the less to *unlearnt instincts*" (Darwin 1989: 107–10). He saw ample empirical evidence that many animals have powers of deliberation and decision making, excellent memories, fertile imaginations, and even moral emotions.

Darwin looked for similarities across multiple species. He pointed out that numerous levels of mental activity are shared by many species close to humans, from basic pain receptors to intentionality. He argued that the moral, physical, and mental qualities of humans evolved through processes similar to those that occur elsewhere in nature. The faculties of reason and speech are comparable in their evolutionary origin to snake fangs, shark fins, and eagles' feet. Moreover,

> The difference in mind between man and the higher animals, great as it is, certainly is one of degree and not of kind . . . If it could be proved that certain high mental powers, such as the formation of general concepts, self-consciousness, etc. were absolutely peculiar to man, which seems extremely doubtful, it is not improbable that these qualities are merely the incidental results of other highly advanced intellectual faculties . . . The half-art, half-instinct of language still bears the stamp of its gradual evolution.
>
> (Darwin 1989: 107–10)

Darwin's theory of evolution challenged the traditional idea that human beings have capacities that give them natural dominance over to the rest of the animal world. He thought we are but one species of rational creature.

The History of Government Codes, Guidelines, and Regulations

Dozens of editions of guidelines and principles of animal care and use for research animal facilities have been issued by governments in the last century or so. As this chapter was being written, the National Health and Medical Research Council of the Australian Government released its eighth edition of its code for the use of animals for scientific purposes, which presents an "ethical framework" whose principles obligate all researchers and teachers in Australia who use animals for scientific purposes (National Health and Medical Research Council 2013).

The history of concentrated attempts at animal welfare protections in the United States can be dated to the previously mentioned 1966 *Animal Welfare Act* legislation. However, the history in some other countries, notably the U.K. among western nations, is much older than either the U.S. or Australia. The British *Animal Welfare Act* 2006 is an Act of the Parliament of the U.K. that dates back to the *Protection of Animals Act* 1911, which it largely replaced. Even earlier, the *Cruelty to Animals Act* of 1876 was passed by Parliament, creating a licensing system for animal experimentation that amended the *Cruelty to Animals Act* of 1849. The U.K.'s history is one of the few truly rich histories of animal research laws and guidelines, and since 1951 significant laws and regulations have continued to be passed in the U.K. almost every decade.

In the U.S. it was not until 1985, when the U.S. Congress enacted the *Improved Standards for Laboratory Animals Act* (Public Law 99-198 1985), that a *major* stride was taken toward government-supported animal research guidelines. This Act came in response to scandals in the use of primates at esteemed research laboratories, one at the University of Pennsylvania and the other at the Institute of Behavioral Research in Maryland. In effect these laboratories had no rules of ethics in place and no knowledge of moral requirements of animal care. Physical treatment of animals was brutal, and behavioral pathologies such as self-injurious behavior were caused during the course of the research.

The 1985 law and subsequent regulations had a profound effect. Suddenly, formal committee review of animal research was a requirement. These review committees had to include non-scientist members, which exposed the work, to a limited extent, to public awareness. Investigators now had to explain, and sometimes defend—as never before—their pain-producing procedures and to reduce the number of animals involved, if possible. Most disturbing to some investigators were new requirements of providing "for a physical environment adequate to promote the psychological well-being of primates" (United States Code (USC), Title 7 § 2143, 2.a.B). This requirement to protect "psychological well-being" was immediately contested by research institutions as too onerous. Struggles over proper criteria of ethologically appropriate conditions and psychological wellbeing have continued from that time to the present (see the section below on "Moral Requirements of Psychological Wellbeing").

In the century-old history of government struggles with animal research guidelines, a key fact is that the responsibilities of research investigators put into effect by governments are matters of both legal and professional *obligations to animals*; they are not merely optional, charitable ideals. However, it would be wide of the mark to regard government guidelines and regulations as merely matters of history. To get a sense of how underdeveloped some of our moral frameworks remain still today, I turn to an uncommon and influential case of government policy that developed between 2011 and 2013.

A Landmark Case in Chimpanzee Research

This case originates in efforts by the U.S. National Institutes of Health (NIH) in 2010 to move 176 NIH-owned chimpanzees from semi-retirement as research subjects at the Alamogordo Primate Facility in New Mexico to a larger, private research facility that engages in invasive research. A public protest erupted over NIH's plan, which was criticized by many animal welfare advocates and by New Mexico Governor Bill Richardson as well as Jeff Bingaman and Tom Udall, the two U.S. Senators from New Mexico. Protesters were concerned about the welfare of chimpanzees in research, and issues were also raised about the risks associated with shipping chimpanzees because some had died in the course of previous transfers (Gray 2011). Virtually all interested parties raised questions about the need for chimpanzees in research, now and in the future. Because most (over 600 of the approximately 950) chimpanzees in U.S. research were owned or financially supported by NIH, its policies had the effect of determining how chimpanzees could be used in about 65 percent of the research population in the U.S.

The two New Mexico senators wrote a letter to NIH Director Francis Collins calling for critical scrutiny by the U.S. National Academy of Sciences of the necessity of chimpanzee research. The NIH then commissioned an Institute of Medicine (IOM) study of the problem (National Institutes of Health Statement on the Alamogordo Primate Facility Chimpanzees 2011). An IOM Committee was formed immediately, almost entirely composed of research scientists. It ultimately released its report in December 2011 (Committee on the Use of Chimpanzees in Biomedical and Behavioral Research 2011: 2).

This striking report surprised almost everyone. The Committee had been expected to endorse NIH's traditionally uncompromising claims of the necessity of animal research, but instead it recommended what are, from an historical perspective, quite demanding guidelines for federally funded research with animal subjects. The

Committee proposed three conditions that must be met for biomedical research on chimpanzees to be justified:

1. The knowledge gained must be necessary to advance the public's health.
2. There must be no other research model by which the knowledge could be obtained, and the research cannot be ethically performed on human subjects.
3. The animals used in the proposed research must be maintained either in ethologically appropriate physical and social environments or in natural habitats.

(Committee on the Use of Chimpanzees in Biomedical and Behavioral Research 2011: 4)

These *principles*, as the Committee designates them, form a framework in the report for ethically permissible use of chimpanzees in research.

These conclusions came as a surprise to most observers because *ethics* had never been an intended target of the investigation by either NIH or IOM. For weeks IOM resisted the idea that the Committee could even discuss the ethics of animal research. Such discussion had never occurred in a policy context at NIH (though conferences on ethics had been held there). However, this committee had a mind of its own and stated firmly that ethics is a significant consideration:

> The committee . . . recognizes that any assessment of necessity for using chimpanzees as an animal model in research raises ethical issues, and any analysis must take these ethical issues into account . . . For the committee, this ethical context is reflected in its assessment of when, if ever, the use of chimpanzees in biomedical research is necessary.
>
> (Committee on the Use of Chimpanzees in Biomedical and Behavioral Research 2011: 4)

The IOM had not taken the term "scientific necessity," in "scientific necessity for using chimpanzees," as a moral notion. The IOM thought the issue was only whether it is, in any given research situation, scientifically necessary to use chimpanzees to achieve desired research results. However, the Committee that IOM had appointed did not see the situation as free of moral considerations. It determined that the term "necessity" (as in "scientific necessity of using chimpanzees") should be analyzed as a necessary condition of *morally justified* use of chimpanzees in research; that is, scientific necessity was analyzed as a *morally necessary*—but *not a morally sufficient*—condition of justified scientific research involving chimpanzees. Put another way, it must be scientifically necessary to use this species to achieve valid scientific results, but this fact does not render the research morally justified because other conditions besides scientific necessity must be met (see the three principles above). What IOM and NIH had viewed as exclusively a scientific question thus became both a scientific and a moral question.

The Committee also recommended that research animals should be allowed to "acquiesce" to participation in research. Here the Committee is expressing its confidence that chimpanzees can act voluntarily to accept or to reject research procedures. The Committee did not conclude that chimpanzees can give an autonomous informed *consent*—an absurdly high-level task. It is revolutionary enough that the Committee judges that chimpanzees have cognitive capacities of voluntary agreement and refusal, not merely submission, fear, and the like. This conclusion acknowledges decision-making capacity, voluntariness, and moral status; it appears to exceed criteria of animal minds and ethics that the NIH had ever contemplated.

Finally, the Committee recommended that chimpanzees be maintained in "ethologically appropriate environments." This recommendation constitutes a demanding requirement in many research settings, requiring in effect that chimpanzees be housed under conditions fundamentally similar to the conditions under which the species is known to flourish—ideally their natural environments.

Unlike virtually all previous federal-level reports regarding the protection of research subjects, this report was immediately accepted as federal policy. The Director of NIH, Francis Collins, stated that "I have . . . decided to accept the IOM Committee recommendations. NIH is in the process of developing a complete plan for implementation of the IOM's guiding principles and criteria." Collins stated that chimpanzees, as our closest relatives, deserve "special consideration and respect" (National Institutes of Health, Office of the Director 2011). NIH had never previously taken a position even approximating this one, and had never before for ethical reasons phased out invasive research on any species, including dogs and cats. These facts alone make this report a landmark that turned NIH policy in a decidedly different direction. But this policy applies only to chimpanzees, not to other species.

In January 2013, a year after the committee submitted its report, an NIH Working Group appointed by Director Collins presented an independent evaluation of the IOM Committee's recommendations (Council of Councils (NIH) 2013). This report heavily supported the original IOM committee's recommendations, principles, and criteria. The Working Group determined that the need (or necessity) for chimpanzee subjects is effectively non-existent for contemporary research on human diseases. It recommended that NIH maintain a population of 50 animals in case an emergency need for chimpanzees should arise, but it also recommended a ban on breeding, which entails that the population would be gradually decreased to zero. As chimpanzees die off, even a small-sized research population will not be available. A later NIH statement endorsed the conclusions of the Working Group (National Institutes of Health 2013).

Animal Minds

The IOM Committee's conclusion that chimpanzees have cognitive capacities of voluntary decision-making, and Darwin's theory of evolution and animal minds, raise ethical and public policy issues as well as questions about the nature of animal minds, including the psychological complexity, cognitive gifts, and social lives of animals.

Close observers of animal behavior today agree that many animals have capacities to understand and have elaborate forms of social interaction and communication. Chimpanzees, for example, have a rich psychology of beliefs, intentional actions, cognitive understandings, structured social organization—and apparently self-awareness as well. Intelligence and adaptation in animal behavior, as explored by ethologists and psychologists, are often inexplicable without acknowledging that animals exhibit understanding, intention, thought, imaginativeness, and forms of communication. These animals therefore have at least some mental properties similar to those of humans.

However, scientists still understand much less about the inner lives of animals than they hope to learn. For example, we have difficulty understanding how to analyze *intention* and *choice* in animals. The behavioral and life sciences together with the philosophy of mind may shed only limited light on animal mental states, but the light increases every year as we learn more about how animals do what they do.

Moral Status

Many writers in animal ethics in the last 35 years have viewed the *moral status* of animals as the major philosophical moral problem of animal ethics. However, it is generally agreed today that many species of animals have some form of moral status. The critical questions are now about what *level* of status they have.

Over the course of human history, vulnerable groups of humans have been refused a significant social status in many countries. Slaves, women, minority groups, and others have been declared to lack some property relevant to their political, legal, or moral status and so have been declared to not qualify for full moral status; but these social norms have also been reconceived in many societies, even though the relevant properties of people in these groups had not changed at all. In this way, slaves, women, and minority groups came to have a full, or at least fuller, moral status in many cultures (Lindsay 2005).

Research animals may be poised for an analogous reconsideration of status, though most species still fail to satisfy reigning criteria of legal status, and confusion persists about their moral status. Traditionally the dominant perspective in animal research laboratories was that protections for research animals are not necessary because they do not have *interests* that carry moral significance, but this thesis is clearly mistaken. Animals certainly have interests. The term "interest" refers to that which is in an animal's interest—that is, what is to the animal's welfare advantage in a given circumstance. Research animals have welfare interests in liberty of action, not suffering physical and psychological harms, a social life, good health, and familiar and clean environments and housing. These interests are the basis of their moral status and of the obligations researchers have to treat animals appropriately, as expressed in the codes and regulations previously discussed.

The cutting edge issues about moral status today are about the level of moral status, the protections that must be provided at that level, and how many interests of animals must be protected. For example, one issue is whether primates must be given a natural habitat free of cages as a basic condition of research involvement. Even among persons who feel strongly that chimpanzees, monkeys, dogs, and even rats deserve moral protections in biomedical research, many regard the interests of these animals as far less significant than the interests of humans. These moral issues will occupy us for the remainder of this essay.

Moral Requirements of Psychological Wellbeing

I start with how animals experience psychological suffering and distress in research, including the semi-hidden suffering that results from maternal separation, captivity, cage confinement and other restraints, social isolation, handling and transportation, and sleep deprivation. Following the *Animal Welfare Act*'s standards for a physical environment sufficient to promote the "psychological well-being of primates" (Committee on Well-Being of Nonhuman Primates 1998), the U.S. Department of Agriculture regulations require use of indices of psychological well-being for primates (U.S. Department of Agriculture 1999). A similar view is endorsed by the American Psychological Association (APA) in its "Guidelines for Ethical Conduct in the Care and Use of Nonhuman Animals in Research" (American Psychological Association 2013).

However, as the APA forthrightly acknowledges in these guidelines, the Association does not attempt to define "psychological well-being" or to provide "specific guidelines for the maintenance of psychological well-being of research animals." It does not even analyze the meaning of "well-being." The reason, it says, is that "procedures that are appropriate for a particular species may not be for others." This default position is disappointing, though fairly typical of literature and guidelines on this subject. A persistent vagueness and absence of adequately specified guidelines has created a lack of understanding of what is ethically required, especially when it comes to the assessment of particular research protocols and housing standards.

Although criteria have been upgraded in recent years—as illustrated by the IOM chimpanzee case—most countries still lack an adequate body of protections of the psychological wellbeing of research animals. In only a few countries are there legal requirements that compel investigators to categorize the invasiveness of their proposed work as to pain, suffering, social deprivation, confinement, and overall social wellbeing.

The Justification of Human Uses of Animals

The single most difficult and the most intractable moral problem about biomedical research with animals is its *justification*. This problem is also the most important, the least carefully investigated, and the most ignored moral issue. When asked to justify their practices with, and beliefs about, the use of animal subjects, investigators have typically not provided a justification. Instead, they note that many examples of successful research show that animals are essential to achieving human health benefits and that many contributions have been made to biological and medical knowledge, even when no direct human medical welfare benefit occurred (cf. Council for the International Organizations of Medical Sciences 2012).

Many of the vaccines, medicines, and other products on the market have been tested on animals and approved by governments on the basis of this testing. However, little investigation has been devoted to the question "How much new knowledge stands to be gained, and does the value of this new knowledge *justify* the harms caused to the animals involved?" It is more assumed than demonstrated or argued that the potential knowledge is sufficient to justify the research. This response begs the critical questions and evades problems confronting an adequate answer to the question.

It becomes increasingly difficult to justify using animals in research as the likelihood of human benefits decreases, as risks of harm increase for animals, and as alternatives to the use of animals become available. Many justificatory appeals are made every week in animal research centers to investigators' conformity to professional ethics and government regulations as a source of justification, but these rules are virtually never themselves the subject of careful ethical scrutiny for adequacy. The IOM Chimpanzee report was a rare case of an exacting, analytical examination of the need to revise traditional rules, regulations, and assumptions. Members of this Committee accepted the fact that there is a possibility that animal research might be necessary and justified under some conditions in order to find a prophylactic vaccine for hepatitis C, but the Committee did not think that this possibility was sufficiently strong to recommend continuing to use chimpanzees (Committee on the Use of Chimpanzees in Biomedical and Behavioral Research 2011: 67). This example is particularly striking because committee members were divided on the scientific promise of the research, but even those who thought chimpanzee use might be justified in the future did not support or recommend new research at the present time.

Every scientific protocol requires a carefully reasoned justification, but there also are troubling problems about how to justify claims regarding what is necessary to medical progress. Despite the many medical success stories in the past, these successes may not be a good predictor of whether continued animal use in any given area of research still shows promise of creating human health benefits. It is widely believed that great discoveries about neurological disorders, heart and blood diseases, pulmonary diseases, infectious diseases, and cancer can now be made if and only if investigators are able to use animals. This claim could be correct; but the promise has to be demonstrated, as must the need for animal research rather than alternative research that does not use animals. When the IOM chimpanzee committee looked closely at claims about past examples of advances made in conquering disease by using research chimpanzees, it found that human subjects could have been ethically used as subjects in many cases and that alternative research models are often available. It appeared that better scientific data could often have been collected if chimpanzees were *not used*. Past examples had been a poor basis on which to justify new protocols with chimpanzees.

The likelihood of human benefits in the future is often either low or uncertain in animal research. Data suggest that the probabilities of a good medical product such as a drug that is approved and marketed resulting from studies *using humans* (starting with phase 1 studies) are somewhere around 8 percent (Wendler 2014). Former Health and Human Services Secretary Mike Leavitt reported that "Currently, nine out of ten experimental drugs fail in clinical studies because we cannot accurately predict how they will behave in people based on laboratory and animal studies" (Food and Drug Administration 2006). Because testing in humans occurs *after* promising animal research has been conducted, the probabilities of successful human medical applications in animal testing prior to use of humans is certainly decreased (even in primate studies), and will be below 1 percent in the use of some species and some forms of research.

There is virtually no way to know whether findings from animal research are applicable to humans until testing has occurred in humans. Interventions that are successful with animals are unsuccessful in many human trials because of high toxicity levels or inefficacy. It seems a prudent principle that the higher the probability of harm to both animals and humans and the lower the probability of health benefits, the more difficult it is to justify use of animals in research. However, practical implementation of such a principle is but a distant hope at the present time.

Committee Review to Control Pain, Suffering, and Distress

The dominant model in most countries of a procedural process to justify, as well as to approve or disapprove, animal research protocols is to establish review committees to examine the protocols to see if they can be improved in various ways, including by reducing or refining animal use. These committees—called Institutional Animal Care and Use Committees (IACUCs) in the U.S. and by different names in other countries—are mandated oversight committees intended to be impartial in their assessments (Whitney 1987). Public Health Service policy in the U.S. requires them for ongoing review of animal care and use, facilities inspection, review and approval or disapproval of research protocols, and the like. Committee review also considers whether immobilization for the animals is necessary and whether tumor burden in cancer research can be reduced. Universities, government facilities, and many corporations in the pharmaceutical, chemical, and cosmetics industries have such committees.

However, the objectives of these committees have proved difficult to achieve in many institutions. Different empirical assumptions are often made about the degree to which animals feel pain or suffer in research; about how to measure pain, distress, discomfort, and suffering; about whether an anesthetic, analgesic, or tranquilizer is adequate for the intended effect; and about whether the animal conceives the experience as agony or torment. In the scientific literature, some assert that animals have different forms of pain reception and many cannot anticipate or remember pain, and therefore suffer less than humans. A contrasting view is that animals suffer more, not less, because they have less understanding of the origin, nature, and meaning of pain. An animal may be a captive of the momentary experience of pain and without the capacity to deal with danger, injury, and the like (Akhtar 2011; Dresser 1988, 1990; Graham 2002).

Review committees are generally given extensive data about proposed *scientific* investigations. The data show intricate planning, probing scientific hypotheses, and familiarity with the relevant literature. Rarely are the committees given comparable detail about *ethics* problems, arguments, and justification issues. Yet, for an adequate ethics review, the ethical problems and reasoning would have to be spelled out, just as the scientific problems and reasoning must be presented. The absence of searching moral examination by these committees has led to widespread suspicion about the quality and worth of the committees' deliberations and conclusions. Many members of these committees would say that framing the issues in this way holds researchers to an unrealistically high ethical standard, but these committees are *ethics* committees, not *scientific* committees, so ethical reasoning needs to be taken with great seriousness.

Should the Ethics of Research with Animals Follow the Example of the Ethics of Research with Humans?

A perspective that may help handle some problems raised in the various sections above is to ask whether animal research ethics should be modeled on human research ethics. Their histories are very different, with markedly dissimilar assumptions about acceptable risk, proper facilities, permission giving, and the like. But why should animal research subjects be governed by rules so unlike those governing human research? An attempt at modeling animal research ethics on human research ethics has never, to my knowledge, been attempted in any country, but as an ideal it makes a great deal of sense. If the two pillars of research ethics (human and non-human) are (1) protection from harm and (2) ethical oversight by committee review, then the human model, which is far more protective of subjects, would seem a good starting model for animal research.

As things now stand, animal subjects have significantly more pain and suffering visited on them than do human research subjects, and pain can also be substantially increased in level with animal subjects far beyond a point that we would allow with human subjects. But human interests and animal interests are relevantly similar in that their welfare is contingent on not being constrained and coerced, not being deprived of basic needs, not experiencing pain and terror, etc. Why, then, are animal interests not treated with similar respect and concern to human interests?

Federal regulations in the U.S. have stringent rules governing use of human research subjects who do not have the ability to consent (for example, children), but no comparable regulations exist for animals. It would be possible to restructure regulations for animal research so that they closely follow regulations for human research with those unable to consent, especially regarding risk of harm. For animals, as for humans, a line of unacceptable risk could be drawn at the point where biomedical research is expected to exceed a threshold or upper limit of pain, suffering, anxiety, fear, and distress. In research with human subjects, it is conventional to insist on thresholds of risk, pain, and discomfort. For such a threshold to be meaningful in research involving animals, careful guidelines would have to be prepared for investigators and review committees, including a grading of research procedures as to their noxious, aversive, and painful properties.

The argument against a firm threshold in our use of animals is that any criterion proposed will be too restrictive and will bring productive research on injury, disease, toxic agents, etc. to a halt. In the end, however, the main problem is less *whether* we should require a threshold in research with animals (it seems clear that we should) than *how and where* to draw the threshold line. The threshold may need to be drawn in different places for different species, but having no threshold at all seems more a case of moral blindness than a morally justified approach.

Finally, human research subjects who cannot give permission for involvement in research not designed to benefit them are heavily protected by mechanisms of informed consent given by parents, guardians, or family members. Requirements of surrogate consent are universally accepted in human research. Animal research could be similarly structured using guardian consent where impartial individuals are charged, as guardians, with protecting the interests of the animals.

Conclusion

We know from excellent data that if human subjects could be substituted for animal subjects in biomedical research, results would be significantly improved. But the painful, invasive, and often lethal character of testing in animal research has long been assessed as presenting insurmountable moral problems for the use of human subjects. The burden of this essay has been to show that, despite scientific and moral advances in recent years, traditional systems that place enormous burdens on research animals are morally flawed and still in need of watchful reform.

Related Topic

Chapter 14, "Biomedical Research Ethics: Landmark Cases, Scandals, and Conceptual Shifts," Jonathan D. Moreno and Dominic Sisti

Note

1 In this chapter the term "animals" refers exclusively to non-human vertebrates, but no assumption is made that questions of research involving invertebrates do not deserve ethical analysis.

References

Akhtar, S. (2011) "Animal Pain and Welfare: Can Pain Sometimes Be Worse for Them Than for Us?" in T.L. Beauchamp and R.G. Frey (eds.) *The Oxford Handbook of Animal Ethics*, New York: Oxford University Press, pp. 495–518.

American Psychological Association (APA), Committee on Animal Research and Ethics (2013) "Guidelines for Ethical Conduct in the Care and Use of Nonhuman Animals in Research," Section 3. Available at: http://www.apa.org/science/leadership/care/guidelines.aspx (accessed July 29, 2013).

Bentham, J. (1996) *An Introduction to the Principles of Morals and Legislation*, J.H. Burns and H.L.A. Hart (eds.), Oxford: Oxford University Press.

Committee on the Use of Chimpanzees in Biomedical and Behavioral Research, Institute of Medicine (2011) *Chimpanzees in Biomedical and Behavioral Research: Assessing the Necessity*, Washington, DC: National Academies Press ("IOM Report").

Committee on Well-Being of Nonhuman Primates, Institute for Laboratory Animal Research, Commission on Life Sciences, National Research Council (1998) *The Psychological Well-Being of Nonhuman Primates*, Washington, DC: National Academies Press. Available at: www.nap.edu/openbook.php?record_id=4909&page=R1 (accessed August 3, 2013).

Council of Councils (NIH), Council of Councils Working Group on the Use of Chimpanzees in NIH-Supported Research (2013) *Report*. January 22, 2013. Available at: dpcpsi.nih.gov/council/pdf/FNL_Report_WG_Chimpanzees.pdf (accessed July 28, 2013).

Council for the International Organization of Medical Sciences (2012) *International Guiding Principles for Biomedical Research Involving Animals*, December. Available at: http://www.cioms.ch/index.php/12-newsflash/227-cioms-and-iclas-release-the-new-international-guiding-principles-for-biomedical-research-involving-animals, http://ora.msu.edu/ICLAS/index.html (accessed August 3, 2013).

Darwin, C. (1989) "The Descent of Man," in T.L. Beauchamp, J. Feinberg and J.M. Smith (eds.) *Philosophy and the Human Condition*, 2nd edition, Englewood Cliffs, NJ: Prentice-Hall, pp. 107–10.

Dresser, R. (1988) "Assessing Harm and Justification in Animal Research: Federal Policy Opens the Laboratory Door," *Rutgers Law Review* 40: 723–95.

Dresser, R. (1990) "Review Standards for Animal Research: A Closer Look," *ILAR News* 32 (4): 2–7.

Food and Drug Administration (2006) "FDA Issues Advice to Make Earliest Stages of Clinical Drug Development More Efficient," News Release, January 12, 2006. Available at: http://www.fda.gov/NewsEvents/Newsroom/PressAnnouncements/2006/ucm108576.htm (accessed July 31, 2013).

Graham, K. (2002). "A Study of Three IACUCs and Their Views of Scientific Merit and Alternatives," *Journal of Applied Animal Welfare Science* 5: 75–81.

Gray, K.L. (2011) "OSU Chimps at Home in Sanctuary," *Columbus Dispatch*, June 5. Available at: http://dispatch.com/content/stories/local/2011/06/05/osu-chimps-at-home-in-sanctuary.html (accessed December 30, 2011).

House of Lords (UK) (2002) "Animals in Scientific Procedures," Session 2001–02, Select Committee on Animals in Scientific Procedures. Available at: http://www.publications.parliament.uk/pa/ld200102/ldselect/ldanimal/150/150.pdf (accessed July 31, 2013).

Lindsay, R.A. (2005) "Slaves, Embryos, and Nonhuman Animals: Moral Status and the Limitations of Common Morality Theory," *Kennedy Institute of Ethics Journal* 15: 323–46.

National Health and Medical Research Council (2013) *Australian Code for the Care and Use of Animals for Scientific Purposes*, 8th edition, Canberra: National Health and Medical Research Council, July. Available at: http://www.nhmrc.gov.au/_files_nhmrc/publications/attachments/ea28_animal_code_130724.pdf (accessed July 25, 2013).

National Institutes of Health (2013) Announcement of Agency Decision: Recommendations on the Use of Chimpanzees in NIH-Supported Research. Available at: dpcpsi.nih.gov/council/pdf/NIHresponse_to_Council_of_Councils_recommendations_62513.pdf (accessed July 28, 2013).

National Institutes of Health, Office of the Director (2011) "Statement by NIH Director Dr. Francis Collins on the Institute of Medicine Report Addressing the Scientific Need for the Use of Chimpanzees in Research," Thursday, December 15, 2011. Available at: http://www.nih.gov/news/health/dec2011/od-15.htm (accessed December 15, 2011).

National Institutes of Health Statement on the Alamogordo Primate Facility Chimpanzees (2011) January 4. Available at: http://grants.nih.gov/grants/policy/air/nih_alamogordo_statement_20110104.htm (accessed January 9, 2012).

Phinizy, C. (1965) "The Lost Pets that Stray to the Labs," *Sports Illustrated*, November 29, 1965. Available at: SI Vault, sportsillustrated.cnn.com/vault/article/magazine/MAG1077956/index.htm (accessed July 30, 2013).

Public Law 99-198 (1985) *Food Security Act of 1985, Subtitle F—Animal Welfare* (*The Improved Standards for Laboratory Animals Act*). December 23. Available at: http://awic.nal.usda.gov/public-law-99-198-food-security-act-1985-subtitle-f-animal-welfare (accessed July 31, 2013).

Regan, T. (ed.) (1986) *Animal Sacrifices: Religious Perspectives on the Use of Animals in Science*, Philadelphia: Temple University Press.

Silva, M. and Wayman, S. (1966) "Concentration Camps for Dogs," *Life* 60 (February 4): 22–9. Available at: books.google.com/books?id=JkwEAAAAMBAJ&pg=PA22&lpg=PA22&dq=life+magazine+concentr

ation+camp+for+dogs&source=bl&ots=i_T7ivGtnV&sig=q5ynlTa6Pa7TPJzDONS7OFWKwiA&hl=en&sa=X&ei=5ABAT93eIeOG0QGlvf3VBw&ved=0CDAQ6AEwAQ#v=onepage&q&f=false (accessed February 18, 2012).

Sorabji, R. (1993) *Animal Minds and Human Morals: The Origins of the Western Debate*, Ithaca, NY: Cornell University Press.

Taylor, K., Gordon, N., Langley, G. and Higgins, W. (2008) "Estimates for Worldwide Laboratory Animal Use in 2005," *Alternatives to Laboratory Animals* 36: 327–42.

United States Code (USC), Title 7 § 2143 (2013) "Standards and Certification Process for Humane Handling, Care, Treatment, and Transportation of Animals." Available at: http://www.law.cornell.edu/uscode/text/7/2143 (accessed July 31, 2013).

United States Department of Agriculture (1999) Animal and Plant Health Inspection Service, Animal Care, "Final Report on Environment Enhancement to Promote the Psychological Well-Being of Nonhuman Primates," Riverdale, MD, July 15. Available at http://www.nal.usda.gov/awic/enrichment/Enviromental_Enhancement_NonHuman_Primates.htm (accessed July 31, 2013).

Wendler, D. (2014) "Should Protections for Research with Humans Who Cannot Consent Apply to Research with Nonhuman Primates?" *Theoretical Medicine and Bioethics*. Forthcoming.

Whitney, R.A. Jr. (1987) "Animal Care and Use Committees: History and Current National Policies in the United States," *Laboratory Animal Science* 37 (spec. suppl. January): 18–21.

Part V

AUTONOMY AND AGENCY

The concept of autonomy has played a central role in contemporary bioethics. It is not the only important moral principle relevant to bioethical debates—notions of beneficence, harm prevention, justice, solidarity, and human rights also play significant roles—but autonomy has arguably been the most salient value across a wide spectrum of bioethical debates, including the foundations of the physician–patient relationship, the ethics of reproduction, research on human subjects, organ transplantation, public health, and so on.

At its Greek linguistic root, autonomy refers to self-government (auto-nomos) or the ability to direct one's actions and life according to one's own values; it thus taps into deep wellsprings of ethical and political thought in both the Western and Eastern traditions. Notwithstanding the great value we all place on individual choice and self-determination, bioethical controversies are often driven by tensions between autonomy and other important values. Within the physician–patient relationship, the patient's autonomous decision-making (e.g., a refusal of treatment) may come into conflict with the physician's obligation to advance her patient's health. In the reproductive arena a couple's autonomous choices (e.g., to determine the sex of their offspring) can on occasion pose a threat to the values of physicians; conversely, sometimes the objectives and routines of reproductive specialists can undermine the autonomy of patients, leaving them with the impression that they "have no choice" but to continue trying to conceive, no matter what the cost in money and/or emotional turmoil. And in the area of public health, autonomous choices (e.g., to avoid vaccination or evacuation) can come into sharp conflicts with communal values of health and safety. How should such conflicts be thought about and resolved?

This section presents several tightly integrated reflections on the theme of autonomy. We begin with Catriona Mackenzie's provision of a helpful analytical framework depicting various competing conceptions of autonomy. In contrast to those who would conceive of autonomy somewhat narrowly—e.g., as restricted to the capacity to make a reasonable choice in a given situation, or to be free of external constraints or coercion—Mackenzie argues that an adequately robust conception of autonomy requires a social context sufficiently endowed with opportunities and the conditions of dignity and self-respect. In other words, in conformity with the overall goal of this volume, she connects autonomy with social justice.

Within the context of the physician–patient relationship, autonomy figures prominently in debates about decision-making capacity or competence. We all agree that autonomous patients should be able to make decisions, but who should count as an autonomous patient? What about children, adolescents, adults institutionalized with a mental disability, or just your everyday confused, anxious, scared and ill-informed patient facing a difficult and risky decision? Jessica Berg and Katherine Shaw Makielski provide both an account of the constituent elements of decision-making capacity/competency and an assessment of the various methods of ascertaining and making judgments of capacity bearing on particular patients. The major focus of their discussion is the tension between respecting patients' autonomy and protecting them from harm.

We often think of autonomous decisions as being entirely self-directed, free from external influences. This is a misleading picture. We live and make decisions within a thick social context, pushed and pulled this way and that by causes and reasons offered up by people and institutional forces within our social environment. Suppose we would like to change our health-related behavior—e.g., with regard to smoking, obesity, avoiding reproduction, accepting vaccination for human papilloma virus (HPV), etc.—but need some additional motivation or reinforcement in order to do what we wish to do. Would it be autonomy-enhancing or autonomy-restricting to offer us incentives of various kinds in order to bring about better states of health? Richard Ashcroft provides a nuanced analysis of this problem, focusing on the sorts of incentives that might be offered, their psychological impacts, and a critical assessment of the reasons often adduced for opposing resort to incentives.

Autonomy also figures prominently in discussions of privacy in the clinical, research, and public health contexts. There are many powerful rationales for the importance of privacy regarding health information, including protection from harm and social stigma, the fostering of trust, and the advancement of public health goals. Alan Rubel contends that the most important defense of privacy rests upon the value of autonomy. Even in those cases where violating our privacy might redound to our personal benefit, Rubel claims that autonomy—i.e., the ability to decide on our own with whom to share our health information—directs us to respect individuals' privacy. Rubel concedes, however, that respect for the privacy of medical information need not always trump other important concerns, such as public health.

James Childress wraps up this section with a careful discussion of tensions between civil liberties, grounded for the most part in the value of autonomy, and public health concerns. While some commentators tend to stress the conflicts between civil liberties and public health, Childress contends that these two sets of values operate for the most part in harmony—i.e., that respecting the autonomy and civil liberties of people will most often redound to the public's trust of medical authorities and thus to the enhancement of the public's health. Although he argues forcefully for a presumption in favor of respecting individuals' civil liberties in public health controversies, Childress concedes that this presumption can be rebutted under certain carefully circumscribed circumstances. Much of his subsequent analysis is addressed to the sorts of particular circumstances that might justify overriding someone's civil liberties, and suggesting ways that advancing the goals of public health might actually be achieved without resort to such violations. In this connection, Childress provides a carefully nuanced discussion of incentives and "nudges" that meshes in interesting ways with the previous reflections of Ashcroft and Rubel.

21
AUTONOMY

Catriona Mackenzie

Introduction

In bioethics, the principle of respect for autonomy is widely understood as the principle that health care professionals have an obligation to respect patients' autonomous choices and decisions about their own health care. Respect for autonomy is a core principle of bioethics, underpinning requirements of informed consent to medical treatment and participation in medical research. It is also of central concern in a number of other areas in bioethics, such as in debates about reproductive choice and end of life decision-making.

Autonomy literally means self-rule or self-governance, reflecting its derivation from the ancient Greek words *autos* (self) and *nomos* (law). In its original usage, the concept was used to refer to the right of sovereign political states to be self-governing. Although this usage still remains, in the modern era the concept has been extended to refer to the authority of individual persons to make decisions of practical importance to their lives and to determine the direction of their lives in accordance with their beliefs, principles, and values. In bioethics, it is this concept of personal or individual autonomy that underwrites the principle of respect for autonomy.

Despite widespread agreement amongst bioethicists about the importance of autonomy, there is considerable disagreement about how the concept and the principle of respect for autonomy should be interpreted. This disagreement reflects, to some extent, two distinct historical influences on contemporary conceptions of autonomy: J.S. Mill's liberalism, which links autonomy to notions of individual self-expression and liberty; and Kant's notion of autonomy as rational self-governance guided by universal moral principles (for discussion, see e.g., O'Neill 2002).

This chapter discusses four different interpretations, or conceptions of autonomy: decisional, conscientious, libertarian, and relational. Each provides a different account of what personal autonomy means, of the conditions that must be met for a person or decision to be considered autonomous, and of the permissions and obligations that follow from the principle of respect for autonomy.

Decisional conceptions understand autonomy as the capacity to make informed, voluntary decisions about health care choices, such as whether to accept or refuse a specific treatment or to participate in a clinical trial. Decisional conceptions thus emphasize two primary conditions for autonomous choice: patient or subject understanding; and voluntariness, or absence of external or internal controlling influences. Respect for autonomy, on this view, gives rise to negative obligations not to unduly influence patients' decisions and positive obligations to ensure patients' decisions are sufficiently informed.

Conscientious conceptions understand autonomy as fidelity to the goals, standards, norms, or principles to which a person is committed and by which she guides her conduct. Conscientious autonomy draws attention to patients' responsibility to themselves and accountability to others, including health professionals, for their ongoing health care practice. Conscientious autonomy interprets the principle of respect for autonomy as an obligation on the part of health care practitioners to foster patients' capacities for conscientious health care management.

Libertarian conceptions equate autonomy with negative liberty; that is, the right to freedom from interference by other persons or the state in one's personal life. Libertarians claim that the principle of respect for autonomy entails obligations to maximize the scope of individual choice and minimize social interference with individuals' choices. In bioethics, libertarian conceptions are particularly influential in debates concerning reproductive and genetic technologies, physical and cognitive enhancement, contested surgical interventions, and markets in organs and tissue.

Relational autonomy is an "umbrella term" (Mackenzie and Stoljar 2000: 4), referring to a cluster of theories of autonomy motivated by feminist concerns about the impacts of oppression and social injustice on women's (and men's) opportunities to lead self-governing lives. While relational conceptions generally understand autonomy as the capacity for competent self-governance and authentic critical self-reflection, their distinguishing feature is that they seek to analyze the relational, social, and political dimensions of autonomy. Relational autonomy theory's focus on the relevance of issues of social justice for autonomy is a salutary counter in many arenas of bioethical debate to the dominance of libertarian autonomy.

The next section provides an account of decisional autonomy and discusses three criticisms of this account, including from the perspective of conscientious and relational autonomy. The following section discusses libertarian autonomy and its limitations. The final section summarizes the distinctive contribution of relational autonomy and its relevance for bioethics.

Decisional Autonomy

In bioethics, the most influential account of decisional autonomy is that of Tom Beauchamp and James Childress (2012). Beauchamp and Childress equate autonomy with informed, voluntary, and competent decision-making. Their account links autonomy closely to legal competence and to informed consent. To count as autonomous, in their view, an action or choice must satisfy three conditions. First, it must be intentional, i.e., planned rather than accidental. Second, the person must be able to understand the particular decision in question. This requires that the person has the requisite competence to understand and make the decision, has sufficient information about the nature of the decision and its import, can give reasons for her decision, and is able to communicate it effectively to others. Third, the person must make the decision voluntarily, that is, not be subject to undue external constraints or controlling influences, such as coercion and manipulation, or to overpowering internal forces, such as addiction, or mental illness.

Beauchamp and Childress stress that both understanding and voluntariness are matters of degree. Their account stipulates that, for a decision to be autonomous, the person must have adequate rather than complete understanding, and not be subject to substantial controlling influences. It follows from this account that the obligations involved in respecting autonomy are of two kinds: negative obligations to refrain from exerting undue influence over another person's actions or choices; and positive obligations to foster the person's capacities for autonomous choice, for example, by taking steps to ensure that the person has sufficient information, is given sufficient assistance (if required) to understand the decision in question, and that the decision is genuinely voluntary.

Decisional accounts of autonomy focus on local as distinct from global autonomy (for discussion, see e.g., Dworkin 1988). To exercise local autonomy is to be autonomous with respect to a particular action, choice, or decision. To exercise global autonomy is to be an autonomous person or to lead an autonomous life. An autonomous person might, temporarily, not be capable of locally autonomous choice, due to severe pain or incapacitating illness. Conversely, a person who is unable to lead an autonomous life, whether due to external constraints or impaired capacity, might nevertheless be able to make locally autonomous decisions, such as whether to accept or refuse treatment.

Beauchamp and Childress claim that decisional autonomy, because it is focused on local autonomy and does not stipulate overly stringent conditions for a decision to count as autonomous, is both maximally inclusive and provides the most appropriate account of autonomy for health care contexts. Their presumption is that most people are able to exercise decisional autonomy in their everyday lives, and that this should also be the default presumption in health care and research contexts, except in cases where patients or research subjects fail to meet the threshold for legal competence. Nevertheless, they acknowledge that there are a number of features of health care contexts that pose challenges for autonomous decision-making. These include patient vulnerability due to pain, illness, and fear; difficulties experienced by some patients in understanding diagnoses and assessing risks, benefits, and probabilities; and differences between health care professionals and patients or research subjects in social power, knowledge, levels of education and professional status, or arising from factors such as age, race, gender, disability, or cultural background. The principle of respect for autonomy imposes ethical obligations on health care professionals and researchers to be attentive to these factors in order to ensure that the conditions are in place for patients or research subjects to make informed and voluntary choices.

The benefit of this inclusive approach to autonomy is that it provides patients and research subjects with important protections against unwarranted medical paternalism, and coercive or manipulative attempts by others (e.g., family members, health care professionals, medical researchers) to influence their decisions. However, critics have questioned whether decisional autonomy does actually provide an adequate account of autonomy for health care contexts, for several reasons. First, decisional theorists of autonomy err in equating autonomy with informed choice; second, this conception does not take sufficient account of social constraints on global autonomy and the effects of these constraints on local autonomy and individual choice; third, an exclusive focus on moments of decision-making overlooks the importance of autonomy in many areas of ongoing health care practice and misrepresents what is involved in exercising autonomy in such contexts.

Beauchamp and Childress provide a nuanced account of the conditions for informed choice. However, there is an important difference between informed choice and autonomy. Two widely accepted conditions for autonomy that distinguish it from informed choice are competent critical reflection and authenticity (for a summary, see e.g., Christman 2009). The critical reflection condition requires that the person in question has competently and critically reflected on the beliefs, desires, values, standards, and commitments guiding her choice; the authenticity condition requires that as a result of such reflection, she regards these aspects of her cognitive and motivational structure as authentically "her own," rather than, for example, uncritically adopted due to her upbringing or socialization.

Beauchamp and Childress reject both requirements as overly onerous and restrictive. Their argument focuses on the influential "hierarchical" theories of Gerald Dworkin (1988) and Harry Frankfurt (1988), which characterize critical reflection as the capacity for second-order reflection on one's first-order preferences, values, or commitments. These count as authentically one's own if the person endorses them in light of such reflection. However, if upon reflection a person feels alienated from her preferences, values, or commitments, she is not autonomous with respect to them. Beauchamp and Childress argue that second-order reflection is not sufficient to secure autonomy because such reflection can sometimes be distorted by overpowering internal forces, such as addictions, and by powerful external influences, such as oppressive socialization. Hierarchical theories therefore lack a plausible account of the difference between competent and distorted forms of critical reflection.

Beauchamp and Childress also reject the authenticity condition on the ground that it seems to require persons to exhibit overly stable motivational and volitional patterns, making it difficult to distinguish failures of autonomy from genuine changes of heart or mind. This condition seems to suggest, for example, that a terminally ill patient, who reverses an earlier decision not to accept highly invasive treatment, is being inauthentic and hence non-autonomous. For this reason, the authenticity requirement "narrows the scope of actions protected by a principle of respect for autonomy" (2012: 103).

These and other objections to hierarchical theories have been extensively discussed in the literature (for a summary, see e.g., Mackenzie and Stoljar 2000). However, these objections do not provide sufficient reason for rejecting the critical reflection and authenticity conditions. In the final section, I discuss alternative accounts of both conditions. Suffice to say here that although it may be difficult to distinguish competent from distorted reflection, and to discern the extent to which a person's decision is fully "her own," health professionals are often called upon to make such judgments. For this reason, both conditions are important.

The second criticism of decisional autonomy is that a focus on local autonomy is overly narrow and does not take sufficient account of the historical and social context of individual decisions, and the effects of social oppression on global autonomy. John Christman's (2009) "historical" theory of autonomy helps to explain this problem. Like relational theories of autonomy, Christman's theory is motivated by the intuition that a person whose endorsement of her current values or preferences is the result of manipulation, oppressive upbringing or environment, or distorted reflection, is not autonomous. His theory highlights the importance of accounting for the historical and social processes by which a person acquired her guiding preferences and values, or came to make a particular decision. Without attending to these processes, he argues, it is often difficult to determine whether or not a particular choice is autonomous.

For example, it would be difficult to determine whether an older person has autonomously chosen to go into a nursing home or whether she has been coerced or manipulated into that decision by family members or health professionals, without some understanding of her personal history, her interests and orienting values, and the nature of her relationships with her family (see e.g., Lindemann Nelson 2001). A further important factor is her emotional attitude to the decision itself or the process by which it was reached. Does she feel distressed, angry, resigned, depressed, or optimistic? And do these emotions persist over time? Christman proposes that a decision counts as autonomous if, in light of sustained reflection upon the decision and the historical process leading up to it, the person would accept the decision without feelings of resistance, rejection, or alienation. Acceptance, or non-alienation, indicates that the decision expresses or is consistent with the person's long-standing practical identity (her self-conception and orienting values), whereas emotions such as anger or depression in the wake of a decision, if sustained over time, are indicative of alienation and hence a decision that is not autonomous.

Decisional theorists such as Beauchamp and Childress are sensitive to the kinds of concerns raised by this example. They acknowledge that the broader context of a decision needs to be taken into account in assessing whether or not it is autonomous, even though the primary focus of their account is the conditions under which specific decisions count as autonomous. They also acknowledge that emotional pressure, manipulation, and coercion are external threats that may undermine autonomous decision-making. And the most recent version of their theory incorporates some of the insights of relational autonomy concerning the importance of social support for autonomous decision-making. Nevertheless, from the perspective of theorists of relational autonomy their theory is still limited in the extent to which it takes account of the effects of social oppression on personal autonomy.

Taking these effects into account requires expanding our understanding of the internal constraints on autonomy, beyond addiction and mental illness, to include the effects of internalized oppression, as I discuss in the final section below. As Susan Sherwin (1998) has argued, it also requires expanding our understanding of the external constraints on autonomy beyond coercion and manipulation to include social and political restrictions on personal liberty, limited opportunities, poverty, and social oppression. Sherwin also urges the importance of considering the impact of social policies, such as welfare or health policies, on the choices available to people, and hence on their local and global autonomy. In relation to the nursing home example, such an expanded analysis would require us to consider whether the lack of affordable, socially supported alternatives, such as regular home visits by a community nurse, is a social injustice that has constrained the older person's global autonomy and her ability to make a locally autonomous decision to remain in her home. Sherwin thus highlights one of the central motivations of relational autonomy, which is to develop a conception of autonomy that is attentive to issues of social justice.

The third criticism, developed by Rebecca Kukla (2005), rejects Beauchamp and Childress' focus on "punctate decisions" and their understanding of autonomy as informed, voluntary, decision-making. Using the example of prenatal care as an illustration, Kukla points out that a major part of effective health care delivery involves forms of health care practice in which patients undertake ongoing self-management in collaboration with health care professionals. To be effective, these practices require that patients exercise autonomy by taking responsibility for diligently monitoring their own health care and holding themselves accountable for doing so to the health care professionals who care for them. These practices cannot be understood, however, as a series of discrete choices or decisions, and for this reason decisional autonomy is an inadequate model of autonomy for many health care contexts.

Drawing on a Kantian conception of autonomy as being bound by commitment to rational norms or principles, Kukla (2005: 39) proposes an alternative notion of conscientious autonomy. Conscientious autonomy "is manifested in actions that express fidelity to goals, principles, values or other normative measures to which the agent is responsibly committed." In exercising conscientious autonomy, patients will often defer to and trust in the authority and judgment of health care professionals, but this is quite different from merely complying with doctors' orders. Conscientious autonomy requires capacities to critically reflect on and articulate the reasons for one's commitments; take responsibility for one's ongoing health care practices; and exercise judgment about when deference and trust in medical authority is appropriate and when it is not. On the basis of this account of autonomy, Kukla suggests that the principle of respect for autonomy should be understood not as a matter of respecting patients' autonomous choices, but rather as an obligation on the part of health care practitioners to foster patients' capacities for conscientious health care management.

The criticisms I have discussed in this section show that while decisional conceptions of autonomy provide a nuanced account of the requirements for informed choice in medical and research contexts, the concepts of informed choice and autonomy, though related, are not equivalent.

Libertarian Autonomy

Libertarian conceptions equate personal autonomy with negative liberty. Libertarian theorists hold that to be autonomous is to be free from unwarranted external interference by other persons or the state with respect to important decisions about one's life (for classic statements of this view in political philosophy, see e.g., Nozick 1974; in bioethics, see e.g., Englehardt 1986). Libertarian conceptions of autonomy are particularly influential in Anglo-American bioethics, especially in debates about contested reproductive and genetic technologies, such as sex selection, cloning or enhancement technologies (Harris 1998; Agar 1998); markets in organs and tissue (Fabre 2006; Radcliffe-Richards 2007; Taylor 2002); and contested surgical interventions, such as cosmetic surgery or demand limb amputation (Bayne and Levy 2005). For example, bioethicists who support individuals' rights to select the sex or to enhance the characteristics of their offspring, or to sell organs, such as single kidneys, or reproductive tissue, usually support these positions on the basis of libertarian autonomy.

Libertarian conceptions are underpinned by several overlapping philosophical justifications. The first is the liberal neutrality thesis. This is the view that in a pluralist society, there is no non-controversial basis for making normative judgments about how people should lead their lives or what values ought to guide their choices. Each individual therefore has a right to live her life as she chooses and to be regarded as the best judge of what is in her interests. The role of the state, on this view, is to secure the social, political, and economic conditions to enable individuals to lead lives of their own choosing. However, the state has no business promoting or supporting particular values or imposing unnecessary restrictions on people's choices.

Second, libertarians regard the main threat to autonomy as coercive or paternalistic interference by others or the state. Such interference can only be justified by Mill's (1962 [1859]) harm principle: the principle that a person's liberty may only justifiably be restricted if the exercise of their liberty threatens to cause harm to others, where harm usually means direct physical harm. Third, libertarians regard freedom of choice as central to autonomy, where choice is understood as satisfaction of a person's subjective preferences, no matter how arbitrary, prejudiced, manipulated, or self-destructive these might be in the eyes of others. On the basis of these justifications, libertarians hold that personal autonomy is best promoted by maximizing the range of choices available to individuals and minimizing regulatory and other forms of constraint on individual choice. Respect for another's autonomy involves refraining from interference with that person's choices, unless those choices threaten to cause harm to others.

The libertarian conception of autonomy seems attractive on a number of grounds. It articulates one of the key ideas underpinning the concept of personal autonomy: that of individual sovereignty with respect to one's own life. At the same time, via the harm principle, it sets clear limits to this sovereignty, thereby distinguishing justifiable (to prevent harm to others) from non-justifiable (coercive or paternalistic) forms of interference. The libertarian conception of autonomy also highlights the important connections among autonomy, freedom, and individual choice. These ideas have played a crucial role in securing political freedoms, such as freedom of religion, or freedom of speech and assembly, that most people in western liberal democracies regard as crucial to their ability to lead autonomous lives. In some jurisdictions, these ideas have also been used to support more controversial personal freedoms, such as women's rights to abortion; the right of terminally ill patients to request voluntary euthanasia; and the rights of those with non-standard sexual or gender identities, such as gays, lesbians, and transgender persons to lead lives of their own choosing, including being able to express their sexual preferences and gender identity without state sanction.

Relational theorists uphold the importance of individual sovereignty with respect to one's life. They also agree that political freedom, personal freedom, and individual choice are important for autonomy. However, they disagree with libertarian interpretations of freedom and individual choice, and reject libertarian conceptions of autonomy on three connected grounds. First, they maintain that negative liberty is insufficient for autonomy. Second, they claim that libertarian autonomy overlooks the social constraints on individual choice. Third, they contend that it pays insufficient attention to exploitation and social injustice.

Why is negative liberty insufficient for autonomy? To exercise autonomy requires both liberty and opportunity. Liberty, or freedom from undue interference, is required because it is difficult for a person to lead a self-governing life if political or personal restrictions prevent her from making choices about matters that are important to her, such as being able to practice her religion, express her political opinions, pursue a career or personal projects, and decide with whom she will have intimate relationships, where she will live, or whether she will have children. However, living an autonomous life or a life of one's own choosing intuitively seems to require more than being free from undue interference by others. It also seems to require access to genuine opportunities, or to a range of significant options (Raz 1986), which means access to social goods such as education, health care, housing, and social support; adequate nutrition, sanitation, and personal safety; opportunities for political participation and paid or unpaid employment; and some degree of mobility. These goods require complex social, economic, and political infrastructures. Relational theorists charge that libertarian autonomy places too much emphasis on the importance of negative liberty or freedom from interference, while overlooking the importance for individual autonomy of access to these social goods and the opportunities they make available.

The second objection, which follows from the first, is that libertarian autonomy pays insufficient attention to the social distribution of opportunities and the social constraints on individual choice. The extent of a person's access to significant options depends both upon their social availability and also on that particular individual's social environment and social relationships. For example, even in societies in which access to a university education is a significant option for many young people, such as Australia, it is unlikely to be a significant option for a young person from a socio-economically disadvantaged background, particularly if he is Aboriginal, who, despite having the native ability to study at university, may have received a poor high school education, may come from a family or community that does not place much value on education, and is unlikely to have been encouraged by his teachers, parents, or peers to consider university as an option (see e.g., Australian Government 2012). In other words, even if there are no formal discriminatory barriers preventing this young man from gaining a place at a university, and even if targeted access programs and financial assistance are available to Aboriginal students, the option to study at university is unlikely to be a significant option for him. One reason for this is what is known as the problem of adaptive preference formation (Elster 1983; Sen 1992). This is the phenomenon whereby persons who are subject to social oppression or deprivation adapt their preferences and goals to their circumstances, eliminating, or failing to form, preferences or goals that cannot be satisfied, and even failing to conceive how these might differ in different circumstances. A young Aboriginal man growing up in circumstances such as those described above, for example, may have little conception of the kind of options that might be available to him or the kind of life he might be able to lead were he able to gain a university education, and so never even forms a preference to undertake university study.

The third objection is that because libertarian autonomy endorses expansions of choice but fails to account for the social distribution of opportunities and the social constraints on individual choice, it can entrench social injustice and overlook exploitation. This is because in contexts of highly constrained choice, it might be rational for persons with significantly reduced options to enter into exploitative personal relationships, or exploitative employment or other commercial arrangements. Bioethicists who endorse libertarian autonomy usually justify such arrangements as freely chosen, advantageous to both parties, and as enhancing the autonomy of the disadvantaged by expanding their option sets. Such justifications therefore assume that any expansion of a person's choices that meets the harm condition (construed minimally) enhances their autonomy. However, according to relational theorists, what such justifications ignore is that some options are unjust and function to entrench or extend existing inequalities, such as inequalities arising from socio-economic status, gender, disability, or citizenship. Rather than enabling a person to lead a more self-governing life, adding these options to her choice set may simply increase the opportunities for others to exploit her. The fact that the option is available may also function as a further constraint, pressuring a person to pursue an option she would not otherwise have chosen, and furthering her disadvantage.

An example from bioethics will help to explain this third objection. Some bioethicists have proposed that in order to meet the increasing demand for organs and shortages in supply, a current market in nonessential or renewable body parts, such as single kidneys, liver lobes, blood, bone marrow, or corneas, should be established (Fabre 2006; Radcliffe-Richards 2007; Taylor 2002). Such proposals are defended on grounds of libertarian autonomy, via two main arguments. First, that people have an autonomy right to determine what happens in and to their bodies, and this includes the right to use their bodies however they choose, including selling body parts and organs for material gain.

Any attempt to limit this right constitutes unjustifiable paternalism. Second, that such markets simply provide prospective donors with extra options. Since nobody is under an obligation to sell their organs if they do not want to, then the availability of this option can only enhance donors' choices and hence their autonomy.

Critics have responded to such arguments by highlighting both the risks to individuals and the broader social harms of organ markets. The trade in body parts is now a global enterprise and those who are most likely to have an interest in selling their organs are the global poor. Since surgical procedures to procure organs are often undertaken in unsafe conditions, individuals who sell an organ such as a single kidney are at risk of suffering a range of harms, including poor health (both short and long term), resulting in consequent loss of employment, and being shamed within their communities (see e.g., Scheper-Hughes 2007). Organ markets, critics claim, therefore exploit people who are vulnerable, disadvantaged, and often desperate, while advantaging the wealthy. Moreover, in doing so they entrench global inequities in the allocation of health care resources (Zutlevics 2001). Critics have also claimed that whereas organ donation involves an altruistic gift of life to another person, organ markets treat the human body and body parts as commodities, thereby undermining respect for human persons (Titmuss ([1970] 1997); Radin 1996).

Bioethicists who defend markets in organs and tissue often acknowledge that such markets may involve the making of exploitative offers to poor, vulnerable, and disadvantaged people, and that those who take up these offers may thereby risk their health and livelihoods. However, these bioethicists argue that if the offer is perceived by the seller as advantageous, if genuine consent has been given in full knowledge of the risks involved, and if the offer makes the seller better off relative to their current situation, then prohibiting the poor from pursuing this option or from pursuing other high-risk opportunities for earning income is unjustifiably paternalistic (see e.g., Radcliffe-Richards 2007; Taylor 2002; Wertheimer 2011). While it is beyond the scope of this article to provide a detailed response to this kind of argument (for a subtle response, see e.g., Radin 1996), one of my concerns is that it effectively ends up defining exploitation away. On this account it is difficult to see how arrangements that seem obviously unjust, such as sweatshop labor, could be classified as exploitative.

The central problem with the libertarian conception of autonomy then, is that it starts from the mistaken premise that autonomy is equivalent to negative liberty and fails to take sufficient account of the effects of social injustice and oppression on individual choice. Despite the influence of libertarian autonomy in bioethics, therefore, I have argued in this section that it does not provide a satisfactory account of personal autonomy.

Relational Autonomy

Relational conceptions hold that autonomy is a complex competence, the development and exercise of which requires ongoing interpersonal, social, and institutional scaffolding. Relational theorists seek to analyze the nature of this competence; to understand the kind of social scaffolding required to develop and exercise it; and to show how autonomy can be thwarted by social oppression and injustice. Relational autonomy theory therefore shares the decisional autonomy theorist's focus on the competences required for autonomy, but develops a richer account of these competences. It shares with the libertarian conception of autonomy a focus on the connections between autonomy, freedom, and individual choice, but develops a more complex social analysis of these concepts and their interconnections. And it shares the conscientious autonomy theorist's focus on the importance for autonomy of critical reflection, responsible judgment, and accountability to others, seeking to analyze the ways such accountability relations are sometimes embedded in oppressive social relationships and institutions.

Relational autonomy theorists such as Diana Meyers (1989) propose that autonomy competence requires a complex repertoire or suite of reflective skills, which may be developed and exercised to varying degrees and in different domains. These skills include but go well beyond the requirements of legal competence—understanding, minimal rationality, and the capacity to communicate one's decision—that are central to Beauchamp and Childress's account of decisional autonomy. They include volitional skills, such as self-control and motivational decisiveness; emotional skills, such as the capacity to interpret and regulate one's own emotions; imaginative skills, required for understanding the implications of one's decisions and envisaging alternative possible courses of action; and capacities to reflect critically on social norms and values. According to Meyers, a person is autonomous, and her choices are authentically her own, to the degree that she has developed these skills and can exercise them in understanding herself (self-discovery), defining her values and commitments (self-definition), and directing her life (self-direction).

Meyers' skills-based theory provides a plausible way of responding to the problem identified by Beauchamp and Childress, concerning how to distinguish authentic from distorted forms of critical reflection, such as in the example of the terminally ill patient who reverses an earlier decision to refuse treatment. Reflection is authentic if a person possesses and can exercise the full repertoire of cognitive, volitional, emotional, and imaginative competences required to direct her life and make choices that express her authentic self-conception. Reflection may be distorted, however, if these competences are under-developed or their exercise is impaired, for example by volitional disorders or social oppression. Meyers' account of critical reflection is procedural or content-neutral. Judgments about whether or not a person's decisions are autonomous do not turn on the specific content of that decision, but on whether or not the person exercises the necessary reflective skills to make a decision that expresses her authentic self-conception.

Meyers' account of autonomy competence, and other relational conceptions of autonomy are relational in four main ways. First, relational autonomy theory emphasizes that autonomy competences emerge developmentally and are sustained and exercised in the context of significant social relationships. Hence, autonomy competence is a relationally, or socially constituted capacity. In contrast to popular conceptions, which equate autonomy with self-sufficient independence, relational theorists stress that an adequate conception of autonomy must be responsive to the facts of human vulnerability and dependency. For this reason, on a relational view, there need be no inconsistency between autonomy and interpersonal relationships of dependence and interdependence. Because relational autonomy starts from a conception of persons as vulnerable and dependent, to varying degrees, it is particularly relevant to health care contexts, where obligations to respond to vulnerability must be balanced with respect for patient autonomy.

Second, relational autonomy theory is premised on a social conception of the self, according to which we constitute our self-identities in relation to social relationships; the specific historical, political, and geographical contexts in which we live our lives; and intersecting social determinants, such as race and gender. This social conception of the self has implications for the notion of authenticity, or what it means for a decision, choice, or action to be "one's own." The notion of authenticity is sometimes interpreted as implying that each individual has a true, deep, or ideal self (see e.g., Wolf 1990). Relational theorists reject such interpretations of authenticity. Autonomy is not a matter of discovering who one essentially is, free from social influence. It is rather a matter of exercising socially acquired reflective skills to determine what one values and how one wants to live one's life. Although this requires some degree of self-knowledge, it is not a solitary exercise, but requires sustained interpersonal and social scaffolding and ongoing dialogical interaction with others, or what Christman (2009) refers to as "socially-mediated self-reflection." Moreover, although some degree of motivational and volitional stability is required for authenticity, relational theorists emphasize that our self-identities are dynamic and changing. Hence the terminally ill patient's change of mind need not impugn her autonomy, so long as she has exercised the relevant reflective skills, has considered the implications of this decision, often in discussion with others, and can give reasons for her decision.

Third, while emphasizing the crucial role of social relationships in shaping our self-identities and developing the skills involved in autonomy competence, relational theorists argue that some social relationships, such as those characterized by domination, abuse, coercion, violence or disrespect, provide hostile conditions for autonomy. These kinds of social relationships, whether in intimate personal and family relationships, institutional care contexts, work environments, between neighbors or friends, and so on, can thwart the development or constrain the exercise of autonomy competence. In accounting for the autonomy-impairing effects of oppressive social relationships, some relational theorists claim that autonomy is both a *capacity* and a *status* concept, and that these two aspects of autonomy are closely intertwined. To lead an autonomous life requires not just possessing and exercising the relevant competences, but also regarding oneself, and being recognized by others, as having the social *status* of an autonomous person (Anderson and Honneth 2005; Benson 2005; Mackenzie 2008; McLeod 2002; Lindemann Nelson 2001; Oshana 2006). Regarding oneself as having the social status of an autonomous person, according to these theorists, requires having positive and appropriate self-evaluative attitudes, in particular attitudes of self-respect, self-trust, and self-esteem. Self-respect involves regarding oneself as the moral equal of others, as having equal standing to have one's views and claims taken seriously. Self-trust is the capacity to trust one's own convictions, emotional responses, and judgments. Self-esteem or self-worth is an evaluative attitude towards oneself, which involves thinking of oneself, one's life, and one's undertakings as meaningful and worthwhile.

McLeod (2002), for example, argues that justified self-trust is required for autonomous choice, judgment, and action. Making autonomous choices requires that a person trusts her own abilities to choose well, to understand the information relevant to that choice, and to discern when it is appropriate (or not) to trust the purveyor of that information. It also requires that she trusts her own judgment that this is the right choice for her to make, given her beliefs and values, and that she trusts in her ability to act on the decision she has made. Similarly, Kukla (2005) argues that justified self-trust is required for exercising conscientious autonomy, that is, for taking responsibility and holding oneself accountable for one's health care practices.

Self-evaluative attitudes such as self-trust, however, are vulnerable to the attitudes of others; that is, to social relations of recognition. Refusals or failures to recognize another person as an autonomous agent, and as deserving respect, are quite typical in social relations involving domination, or inequalities of power, authority, or social and economic status. McLeod (2002) and other relational autonomy theorists claim that the internalization of oppressive social relations and stereotypes can corrode a person's sense of self-respect, self-trust, and self-esteem, thereby impairing her autonomy.

In health care contexts, patients' self-evaluative attitudes are particularly vulnerable not only to the effects of illness or disability, but also to the attitudes, judgments, and styles of communication and interaction on the part of clinicians. For example, a parent's sense of self-respect and confidence in her judgment can be undermined if health care professionals dismiss her concerns about her child's health or ignore her reports of the child's symptoms; convey attitudes of disrespect or disinterest; make stereotypical judgments based on the parent's gender, religion, occupation, or cultural background; or communicate using medical terms she does not understand without explanation. As a result, she may feel (rightly) that her autonomy has been overridden and her judgment impugned if she ends up agreeing that there is nothing wrong with her child when she knows that he is ill, or agreeing to treatment plans that she suspects may be useless or harmful.

Finally, relational autonomy theory focuses attention on the impact of social oppression and injustice on individuals' capacities to lead autonomous lives and to make autonomous choices. Relational autonomy theorists agree with libertarians that there is an important connection between freedom, choice, and autonomy, and that constrained option sets can compromise a person's ability to lead an autonomous life. However, they argue that what matters for autonomy is not the mere proliferation of choice, but the range of significant options that are available to a person or social group. If we are interested in promoting autonomy we therefore need to be concerned with the social distribution of opportunities; that is, with questions such as whether there are significant inequalities in the opportunities available to members of different social groups, and whether these inequalities perpetuate injustice and enable exploitation. For relational theorists, then, an interest in promoting autonomy goes hand in hand with an interest in promoting social justice.

This aspect of relational autonomy is particularly pertinent to public health ethics (Baylis et al. 2008; Faden and Powers 2006). Public health is focused on what societies collectively can do to promote the health of the population and to reduce health inequalities and inequities among individuals and social groups. It is fundamentally concerned with issues of social justice, in particular with the social determinants of health. This refers to the impact on health, at both the individual and population levels, of patterns of systematic disadvantage, due to factors such as socio-economic inequality, geographical location, gender, race, or disability. Relational conceptions of autonomy are particularly relevant to public health because their attention to the social constraints on individual choice and the social distribution of opportunities can help focus attention on the background conditions that shape individual health choices. For example, in poor communities, food choices, such as high levels of consumption of fast food, are often shaped by factors such as the low cost and ready availability of fast food compared with fresh fruit and vegetables, insufficient education concerning nutrition, and time poverty due to long working hours. Relational conceptions also focus attention on the way that health and social policy decisions can limit or expand the options available to people and may affect different social groups in different ways (Baylis et al. 2008: 202).

An objection that has been raised against relational conceptions of autonomy is that highlighting the social constraints on individual choice and the autonomy-impairing effects of social oppression may invite disrespect towards persons who may already be socially marginalized. As a result, relational conceptions may sanction unwarranted paternalistic interference with their choices (Christman 2005; Holroyd 2009). In response, I would argue that this objection misidentifies the critical target of relational conceptions, which is unjust and oppressive social relationships and institutions that impair individuals' capacities for autonomous agency and choice. The kinds of interventions that relational autonomy theorists would sanction are regulatory interventions aimed at preventing exploitation, coercion and abuse, or expanding the significant options available to individuals from oppressed or disadvantaged social groups. However, it does not follow from recognizing that a person's autonomy may be impaired to some degree that disrespect and paternalistic interference with that individual's choices are thereby licensed. Rather, relational autonomy theorists emphasize the importance of providing forms of social support that scaffold individuals' capacities for autonomy. In clinical contexts this might mean adopting approaches to clinical care that facilitate dialogical interaction between clinicians and patients, or providing assistance to patients who find it difficult to implement treatment regimes. In public health contexts it might mean developing targeted programs to improve knowledge about nutrition, or how to avoid infection, while taking care to avoid stereotyping of targeted social groups. For relational autonomy theorists then, respecting autonomy requires more than respecting an individual's autonomous choices; it means promoting the kinds of social relationships and institutional structures that enable people to lead self-governing lives.

Related Topics

Chapter 24, "Privacy, Surveillance, and Autonomy," Alan Rubel
Chapter 25, "Public Health and Civil Liberties: Resolving Conflicts," James F. Childress
Chapter 33, "Alzheimer's Disease: Quality of Life and the Goals of Care," Bruce Jennings

Acknowledgments

Thanks to John Arras, Rebecca Kukla, and Wendy Rogers for extremely helpful comments on earlier versions of this chapter.

References

Agar, N. (1998) "Liberal Eugenics," *Public Affairs Quarterly* 12 (2): 137–55.

Anderson, J. and Honneth, A. (2005) "Autonomy, Vulnerability, Recognition and Justice," in J. Christman and J. Anderson (eds.) *Autonomy and the Challenges to Liberalism*, Cambridge: Cambridge University Press, pp. 127–49.

Australian Government, Department of Industry, Innovation, Climate Change, Science, Research and Tertiary Education (2012) *Report of the Review of Higher Education Access and Outcomes for Aboriginal and Torres Strait Islander People*. Available at: www.innovation.gov.au/higher education/Indigenous Higher Education (accessed August 26, 2013).

Baylis, F., Kenny, N. and Sherwin, S. (2008) "A Relational Account of Public Health Ethics," *Public Health Ethics* 1 (3): 196–209.

Bayne, T. and Levy, N. (2005) "Amputees by Choice: Body Integrity Disorder and the Ethics of Amputation," *Journal of Applied Philosophy* 22 (1): 75–86.

Beauchamp, T. and Childress, J. (2012) *Principles of Biomedical Ethics*, 7th edition, New York: Oxford University Press.

Benson, P. (2005) "Taking Ownership: Authority and Voice in Autonomous Agency," in J. Christman and J. Anderson (eds.) *Autonomy and the Challenges to Liberalism*, Cambridge: Cambridge University Press, pp. 101–26.

Christman, J. (2005) "Relational Autonomy, Liberal Individualism and the Social Constitution of Selves," *Philosophical Studies* 117: 143–64.
Christman, J. (2009) *The Politics of Persons: Individual Autonomy and Socio-historical Selves*, Cambridge: Cambridge University Press.
Dworkin, G. (1988) *The Theory and Practice of Autonomy*, New York: Cambridge University Press.
Elster, J. (1983) *Sour Grapes*, Cambridge: Cambridge University Press.
Englehardt, H.T. Jr (1986) *The Foundations of Bioethics* (1st edition; (1996) 2nd edition), New York: Oxford University Press.
Fabre, C. (2006) *Whose Body Is It Anyway? Justice and the Integrity of the Person*, Oxford: Oxford University Press.
Faden, R. and Powers, M. (2006) *Social Justice: The Moral Foundations of Public Health and Health Policy*, New York: Oxford University Press.
Frankfurt, H. (1988) "Freedom of the Will and the Concept of a Person," in *The Importance of What We Care About*, Cambridge: Cambridge University Press.
Harris, J. (1998) *Clones, Genes and Immortality*, Oxford: Clarendon Press.
Holroyd, J. (2009) "Relational Autonomy and Paternalistic Interventions," *Res Publica*, 15 (4): 321–36.
Kukla, R. (2005) "Conscientious Autonomy: Displacing Decisions in Health Care," *The Hastings Center Report* 35 (2): 34–44.
Mackenzie, C. (2008) "Relational Autonomy, Normative Authority and Perfectionism," *Journal of Social Philosophy* 39: 512–33.
Mackenzie, C. and Stoljar, N. (2000) "Introduction: Autonomy Refigured," in C. Mackenzie and N. Stoljar, *Relational Autonomy: Feminist Perspectives on Autonomy, Agency and the Social Self*, New York: Oxford University Press.
McLeod, C. (2002) *Self-trust and Reproductive Autonomy*, Cambridge, MA: MIT Press.
Meyers, D. (1989) *Self, Society and Personal Choice*, New York: Columbia University Press.
Mill, J.S. (1962 [1859]) *On Liberty*, in M. Warnock (ed.) *Utilitarianism, On Liberty and other Essays*, London: Fontana, pp. 126–250.
Nelson, H. Lindemann (2001) *Damaged Identities, Narrative Repair*, Ithaca, NY: Cornell University Press.
Nozick, R. (1974) *Anarchy, State, and Utopia*, New York: Basic Books
O'Neill, O. (2002) *Autonomy and Trust in Bioethics*, Cambridge, UK: Cambridge University Press.
Oshana, M. (2006) *Personal Autonomy in Society*, Aldershot, UK: Ashgate.
Radcliffe-Richards, J. (2007) "Selling organs, gametes and surrogacy services," in R. Rhodes, L. Francis and A. Silvers (eds.) *The Blackwell Guide to Medical Ethics*, Malden, MA: Wiley-Blackwell, pp. 254–68.
Radin, M. (1996) *Contested Commodities: The Trouble with the Trade in Sex, Children, Body Parts, and Other Things*, Cambridge, MA: Harvard University Press.
Raz, J. (1986) *The Morality of Freedom*, Oxford: Clarendon Press.
Scheper-Hughes, N. (2007) "Illegal Organ Trade: Global Justice and the Traffic in Human Organs," in R.W.G. Gruessner and E. Beneditti (eds.) *Living Donor Organ Transplants*, New York: McGraw-Hill, pp. 106–21.
Sen, A. (1992) *Inequality Reexamined*, Cambridge: Cambridge University Press.
Sherwin, S. (1998) "A Relational Approach to Autonomy in Health Care," in S. Sherwin and the Feminist Health Care Ethics Research Network (eds.) *The Politics of Women's Health: Exploring Agency and Autonomy*, Philadelphia: Temple University Press, pp. 19–47.
Taylor, J.S. (2002) "Autonomy, Constraining Options, and Organ Sales," *Journal of Applied Philosophy* 19 (3): 273–85.
Titmuss, R. ([1970] 1997) *The Gift Relationship: From Human Blood to Social Policy*, expanded and updated edition, A. Oakley and J. Ashton (eds.), London: New Press.
Wertheimer, A. (2011) *Rethinking the Ethics of Clinical Research: Widening the Lens*, New York: Oxford University Press.
Wolf, S. (1990) *Freedom within Reason*, Oxford: Oxford University Press.
Zutlevics, T. (2001) "Markets and the Needy: Organ Sales or Aid?" *Journal of Applied Philosophy* 18 (3): 297–302.

22

CAPACITY AND COMPETENCE

Jessica Berg and Katherine Shaw Makielski

Introduction

The validity of a patient's informed consent to medical treatment depends on several factors, including the topic of this chapter: competency. While competent patients may make any reasonable or unreasonable choices with regard to their health care, a determination of incompetence—even temporary—severely limits a person's ability to exercise self-determination. Incompetence is sometimes referred to as a formal exception to informed consent (e.g., informed consent does not need to be sought from an incompetent patient), and other times competence is considered simply to be a core requirement for a valid consent (i.e., patients must be competent to make an informed decision). From either perspective, competence is a crucial aspect of autonomy, a term which, in the context of informed consent, may be defined as the highly valued and protected right to make independent decisions about one's body and health care. But competence is not the only determinant of autonomy. An individual may have all the capacities necessary to make an informed decision, but fail to exercise autonomy because of coercive forces that interfere with voluntariness, or due to lack of pertinent information. It is capacity, however, not other limitations of autonomy, which is the focus of this chapter.

While a competent patient may make a wide range of choices, reasonable or otherwise, with regard to his health care, a determination of incompetence—even temporary—severely limits a person's ability to exercise self-determination and make an autonomous choice. This is because the concept of autonomy requires that an individual who possesses the ability to recognize and act upon his own interests must be given the freedom to act upon those interests (or not, should he so choose). The lack of certain abilities, or capacities, interferes with the exercise of autonomy by preventing the individual from knowing his interests, from knowing the scope or import of the decision in question, or actually making a choice. There are two fundamental concerns here: identification of the abilities or capacities necessary to exercise autonomy; and identification of the means or tests by which to determine the presence of those capacities. Beyond these two questions, there are also practical issues related to applying various tests of capacity, and what to do when someone is found to lack capacity. This chapter outlines basic concepts for understanding patient competence and incompetence, and explores some key areas of ongoing debate, including setting competence standards, identifying mechanisms for determining capacity in different situations, and recognizing the capacity of minors. It focuses on competence to consent to medical treatment, rather than research participation. The underlying concepts are the same, but the research area is governed primarily by federal regulations.

Terminology

It is important to distinguish between two often confused and interchangeably used terms: competence and capacity. Competence, a legal construct, refers to a court's determination of whether a patient possesses the requisite capacities to make a medical decision. Capacity, however, is assessed by medical or mental health professionals in the clinical setting (Berg et al. 2001). Decision-making capacity falls along a continuum; competence, however, is a binary category—a court must judge a person either competent or not. The two concepts are interrelated; judicial determinations of competence generally rest on the clinician's evaluations of capacity.

In practice, clinicians act as the "first line of defense" in determining whether a patient is capable of consenting to treatment. If a physician finds that a patient lacks capacity to make an informed choice, then he or she consults a surrogate decision-maker (often one or more family members). This approach renders the patient *de facto* incompetent: incompetent in fact, but not legally adjudicated as such. Courts, however, may be called upon to formally adjudicate competence in a variety of situations involving different kinds of patients, including adult patients with permanent impairments in capacity (e.g., developmental or psychiatric disabilities), when family members and/or surrogates cannot agree on the course of treatment, where specific legal liability concerns exist based on the treatment decision in question, or when a patient with uncertain capacity refuses a recommended treatment plan (Appelbaum 2010; Berg et al. 2001). Capacity determinations are made daily by health professionals. Often mental health professionals are called upon to provide more extensive evaluations, or to assist with a difficult determination. By contrast, court determinations of competence are relatively rare. Because a judicial determination can only be changed through another judicial hearing, formal competence proceedings should be used sparingly. In most cases informal determinations of incapacity will be sufficient and are preferable as they can more easily accommodate the normal fluctuations in patient decision-making abilities.

While courts can determine a person generally incompetent for all decisions and purposes (global incompetence), this is becoming less common. More often a court will rule a person incompetent for a specific decision or for limited purposes (specific incompetence) (Berg et al. 2001). For example, courts almost always distinguish a person's competence to make medical decisions from competence to make financial or other life decisions. A competence determination can even be specific to certain types of medical decisions, although this is more likely to occur via an informal capacity evaluation than through a formal competence adjudication. Thus, a patient may have the capacity to make a less complex treatment decision such as whether to take a daily aspirin, but not to make a more complex treatment decision such as whether to consent to open-heart surgery. The idea of different levels of competence required for different types of decisions seems intuitive, but is not well codified in law. We will return to this point later.

Presumption of Competence

Adults are presumed competent unless evidence indicates potential problems. Minors—a legal category that can vary according to state but usually refers to those under 16–18 years of age—are presumed incompetent, although there is increasing effort to include minors in medical decision-making (see discussion of minors below). The presumption of competence for adults remains even where a court previously deemed a person incompetent in another setting (Fisher 2009; Berg et al. 1996). Moreover, the presumption of competence is not automatically defeated with diagnosis of a mental illness or commitment, whether voluntary or involuntary, to a mental health facility.

As testament to the emphasis placed on the right to be presumed competent, several states have laws protecting the presumption in situations where people may be especially vulnerable (Fisher 2009). For example, Alaskan law states that even people with court-appointed guardians may not be presumed incompetent as a result of a guardianship, and further specifies that all rights not explicitly granted to the guardians remain with the individuals (Alaska 2012). California requires (1) that people retain their presumption of competence following treatment or evaluation for either mental illness or chronic alcoholism, and (2) that individuals be notified of their protected status upon leaving a mental health facility where services were sought (California 2012). Finally, Texas law specifically enumerates the rights of people with mental retardation, including the right to be presumed competent (Texas 2011).

Any limitation of decision-making authority (even requiring an evaluation of capacity before accepting a decision) restricts an individual's freedom. Because we want to be especially careful about imposing such limits in the absence of a clear indication of impairment, the law recognizes a general presumption in favor of competence. Just the act of questioning someone's capacity may limit their autonomy in some sense; a person whose capacity has been questioned is no longer able to make a decision without any interference until a determination has been made. We may accept this burdensome effect of questioning another's capacity because of the importance of assuring that certain decisions, such as those that deal with one's body and health care, are made by capable, and thus fully autonomous, patients.

But it is worth noting that not all decisions are of such import that we must ensure they are fully autonomous. We do not question an adult's freedom to make a multitude of choices throughout the day (what to wear, what to eat, where to go, what to buy, whom to marry, etc.). Nonetheless, many of these day-to-day decisions are likely made with varying levels of capacity (and therefore autonomy). For practical reasons we do not interfere with such decisions, even to assure ourselves the choices are completely autonomous and made by completely competent individuals. In this way, we also limit the extent to which we interfere with overall autonomy to make decisions free from the interference of others.

Elements of Capacity and Standards of Competence

As mentioned previously, competence standards should be based on those capacities necessary to make an autonomous decision. While there may be disagreement about the extent of capacity necessary in a specific context, there are some basic abilities that should be included in all situations. For example, someone who cannot communicate at all, or is generally unaware of their situation (e.g., someone who is unconscious) does not have the capacity to exercise any autonomy. In addition, someone who lacks the ability to understand the decision at hand, or information related to the decision, likely also lacks the capacity to make an autonomous decision. In fact, understanding is the most common capacity requirement. Beyond this, however, there is some debate.

Legal standards for competence vary by jurisdiction (Berg et al. 1996). Courts look to the relevant state law to determine which capacities are required for a ruling of competence, and evaluate medical findings and witness testimony accordingly. Although there is variation between jurisdictions, in general competence standards use some combination of four components: (1) the ability to communicate a choice; (2) the ability to understand relevant information; (3) the ability to appreciate the nature of the situation and its likely consequences; and (4) the ability to manipulate information rationally (Berg et al. 1996). There are a few outlier statutes that use vague standards such as "ability to make an intelligent choice"; ideally, however, the laws use language that can be more readily linked to specific capacities.

The first component, ability to communicate a choice, is the least stringent requirement. Clearly someone who cannot communicate a choice at all should not be considered competent. Patients who speak other languages, or who need to communicate through non-verbal means, however, do not lack the ability to communicate a choice. In contrast, a patient who can communicate but who cannot reach a decision, or who changes his mind so rapidly as to make it impossible to settle on one option, would fail this standard. This is a trickier situation than the person who simply fails to communicate at all. While the communication component often marks the lower threshold of capacity, it rarely stands alone in determining competence. It is a necessary, but not a sufficient, element. Thus, courts and legislatures usually apply the communication component in conjunction with one or more other components.

The second component, the ability to understand relevant information, is the most commonly used and most heavily weighted element of capacity. It requires that a patient understand specific information related to the decision at issue. Because of this, the informed consent disclosure itself is often used to test understanding. A patient may be provided the relevant information to make the decision and then asked whether she understands the key concepts and issues. Patients are not necessarily required to comprehend the situation as a whole, but rather the specific issues pertaining to informed consent disclosures. Scholars point out that this type of abstract understanding should be distinguished from appreciation, which is sometimes referred to as "deep understanding."

This third component, the ability to appreciate the nature of the situation and its likely consequences, focuses on a patient's ability to apply the abstractly understood information to his own situation. In some cases a patient may understand generally the procedure or diagnosis and thus meet the basic understanding component, but fail to appreciate how this information relates to her specific situation (i.e., fails to demonstrate appreciation or "deep understanding"). For example, a patient may understand that a positive antibody test means someone has contracted the human immunodeficiency virus (HIV), but later refuse to acknowledge she has HIV despite repeat positive test results from the patient's blood samples. In such a case, the patient may be found incompetent because she failed to appreciate the nature of her specific situation or the future implications. Distinguishing between understanding and appreciation may be difficult in practice, and capacity evaluations may conflate the two concepts. But from an ethical perspective it is important to separate out the two. A failure of understanding may stem from a cognitive deficit, but in some cases can be remedied by focusing on the mechanism, timing, or amount of information disclosure. A failure of appreciation may stem from less easily addressed impairments or barriers, such as the inability or even refusal to accept longer-term consequences.

Several states appear to require both appreciation and understanding in their standards for competence. In Massachusetts, for example, the Supreme Judicial Court held a man incompetent when physicians diagnosed him with schizophrenia, but he denied he suffered from mental illness and accordingly refused to take antipsychotic medication (*In re Roe* 1992). In the case, the man *understood* the risks associated with taking the prescribed antipsychotic medicine, but, as the court stated, "he clearly [did] not *appreciate* the risks associated with refusing it." In other words, the court deemed the man unable to appreciate the need to control this illness with antipsychotic medication. This case provides an example of how the distinct qualities of understanding and appreciation work in tandem to demonstrate competence. Using understanding alone, the state would have deemed this man competent because he understood the factual risks of taking the medicine.

Simply refusing treatment does not render a person incompetent. Indeed, the law allows competent people to make any decision, reasonable or not, when it comes to controlling their health care. In another Massachusetts case, the appellate court upheld a woman's right to refuse amputation of her gangrenous leg (*Lane v. Candura* 1978). Because the woman appreciated both that her leg was infected with gangrene and that she would likely die without amputation, the court found the woman to be competent. As a competent patient, the woman was free to refuse even life-saving treatment.

By requiring appreciation, legislatures and courts recognize that delusional beliefs affect competence only if those delusions interfere with a patient's ability to appreciate the nature of his or her own situation and likely consequences. But that nuanced recognition depends largely on the language contained in a state's law and how state courts interpret that language. For example, in Vermont, the law states that "[i]n determining whether or not the person is competent to make a decision regarding the proposed treatment, the court shall consider whether the person is able to make a decision and appreciate the consequences of that decision" (Vermont 2012). So when a trial court deemed a man incompetent simply because he had delusions and other mental health symptoms, the Supreme Court of Vermont reversed and sent the case back for further review (*In re L.A.* 2006). Instead of merely listing the patient's symptoms—which frequently occurs in cases where parties seek involuntary medication—the trial court needed to look further to determine if and how the patient's symptoms affected his ability to make the decision in question and to appreciate the consequences of that decision.

The final component, the ability to manipulate information rationally, focuses on the patient's ability to reason. Sometimes difficult to evaluate objectively or with quantitative measures, this criterion is sometimes excluded from states' legal competence standards. There is also some concern that the component will be improperly applied to evaluate the rationality of the final decision, rather than the decision-making process. The requirement is not that a patient makes a correct, conventional, or even reasonable decision, but that he follows a rational process to arrive at the final decision (based on those factors which the patient himself finds to be most relevant). For example, someone who states that it is important to choose a treatment option that does not take him away from his small children for any period of time, but then chooses a surgical option which involves a considerable hospital stay instead of an outpatient medical option, without any explanation of why, may fail this component. The rational manipulation component, like the communication criterion, is not used as a standalone test for competence. Just as someone can communicate a choice without understanding or appreciation, a person can reason and manipulate facts without actually understanding or appreciating them. Thus a patient who believes (based on lack of understanding) that sunlight will kill a staph infection may take reasonable steps to increase exposure to sunlight, and make medical (and other) decisions to facilitate that exposure.

Courts sometimes struggle with the application of the reasoning component. For example, California competence law includes two distinct elements: (1) the ability to understand and appreciate the consequences of decisions (and mental illness can only be considered if it significantly interferes with the patient's ability to do so); and (2) the ability to participate in a treatment decision through a rational thought process (*In re Conservatorship of Burton* 2009). These requirements were at odds in *Burton* because the patient understood and appreciated the consequences of going on a hunger and medication strike (which could be grounds for finding him competent under the first requirement) but based his decision on psychotic delusions (which could be grounds for finding him unable to participate in a rational decision-making process under the second requirement). The court resolved the conflict by holding that the second requirement, the ability to engage in a rational decision-making process, was meant to stand alone and thus superseded the language limiting consideration of psychotic symptoms. In the court's view, appreciating the consequences that could result from an irrationally reasoned decision does not render a patient competent. Thus, even though the patient argued that his delusion did not interfere with his ability to appreciate the consequences of his hunger strike, the court ruled the patient incompetent with regard to that decision because his delusions prevented him from participating in a rational decision-making process in the first place.

Perhaps most difficult from both the legal and ethical perspectives are the cases which are based on contested religious beliefs such as faith healing. Patients in these cases follow a rational decision-making process refusing medical care and seeking help from faith healers. While parents may not be allowed to rely on faith healing for their minor children, it is less clear whether adults should be allowed to rely on it for themselves. Faith healing is one of the more extreme situations, but these debates about allowing refusal of treatment also arise in other contexts such as those involving Scientologists and Jehovah's Witnesses.

Applying the Standards

Courts and legislatures employ various combinations of these four components in their legal competence standards. Although the requisite capacities differ by jurisdiction, the goal of these standards remains constant: to determine as accurately as possible who is capable of making autonomous medical decisions and who requires a surrogate decision-maker. There remain various questions related to the application of the standards, including the scope of information that should be used to demonstrate capacity and the means by which capacity should be tested.

First, if understanding is a necessary element of capacity, what information must be offered and understood in a specific context? There are two aspects of this inquiry—quantitative and qualitative. From a quantitative standpoint, should there be a threshold amount of information that must be understood for a patient to be considered competent? If so, would it be 50 percent of the information disclosed, 75 percent, 90 percent, or more? From a qualitative standpoint, are there specific facts that must be understood no matter how much other information is understood? For example, for a surgical procedure, should we require a full understanding of the risks and implications of general anesthesia (qualitative), regardless of whether the patient understands 95 percent of the remaining overall information (quantitative)? Importantly, standards should not be set so high as to exclude the majority of the population from making their own decisions. That is to say, we should not require levels of autonomous decision-making that are beyond most people's capacity levels. Thus, some empirical work may be needed to understand the range of abilities in the general population.

There are few direct requirements regarding what specific information to put into an informed consent disclosure. A few hospitals provide checklist consent forms for physicians. Laws in some states require specific disclosures for certain procedures, although this is rare. For example, a handful of states define by statute specific information that must be disclosed related to breast cancer screening and treatment options. Rather than provide specific requirements, most states use general standards for disclosure, requiring at least that information which a "reasonable patient" would want to know, or that a "reasonable professional" would disclose. In practice, now, the two standards result in similar, if not identical, disclosures (i.e., most reasonable professionals disclose what reasonable patients would want to know). These standards, however, do not speak to the quantitative or qualitative questions raised above.

One approach to the quantitative question is to have a set standard for all decisions (e.g., everyone must understand 80 percent of the information disclosed), another is to allow a sliding scale based on the importance of the decision in question (e.g., 75 percent for simple decisions and 90 percent for complex ones). There are also suggestions that the issue is not complexity, but riskier decisions should require greater levels of capacity. Sliding scales are likely to be difficult to apply in practice. Moreover, it may prove hard to distinguish "simple" from "complex" decisions, or between levels of risk. The real concern is the consequence of a wrong determination of competence. We are often less concerned about a person who is incompetent consenting to a medically recommended treatment, than refusing such treatment. This is because we assume (rightly or wrongly) that the consequences of an incompetent consent are usually less momentous than an incompetent refusal; we may weigh beneficence in these situations more heavily than autonomy. But there are numerous medical decisions that fail to fall easily into a simple or complex category, and for which a medically "recommended" option may not be identified readily. And perhaps more importantly, beneficence is hard to separate from autonomy; one important point of respecting autonomy is to recognize that the patient is often a better judge of what treatments are in his or her benefit (since "benefit" is broader than simply medical benefit). The best approach may not be to use different standards for different types of decisions, but to allow these other factors to trigger more scrutiny of patient capacity. As noted previously, the default is a presumption of capacity. Even questioning a patient's capacity is an imposition on autonomy—better avoided if there is no reason to interfere. This is not to say that we should not be concerned with incompetent consents to treatment, but that we should consider a range of factors in deciding whether to examine capacity more closely. A refusal of treatment is one element (in the past, a refusal alone was often wrongly equated with incapacity). Failing to understand a crucial fact (the qualitative factor above) is another. A lower percentage of understanding (the quantitative factor above) is a third. Any or all of these elements may trigger additional evaluation of capacity by medical professionals, or weigh into a court's determination of competence. None should result in automatic determinations of incompetence.

Besides types of questions about applying the standards, there are also questions about how to engage in a capacity evaluation. Should a standardized capacity tool be used, or should informal mechanisms be employed? As noted earlier, the best solution is to use the informed consent disclosure itself to test capacity, rather than an abstract capacity tool. We are concerned with the patient's ability to understand, appreciate, and rationally manipulate information related to the decision at hand, not necessarily whether they can remember a stream of numbers or be perfectly oriented to time or place. These latter tests may be good triggers for additional capacity evaluations, but should not be a sufficient basis for determining competence. In contrast, the MacArthur Competence Assessment Tool for Treatment (MacCAT-T)—the most widely used capacity assessment instrument—incorporates specific details of the patient's pending medical decision, thus making the assessment more akin to an informed consent disclosure than a separate screening test. The MacCAT-T uses a structured interview process, which can be administered in approximately 15–30 minutes (Dunn et al. 2006; Appelbaum 2007). It assesses communication, understanding, appreciation, and rational manipulation through a series of physician-facilitated questions. To help ensure accurate and reliable findings by clinicians, the MacCAT-T offers extensive training materials, including both a manual and video.

Surrogate Decision-Making

Unlike other exceptions to informed consent, a finding of incapacity or incompetence does not relieve the health care professional of disclosure obligations, nor does it avoid the need to identify a decision-maker with legal authority to make the treatment choice. This decision-maker is called a "surrogate," and he or she is entitled to all informed consent information that would have been shared with the patient. There are different types of surrogates: guardians or conservators, who are legally designated through a judicial process; health care proxies, who are legally designated by the patient in a living will or health care power of attorney; and informal surrogates (family members or close friends) identified by health care professionals. Some states have statutes that specify a hierarchy of surrogate decision-makers to be consulted in cases of incapacity, and many health care institutions have policies that govern these interactions.

Surrogates make decisions based on one of two standards: substituted judgment or best interests. A substituted judgment standard is designed to have the surrogate determine what decision the patient would have made if he or she were competent. This is, of course, not an easy task and in many cases there may be limited evidence to help identify the appropriate choice. A best interests standard is used when there is little or no indication of the patient's preferences, or when the patient has never been competent. Decision-making for children and for developmentally disabled adults almost always uses a best interests standard. There are many complexities involved in the application of the standard and debates about the appropriate scope of surrogate decision-making, particularly in the end-of-life context. But these are beyond the scope of this chapter. One point that should be emphasized, however, is the importance of determining the capacity of the surrogate to make decisions. Like the patient, a surrogate must be competent and the norms described previously apply to the surrogate in cases of patient incapacity.

Capacity of Minors

The principle of respect for autonomy is less clearly applied to children than to adults (Goodlander and Berg 2011). Children develop the capacity for autonomous decision-making as they age, but there is wide variation among children even of the same age and significant disagreement about how much children should be involved in medical decision-making. The developmental literature provides some rough guidelines. Children under the age of 7 rarely have the capacity to make autonomous decisions. Children between 7 and 13 are developing the relevant capacities for autonomous decision-making. Children over the age of 14 usually demonstrate the same decision-making capacities as young adults between the ages of 18 and 21. Even at these later ages there are some developmental limitations in decision-making. For example, most individuals in these age groups lack significant life experiences; there is also some empirical evidence that the ability to evaluate long-term risks (particularly risks of death) are impaired in teens and juveniles. Nonetheless, all states set the age of majority for decision-making between 16 and 18, and some allow certain decisions before this cut off. It is important to remember that the age of majority is just the age at which the presumption of competence shifts. Before that age, the presumption is that the individual does not have capacity, and after that age the individual is presumed to have capacity. Evidence in a particular case may show either presumption to be incorrect (Blustein et al. 1999).

Because capacities are developing and should be respected, and because autonomy is valued at all stages, minors should be involved in decision-making to the extent they are able. In some cases a minor's assent to treatment will be sought (instead of a formal informed consent). In other cases a minor will be given full decision-making authority. Informed consent laws in different states recognize legal status such as mature minors and emancipated minors, and also grant decisional authority over certain types of care, such as those relating to birth control, treatment of sexually transmitted infections, and mental health or substances abuse treatment (Goodlander and Berg 2011). These latter statues are based mainly on public health rationales (e.g., it is better to allow access to the treatments in question regardless of autonomy), rather than a recognition of the minor's decision-making capacity. The laws in this area are silent on the question of whether to accept a minor's decision where there is clear evidence of incapacity either due to age or due to impairments. In other words, should the laws be viewed as simply shifting the presumption of capacity, as it is for adults, rather than granting legal authority regardless of capacity? For emancipated minors (i.e., a minor who has been determined by a court to meet specific statutory requirements for emancipation, based, for example, on marriage or participation in the armed forces), the legal presumption shifts, an emancipated minor who demonstrates impaired capacity should no more be permitted to make a decision than a legal adult who lacks capacity. The public health situations are trickier. The recognition of the public health goals may weigh in favor of a fairly low standard for capacity at least when making decisions in favor of treatment. Thus we may not scrutinize capacity for those minors who make decisions in favor of treatment to the same extent we do those who refuse recommended treatment. Essentially that is what the laws granting decisional authority are designed to do. As a practical matter, however, minors who chose not to seek treatment at all will not have their capacity evaluated. Those that do seek treatment may be more inclined to consent, so the distinction may have little impact. Moreover, there are various protections of minors' privacy and confidentiality that sometimes apply along with the grant of legal authority to consent. Thus, surrogate decision-making in these contexts may be more complex than the usual default of parental decision-making. This is an area that needs additional research.

Conclusion

Autonomy, particularly the right to make decisions as to one's body and health care, is deeply valued in American society. Promotion of autonomy requires that decisions be made by informed patients with sufficient decision-making capacity. Because the law protects a competent person's right to make a wide range of choices, it is important that competence determinations be based on more than just refusal to follow a physician's recommended treatment course. Instead, state legislatures (through statutes), courts (through competence hearings), and health care professionals (through clinical assessment of capacity) evaluate multiple aspects of decision-making ability. The abilities most often included in such evaluations include communication, understanding, appreciation, and rational manipulation. Adults are entitled to a strong and sometimes statutorily protected presumption of competence. Questions remain, however, regarding a number of points, including the best way to assess an individual's decision-making capacity; whether a threshold level of ability must be met on any aspect under evaluation (either qualitatively or quantitatively); and, in the case of minors, how to balance concerns about providing adequate protection, ensuring access to confidential treatment, and recognizing minors' varying development rates.

Fundamentally, informed consent represents a basic tension between our interests in promoting autonomy and protecting individuals from harm. Autonomy wins in most situations since the individual is generally best situated to determine their interests and thus maximize beneficence. But there are clearly cases in which patients are making choices that a treatment team and even family members believe are not in the patient's interest. In the absence of evidence of defects in capacity, voluntariness, or information disclosure, we may be limited in our legal ability to intervene. But ethics does not require we remain neutral in these situations; in certain cases it is appropriate to encourage patients to reconsider even fully autonomous decisions.

Related Topics

Chapter 16, "The Future of Informed Consent to Research: Reconceptualizing the Process," Paul Appelbaum
Chapter 21, "Autonomy," Catriona Mackenzie
Chapter 33, "Alzheimer's Disease: Quality of Life and the Goals of Care," Bruce Jennings

Bibliography

Alaska Statutes, annotated (2012) Section 13.26.0900: "Purpose and basis for guardianship." West.

Appelbaum, P.S. (2007) "Assessment of Patients' Competence to Consent to Treatment," *New England Journal of Medicine* 357: 1834–40.

Appelbaum, P.S. (2010) "Consent in Impaired Populations," *Current Neurology and Neuroscience Reports* 10: 367–73.

Berg, J.W., Appelbaum, P.S. and Grisso, T. (1996) "Constructing Competence: Formulating Standards of Legal Competence to Make Medical Decisions," *Rutgers Law Review* 48: 345–96.

Berg, J.W. Appelbaum, P.S. and Lidz, C.W. (2001) *Informed Consent: Legal Theory and Clinical Practice*, 2nd edition, New York: Oxford University Press.

Blustein, J., Levine, C. and Dubler, N. (eds.) (1999) *The Adolescent Alone: Decision Making in Health Care in the United States*, Cambridge: Cambridge University Press.

Buchanan, A.E. and Brock, D.W. (1989) *Deciding for Others: The Ethics of Surrogate Decision Making*, Cambridge: Cambridge University Press.

California Welfare and Institution Code, annotated (2012) Section 5331: "Evaluation on competency; effect; statement of California law."

Dunn, L.B., Nowrangi, M.A., Palmer, B.W., Jeste, D.V. and Sakes, E.R. (2006) "Assessing Decisional Capacity for Clinical Research or Treatment: A Review of Instruments," *American Journal of Psychiatry* 163: 1323–34.

Fisher, Jr., M.S. (2009) "Psychiatric Advance Directives and the Right to be Presumed Competent," *Journal of Contemporary Health Law and Policy* 25: 386–405.

Freedman, B. (1981) "Competence: Marginal and Otherwise," *International Journal of Law and Psychiatry* 4: 53–72.

Goodlander, E.C. and Berg, J.W. (2011) "Pediatric Decision-Making: Adolescent Patients" in *Clinical Ethics in Pediatrics, Section 1: Core Issues in Clinical Pediatric Ethics*, Cambridge: Cambridge University Press.

In re Conservatorship of Burton (2009) 88 Cal. Rptr. 3d 524 (Cal.).

In re L.A. (2006) 912 A.2d 977 (Vt.).

In re Roe (1992) 583 N.E.2d 1282 (Mass.).

In re Conroy (1985) 486 A.2d 1209 (N.J.).

Jones, R.C. and Holden, T. (2004) "A Guide to Assessing Decision-Making Capacity," *Cleveland Clinic Journal of Medicine* 71 (12): 971–5.

Lane v. Candura (1978) 376 N.E.2d 1232 (Mass. App. Ct.)

Texas Statutes and Codes, annotated (2011) Health and Safety Code Section 592.021: "Additional Rights." Vernon.

Vermont Statutes, annotated (2012) Section 7625: "Hearing on petition for involuntary medication; burden of proof." West.

White, B.C. (1994) *Competence to Consent*, Washington, DC: Georgetown University Press.

23
INCENTIVES IN HEALTH
Ethical Considerations

Richard Ashcroft

Introduction

The use of incentives is an increasingly popular technique in health promotion (Oliver and Brown 2012). The central idea is this. A person currently has a pattern of behavior which has an impact on their current or future health. Although adopting a different "health behavior" would improve their current or future health, they are unwilling or unable to do so. Other methods of changing this behavior (typically, advice and information-giving, or personal resolution-making) may have been tried but without any, or without consistent, success. The behavior itself may involve no direct harm to others, so that direct coercion may not be permissible. The behavior is sufficiently under the voluntary control of the person that a "hard paternalist" justification for forcibly changing the person's behavior for their own sake (as opposed to for the prevention of harm to others) is also lacking. Under these circumstances, an incentive may be offered to the person, in the hope that their desire for the incentive is sufficiently strong that they will change their behavior in order to earn the incentive. And further, having changed their behavior, and earned the incentive, their behavior will now not revert to the previous, undesirable behavioral pattern. Although this account of incentives gives a good indication of why incentives in health behavior change may be a good idea, there are some frequently identified moral problems which may afflict incentive schemes, at least sometimes. They may be coercive (the idea of "the offer you cannot refuse"); they may be corrupting (if people are induced by the offer of an incentive to act against their own principles or to seek to be paid where they should act from duty); they may be unfair (if some people are "rewarded" for a change in behavior but others are not, or if certain kinds of people are unfairly singled out for intervention where others are left alone).

Examples

This sketch is rather schematic, so here are some examples of practical incentives in healthcare. The standard case is smoking cessation. If I am a smoker, while there are a variety of reasons to limit my smoking where it imposes harm on others, few would argue that I should be prevented from smoking altogether, if I wish to smoke. But there is a weak public interest in encouraging me to give up smoking (because of the long-term costs my smoking imposes on the health system), and a soft paternalist reason to discourage me from smoking for my own sake (I may be irrationally discounting the future harms to my own health or simply unaware of them). Absent a notion that we have a duty to the commonweal to be as healthy as possible, these public good and soft paternalist reasons may warrant no more than informing and seeking to persuade me of the hazards of smoking and the benefits of quitting. However, most confirmed, habitual smokers do want to give up smoking. They fail to do so for many reasons, ranging from addiction, to social reinforcers that make smoking attractive (peer pressure, for instance), to the pains of withdrawal. In particular, while the health benefits of not smoking extend over one's whole lifetime, these are in an important way non-experiential. Being healthy is, for the most part, a state of *not* feeling ill. Illness has a rich phenomenology of pain, discomfort, impairment, and so on; whereas health only intermittently expresses itself as felt wellbeing and then usually only in contrast to recalled or anticipated illness or discomfort. The pains of quitting smoking are real, however, and are experienced directly; and so is the sense of desire and frustration which go along with wanting to smoke and trying not to give into that want. These pains and wants continue for quite a long time. Informally, smoking cessation experts say that it takes up to a year of confirmed non-smoking for a once-habitual smoker to become unlikely to start again.

A number of health promotion schemes have experimented with the use of incentives to help people quit smoking. Usually these are restricted to people who have already consulted smoking cessation services and have tried and failed to give up smoking for more than a few weeks. The incentive scheme usually works by offering small money payments at staged intervals over six to twelve months, with a relatively large completion incentive if the participant successfully quits smoking for the whole course of the scheme. Some schemes rely on self-reported non-smoking, but others use physiological tests to check whether the participant has smoked in the recent past. The total sums participants stand to gain are usually no more than a few hundred dollars, and it should be noted that these are usually much less than the money they will have saved by not purchasing tobacco products over the time they are participating in the scheme (Volpp et al. 2009).

The smoking cessation case is an example of an incentive offered to someone who wants to stop doing something, finds it hard to do so, and is seeking help. A different kind of incentive scheme is represented by an intervention tried in the UK to encourage teenage girls to undergo human papilloma virus (HPV) vaccination. In this case participants were offered a low-value shopping voucher, with receipt contingent on completing the vaccination schedule. HPV vaccination involves presenting on three occasions a few days apart to receive an injection of a vaccine, which is considered to be safe and effective in preventing HPV infections, which have been associated with an increased lifetime risk of cervical cancer. Because HPV is often transmitted sexually, it is thought that vaccinating teenagers before they become sexually active will confer the greatest benefit in terms of reducing their risk of infection. The nature of the vaccination is such that teenagers will typically be competent to consent to the vaccination, but being teenagers may be relatively risk prone, less likely than an adult to give thought to their lifetime health and the long-term consequences of their decisions, and so less than ideally likely to participate in a vaccination scheme merely because it is a good idea. Thus, participation rates will be lower than public health professionals would like, both in terms of individual protection and in terms of "herd immunity." As with smoking, the benefits of vaccination are remote in time; unlike smoking, the harm and discomfort associated with the intervention is rather small; and unlike smoking, to be successful the participant only needs to do something three times rather than adopt a whole new lifestyle. An incentive scheme like this one seeks to promote uptake of a beneficial service rather than long-term behavioral change (Mantzari et al. 2012).

Incentives can take many and various forms, and the debates can quickly become quite confusing. The type I have discussed in these two examples involves making small, definite positive payments to people to do something that is in their own interest, and is acknowledged by participants as being in their own interest, as a way of overcoming barriers to achieving people's own goals which reflect neither their own preferences nor rational choice. However, incentives may take a negative form: In so-called "pre-commitment" contracts, for example, someone may place a sum of money in trust for a set period, and if they fail to adhere to a planned change of behavior, they will lose that money (Karlan and Appel 2011). Incentives can also be uncertain: Many schemes offer people a lottery ticket rather than a definite sum of money (a chance of winning $500 rather than a certainty of winning $5). Incentives are not always targeted at the service user or citizen personally—many schemes involve making conditional payments to professionals, who must meet some service uptake or usage or measurable outcome target. And incentives can be hard to distinguish from schemes such as "conditional cash transfer" schemes in education or social policy, which combine elements of behavior change and welfare benefits in ways which have been quite controversial in the debates around welfare reform (*Journal of Applied Philosophy* 2004). For the purposes of this chapter I will concentrate on incentives to individuals who are seeking to change their own behavior, for health-related reasons, where these incentives are offered in a healthcare setting, rather than via other types of public or private service setting. For practical purposes it makes sense to call these individuals "patients," even when they may be neither ill nor consulting a healthcare professional at the point when they encounter the incentive scheme. We will assume that the incentive scheme is focused on health, and that it is operated and supervised by health professionals, be those doctors, nurses, midwives, or public health professionals.

Autonomy and Incentives: Coercion

In introducing incentives, I described a space in between the free, deliberate, and more or less unmediated decision of the individual and the forced choices or behaviors under coercion or hard paternalism. Here the person is the author of their own behavior but that behavior is influenced by the offer of an incentive (or series of incentives in a structured scheme) by a second party. Many of the moral issues arising in the use of incentive schemes turn on the autonomy-related questions arising in this space.

One straightforward question is whether incentives are coercive. Most readers will be familiar with the idea of an "offer you can't refuse," which apparently confers some benefit on the recipient, but on very disadvantageous terms, and in a form and in a context where there is no alternative but to accept. An incentive has the form of an offer, which requires a choice by the recipient: If you act in a certain way, you will gain the incentive; if you don't, you will not; but it is up to you whether or not to act in this way. However, although the incentive has the form of an offer, some offers will be instances of exploitation, others will be straightforward threats dressed up as offers. Three responses to this question come immediately to mind. The first is to accept that some incentives, or some schemes, or some incentives offered to people in some particular situations, may in fact be coercive. But unless we simply stipulate that coercion is always wrong, this simply redefines the problem as one of stating whether or not such incentives are unjustifiably coercive. It is the justification that will matter, rather than the coerciveness. The same applies to attempts to dismiss incentives as paternalistic: so they may be, but paternalism is sometimes justified. The second is to deny that incentives, when properly understood and properly formulated, are coercive in any reasonable sense of that term. The third is to hold that the claim that incentives are coercive is not so much wrong as misconceived.

The response that incentives are sometimes coercive, but that sometimes this coercion may be justified, is commonly mentioned, especially in media discussions of incentives (Parke et al. 2013; Promberger et al. 2011). As its features of interest depend on debates about justified coercion (and, relatedly, justified paternalism) that are outside the scope of this chapter, I set it aside (for a discussion of justified coercion, see Lamond 2001). The second response is more specific to incentives. Here the argument is that in its proper sense, an incentive must satisfy certain conditions if it is to be distinguished from a payment, a bribe, or an unfair inducement (much as we try to distinguish reasonable wages from tips, bribes and unfair exploitation). One element of an incentive is that it must be offered in a context where the recipient has an occurrent or potential desire to change their behavior in the direction signaled by the incentive, and that this desire is occurrent or potentially so in the absence of that incentive. Thus, the smoker must wish to give up smoking; the teenager would, other things being equal, wish to be vaccinated against HPV. The incentive should not be of a size or type, or offered in a context, such that it changes the desires of the recipient, or somehow overrides them, in a way which, absent the incentive, they would not endorse. If we accept this condition, then it is hard to see how an incentive could be coercive. What it may do is strengthen the determination to act on one's occurrent desire to quit smoking, or to consider one's preferences in such a way that one's potential desire to be vaccinated against HPV becomes occurrent. The HPV case is somewhat more difficult to defend than the smoking case, as the argument rests on a potential or all things considered desire in a set of circumstances where that desire is not occurrent or all things have not been considered (we are thinking of teenagers here!). It must be acknowledged that there is an element of paternalism here that will not go away, no matter how much we frame things in terms of autonomy and choice: We are only offering the incentive because, like the offer of HPV vaccination itself, we think it is a good thing, and it would be wise to take it up. Prior to the offer, the recipient may not have thought about HPV vaccination at all, or not have made up her (or, more recently as HPV vaccination has been opened to boys too, his) mind about it. But though the offer may have a paternalistic inspiration, the form of the offer, which permits refusal, and where the sums of money are small and refusable themselves should the individual actually prefer not to be vaccinated, is autonomy respecting. I do not propose to give a full set of necessary and sufficient conditions for an incentive to be non-coercive. The sketch of the argument is simply to show one illustrative way in which the characterization of incentives as coercive in form and essence may fail.

Turning to the third response to the coerciveness claim, the misconception argument, the main line of argument here is psychological. The thought is this: The argument from coercion sees the free and autonomous subject not doing something (being vaccinated) or doing something we think they should not (smoking); they do not respond to information, argument, or persuasion; so we offer an incentive, and lo! They change their behavior. This must be evidence, prima facie, of force. First, to head off one natural skeptical challenge to this argument, responding to an incentive rather than to a (verbal) reason looks like economic behavior rather than health behavior. It looks as if I was just waiting to see how much you will pay me to quit smoking, rather than making a decision to quit smoking because it is a good idea for me to quit smoking. So if I am quitting smoking for that sort of reason, it must be because your offer of an incentive is crowding out my underlying preference to smoke. It can be assumed that this is "really" my preference, because, absent your incentive, I *actually* carry on smoking, notwithstanding my *saying* that I really don't want to smoke. And in this line of thought it is assumed that once you take the incentive away, my real preference (for smoking) will reassert itself. This again is evidence that while I was not smoking it was due to your coercion, because as soon as you stop forcing me not to smoke, I start smoking again. Furthermore, the skeptical challenge goes, this is also evidence that incentive schemes don't even work because they don't really *reinforce* some hypothetical better self that really wants me to stop smoking. They simply "artificially" prevent me from smoking.

This skeptical argument appears quite ingenious: Some libertarians would favor incentives over legal prohibition or compulsion, because they leave room for choice. But the argument suggests that some incentives are coercive in a rather subtle way—the evidence for them being coercive is that once they are taken away, the behavior reverts to its former pattern. The misconception argument itself has two elements. The first is conceptual. It says that the reason the coercion argument here sketched fails is that people are not free autonomous subjects with reasonably robust sets of preferences that exist prior to our engagement with them. This model of psychological autonomy is incoherent. It depends on a model of the self which, since David Hume and Immanuel Kant, no philosopher can seriously subscribe to. I am not my preferences, nor are my preferences somehow constitutive of me and prior to my engagement in the social world. I have certain habitual traits and patterns of behavior and so on, but these are dynamic and shifting. There is no "authentic" self being traduced by these offers of incentives. To defeat the conceptual version of the misconception argument we need to supply an argument about the narrative coherence of the self which shows how a certain consistency in the stories we tell of ourselves is important morally, metaphysically, and practically (Korsgaard 2009).

This takes us to the second part of the misconception argument, which is empirical. Rather than theorizing about whether incentives normatively are coercive, and how people's preferences and behaviors change in the presence or absence of incentives of a certain kind, the claim here is that we need to do psychological experiments and build on psychological research which examines both what people actually do say about incentives, both as offered to themselves and as they are perceived when offered to third parties (in reality or hypothetically), and more importantly what they actually do in the context of incentive schemes and their alternatives. The flourishing emerging sciences of behavioral economics and experimental choice and decision theory are rich in such studies, though they are in the early days and most of the well known studies have rarely if ever been replicated. In a sense that point is *not* what these studies currently show, but rather that it is an empirical question, not a theoretical one, whether or not incentives are coercive; that is to say, whether they work through the same psychological mechanisms as paradigm cases of coercion. So far we have no reason to think that they do (Kahneman 2011).

Before moving on from coercion, we need to briefly consider incentives in the light of other more subtle kinds of influence: manipulation, persuasion, and nudging

(Wilkinson 2013). While the literature on the psychology and ethical issues relating to these kinds of influence is rich and growing, they are to some extent a distraction in the debate around incentives. To the extent that manipulation and nudging are attempts to trick subjects, to exploit their non-rational or imperfectly rational decision-making processes, incentive schemes are for the most part direct addresses to the person. The mode of address is essentially, "Here is something you want to do, but find difficult: How can we help?" In all the incentive schemes in health promotion that I have seen, there is a strong commitment both to explicit description of what the health behavior change sought is, why it is being sought, and the benefits and costs to the patient, and also of the incentive scheme itself, its structure, and how it is meant to assist the patient in changing his or her behavior. Informed consent *both* to the behavior change *and* to the incentive scheme is a central element.

There are two cases that do give us more pause for thought, however, and these relate to the relationship between incentives and persuasion. Persuasion seeks to influence the patient's thinking and behavior by giving explicit reasons, and seeking to have the patient take these up as her or his reasons for action (or desisting from action). As is well known, persuasion comes in many forms, and philosophers in particular are taught to be wary of rhetorical (as somehow distinguished from rational) persuasion. This can create difficulties when the patient's reasoning is either underdetermined or subject to strong non-rational influences. Consider the use of incentives in drug treatment (where it is more commonly known as "contingency management"). Here, a drug user will receive small payments each time he or she presents to treatment with a clean drug-testing sample, and a somewhat larger payment on successful completion of the program (rather like smoking cessation, but with the more complex social, legal, and psychological difficulties associated with unlawful drugs). Particularly for addictions to heroin and crack cocaine, the imperative to get hold of one's drug of choice can be very strong, and the person in treatment may be struggling rather desperately to stay clean and in treatment. It is often far from clear which of the patient's occurrent desires (to stay clean or get a fix) is predominant at any given time. He or she may seek the incentive both as a motivational aid to staying in treatment but also as a quick way to get money so as to get drugs (and thus drop out of treatment). The way the incentive tips and the impact it has in the context of the relationship with his or her clinician, are quite unpredictable. In this state of flux, it is not clear that the incentive acts as a reason or rational motivation in the right way.

Similarly, incentive schemes also exist to aid in keeping people with schizophrenia who live in the community in treatment; they can be offered small sums of money to attend clinics to receive depot injections of antipsychotic medication. The problem here is that they may be undecided as to whether they prefer the benefits of treatment over the harms of the side effects of treatment. The incentive may function as a way of stiffening their resolve to stay in treatment if they have decided that these benefits are what is important to them; or it may be that they tip their judgment in favor of treatment when the side effects are genuinely bad and they might otherwise drop out. The incentive acts to persuade them of the overall benefit of treatment. There is also the signaling effect: My clinician wishes me to stay in treatment and is giving me money to do so. The meaning of this in the context of the clinical relationship is subtle and complex. So in the drug treatment case, we may have situations where decision-making is less than rational, and the incentive is then processed in that unstable context; and in the schizophrenia treatment case it may resolve a conflict of values in a somewhat problematic way. The point is that *if* there is a conflict of values, would we be happy that the incentive could be the tie-breaker? The defense of incentives is that they are intended to aid someone in sticking to a decision once they've made it. But does this defense carry over to the case where the incentive feeds into the decision itself (Szmukler 2009)?

Autonomy and Incentives: Dignity

Bearing this discussion in mind, we now turn to another dimension of autonomy. This is not the psychological dimension of autonomy given prominence in Mill and liberal moral theory, but the moral dimension of autonomy given prominence by Kant. The concept here is not autonomy as freedom, so much as autonomy as dignity (Korsgaard 2009). The central thought here is that what matters in autonomy is moral responsibility for one's own actions and behavior. In particular, we need to pay close attention to *doing the right thing for the right reason*. Consider our patient with schizophrenia, who is currently taking antipsychotic medication and is, in psychiatric terms, "well," but who is suffering from medication side effects, and is genuinely in doubt as to whether he or she prefers being "well" with side effects or "ill" without. He or she may consider that even when "ill" he or she is not all that ill, and so medication is at best a mixed blessing, and at worst an unnecessary harm. Participation in an incentive scheme is offered to aid in keeping patients in treatment. The explicit logic of the scheme is that patients in the community may forget to attend clinics, lead chaotic lifestyles, or otherwise drop out of treatment for lifestyle reasons. Our patient decides all things considered to participate in the scheme and continue in treatment. The incentive has resolved the conflict of values and decision-making uncertainty. Two questions of reason-giving arise here. The first is whether the incentive is the *patient's* reason or whether patient has, heteronomously, acted on someone else's reason or perhaps failed to act on a moral reason at all and simply given into a desire (here, for the money incentive). The second concerns whether, if we accept that the patient has acted on a reason, it is the right *kind* of reason.

I propose that we set aside the question of heteronomy. In this scenario, the role of trust, the clinician–patient relationship, the decision-making capacity of the patient, and the background conditions of potential coercive treatment (the patient could be subject to compulsory treatment under law if her or his behavior warranted it) are such that these fall under quite general questions of coercion and paternalism in medical and psychiatric care. Incentives are not a particularly illuminating detail in those debates. In a context in which medical care may be inherently coercive (as much psychiatric treatment is), incentives in themselves may be more or less coercive than other kinds of treatment, but only marginally so. Compulsory detention or long-acting drug implants are more coercive than an offer of money, even if that offer is perceived as being coercive other things being equal. We have already touched on these issues above. So to develop our understanding of the morality of incentives, it is more interesting to look at the second issue: From the point of view of law and psychology the patient is choosing autonomously; but from the point of view of morality, there is a difficult question about the relevance of kinds of reason to the moral evaluation of a course of action.

Recent philosophical scholarship has revisited this question quite forcefully (Crisp 2006). In particular, the idea is that there are certain kinds of decision in which money can and does play a part, but it should not. Thus, if I have a wealthy relative whom I do not much love, but who gives me cash presents when I visit, the moral quality of my decision to visit him is diminished by the thought that it is the money, rather than the family bond, which motivates me to go. This argument has two basic forms. One is act-specific. The act itself is spoilt or corrupted by my offer or receipt of money where it does not belong. The other concerns the practice of which the act is an instance. By introducing money into a practice we corrupt the practice itself. No individual act may be corrupted, so to speak, but taken altogether, the set of acts constitutes the practice, and the practice loses or changes its moral quality. Take our HPV vaccination example for instance. One might feel that there is no particular wrong involved in offering a small incentive to any particular teenager to get vaccinated. However, if we come to expect that teenagers (and maybe others as well) will receive payments to be vaccinated, then the vision of vaccination as something which I do to protect myself, first of all, for my own sake, and second of all, to do my bit to promote the collective public health may be lost. It becomes something I do not want to do, and only do under sufferance, for a fee.

Some prominent commentators on incentives take this objection very seriously (for instance, Sandel 2012). However, it is very hard to substantiate. First of all, we can highlight an important feature of incentive schemes, which is that they carry meanings, and it is the meaning which is part of the mechanism. Consider smoking cessation schemes involving incentives. If they were simply "paying people to give up smoking," we have no reason to think that they would either be legitimate or justifiable. But, more importantly, there is no reason to think that they would work. There is no good reason to think that quitting smoking because I am paid to quit would be any more likely to succeed than quitting smoking because of the money I save by not smoking, or than simply trying to form my will not to smoke. Instead, we have to consider the form of the incentive and the way it works with the grain of individual psychology. An analogy can be made with going for a long run. I may set out to run a marathon. But a marathon is a long distance, and it takes a long time to complete. The pain and discouragement are present and real, the reward and pride are remote and imaginary. So, what many runners do is break down the distance into sections (quarter distance, half distance, laps, the distance to the next landmark, etc.) and focus on making it to the next waypoint, and then the next, until the race is run. Similarly, with smoking cessation, what incentives can do is set "waypoints" and small rewards to look forward to with an external party being responsible for confirming whether or not I've made it. It is the psychological structure which matters here, more than the money payments as such. The meaning of the payments and the way they fit into the resolve to quit smoking is more subtle than the critic has allowed, and it is not clear that, with this meaning in mind, the "practice" of smoking cessation has been corrupted.

Thus, while the corruption argument is telling and important, it is not general to all incentive schemes, from a conceptual point of view. Nor is it an a priori argument: It is an empirical one. It is a question of empirical sociology whether or not the introduction of incentive schemes in health promotion does have the consequences feared or not. This is a hard question to answer, either experimentally or using qualitative and historical methods. Insofar as empirical evidence exists, much of it is highly theory-laden in a non-trivial way (most studies rely rather uncritically on a distinction between intrinsic and extrinsic motivation which has rarely been articulated in any detail), and at least some points in the opposite direction. For example, "money" is not just one thing, with just one social significance; we have subtle ways of distinguishing gifts, tips, fees, or wages which depend on the context of giving, the identity and role of the donor, the scale of the sum involved, and so on (Zelizer 2011). It can be true that paying incentives to people can be a way to "govern" people, as Ruth W. Grant has suggested (Grant 2012). But it is not always true. And we don't currently have robust ways of sorting out good from bad incentives as a matter of principle. This throws us back on context, and on local ideas of acceptability, and on concrete evidence of effectiveness and specific mechanisms of action. The impact of incentives on the clinician–patient relationship are complex, for instance: As with any other kind of intervention, incentives must be offered in ways consistent with good medical practice and medical ethics. What we need not assume is that incentives are *inherently* destructive of good clinical relationships or necessarily a poor *substitute* for such relationships, although of course they could, under the wrong circumstances, be both.

Fairness

Beyond the moral effects on the recipient of the incentive (and on the donor), arguments from fairness are important. Incentives in health behavior change might be *distributively* unfair. Some people either never practice the (adverse) health behavior in question, or take responsibility for their (positive) health behaviors, without the need to be incentivized. Yet because of this, they are not eligible for incentivization. Symmetrically, if the incentive were actually universal, so that everyone gets the incentive *unless* they fail to quit smoking or get vaccinated, we could make an argument from the unfairness of using an incentive as a penalty. In the former, limited incentive case, we might argue that those who need to benefit from the incentive scheme are being rewarded for "bad" behavior or weakness of will, and we might be concerned that we are creating a perverse incentive to take up a bad behavior in order to get the incentive. In the latter, universal but conditional incentive case, we might argue that those who fail to meet the condition are more likely to be seriously ill or socially vulnerable and we are reinforcing that vulnerability both by stigma and by denial of what is otherwise a universal benefit. Interestingly, some critics of targeted incentives also level this criticism: Incentive schemes for some kinds of health behavior change (e.g. smoking cessation in pregnancy) may be criticized for focusing on the relatively poor, and thus stigmatizing them, giving them money which it may be relatively hard to refuse because of their low baseline income, and labeling the behaviors of the poor as something in which the State will take an interest while leaving behaviors of the rich untouched. While there is something to this (if we think of the way smoking is now much more common in low-income groups than in high-income groups across the West), it is also the case that the State has a legitimate interest in trying to relieve inequalities in health, as it does in trying to relieve inequalities in status, opportunity, and wealth (Oliver and Brown 2012).

One way to answer these objections is to argue that incentives are not different from medicines: They are offered as an intervention to improve health. They are not properly analogous to welfare benefits, and the arguments about conditionality and distribution which arise in the welfare context do not apply. Moreover, the scale of incentives is not usually such that forgoing them represents a significant loss to the individual (in comparison with the costs of continuing to purchase cigarettes, for instance). The specific fairness objections relating to varieties of moral hazard depend in part on whether they *actually* happen, and moreover if someone is irrational enough to change their behavior in a direction which is harmful to them in order to benefit from small cash payments they would be eligible to receive if they (successfully!) change their behavior back, then it is the irrationality, rather than the unfairness, which is probably of more concern from a health promotion point of view. Finally, it is worth noting that in the limited social surveys which have been done on incentives in behavior change, most respondents place more emphasis on the difficulty of achieving health behavior change than on the potential unfairness of making payments to people as a method for helping to bring about this change. So far as public acceptability is concerned, at least, it is more important to help people beat addictions (or serious mental health problems, or dangerous infectious diseases) with which they may need help than it is to worry about the relative *fairness* of different methods. Autonomy, however, remains central to any moral evaluation of incentives and indeed of behavior change programs more broadly (Promberger et al. 2011).

Related Topics

Chapter 19, "The Ethics of Incentives for Participation in Research: What's the Problem?" Alan Wertheimer
Chapter 21, "Autonomy," Catriona Mackenzie
Chapter 22, "Capacity and Competence," Jessica Berg and Katherine Shaw Makielski

References

Crisp, R. (2006) *Reasons and the Good*, Oxford: Oxford University Press.

Grant, R.W. (2012) *Strings Attached: Untangling the Ethics of Incentives*, Princeton, NJ: Princeton University Press.

Journal of Applied Philosophy (2004) Special Issue: Philosophical Justifications of Workfare, 21 (3): 239–320.

Kahneman, D. (2011) *Thinking, Fast and Slow*, London: Allen Lane.

Karlan, D. and Appel, J. (2011) *More Than Good Intentions: How a New Economics Is Helping to Solve Global Poverty*, New York: Dutton.

Korsgaard, C.M. (2009) *Self-Constitution: Agency, Identity and Integrity*, Oxford: Oxford University Press.

Lamond, G. (2001) "Coercion and the Nature of Law," *Legal Theory* 7: 35–57.

Mantzari, E., Vogt, F. and Marteau, T.M. (2012) "Using Financial Incentives to Increase Initial Uptake and Completion of HPV Vaccinations: Protocol for a Randomized Controlled Trial," *BMC Health Services Research* 12: 301–7.

Oliver, A. and Brown, L.D. (2012) "A Consideration of User Financial Incentives to Address Health Inequalities," *Journal of Health Economics, Policy and Law* 37 (2): 201–26.

Parke, H., Ashcroft, R.E., Brown, R.C.H., Marteau, T.M. and Seale, C. (2013) "Financial Incentives to Encourage Healthy Behaviour: An Analysis of UK Media Coverage," *Health Expectations* 16 (3): 292–304.

Promberger, M., Brown, R.C.H., Ashcroft, R.E. and Marteau, T.M. (2011) "Acceptability of Financial Incentives to Improve Health Outcomes in US and UK Samples," *Journal of Medical Ethics* 37: 682–7.

Sandel, M. (2012) *What Money Can't Buy: The Moral Limits of Markets*, London: Allen Lane.

Szmukler, G. (2009) "Financial Incentives for Patients in the Treatment of Psychosis," *Journal of Medical Ethics* 35: 224–8.

Volpp, K.G., Troxel, A.B., Pauly, M.V., Glick, H.A., Puig, A., Asch, D.A. et al. (2009) "A Randomized, Controlled Trial of Financial Incentives for Smoking Cessation," *New England Journal of Medicine* 360: 699–709.

Wilkinson, T.M. (2013) "Nudging and Manipulation," *Political Studies* 61: 341–55.

Zelizer, V.A. (2011) *Economic Lives: How Culture Shapes the Economy*, Princeton, NJ: Princeton University Press.

24
PRIVACY, SURVEILLANCE, AND AUTONOMY

Alan Rubel

Introduction

We all like at least some privacy, and there isn't much dispute that privacy in health and medical information matters. This is for a variety reasons. One is that support for privacy protections is strong; public opinion research consistently indicates that persons care deeply about health privacy. Another is that health privacy has significant historical roots, dating back to the provisions for physician–patient confidentiality in the Hippocratic Oath. The popular appeal and historical protections for health privacy make sense because privacy implicates important interests. Information about a person's health can be used to deny that person employment, financial, or other opportunities; and learning about a person's medical condition may lead others to define or view that person disproportionately in light of that condition. Accordingly, there are a variety of legal protections for health information privacy. In the U.S., these include the *Health Insurance Portability and Accountability Act*, the *Genetic Information Nondiscrimination Act*, and the *Common Rule* covering certain human subjects research.

But the sheer usefulness of health information creates enormous pressure for access. Information about disease incidence aids in protecting public health; information about the behavior of patients is useful in providing care; information about drug prescribing and use can help in enforcing drugs laws; and many kinds of health information can serve as data for research. Health information can also be important for democratic governance: Health information may be relevant in determining candidates' fitness for public office, and government transparency may require that people have access to information about government-provided health services, even where that information contains individually identifiable information.

The importance of health privacy and the usefulness of individual health information give rise to a variety of conflicts about the extent to which it is justifiable to collect and disseminate health information. In order to make sense of these conflicts, it will be useful to first examine what privacy is and why it is valuable (*if* and *when* it is valuable).

What Is Privacy?

There are a number of different accounts of the nature of privacy. One important divide in the literature is whether privacy is primarily about others' access to one's personal information or whether it is primarily about one's control over personal information. On access views, a person has privacy with respect to one's information just in case others are unable to learn of, physically obtain, or otherwise have that information (Allen 1988: 15; Gavison 1984: 347). There is a dispute about what the nature of that access is. Is another person's physical access to information enough for there to be a privacy loss, such that a person who can physically examine another's personal information, but doesn't, diminishes the privacy of those persons with information in the database? Or is it instead that *cognitive* access is required, such that one must actually learn information about the individuals (Powers 1996)? Must another person know some *fact* about another for her to lose privacy, or is it enough that she have a reasonable belief about her (Parent 1983; Rubel 2011: 280–4)? Regardless, the key to any of these access views is that privacy turns on what other persons are able to do with one's information, and not on one's own power to act.

In contrast, control accounts emphasize one's ability to make decisions about one's information. On these views, one has privacy only if she can actually exercise power over her information, for example by granting or denying others access (Westin 1967: 7; Inness 1992: 41–55; Fried 1970: 140–1). To see the difference, consider the case of a person leaving a version of his medical record on the seat of a city bus. On control views, he has lost privacy with respect to that record regardless of whether anyone actually picks up the record and examines it. On access views, that loss of control does not entail that his privacy is diminished.

Whether or not one controls information will on most accounts matter morally; we often care about protections for personal information because we want the power to choose who can access it. This points to a different divide regarding the nature of privacy: Morally neutral (descriptive) accounts and normative accounts. In her influential book, Judith DeCew maintains that privacy pertains to information that "is not generally—that is, according to a reasonable person under normal circumstances . . . a legitimate concern of others" (DeCew 1997: 58). This view builds in the idea of *legitimate* concern into privacy, and hence privacy is by definition morally weighty. Morally neutral accounts allow that one can have privacy even in information that is mundane, such as one's location when he walks down a public street, or that is the legitimate concern of others, such as whether one committed a crime. On these views, the moral question comes in determining what sort of information one has a claim or legitimate interest in keeping private (Moore 2010: 26–7).

For our purposes here, it is useful to navigate these conflicting accounts by stipulating several things. First, privacy concerns access to information. Second, only some information is weighty enough that one could have a legitimate claim to prevent others from having access to it. And control of one's information, or control over that information that one has a legitimate interest in keeping others from accessing, is at least prima facie morally important. This leaves open the question of what information one can legitimately prevent others from accessing. To answer that question requires looking at underlying moral justifications for privacy and specifically health privacy.

Why Health Privacy?

Why should we protect privacy in health information at all? That is, why should we consider the ability to restrict others' access to individuals' health information morally important? To begin, it's at least intuitively plausible that persons have a claim to limit others' access to their health information; otherwise, it would be utterly unproblematic for physicians, insurers, records managers, researchers, and so forth to share indiscriminately all of one's test results, records of doctor visits, prescription information, and so forth. But to make the case that privacy protections are justified, we will need a fuller explanation.

One possibility is that privacy protections are justified by the potential negative effects of information disclosure on persons' welfare. For example, a lack of privacy may undermine persons' healthcare: Where individuals worry about privacy regarding their medical information, they are likely to engage in "privacy protective" behaviors, such as lying to their care providers, seeing multiple providers, using different pharmacies, not participating in research, and paying in cash rather than using insurance (Goldman 1998: 49; California Healthcare Foundation 2010: 20). Likewise, privacy may increase or protect one's opportunities. Information about a person's health status, medical history, or genetic attributes may undermine her employment prospects, insurance eligibility, financial backing, promotion potential, or opportunities for positions of responsibility. Privacy may also protect people from stigma. Some may believe that aspects of a person's health and medical status reflect negatively on that person (for example, sexually transmitted infections, mental illnesses, some chronic diseases). Hence, where others learn that one has such a condition, she may lose some degree of social esteem.

Although the possibility of negative effects on persons' welfare provides a plausible ground for protecting health privacy, it has important limitations. The fact that people engage in privacy protective behaviors when they worry about health privacy is a reason to protect privacy only on the assumption that doing so will engender trust among patients and lead them to optimize care decisions. Trust, however, is based on *beliefs* about information privacy and security. Suppose that instead of working to secure persons' health information, we sought merely to deceive them about potential negative consequences of disclosing their health information and convincing them that their information is far more secure than it actually is. By doing so we might achieve the result of people optimizing their care and therefore having better results. Surely, though, it is wrong to mislead people about such important matters. The wrongness cannot be attributed to the negative effects on persons' welfare—the effects of the deceit are actually beneficial to persons' welfare.

Rather, the wrongness is based on deceit, which is an affront to their *autonomy*. Autonomy is a complex concept, and there are a number of controversies about its nature, scope, and moral weight, as discussed in several chapters in this volume (see "Related Topics" at the end of this chapter). Nonetheless, autonomy at least includes the ability to govern oneself and make important decisions according to one's own reasons and values, to the extent that one sees fit. Deceit is an affront to autonomy because it short-circuits a person's decision-making capability and her ability to act according to her own reasons. Thus, deceiving persons regarding the status of their health information might have beneficial consequences for their welfare but be morally unjustifiable because it impinges their autonomy.

Consider next the possibility that persons could lose some opportunity or suffer some material harm by disclosure of health information. Certainly that would be a negative effect from the standpoint of the person whose information is disclosed, but it is not clear that such consequences could justify privacy protections as a general matter. Richard Posner has famously argued that insofar as individuals seek to protect from disclosure only "discrediting" information (that is, people tend to advertise information favorable to their prospects and conceal information that is unfavorable), it is likely more efficient from the standpoint of social welfare to not protect individual privacy in most cases (Posner 1984). Posner's argument turns on the difference between consequences for an individual—perhaps loss of some opportunity—and overall consequences for society. It could be the case that if employers, financiers, insurers, and so forth had more information that was disadvantageous to some individuals, they could make better decisions, and aggregate social welfare would increase through better employment decisions, sounder financing schemes, lower insurance premiums, and the like (though at the expense of those persons who lose out on opportunities).

One might doubt whether this would actually come to pass—decision-makers might give undue weight to medical information. Alternatively, one might doubt that the proper measure for determining whether privacy protections are justified is aggregate social welfare. Perhaps instead the right question to ask is whether denying persons opportunities on the basis of health information is *unfair* or *discriminatory*. Such an argument based on unfairness or discrimination can be understood as an appeal to autonomy. The ability to self-govern includes the ability to exercise a degree of choice over important aspects of one's life and to navigate one's life according to values that are one's own. Whether one can secure employment, financial backing, insurance, or positions of responsibility are important in modern society, and it is exceedingly difficult to participate as a full member of society if one is precluded from these opportunities. Having one's ability to participate as a full member of society restricted for reasons that are largely out of her control—for example because of information regarding her health—therefore imposes an important limit on one's ability to exercise choice over her life and to navigate her life according to her values. As such, it is a limitation on a person's autonomy. There remain questions about whether it is the responsibility of employers, financiers, and others to ensure availability of opportunities. Nonetheless, if privacy is to be justified on the grounds of preserving opportunities, it is at least partially a matter of autonomy rather than overall welfare.

So, while appealing to welfare can provide some grounds for privacy protections, welfare-based protections are buoyed by the value of individual autonomy. Privacy protections may also be justified by direct appeal to individual autonomy, either insofar as privacy is an important object of autonomous choice or insofar as privacy is an important condition for exercising autonomy. These views are sometimes referred to as "personhood" or "personal dignity" accounts of privacy's value (Allen 1988: 43).

Privacy is an object of autonomous choice to the extent that individuals value privacy and conceive of their goals and projects as being their own, and not for others' observation. Persons are capable of choosing for themselves what is of value in their lives. In many cases what people value will include existing, acting, and making decisions privately, without the scrutiny of others. That valuation provides a reason for respecting privacy, at least with respect to self-regarding actions. Moreover, others' knowledge of important facts about a person affects the nature and meaning of the choices she makes (Benn 1984: 228–9). That is, whether one engages in an action might have a different meaning to her depending on whether she believes it is done without others' knowledge or with others' knowledge. In other words, privacy is important to individuals and is a constituent part of the actions and projects they choose. Note that the way privacy is incorporated into one's values is independent of any harms or negative effects that might result from information disclosure. One might want her medical records to remain private with respect to her employers, business investors, or the general public even if the information in those records were *beneficial*—for example if her records showed her to be the very picture of good health. Where one values having privacy, and where privacy is an important element of the life one wishes to lead, privacy is valuable not because it increases one's welfare—perhaps it does, perhaps it doesn't. Rather, it is valuable because it is a constituent part of the sort of life that she considers valuable (see Raz 1988: 200–1 for an account of constitutive value). Failure to give weight to that value results in a failure to give weight to autonomy.

There is ample reason to think people place this sort of value on health information privacy. As noted, there is evidence that people engage in privacy-protective behavior when they worry about disclosure of health information. Focus group research conducted in numerous cities has revealed that concerns about privacy form an important barrier in getting people to participate in large cohort medical research (Krane 2007; Williams et al. 2009). A study conducted by the Gallup Organization (2000) found that almost 80 percent of its respondents were concerned about their medical information privacy, and over 90 percent thought that genetic research was particularly important from the standpoint of privacy. And public opinion surveys regarding biobank research indicate that a majority of respondents would participate in biobank research, but 90 percent would have concerns about their privacy (Kaufman et al. 2009).

A different way that privacy is relevant to autonomy is that privacy can be a *condition* for autonomy. Others' scrutiny of one's opinions, aspirations, and feelings can have a leveling or homogenizing effect, such that important decisions are less the product of one's own values and deliberations. Implicitly incorporating others' views into one's important, self-regarding choices diminishes the extent to which those choices are the agent's own (Bloustein 1964: 187–8; see also Reiman 1976). More important in this regard is that privacy protections create the conditions necessary to exercise autonomy in human relationships. People maintain many, highly varied relations, ranging from deeply intimate friendly and familial relationships to arm's length business relationships. Appropriate information disclosure is important to each (Fried 1970: 140–4; Rachels 1975: 326). For example, part of what it means to be a close friend is choosing to share important information; it would be difficult to say that a person is a close friend if one never shared anything important and personal with that person. In contrast, keeping the appropriate distance in business relationships involves limiting disclosures of personal but irrelevant information.

The inability to choose what information to share with friends or choose the information available to business relations makes one less able to steer those relationships. Moreover, the relationships individuals enter and how they decide to navigate those relationships are among the most important ways we use our values, goals, and projects to steer the course of our lives. Selective disclosure of information in the context of relationships is vital to exercising autonomy. And where one cannot selectively choose to disclose important information in entering many and varied relationships, autonomy is circumscribed. Hence, privacy protections for important information, which allow individuals to decide when, how, and with whom to share information, are thus important in their exercising autonomy over a fundamental aspect of life. Privacy with respect to health information is crucial here, as it is often the case that sharing or not sharing health information is part of what defines one's relationships.

Health Privacy Disputes

The tensions between desire for privacy, underlying justifications for privacy protections, and usefulness of health information become clearer when we examine health information and privacy in several controversial contexts.

Public Health Surveillance: Overriding Autonomy Interests for General Welfare

One conflict concerns health information in which individuals have an autonomy interest, but which is particularly important for social welfare. Consider public health surveillance.

Surveillance is central to efforts of public health organizations in assessing the status of public health, establishing priorities, detecting epidemics, monitoring disease, and assessing programs (Thacker et al. 2003). Some data collected for the sake of public health, such as vital statistics and environmental data, do not have serious health privacy implications. But public health surveillance also includes mandatory, named reporting of various diseases and development of disease registries that track individuals with certain conditions over time. In the U.S., individual states require care providers and laboratories to report cases of (among other things) infectious diseases such as tuberculosis (TB), HIV/AIDS, and syphilis. In addition, there are registries for non-infectious diseases, including cancer, occupational disease, and lead poisoning in children (Fairchild et al. 2007; Chamany et al. 2009: 561). A particularly controversial case is New York City's recent mandate that city laboratories report by name results of A1C (blood glucose) tests in an effort to address the growing diabetes problem. The reporting is coupled with a pilot program in which residents of certain areas with particularly high rates of diabetes will have their providers notified when test results are elevated (Fairchild and Alkon 2007; Goldman et al. 2008).

Mandatory, named reporting of diseases to public health entities clearly conflicts with individual privacy regarding health information. Surely, though, at least some types of public health surveillance are morally justified. Consider TB, which is infectious, largely treatable with antibiotics, serious and potentially fatal without treatment, and historically lethal. If mandatory reporting of TB (including multiple-drug resistant strains, which are particularly worrisome from the standpoint of public health) is an effective part of efforts to prevent others from becoming infected (and preventing some from dying), it is hard to see how persons' autonomy interests in privacy could provide a compelling case against reporting. The difficulty comes in determining how to resolve cases that are less clear cut. The approach currently employed by the U.S. Centers for Disease Control and Prevention and by state and local health departments is to distinguish between public health research, for which there should be privacy protections such as those required for all health research, and public health practice, which warrants less privacy protection (Gostin 2008: 309). This approach is problematic for several reasons, including the difficulty of distinguishing research and practice and the distinction's failure to track anything of independent moral importance (Fairchild and Bayer 2004; Mariner 2007: 374; Rubel 2012: 6).

Another possibility is to turn to moral principles underwriting public health surveillance and protections for individual medical privacy. Public health entities are centrally concerned with health issues at the population level, in contrast to clinicians who have responsibilities to individual patients and researchers who have responsibilities to protocols and the scientific enterprise (Rothstein 2002: 145; Institute of Medicine 1988: 19). Public health surveillance may therefore be understood as a mechanism of protecting overall health and welfare (see Parmet 2009), and surveillance efforts will be justified to the extent that they lead to greater, aggregated health of the members of a population.

But how should we justify privacy protections—should *any* increase in aggregate welfare warrant surveillance efforts? Consider first the view that privacy protections should be based on consequences for persons' welfare. Where individuals are likely to engage in the sorts of privacy-protective behaviors discussed above, surveillance efforts might have deleterious effects on their health and in the case of infectious disease, the health of others. For example, in the early days of HIV/AIDS testing in the U.S., many activists and public health officials opposed mandatory reporting of the names of infected individuals to confidential state registries for fear that it might dramatically reduce voluntary testing and counseling, and hence would increase infection rates (Bayer 1991). Those effects, however, fit easily within the view that public health should promote aggregate health within the population. That is, if the effects are large, and lots of people avoid care, then they would undermine the very rationale justifying the surveillance in the first instance.

A different welfare argument for protecting privacy is that if others were to learn the identities of persons with reportable diseases, it could harm their employment, social, financial, and other prospects. Protecting individuals from harms to opportunities can be addressed within the context of public health surveillance by placing restrictions on those who can access information in disease registries. This seems to be the strategy employed by the New York City public health department in its diabetes surveillance initiative. In defending the initiative, department members have pointed out that information collected is more difficult to access than information collected for other disease registries (Chamany et al. 2009: 560).

But neither of these rationales accounts for persons' autonomy interests in privacy regarding health information. A different approach is to take seriously the idea that persons have important autonomy interests in privacy and then consider the conditions under which it is justifiable for a society to subordinate that autonomy interest. One possible dividing line is where a person's maintaining privacy in her health information unreasonably threatens others' health, for example by making it likely that they will become seriously ill or die (Rubel 2012). On this view, mandatory reporting of serious infectious diseases would be justified because keeping private the fact that one has such a disease makes it likely that others will contract the disease and become seriously ill or die. Likewise, reporting of diseases could be justified if the knowledge obtained is necessary for controlling the disease. However, where the reporting primarily redounds to the benefit of the person whose information is reported, it is more difficult to see how it can be justifiable to subordinate persons' autonomy interests in keeping the information private. Of course, the information could be collected *voluntarily*, for that would be a means of allowing persons to make the reporting decisions according to their own reasons and values.

Whole Genome Sequencing: Autonomy and the Ability to Share

Respect for autonomy does not always weigh in favor of greater privacy protections. As discussed, privacy protections are either buoyed by autonomy, the object of autonomous choices, or a condition of autonomous choice. But because autonomy includes the ability to act according to one's reasons and values as one sees fit, one may choose to diminish one's own privacy by sharing information. Prohibiting outright persons from sharing their health information would likewise restrict persons' autonomy by preventing them from sharing information where doing so comports with their values and reasons.

Consider the case of whole genome sequencing in the context of medical research and in clinical practice. Since the human genome was first sequenced in the early 2000s, there have been substantial advances in genomic research. One such advance is the capacity to sequence individuals' entire genomes. It is projected that sequencing a single person's entire genome will soon cost as little as $1000 (PCSBI 2012: 22). The ability to store entire genomes, correlate them with health conditions, and compare the genomes of a growing number of people promises significant advances for medical research and clinical practice. Whole genome sequencing has already aided care providers in identifying and treating rare diseases, and the hope is that it will lead to greater personalization of medicine (e.g., by identifying promising interventions based on individuals' genomes) and identification of genetic variants that correlate with specific diseases (PCSBI 2012: 19–20). For example, discoveries of genetic variants that make one more susceptible to diseases like diabetes, Alzheimer's disease, cancer, and heart disease may lead to better clinical outcomes.

However, as the predictive value of whole genome sequencing rises—that is, as the number of conditions known to correlate to particular gene variants grows—there is greater potential harm to individuals who have their genomes sequenced. If others have access to an individual's genomic information, they may be able to make inferences about that person's health prospects. This has important implications for persons' welfare, for the reasons discussed above. It is also important insofar as there is the potential for persons to experience psychological harms should they learn that they have variants associated with diseases that will become manifest in the future (Powers 2008).

It would seem that protecting genomic information as a general matter is important for preventing such potential harms. Doing so would also give persons the opportunity to disclose their own information selectively, according to their values as they see fit. In light of vast and growing amount of information shared via social networks, and the widespread appeal of participating in such networks, it is plausible that many people will value the opportunity to share genomic information. That is, they could exercise autonomy in deciding to share their information as part of the research enterprise, to aid clinicians in their care, and potentially with others sharing similar conditions in order to build community. But the case for autonomy-based sharing is not clear cut. For one, the degree to which persons' decisions to share information would be autonomous is unclear. The potential of whole genome sequencing is largely unrealized, and we cannot anticipate just what research will reveal (PCSBI 2012: 18). This uncertainty undermines the degree to which consent to information sharing is informed, and hence the degree to which it is autonomous.

Moreover, there are cases where it is justifiable to limit persons' exercise of autonomy for paternalistic reasons. Anita Allen has argued that if privacy is important enough, it is justifiable to paternalistically protect privacy, which could include preventing certain types of information disclosures (Allen 2011). Note, too, that there may be negative consequences should people extensively exercise choice regarding use of their information. For example, if people can control what types of research to which they will contribute information, or if they can withhold information from endeavors that benefit from large datasets, they could undermine research results and hinder public benefits (Gostin 2009).

Exercising autonomy by sharing genetic information carries different sorts of risks than participating in other sorts of research. By sharing genetic information, one also shares information about one's family members. Hence, the risks of stigma, discrimination, and psychological stress extend to others. A related issue has to do with discrete groups of people who share genetic traits. One famous example regards DNA samples collected from members of the Havasupai Tribe in the Southwest U.S. for the purpose of diabetes research (see Chapter 17 in this volume). These samples were subsequently used without further consent for different research, including studies on schizophrenia, historic migration patterns, and inbreeding (Lee et al. 2009). Because such research bears upon all members of the group, the decision to share information implicated the interests of many persons other than those who agreed to share information. Note that determining what consent procedures are appropriate in such circumstances is particularly difficult.

In the final analysis, it may be that persons should be able to choose to share their genomic information. That is the conclusion of the Presidential Commission for the Study of Bioethical Issues, which has recommended that persons have the opportunity to share their information, though noting that such sharing should occur only with robust consent procedures and against a background of strong privacy protections (PCSBI 2012: 74, 91). Nonetheless, because knowledge of what genomic research will uncover is limited and because decisions to disclose directly implicate others, the autonomy issues surrounding privacy in genomic information are not clear cut.

Privacy and Democratic Principles

Privacy protections for health information can also conflict with democratic principles, which are on many accounts justified by autonomy. For example, health information may be relevant to electoral decisions. It may also be part of government records to which the public should have access.

Suppose that a candidate for public office has been diagnosed with a terminal disease, and it is likely that she will not survive her first year in office. A different candidate has a family history of heart disease, but is himself in good health. It would seem unfair and distracting to make the second candidate's medical record (including his family history) available to the public and hence a campaign issue. However, it also seems reasonable that the health information about the first candidate is relevant and important for voters to know. But is that correct? Why should candidate health information matter at all, and why should voters have access to any information? Addressing the issue will pit candidates' autonomy interests in health privacy against voter autonomy interests based in democratic principles.

Democratic theory relies on individual autonomy in the practice of political representation and in the right to vote, which are essential to any plausible conception of democracy. There are competing views of why liberal democracy is a justified form of government. Some accounts maintain states are legitimate, and can command authority, only insofar as they enjoy the consent (either explicit or tacit) of the governed (Locke 2009; Estlund 2008). Others locate the legitimacy and authority of democratic, representative government in its consequences; such a government leads to better outcomes for persons living under it (Mill 1859; Raz 1988). But in either case, exercising the right to vote is important insofar as it allows persons to exercise their wills in political processes, and this requires persons do so autonomously (Schauer 2000: 307–8). After all, coerced and purchased votes are under no plausible view legitimate. And adequate information is required to ensure that votes are actually cast autonomously. Without good information, an electoral choice may not be based on a person's own values and reasons, much as a person's consent to a medical procedure is inadequate where she is not provided important, relevant information.

The question here is when, and to what degree, persons' health and medical information should be disclosed based on liberal, democratic principles. In at least a few cases, it would appear that some medical information about candidates for elected office is important in order to ensure that votes for that candidate are based on sufficient information that they are cast autonomously. Consider that several U.S. presidential candidates, including John F. Kennedy, have had health risks that they have kept secret from voters; in some cases those risks have been serious enough that there was a substantial risk that they would be unable to fulfill the tasks of office. This possibility raises several questions. First, do candidates for office have some duty to disclose serious medical conditions to the electorate? Streiffer et al. (2006) argued that there *is* such a duty for presidential candidates where the condition is likely to undermine the candidate's ability to complete the "core functions" of office. That duty is based on persons' rights in a liberal democracy to be governed with their consent.

A further question is whether laws can be justified requiring candidates to disclose serious medical conditions to voters or representatives upon seeking office. This is a more difficult question. Such a requirement might undermine its very purpose by deterring good candidates from seeking care for health issues, thereby jeopardizing their ability to fulfill the responsibilities of office (Annas 1995: 948). Also problematic is that disclosure requirements could serve to derail campaigns, causing them to focus on claims about candidates' health rather than on more substantive issues (Annas 1995: 948). But what, if any, health information is actually relevant to persons' decisions about voting? Frederick Schauer argues that people in a democracy have not only the right to make electoral decisions autonomously, but also the right to decide what information is a relevant basis for that choice (Schauer 2000: 303–6). This would appear to imply that any health information about any candidate could be relevant. Surely, though, some medical information is either unrelated to the ability to perform the functions of office (prior minor illnesses, ancestry) or important only in light of unreasonable prejudices (sexual history, minor mental health issues) such that disclosure is not warranted by autonomy interests. Finally, if there is a duty to disclose, and if it is justifiable to require disclosure, there remains a question as to how broadly that requirement ought apply. The President of the United States, for example, is in many ways a special case due to the scope of presidential power. The extent to which disclosure and disclosure laws are appropriate for that office need not apply to positions where the consequences for health problems are not as great.

A different health privacy issue concerns the democratic principle of open government, or the idea that governments ought to be transparent about their policies and workings. Transparency is encoded in a variety of laws requiring that government bodies meet in public, that information collected and held by state actors be accessible to the public, and that members of the public have the right to speak freely about government information. This principle of publicity can be justified both on consequentialist grounds (publicity helps ensure good government) and on autonomy grounds (publicity of government policies and information is necessary to secure either tacit or explicit consent) (Gutmann and Thompson 1996: 97–101).

This creates a conflict when state actors provide key medical services. Consider, for example, state coordination and provision of emergency medical services. In the U.S. and elsewhere, emergency medical services (along with other emergencies, such as police and fire protection) originate with calls to a centralized number (9-1-1 in the U.S.). Dispatchers collect information from a caller and relay it to others who respond to the emergency. Calls to 9-1-1 are generally recorded, and in most states these recordings are public records. Hence, they are available to the public by request. Because such calls often contain personal health information—names, addresses, symptoms, history, and so forth—there is a conflict between interests in open government and interests in health information privacy. It is easy to see why such information would be important from the standpoint of transparency. People may wish to know how responsive emergency services are to different locations and different conditions, or to hear how personnel respond to particular, important cases. Investigating such issues is surely part of exercising one's autonomy within a democratic society. But whether that interest suffices to override persons' privacy interests, also grounded in autonomy, is unclear.

Conclusion

Regardless of the particular conception of privacy, the moral importance of health information privacy depends on autonomy, either in support of welfare-based justifications for privacy, as an object of autonomous values, or as a condition for autonomy. But that only goes so far in determining what privacy protections are justified. Privacy in health information may conflict with others' welfare, as illustrated by the public health surveillance issue. The choice to share information may be important enough or implicate others' interests sufficiently that we might consider constraints on sharing, as illustrated by the whole genome sequencing case. And privacy protections, themselves based on autonomy interests, may frustrate others' autonomy in a democratic state. There are myriad other health privacy issues out there, such as the moral basis for physician–patient confidentiality, the relation between privacy regarding information and privacy of health decision-making, and the testing of students, athletes, and employees for drug use. Nonetheless, these issues often track the same conflicts—between others' welfare and individuals' autonomy interests, between an individual's autonomy interest and her own welfare interest, and between one's autonomy interest in privacy and others' autonomy interest in information.

Related Topics

Chapter 17, "Ethical Issues in Genetic Research," Dena S. Davis
Chapter 21, "Autonomy," Catriona Mackenzie
Chapter 25, "Public Health and Civil Liberties: Resolving Conflicts," James F. Childress

References

Allen, A.L. (1988) *Uneasy Access: Privacy for Women in a Free Society*, Totowa, NJ: Rowman & Littlefield.

Allen, A.L. (2011) *Unpopular Privacy: What Must We Hide?* New York: Oxford University Press.

Annas, G.J. (1995) "The Health of the President and Presidential Candidates: The Public's Right to Know," *New England Journal of Medicine* 333: 945–9.

Bayer, R. (1991) "Public Health Policy and the AIDS Epidemic," *New England Journal of Medicine*, 324: 1500–4

Benn, S.I. (1984) "Privacy, Freedom, and Respect for Persons," in F.D. Schoeman (ed.) *Philosophical Dimensions of Privacy: An Anthology*, New York: Cambridge University Press.

Bloustein, E. (1964) "Privacy as an Aspect of Human Dignity: An Answer to Dean Prosser," *New York University Law Review* 39: 962–1007.

California Healthcare Foundation (2010) *Consumers and Health Information Technology: A National Survey*. Available at: http://www.chcf.org/publications/2010/04/consumers-and-health-information-technology-a-national-survey (accessed June 7, 2011).

Chamany, S., Silver, L.D., Bassett, M.T., Driver, D.R., Berger, D.K., Neuhaus, C.E. et al. (2009) "Tracking Diabetes: New York City's A1C Registry," *Milbank Quarterly* 87 (3): 547–70.

DeCew, J.W. (1997) *In Pursuit of Privacy: Law, Ethics, and the Rise of Technology*, Ithaca, NY: Cornell University Press.

Estlund, D.M. (2008) *Democratic Authority: A Philosophical Framework*, Princeton, NJ: Princeton University Press.

Fairchild, A.L. and Alkon, A. (2007) "Back to the Future? Diabetes, HIV, and the Boundaries of Public Health," *Journal of Health Politics, Policy & Law* 32: 561–93.

Fairchild, A.L. and Bayer, R. (2004) "Ethics and the Conduct of Public Health Surveillance," *Science* 303: 631–2.

Fairchild, A.L., Bayer, R. and Colgrove, J.K. (2007) *Searching Eyes: Privacy, the State, and Disease Surveillance in America*, Berkeley, CA: University of California Press.

Fried, C. (1970) *An Anatomy of Values: Problems of Personal and Social Choice*, Cambridge, MA: Harvard University Press.

Gallup Organization (2000) "Public Attitudes Toward Medical Privacy." Available at: http://www.forhealthfreedom.org/Gallupsurvey/IHF-Gallup.html#Sect2 (accessed July 19, 2014).

Gavison, R. (1984) "Privacy and the Limits of Law," in F.D. Schoeman (ed.) *Philosophical Dimensions of Privacy*, Cambridge: Cambridge University Press, pp. 346–402.

Goldman, J. (1998) "Protecting Privacy to Improve Health Care," *Health Affairs*, 17: 47–60.

Goldman, J., Kinnear, S., Chung, J. and Rothmann, D.J. (2008) "New York City's Initiatives on Diabetes and HIV/AIDS: Implications for Patient Care, Public Health, and Medical Professionalism," *American Journal of Public Health* 98: 807–13.

Gostin, L.O. (2008) *Public Health Law: Power, Duty, Restraint*, 2nd edition, Berkeley: University of California Press.

Gostin, L.O. (2009) "Privacy: Rethinking Health Information Technology and Informed Consent," in M. Crowley (ed.) *Connecting American Values with Health Reform*, Garrison, NY: The Hasting Center, pp. 15–17.

Gutmann, A. and Thompson, D. (1996) *Democracy and Disagreement*, Cambridge, MA: Belknap Press.

Inness, J.C. (1992) *Privacy, Intimacy, and Isolation*, New York: Oxford University Press.

Institute of Medicine (1988) *The Future of Public Health*, Washington, DC: National Academy Press.

Kaufman, D.J., Murphy-Bollinger, J., Scott, J. and Hudson, K.L. (2009) "Public Opinion about the Importance of Privacy in Biobank Research," *The American Journal of Human Genetics*, 85: 643–54.

Krane, D. (2007) *Many U.S. Adults Are Satisfied with Use of Their Personal Health Information*, Harris Interactive. Available at: http://www.harrisinteractive.com/vault/Harris-Interactive-Poll-Research-Health-Privacy-2007-03.pdf (accessed June 8, 2011).

Lee, S.S.-J., Bolnick, D.A., Duster, T., Ossorio, P. and Tallbear, K. (2009) "The Illusive Gold Standard in Genetic Ancestry Testing," *Science* 325: 38–9.

Locke, J. (2009) *Second Treatise of Government*, New York: Classic Books America.

Mariner, W.K. (2007) "Mission Creep: Public Health Surveillance and Medical Privacy," *Boston University Law Review*, 87: 347–95.

Mill, J.S. (1859) *On Liberty*, London: John W. Parker and Son, West Strand.

Moore, A.D. (2010) *Privacy Rights: Moral and Legal Foundations*, University Park, PA: Pennsylvania State University Press.

Parent, W.A. (1983) "Privacy, Morality, and the Law," *Philosophy and Public Affairs*, 12: 269–88.

Parmet, W. (2009) *Populations, Public Health, and the Law*, Washington, DC: Georgetown University Press.

PCSBI (Presidential Commission for the Study of Bioethical Issues) (2012) *Privacy and Progress in Whole Genome Sequencing*, Washington, DC. Available at: http://bioethics.gov/cms/sites/default/files/Privacy-and-Progress_PCSBI.pdf (accessed October 11, 2012).

Posner, R.A. (1984) "An Economic Theory of Privacy," in F.D. Schoeman (ed.) *Philosophical Dimensions of Privacy*. Cambridge: Cambridge University Press, pp. 333–45.

Powers, M. (1996) "A Cognitive Access Definition of Privacy," *Law and Philosophy* 15: 369–86.

Powers, M. (2008) "Privacy and Genetics," in J. Burley and J. Harris (eds.) *A Companion to Genethics*, Oxford: Blackwell Publishing, pp. 364–78.

Rachels, J. (1975) "Why Privacy Is Important," *Philosophy and Public Affairs*, 4: 323–33.

Raz, J. (1988) *The Morality of Freedom*, Oxford; New York: Clarendon Press; Oxford University Press.

Reiman, J.H. (1976) "Privacy, Intimacy, and Personhood," *Philosophy and Public Affairs* 6: 26–44.

Rothstein, M. (2002) "Rethinking the Meaning of Public Health," *Journal of Law, Medicine & Ethics* 30: 144–9.

Rubel, A. (2011) "The Particularized Judgment Account of Privacy," *Res Publica* 17: 275–90.
Rubel, A. (2012) "Justifying Public Health Surveillance: Basic Interests, Unreasonable Exercise, and Privacy," *Kennedy Institute of Ethics Journal*, 22: 1–33.
Schauer, F.F. (2000) "Can Public Figures Have Private Lives?" in E.F. Paul, F.D. Miller and J. Paul (eds.) *The Right to Privacy*, Cambridge, UK; New York: Cambridge University Press, pp. 293–309.
Streiffer, R., Rubel, A. and Fagan, J.R. (2006) "Medical Privacy and the Public's Right to Vote: What Presidential Candidates Should Disclose," *The Journal of Medicine and Philosophy* 31: 417–39.
Thacker, S.B., Stroup, N.E. and Dicker, R.C. (2003) "Health Data Management for Public Health," in F.D. Scutchfield and C.W. Keck (eds.) *Principles of Public Health Practice*, Stamford, DT: Cengage Learning, pp. 223–52.
Westin, A.F. (1967) *Privacy and Freedom*, New York: Atheneum.
Williams, S., Scott, J., Murphy, J., Kaufman, D., Borchelt, R. and Hudson, K. (2009) *The Genetic Town Hall: Public Opinion about Research on Genes, Environment, and Health*, Genetics & Public Policy Center, Johns Hopkins University. Available at: http://www.dnapolicy.org/pub.reports.php?action=detail&report_id=27 (accessed June 8, 2011).

25
PUBLIC HEALTH AND CIVIL LIBERTIES

Resolving Conflicts

James F. Childress

Introduction

This chapter considers public health ethics in a particular context—a liberal, pluralistic, democratic society that maintains explicit commitments to several basic civil liberties: Bodily integrity, privacy, freedom of movement, freedom of association, and freedom of religion and conscience (Gostin 2008). In addition to functioning as sociocultural norms, these liberties are embedded in legal and, in some cases, constitutional rights. They are also incorporated into international human rights documents and discourse. Beyond these civil liberties, there are several basic economic liberties, including freedom of contract and uses of property, which this chapter does not address. Nor is this the place to offer a theoretical defense of a liberal, pluralistic, democratic society; I assume this as the context for these reflections about public health ethics.

Examinations of the relations between public health and civil liberties are often framed by one of two major perspectives: conflict or concord. These differ according to whether they hold that conflict between public health and civil liberties is more fundamental and prevalent than their harmony. Of course, both perspectives acknowledge that conflicts do arise between public health and civil liberties, but their starting assumptions differ greatly. One views conflicts as common and inevitable, and trade-offs as unavoidable (Gostin 2002, 2003), while the other views conflicts as occasional, even rare, and trade-offs as generally avoidable (Annas 2002a, 2002b, 2007). The conflict perspective is also captured in the language of "inherent tensions" between public health and civil liberties "across the spectrum of threats to public health" (Bayer 2007). The concord perspective stresses that respect for civil liberties and rights constitutes an important part of public health policy and practice and is essential for voluntary public cooperation with public health authorities. The dominance of conflict or concord perspectives varies in different sociocultural contexts and over time.

The perspective of this chapter, which its overall argument supports, is that concord is more basic than conflict. However, difficult conflicts do sometimes erupt, and public health officials, invoking the "police power" of the state, sometimes rightly believe they must restrict civil liberties in order to protect or promote public health. In this chapter, I argue that:

- When conflicts do emerge, a presumptivist framework is more defensible and helpful than an absolutist or a contextualist one for determining appropriate public health interventions, some of which may infringe civil liberties.
- The presumptivist framework involves specifying public health ends and goals and viewing civil liberties, also specified, as presumptive directions for and constraints on measures to accomplish those ends and goals.
- The presumptivist framework operates with several conditions for rebutting the presumption, in some circumstances, against interventions that infringe civil liberties.
- Often, rebutting the presumption against infringing civil liberties is not necessary because it is possible to obtain voluntary cooperation and compliance. The metaphor of the intervention ladder from the Nuffield Council on Bioethics allows us to explore different ways to secure individuals' cooperation and compliance with public health measures without infringing their civil liberties.

I focus my discussion on a few civil liberties—freedom of movement and association and freedom from intrusions on bodily integrity—and I mainly draw examples from vaccinations, directly observed therapy (DOT) for tuberculosis (TB), and quarantine following probable infectious disease exposure.

Frameworks of Ethical Analysis of Conflicts between Civil Liberties and Public Health

If conflicts emerge between public health and civil liberties, how should they be adjudicated? Among three possible frameworks for adjudication, I argue that a presumptivist framework is preferable to either an absolutist or a contextualist framework (for a fuller discussion, see Childress and Bernheim 2003, 2008; Bernheim et al. 2014).

An absolutist framework holds that a certain value has absolute priority over some or all conflicting values. It is not plausible in public health ethics to take an absolutist approach, whether the absolute value is liberty or public health. Only an extreme libertarian position—verging on anarchism—could assign absolute priority to liberty in the face of, say, a major pandemic that threatens a country's survival. Most libertarians recognize warrants for overriding liberty in such cases—for instance, David Boaz, an influential libertarian, concedes that forcible quarantine, exercised with "great caution, and with appropriate safeguards for due process" appeared to be a "necessary" step in response to the outbreak of SARS (Severe Acquired Respiratory Syndrome) which is known to have infected over 8,000 persons worldwide and killed 775 of them in 2002–3 (Boaz 2003). Similarly, only an extreme communitarian position—verging on totalitarianism—could assign absolute priority to public health. Most communitarians recognize some liberties as communal values, along with public health and other values.

At the other end of the spectrum is a contextualist approach that refrains from assigning advance weights to either public health goals or civil liberties. Instead, it considers all of them equally in particular contexts. The dominant metaphors are "weighing" and "balancing." For instance, Amitai Etzioni (2002: 102) holds "that individual rights and social responsibilities, liberty and the common good, have equal standing; that neither should be assumed *a priori* to trump the other; and that we need to seek a carefully crafted balance between these core values."

It is common for governmental officials to describe their reasoning as *balancing* public health and civil liberties. Often, this focuses on public health and liberty as abstract concepts, as though all public health goals are equally significant and all civil liberties are equally important. Attending to particular contexts offers at least a partial corrective, but this approach still fails to provide an adequate structure for moral reasoning and relies too much on bare intuition. Furthermore, it fails to capture a key commitment of liberal societies to assign presumptive priority to means in public health and elsewhere that respect civil liberties and voluntary choices. It tends to reduce all judgments to proportionality, failing to see that even policies that pass an overall balancing test still need to be necessary, the least restrictive, the least intrusive, and so forth.

A presumptivist approach, by contrast, requires specification of the public health ends or goals that are sought and then assesses the range of potentially useful and available means. In pursuing public health goals, it starts from a presumption in favor of interventions that respect, and against measures that violate, basic civil liberties. To be sure, this presumption can sometimes be rebutted, but this rebuttal process requires a more precise and nuanced analysis than is available to the contextualist.

The presumptivist framework avoids pitfalls that trouble both absolutist and contextualist approaches. It avoids the extreme and implausible absolutist positions—that public health always trumps liberty/ies or that liberty/ies always trump public health. It is closer in spirit to the contextualist approach but provides a needed and helpful structure for moral reasoning about public health interventions. The presumptivist framework assigns presumptions, starting points, and burdens of proof in deliberation about interventions that could be used to realize the goals of public health. The presumption favors those that do not infringe civil liberties.

Goals of Public Health

The first task in justifying interventions is to identify, specify, and justify the assignment of weights to the goals of public health. Too often "public health" is presented as a univocal and sufficient goal even though it is too broad without further specification. Here I focus on five general types of goals offered as justification for public health interventions.

Public health has historically encompassed actions that individuals cannot perform entirely for themselves, for instance, when collective action is required in public sanitation and in preventing the spread of communicable diseases. The major justification for liberty-limiting interventions is the "harm-to-others principle," presented in John Stuart Mill's *On Liberty* (Mill 1975). This principle authorizes the society's intervention into individuals' other-regarding actions, that is, actions that harm others or put them at risk of harm. A version of what Mill calls societal "self-protection" appears in the early twentieth century U.S. Supreme Court decision, *Jacobson v. Massachusetts* (1905), which upheld a mandatory vaccination law: "Upon the principle of self-defense, of paramount necessity, a community has the right to protect itself against an epidemic of disease which threatens the safety of its members."

A second goal is protecting people who lack the capacity to protect themselves, even from effects of their own actions (Gostin 2008). In *On Liberty* Mill gives an example of a person about to cross a dangerous bridge and there is "no time to warn him of his danger." In such a case, Mill said, it would be ethically acceptable to "seize him and turn him back, without any real infringement of his liberty" on the assumption that he does not want to fall into the river (Mill 1975: 89). In such a case, a person's lack of information or, as we might broaden this, lack of capacity, combined with the risk to him or her, warrants the intervention. This is a form of weak or soft paternalism that is unobjectionable from the standpoint of civil liberties if it is exercised in good faith (Childress 2007; Beauchamp and Childress 2013).

A third possible goal is protecting an individual's health interests even if she is competent, has adequate information, and voluntarily rejects the intervention on her behalf. This is strong or hard paternalism. Mill (1975) argued for an absolute prohibition of coercive interventions in an individual's self-regarding actions, i.e., actions with adverse effects that fall only on the autonomous individual herself or also on others with their consent. Such strong or hard paternalism is very difficult to defend as a warrant for breaches of civil liberties.

A fourth possible goal employs an expanded notion of "harm to others." It rejects Mill's sharp distinction between self-regarding and other-regarding conduct and contends that some apparently paternalistic interventions may be primarily, or at least significantly, aimed at protecting others. Such expansionist views of *public* health hold that in the modern welfare state, so different from Mill's context in the mid-nineteenth century, some apparently self-regarding conduct is now other-regarding in its effects if not in its intention.

Consider the following example: Arguments for mandatory motorcycle helmet laws appear paternalistic in nature, having only the goal of protecting motorcyclists themselves from severe head injuries or death. However, some other arguments focus on the increased risks, burdens, and costs to other individuals and to the society. Such an extension of the harm-to-others principle appears in a Massachusetts court decision:

> From the moment of the injury, society picks the person up off the highway; delivers him to a municipal hospital and municipal doctors; provides him with unemployment compensation if, after recovery, he cannot replace his lost job; and if the injury causes permanent disability many assure the responsibility for his and his family's continued sustenance . . . We do not understand a state of mind that permits a plaintiff to think that only he himself is concerned.
>
> (quoted in Bayer 2007: 1102)

A fifth possible goal under the rubric of public health is *population health*. A healthy population is a worthy societal goal in and of itself. It also provides human capital for a more productive society, more capable of competing in the global arena and defending itself from external enemies. Even if individuals' health-damaging actions appear to affect only themselves, they are at the same time depriving society of fully capable and productive citizens. This goal also allows the society to target chronic conditions such as diabetes and/or obesity in its public health programs. Its logic is similar, on a larger scale, to the logic of the expanded "harm-to-others" principle. For instance, after arguing for paternalistic regulation of individuals' conduct in order to protect the individuals themselves, Ronald Bayer adds "because such [paternalistic] efforts can have a broad and enormous impact at a population level" (Bayer 2007: 1102). This joins a paternalistic rationale with the societal benefit of population health.

A sixth possible goal also attends to population health but from a distributive rather than an aggregative perspective. This goal, resting on egalitarian conceptions of social justice, involves efforts to close the health gaps between the better off and the worse off in the society. Over the last several decades, for example, this goal has been clearly evident in mandatory vaccination laws, tied to school attendance, that seek to "foster the equitable distribution of the benefits of vaccines, especially among children whose life circumstances make them less likely to be fully immunized" (Colgrove 2010).

Of course, it is possible—and common—to combine several of these goals as warrants for policies and practices that limit or override civil liberties. Strong (but not necessarily overriding) unmixed goals, when the proposed interventions conflict with civil liberties, are the first, second, and sixth; the third is the most controversial in a liberal society but has its defenders (Bayer 2007); the fourth and fifth are commonly invoked but require close attention to the actual effects of individuals' actions on others and on the society before they can override civil liberties. Under these six broad goals, under the rubric of public health, we need to formulate and deliberate about specific, concrete goals.

Justificatory Conditions for Liberty-Limiting Public Health Measures

A presumption in favor of interventions that respect civil liberties in the pursuit of public health goals can be rebutted under some conditions, and it is important to delineate these rebuttal conditions. We can call them *rebuttal conditions* because they specify conditions for rebutting the presumption in favor of respecting specific civil liberties, or we can call them *justificatory conditions* because they specify conditions for justifying infringements of specific civil liberties. (For other versions of these conditions, see Childress et al. 2002; Childress and Bernheim 2003, 2008.)

The presumption-rebuttal or justification process occurs in particular contexts when measures that limit, infringe, or violate civil liberties are being considered as possible ways to achieve specific public health goals. The process should be directed at all stakeholders.

The first task of this process, as we noted above, is to specify and weight the public health goals, and so the first rebuttal condition focuses on the following question: Is there a legitimate and important public health end or goal? The other justificatory conditions kick in once there is a specific, legitimate, and important public health goal and some of the possible interventions involve limiting liberties. It is not sufficient merely to assert that public health is at stake. As we have seen, some of the general types of goals are weaker than others in justifying infringements of civil liberties.

Second, would the proposed liberty-limiting measure probably be effective in achieving an important public health goal? If there is no reasonable chance that the liberty-limiting measure—such as forcible quarantine—would achieve its goal, then it is both unwise and unethical. A reasonable prospect of success is a condition for rebutting the presumption in favor of civil liberties of movement and association.

Third, is the proposed liberty-limiting measure necessary? We can imagine circumstances in which liberty-limiting measures, such as forcible quarantine or mandatory vaccination, would be effective but nonetheless ethically unjustifiable because they are not necessary to realize the public health goal being sought. It is often, though not always, possible to secure individuals' voluntary adherence to public health measures without coercion or threat of coercion. Moreover, the logic of presumptive principles or values compels us to seek alternatives before we can justifiably override them. A liberty-limiting measure is necessary only if other measures have failed or have been determined to have no reasonable chance. Only then is it a last resort.

Some frameworks do not include necessity as a justificatory condition, holding instead that it is incorporated into the fifth condition of proportionality. However, it serves as a valuable reminder that consequentialist considerations, such as effectiveness and proportionality, which would also include cost-effectiveness and a wide range of consequences, do not exhaust our moral concerns in public health.

Fourth, is the proposed infringement of liberty the least restrictive or least intrusive means available? In some interpretations, this justificatory condition is simply a corollary of the previous one, necessity. If liberty-limiting measures are necessary, the degree of infringement, as well as the kind of infringement, should be necessary. Nevertheless, it is also useful to consider this condition as a specific requirement of the logic of presumptive principles or values—to minimize the restrictiveness, intrusiveness, and invasiveness of justified infringements, such as infringements of freedom of movement and association and protections of bodily integrity, and to narrow their scope as much as possible. If, for example, public health officials have determined that forcible quarantine is necessary to control a SARS outbreak, they should employ the least restrictive, intrusive, and invasive measures and aim at the narrowest range of possible targets of quarantine consistent with achieving the public health goal being pursued. They might, for instance, select quarantine in home rather than in a hospital or in jail; of course, other factors such as cost will enter into these deliberations too.

Fifth, is the proposed liberty-infringing measure proportionate? From one standpoint, if a proposed limiting-infringing measure is effective, necessary, the least intrusive, etc., then it is proportionate in the sense of being appropriate and fitting (see Working Group 2003). In this chapter, proportionality involves the kind and range of balancing featured in contextualist analyses. It considers not only the probable benefits of the proposed measure, weighed against the relevant liberty interests, but also attends to the probable overall balance of good and harmful short- and long-term effects of the proposed liberty-limiting interventions.

Sixth, is the proposed liberty-limiting measure impartially applied? In a seminar on "Confronting Epidemics: Historical and Contemporary Perspectives," which I co-taught several times with a colleague in law and public health, we were initially surprised to see how often liberty-limiting measures were imposed unfairly, based on race, ethnicity, and social class, among other characteristics. Discrimination based on such characteristics is common in epidemics, particularly in singling out some victims for blame. In the 2003 SARS outbreak in Canada, Asian persons in Toronto experienced stigmatization and discrimination (Schram 2003).

There are concerns that presumptions and rebuttal or justificatory conditions, such as those just delineated, too often stand in the way of effective measures for reaching public health goals. Some advocates for public health worry that these presumptions and rebuttal conditions erect barriers to public health by requiring that liberty-limiting measures pass excessively stringent tests (Gostin 2002; Etzioni 2002). And yet if the commitment to civil liberties in a liberal, pluralistic, democratic society is meaningful, it at least sets a (rebuttable) presumption against infringements of civil liberties. Moreover, such criticisms fail to note that safeguarding civil liberties regularly goes hand in hand with protecting and promoting public health, in part because of the need for public trust and cooperation. Finally, as I have suggested and elaborate in the next section, respect for civil liberties can often be maintained by persuading or nudging individuals voluntarily to accept and act on public health measures, such as vaccination or quarantine or directly observed therapy (DOT) for TB. Hence, the justificatory conditions compel public health officials to seek measures that may elicit voluntary cooperation before resorting to infringements of civil liberties.

The Intervention Ladder

The metaphor of an "intervention ladder," introduced by the Nuffield Council on Bioethics (2007), helps us think about a range of interventions that may secure the public's cooperation with public health measures without infringing civil liberties. The interventions higher on this ladder are considered to be more intrusive and thus to require a stronger justification (Nuffield Council 2007). In line with a presumptivist approach, the justificatory burden increases as higher rungs of the ladder, involving infringements of liberty, are reached. Not every rung is available for every public health measure. My primary examples, as earlier, are vaccinations, DOT for TB, and quarantine for infectious diseases (Figure 25.1).

This ladder is not complete, there is overlap among the rungs, and each covers several possible kinds of policies and practices. In some contexts, some of the lower rungs may be unjustifiable for reasons other than infringement of civil liberties—indeed, for the most part, the lower rungs do not infringe civil liberties. Doing nothing—or monitoring the situation (1)—may seem unproblematic, but if, for example, serious illnesses or deaths are occurring while vaccination rates are being monitored, without any interventions, then it too requires solid ethical justification in view of the risks involved.

Providing accurate and truthful information (2) also appears ethically unproblematic, whether the goal is to ensure informed choices or to convince citizens and residents to act in certain ways, for instance, to accept certain vaccinations. Ethical issues do arise in efforts to motivate individuals through presenting graphic images, appealing to emotions, stigmatizing conduct, shaming failures to comply with social norms, and the like. Most governments have relied mainly on persuasion and motivation through a variety of educational and advertising campaigns to promote needed vaccinations, but they have employed other interventions as well.

Intervention Ladder
8. Eliminate choice
7. Restrict choice
6. Guide choice by disincentives
5. Guide choice by incentives
4. Guide choice by changing the default policy
3. Enable choice
2. Provide information
1. Do nothing

Figure 25.1 Intervention ladder

Source: This figure was prepared by the author from the Nuffield Council on Bioethics report (2007)

A policy or practice of enabling choices (3) seeks to secure compliance with public health measures by providing resources or otherwise increasing individuals' capacities to act in certain ways. It does not violate civil liberties to enable people to exercise those liberties in particular ways or to choose to waive their liberties. Enabling choices may involve removing financial, logistical, and other disincentives, obstacles, or barriers. These could be as straightforward as providing free fresh fruit for students or constructing lanes for bicyclists.

Consider the following scenario: Public health officials may believe that a particular individual who has TB should be in a DOT program until non-contagious or even cured in order to protect others and to reduce the chances of multidrug-resistant TB with its serious risks and huge costs to the individual and the society. It may be possible to secure that individual's compliance by providing vouchers for transportation to a center for DOT along with free care. In this case, the individual's failure to comply may not reflect a lack of will but rather a lack of resources for easy and non-burdensome compliance. Similarly, programs to increase access to vaccinations and to reduce or eliminate parents' out-of-pocket costs for getting their children vaccinated, according to the recommended schedule, have also been effective (Community Preventive Services Task Force 2008). Such programs do not infringe civil liberties and hence are unobjectionable from that standpoint.

For some public health measures, it may be possible and ethically justifiable to take another step and to guide individuals' choices by altering defaults (step 4 on the intervention ladder) or using other nudges. This is attractive because it maintains individuals' liberties while gently pushing their choices in certain directions. As Richard Thaler and Cass Sunstein argue in *Nudge: Improving Decisions about Health, Wealth, and Happiness* (2008), a "nudge" is an aspect of a society's "choice architecture" that seeks to change what people do without prohibiting any of their options and without significantly modifying their economic incentives. A mere nudge must not be difficult or costly to avoid. Changing the default in an organ donation system from opt in, as is current in the U.S., England, and Australia, to opt out, as is common in a number of European countries, selects one nudge over another in an effort to increase the rates of organ donation. Placing fruit, rather than less healthy foods such as potato chips, at students' eye level in a school cafeteria counts as a nudge, in contrast to banning junk food altogether from the choices in the cafeteria (Thaler and Sunstein 2008).

I briefly consider the role of nudges in one part of mass mandatory immunization programs. It is worth noting that immunization programs in about half of the countries in the European Union do not have any mandatory vaccinations, only recommended ones, while the other countries include at least one mandatory vaccination (Haverkate et al. 2012). Many of the countries only recommending vaccinations have high coverage nonetheless (Haverkate et al. 2012; specifically for the U.K., see Salmon et al. 2006). Immunization programs generally aim at herd or population immunity, which does not require universal immunization. Governments that mandate vaccinations generally exempt some individuals from the requirements. On the one hand, some children and adults have medical conditions that put them at risk from particular vaccinations; all states in the U.S. recognize medical exemptions. On the other hand, mandatory vaccination programs threaten another civil liberty, freedom of religion or, more broadly, freedom of conscience. Freedom of religious/conscientious action is generally more limited than freedom of belief. However, only two states in the U.S. do not allow exemptions from immunizations to religious objectors, and nineteen states also allow exemptions to persons (or to parents or guardians of minors) with philosophical, personal, moral, or other objections (National Conference of State Legislatures 2012). In the U.S., such non-medical exemptions are not deemed to be constitutionally required, and they may legitimately be overturned in a declared public health emergency or epidemic.

Not only is there a question about whether non-medical exemptions should be allowed, but there are also questions about how to exempt particular objecting individuals. States have had to consider whether to grant these non-medical exemptions upon request or also to require further steps and formal review. This has become an important question because outbreaks of communicable diseases, particularly pertussis (whooping cough) in some states, have resulted in part from the increased numbers of exemptions (Omer et al. 2006). Some states have responded by introducing such formal requirements as an annual written request for exemption followed by a review. The available evidence suggests that such nudges can effectively reduce the number of requests for exemptions (Salmon and Siegal 2001; Salmon et al. 2006). The explanation is simple: Parents or guardians whose children have fallen behind on their immunization schedules may find it much easier to request an exemption, in the absence of nudges and slight hurdles, than to complete the immunizations. These nudges and slight hurdles may also serve as a limited test of objectors' sincerity. In any event, they represent only minor and justifiable encumbrances of freedom of religion and freedom of conscience without violating those fundamental civil liberties.

Nudges work for several reasons (Thaler and Sunstein 2008; Johnson and Goldstein 2003). One factor is the cost of acting against the nudges, for instance, by taking the non-default option, especially when the default option is recommended by public health officials and is considered socially normative. However, to count as a mere nudge, an option's cognitive, psychological, or other costs must be insignificant. If they are significant, then (4) is indistinguishable from (5) and (6), guiding individuals' choices by incentives or by disincentives. To return to our example of ensuring adherence to DOT by a person with TB, providing vouchers for transportation (an instance of (3)) may not be sufficient to secure his or her compliance. It may also be possible and desirable to provide incentives, such as additional money, to motivate compliance. A small incentive, such as money for an inexpensive lunch, could count as a nudge whereas a more substantial amount would fall under (5).

What evidence do we have for the effectiveness of incentives? The Community Preventive Services Task Force (2011a), a body of independent, non-federal, unpaid experts in prevention and public health, established by the U.S. Department of Health and Human Services, looked at studies from Australia and the U.S. of the use of several types of positive incentives, which it labels "incentive rewards," for vaccinations: One time payments; child care assistance; lottery prizes (grocery vouchers and monetary prizes); gift cards (for baby products); food vouchers; and baby products. It concludes that, based on the solid evidence of effectiveness of such incentive rewards in increasing the vaccination rates of both adults and children, there is warrant to recommend their use either alone or conjoined with other interventions (Community Preventive Services Task 2011a; for more on the positive effects of incentives on vaccination rates in Australia, see Salmon et al. 2006).

According to some critics, incentives, especially larger and more significant incentives, are potentially coercive. For instance, one such critic objects to paying people to take care of their health: "Cash might coerce some people into changing behavior . . ." (Popay 2008). By contrast, I take the view that providing incentives is not coercive because it expands rather than restricts personal options (Hawkins and Emanuel 2005). However, providing incentives still needs ethical scrutiny in order to avoid either exploitation or undue inducement and in order not to stigmatize disadvantaged persons through cash transfers conditional on their behavioral changes.

Some critics point to incentives' deeper potential harms to individuals (and ultimately to public health). Incentives target individuals' conduct, usually in the short run, but may damage their overall motivational structure and character in the long run. Hence, these critics sound a strong cautionary note (Grant 2012). Sometimes, however, it is important to achieve short-term public health goals through altering conduct—for instance, using incentives to get individuals to undergo DOT or to receive vaccinations—even if their motivational structure or character is not improved and perhaps even slightly damaged. Claims of character damage through such incentives are difficult if not impossible to substantiate. As a result, we can make judgments about effectiveness and cost-effectiveness, in light of an important public health goal, but judgments of proportionality will be incomplete because of missing information and evidence about possible threats to character.

The final three rungs on the intervention ladder introduce more liberty-limiting and coercive policies than the ones below them; they thus stand in greater tension with civil liberties. Policies at rung 6 on the intervention ladder significantly shape individuals' choices through the imposition of disincentives, including but not limited to financial disincentives. Substantially increasing taxes on harmful products, such as cigarettes, is one example. Another is fining people who seek to avoid mandatory vaccinations. In *Jacobson v. Massachusetts* (1905), the U.S. Supreme Court upheld Massachusetts' imposition of a fine for failing to accept a vaccination in a smallpox outbreak and imposition of a jail term for failing to pay the fine (Willrich 2011).

Despite *Jacobson*, vaccination policy in the U.S. has historically relied mainly on persuasion rather than coercion. However, in the late 1960s, efforts to eradicate—and not merely to control—infectious disease, in the context of a campaign against measles, more states adopted laws requiring children to be immunized in order to attend school (Colgrove 2006, 2010). These laws, which had already been upheld by the U.S. Supreme Court in 1922, represent a significant non-monetary disincentive or sanction to ensure the vaccination of school-age children; they may also have monetary effects if parents have to resort to home schooling. Even so, the assumption was that parents are basically willing to have their children vaccinated but may need this "special stimulus" (Colgrove 2010). Moreover, the use of school attendance laws to ensure vaccinations was based in part on the egalitarian value of increasing children's access to conditions for healthy lives. Some supporters viewed these laws "as a kind of societal safety net to catch the children of the 'hard to reach'" (Colgrove 2010: 12). The laws also had the benefit of protecting other children in interactions at school.

More problematic is applying certain monetary disincentives or sanctions when parents or guardians do not adhere to the official public health schedule for children's vaccinations. Particularly troubling is withholding or reducing food vouchers (e.g., providing food vouchers for one month rather than for three months) or other welfare benefits to families, thus potentially damaging children's health by reducing their available nutrition. Even though a few studies indicate that such financial disincentives or sanctions may be somewhat effective in the short term (Hoekstra et al. 1998; Kerpleman et al. 2000), critics have rightly challenged them as unfair and potentially harmful to children (Wood and Haflon 1998; Minkovitz and Guyer 2000; Davis and Lantos 2000).

Even their effectiveness is not clear cut. Based on its review of a range of recent studies, the Community Preventive Services Task Force (2011b) found "insufficient evidence to determine the effectiveness of monetary sanction policies to increase vaccination rates in children of families on government assistance." The finding of "insufficient evidence" reflects the limited number of studies testing different sanctions and reaching inconsistent results. The Community Preventive Services Task Force (2011a) also noted the "limited information on potential harms of these policies."

Starting from a baseline of eligibility for food vouchers or other welfare benefits for preschool-aged children and then threatening to stop those benefits in an effort to motivate parental or guardian behavior is arguably unfair and harmful to the children as well as coercive to the parents or guardians. It may be unreasonable to reject such sanctions altogether, but they should be used, in line with our justificatory conditions, only as a last resort when persuasion, removal of disincentives, provision of positive incentives, and nudges fail to work, and only when children's nutritional status and other health indices can be maintained.

The final two rungs (7 and 8) of the intervention ladder involve restricting choice or eliminating choice. Examples of restricting choice include legal requirements that food producers remove certain unhealthy ingredients from their food products and former New York City Mayor Michael Bloomberg's proposed ban on the sale of sugared drinks over sixteen ounces in certain settings. Both would make it more difficult, to different degrees, for consumers to partake of unhealthy foods. Some of what we discussed under step 6 related to disincentives and sanctions for vaccinations would also fall here, for instance, not allowing children to attend school if they have not been vaccinated.

Step 8 goes farther to eliminate choice, sometimes even by forcible confinement. An obvious example is forcibly quarantining individuals who have been exposed to certain communicable diseases, such as SARS, and who do not voluntarily comply with a quarantine order. Another example is forcibly detaining a person with TB who, after efforts to secure his or her cooperation with DOT, still refuses to adhere to the protocol. Among infringements of civil liberties, forcible detention, as a restriction of free movement and association, is easier to justify than forcible administration of the required medication through an invasion of the uncooperative person's body. Indeed, the Nuffield Council on Bioethics (2007) indicates that it is "not aware of any countries that go so far as to force individuals to be vaccinated."

Some public health measures on the final three rungs of the intervention ladder are or may be coercive. In general, they need to pass a higher bar of justification because of their threats to civil liberties. But they can sometimes meet our several justificatory conditions and thus rebut the presumption against their use. Often, however, interventions that stop short of coercion can secure individuals' cooperation without violating their liberties. In such cases individuals voluntarily comply with the recommended public health measures, such as quarantine, vaccinations, or DOT, whatever their motivations for doing so as a result of other interventions. These interventions, as we have seen, may not be objectionable from the standpoint of civil liberties themselves, but they may raise other ethical issues that need attention and resolution in particular circumstances.

Conclusion

In conclusion, we should not overlook, but also should not overemphasize, liberty-limiting interventions in the pursuit of effective public health measures. In public health, concord with civil liberties is more basic than conflict. However, conflicts do emerge, and several rebuttal conditions, or justificatory conditions, need to be met to justify liberty-limiting interventions. The presumptive limits set by civil liberties can often direct public health officials to find ethically preferable interventions that do not sacrifice effectiveness in the pursuit of important public health goals. Focusing mainly on examples from vaccination, DOT for TB, and quarantine, this chapter has considered a variety of interventions, stressing possible ways to secure individuals' compliance with important public health measures without breaches of civil liberties. In many contexts, individuals voluntarily choose to exercise their civil liberties, such as freedom of movement and association, or waive their rights to civil liberties, such as freedom from intrusion on bodily integrity. In those cases, it is not necessary for public health officials to infringe those liberties.

A distinction between *imposing* community and *expressing* community is useful (Childress 1997). Certainly, in some cases, it is ethically justifiable to impose community, in the sense of enforcing communal responsibilities and obligations, in order to protect or promote public health. However, public health officials can generally avoid imposing community by using the various non-coercive interventions discussed in this chapter. This outcome is more likely if the society has also expressed community by displaying solidarity with and respect for all its citizens and residents. This expression of community, which includes respecting civil liberties and rights and providing adequate resources, can usually generate trust and voluntary cooperation through such measures, coupled with truthful public communication and active public engagement.

Related Topics

Chapter 23, "Incentives in Health: Ethical Considerations," Richard Ashcroft
Chapter 24, "Privacy, Surveillance, and Autonomy," Alan Rubel

Bibliography

Annas, G.J. (2002a) "Bioterrorism, Public Health, and Civil Liberties," *The New England Journal of Medicine* 346: 1337–42.

Annas, G.J. (2002b) "Bioterrorism, Public Health, and Human Rights," *Health Affairs* 21: 94–7.

Annas, G.J. (2007) "Your Liberty or Your Life: Talking Point on Public Health Versus Civil Liberties," *EMBO Reports* 8 (12): 1093–8.

Bayer, R. (2007) "The Continuing Tensions between Individual Rights and Public Health: Talking Point on Public Health versus Civil Liberties," *EMBO Reports* 8 (12): 1099–103.

Bayer, R. and Colgrove, J. (2002), "Bioterrorism, Public Health, and the Law," *Health Affairs* 21: 98–101.

Beauchamp, T.L. and Childress, J.F. (2013) *Principles of Biomedical Ethics*, 7th edition, New York: Oxford University Press.

Bernheim, R.G., Childress, J., Melnick, A. and Bonnie, R. (2014) *Essentials of Public Health Ethics*, Boston, MA: Jones and Bartlett Learning.

Boaz, D. (2003) "SARS and the Bureaucratic Creep of 'Public Health,'" Commentary, Cato.org, June 18. Available at: http://www.cato.org/publications/commentary/sars-bureaucratic-creep-public-health (accessed July 11, 2013).

Childress, J.F. (1997) *Practical Reasoning in Bioethics*, Bloomington, IN: Indiana University Press.

Childress, J.F. (2007) "Paternalism in Health Care and Public Policy," in R.E Ashcroft, A. Dawson, H. Draper and J. McMillan (eds.) *Principles of Health Care Ethics*, 2nd edition, Chichester, UK: John Wiley & Sons, pp. 223–31.

Childress, J.F. and Bernheim, R.G. (2003) "Beyond the Liberal and Communitarian Impasse: A Framework and Vision for Public Health," *Florida Law Review* 55 (5): 1191–219.

Childress, J.F. and Bernheim, R.G. (2008) "Public Health Ethics: Public Justification and Public Trust," *Bundesgundheitsblat: Gusundheitsforschung, Gesundheitsschutz* 51 (2): 158–63.

Childress, J.F., Faden, R.R., Gaare, R.D., Gostin, L.O., Kahn, J., Bonnie, R.J. et al. (2002) "Public Health Ethics: Mapping the Terrain," *Journal of Law, Medicine & Ethics* 30 (2): 169–77.

Colgrove J. (2006) *State of Immunity: The Politics of Vaccination in Twentieth-Century America*, Berkeley, CA: University of California Press; New York: Milbank Memorial Fund.

Colgrove, J. (2010) "The Coercive Hand, The Beneficent Hand: What the History of Compulsory Vaccination Can Tell Us About HPV Vaccine Mandates," in K. Wailoo, J. Livingston, S. Epstein and R. Aronowitz (eds) *Three Shots at Prevention: The HPV Vaccine and the Politics of Medicine's Simple Solutions*, Baltimore, MD: The Johns Hopkins University Press.

Community Preventive Services Task Force (2008) *Guide to Community Preventive Services: Universally Recommended Vaccinations: Reducing Clients Out-of-Pocket Costs for Vaccinations*. Review completed October 2008. Available at: www.thecommunityguide.org/vaccines/universally/index.htm (accessed July 12, 2013).

Community Preventive Services Task Force (2011a) *The Community Guide: Universally Recommended Vaccinations: Client or Family Incentive Rewards*. Review completed April 2011. Available at: http://www.thecommunityguide.org/vaccines/universally/clientoutofpocketcosts.html (accessed August 6, 2012).

Community Preventive Services Task Force (2011b) *The Community Guide: Universally Recommended Vaccinations: Monetary Sanction Policies*. Review completed April 2011. Available at: http://www.thecommunityguide.org/vaccines/universally/MonetarySanctions.html (accessed August 6, 2012).

Davis, M.M. and Lantos, J.D. (2008) "Ethical Considerations in the Public Policy Laboratory," *Journal of the American Medical Association* 284: 85–7.

Etzioni, A. (2002) "Public Health Law: A Communitarian Perspective," *Health Affairs* 21: 102–4.

Gostin, L.O. (2002) "Public Health Law in an Age of Terrorism: Rethinking Individual Rights and Common Goods," *Health Affairs* 21 (6): 79–93.

Gostin, L.O. (2003) "When Terrorism Threatens Health: How Far Are Limitations on Personal and Economic Liberties Justified?" *Florida Law Review* 55: 1105–70.

Gostin, L.O. (2008) *Public Health Law: Power, Duty, Restraint*, revised and expanded 2nd edition, Berkeley, CA: University of California Press; New York: The Milbank Memorial Fund.

Grant, R.W. (2012) *Strings Attached: Untangling the Ethics of Incentives*, New York: Russell Sage Foundation; Princeton, NJ: Princeton University Press.

Haverkate, M., Ancona, F.D., Gimabi, C., Johnansen, K., Lopalco, P.L., Cozza, V. et al. (2012) "Mandatory and Recommended Vaccination in the EU, Iceland and Norway: Results of the Venice 2012 Survey on the Ways of Implementing National Vaccination Programs, Eurosurveillance 17 (22). Available at: http://www.eurosurveillance.org/images/dynamic/EE/V17N22/art20183.pdf (accessed July 17, 2013).

Hawkins, J.S. and Emanuel, E.J. (2005) "Clarifying Confusions about Coercion," *Hastings Center Report* 35 (5): 16–19.

Hoekstra, E.J., LeBaron, C.W., Megaloeconomou, Y., Guerrero, H., Byers, C., Johnson-Parlow, T. et al. (1998) "Impact of a Large-Scale Immunization Initiative in the Special Supplemental Nutrition Program for Women, Infants, and Children (WIC)," *Journal of the American Medical Association* 280: 1143–7.

Jacobson v. Massachusetts, 197 U.S. 11 (1905).

Johnson, E.J. and Goldstein, D. (2003) "Do Defaults Save Lives?" *Science* 302 (5649): 1338–9.

Kerpelman, L.C., Connell, D.B. and Gun, W.J. (2000) "Effect of a Monetary Sanction on Immunization Rates of Recipients of Aids to Families with Dependent Children," *Journal of the American Medical Association* 284: 53–9.

Mill, J.S. (1975) *On Liberty*. D. Spitz (ed.), New York: W.W. Norton & Company, Inc.

Minkovitz, C.S. and Guyer, B. (2000) "Effects and Ethics of Sanctions on Childhood Immunization Rates," *Journal of the American Medical Association* 284: 2056.

National Conference of State Legislatures (2012) *States with Religious and Philosophical Exemptions from School Immunization Requirements*. December. Available at: http://www.ncsl.org/issues-research/health/school-immunization-exemption-state-laws.aspx (accessed March 22, 2013).

Nuffield Council on Bioethics (2007) *Public Health: Ethical Issues*, London: Nuffield Council on Bioethics. Available at: www.nuffieldbioethics.org (accessed January 17, 2013).

Omer, S.B., Pan, W.K.Y., Halsey, N.A., Stokley, S., Moulton, L.H., Navar, A.M. et al. (2006) "Nonmedical Exemptions to School Immunization Requirements: Secular Trends and Association of State Policies with Pertussis Incidence," *Journal of the American Medical Association* 296: 1757–63.

Popay, J. (2008) "Should Disadvantaged People be Paid to Take Care of Their Health? No," *British Medical Journal* 337: 141.

Salmon, D.A and Siegel, A.W. (2001) "Religious and Philosophical Exemptions from Vaccination Requirements and Lessons Learned from Conscientious Objectors from Conscription," *Public Health Reports* 116: 289–95.

Salmon, D.A., Teret, S.P., MacIntyre, C.R., Salisbury, D., Burgess, M.A. and Halsey, N.A. (2006) "Compulsory Vaccination and Conscientious or Philosophical Exemptions: Past, Present, and Future," *The Lancet* 367: 436–42.

Schram, J. (2003) "Personal Views: How Popular Perceptions of Risk from SARS are Fermenting Discrimination," *British Medical Journal* 326: 939.

Thaler, R.H. and Sunstein, C.R. (2008) *Nudge: Improving Decisions about Health, Wealth, and Happiness*, New Haven, CT: Yale University Press.

Willrich, M. (2011) *Pox: An American History*, New York: Penguin Press.

Wood, D. and Halfon, N. (1998) "Reconfiguring Child Health Services in the Inner City," *Journal of the American Medical Association* 280: 1182–3.

Working Group of the University of Toronto Joint Centre for Bioethics (2003) *Ethics and SARS: Learning Lessons from the Toronto Experience*, Toronto, Canada: The University of Toronto Joint Centre for Bioethics. Available at http://www.yorku.ca/igreene/sars.html (accessed July 31, 2007).

Part VI

REPRODUCTION

Beginning-of-life decision-making represents a major field of contemporary bioethical interest. While it may be tempting to construe this area as primarily asking questions about abortion and contraception, the authors in this section reflect the variety of issues at stake with respect to reproduction. These topics, ranging from assisted reproductive technologies (ARTs) to population control to disability, demonstrate the complicated relationships between individuals and groups that pose some of the crucial ethical dilemmas in this literature.

As is evident from the previous section on autonomy and agency, the ideal of self-governance is immensely important not only for bioethics, but for Western social and political culture writ large. However, the reproductive domain inherently implicates multiple moral agents, including potential parents, families, gamete donors or surrogates, medical practitioners, members of social groups, as well as the new entity (or entities) being conceived (the moral status of which has been hotly contested). These relationships between individuals involved in the reproductive process raise questions about the extent to which one person's autonomy can or should be privileged in the face of countervailing interests, especially in such cases where moral obligations to others are far from clear.

Carolyn McLeod and Chloë FitzGerald speak to this very question when considering the legitimacy of conscientious refusal to provide reproductive health services, such as abortions or contraceptives. Because such services are legal in many jurisdictions, one might suppose that their citizens ought to have ready access to them if they so choose. However, many bioethicists agree that conscientious refusal is permissible in some cases on the ground that requiring medical professionals to provide services that contravene their deeply held moral convictions could be seen as a violation of individual autonomy. In reviewing the literature in support of conscientious refusal, McLeod and FitzGerald argue that even a restricted scope of refusal runs the risk of significantly interfering with women's reproductive autonomy, while relying on a construal of conscience that is difficult to defend. On their view, an adequate account of acceptable refusal must focus more on potential harms to patients, particularly when the implications of refusal have a disproportionate likelihood of harming women and thus have downstream consequences for justice.

While some women are faced with concerns about the availability of abortions or contraceptives, other women struggle to conceive, and so avail themselves of in vitro fertilization (IVF) or other ARTs to try to become pregnant. However, the production of embryos outside of the body raises questions about what ought to be done with the embryos that are not needed for reproductive objectives. Can such embryos legitimately be used for research without harming those who helped to produce them? Can scientists legitimately produce embryos solely for the purpose of research? Françoise Baylis considers the various claims regarding the moral status of embryos, and the harms that can accrue as a result of the overproduction of ova, for whatever purpose. Because of the increasing popularity of IVF and the need for scientific research on the early phases of human embryonic development, Baylis advocates for a nuanced view of embryo use that can support both reproductive and scientific aims.

The legitimacy of the scientific use of embryonic materials can be seen as a question stemming from broader considerations about the regulation of reproductive technology. No matter the ultimate consensus on experimentation, regulation regarding ARTs has powerful consequences, as laws regarding when and where ARTs can be used impact not only reproductive autonomy, but also help steer social norms of reproductive behaviors. Isabel Karpin takes as case studies the regulations of several nations governing ARTs, and suggests that the liberal legal notion of a bounded individual is intrinsically threatened by pregnancy, which muddles straightforward notions of where one body ends and another begins. Karpin proposes an understanding of the pregnant body as "not-one-but-not-two" in order to capture the relationality inherent in any conception of reproduction, and suggests that an understanding of autonomy as relational can be applied even to cases where the embryo exists outside of the human body. In so doing, she aims for an embodied, feminist analysis of reproductive regulation.

Reproduction as understood in this section involves not only biological reproduction (i.e., conception), but also social and ethical reproduction (for example, the ongoing process of raising and socializing children). An important element of this latter form of reproduction is assuring children's health, a role obligation typically seen as part and parcel of parenthood. Even while parents may rightly be supposed to have responsibility for the health of their children, Amy Mullin suggests that non-parental actors also have legitimate interests in ensuring the health of children in their communities. However, the standard of health cannot be too onerous, as all interests concerning the community must be weighed against others. Mullin uses the capability approach to argue for a right to minimally decent care for children, while illustrating that this standard cannot be met without support from both parents and the state. By identifying children as members of social communities with independent moral status, Mullin can be seen as expanding upon the notion of relationality introduced earlier in this section.

Relationality is salient for autonomy not only among individuals or between individuals and communities, but also between communities themselves. In an increasingly globalized world with variable laws and social mores, it is becoming more and more commonplace to see citizens of one country travel to another for reproductive services unavailable in their own jurisdictions. While such international movement can allow individuals to make reproductive decisions that would be impossible in their home countries, such "reproductive travel" can have problematic consequences. While this practice may enhance reproductive autonomy for would-be travelers, G.K.D. Crozier cautions that this enhancement is not available in an egalitarian way, and can lead to exploitation of foreign gamete providers as well as unacceptably permissive reproductive legislation. Crozier makes clear the intersection of reproductive travel with other bioethical concerns discussed throughout this volume, including medical tourism, the sale of biological materials, and the need to weigh concern for autonomy with justice and egalitarianism.

The international arena is salient for reproduction not only with respect to the kinds of pregnancies made possible by globalization, but also the overall quantity of pregnancies worldwide. Since 1959, the global population has more than doubled, while economic and industrial development has led to the unprecedented use of resources to support human life. This has led to widespread environmental concerns about the carrying capacity of the planet, and activist efforts to minimize rapid population expansion to a leveling-off point, where reproduction is no longer potentially perilous on a global scale. If limiting reproduction is imperative to saving the planet, this will undoubtedly have implications for justice, since fair policies must be articulated that determine who can reproduce and how often. Margaret P. Battin considers the impacts previously imposed regulations have had in the developing world, and suggests that family planning mandates, like those of India's vasectomy program and China's one-child policy, can have negative repercussions for autonomy by introducing state coercion into reproduction, which has been criticized on both feminist and religious grounds. However, the epistemological uncertainty underpinning any future projections about population results in Battin's thoughtful—yet measured—proposal to consider how we might address population concerns in an ideal world while still protecting reproductive rights.

Finally, Adrienne Asch and David Wasserman consider justice and population from a different vantage point; one that returns to the issues of ARTs discussed earlier in this section. While technologies like IVF have enabled otherwise infertile couples to conceive, other advancements in the technology of reproduction have generated means to avoid the reproduction of certain traits. Prenatal genetic testing has enabled couples to find out if their children will be (or will be likely to be) born with certain disabilities, which enables parents to decide whether they are willing to parent disabled children. Such a decision, Asch and Wasserman argue, is incompatible with a view that considers the lives of the disabled to be equally valuable or worthwhile compared with the lives of the able-bodied, and ignores many first-person accounts of the quality of life with a disability. While it might be supposed that the possibility of terminating an impaired pregnancy increases reproductive options, Asch and Wasserman point out that, in fact, biases against the disabled often lead to pressures that preclude the possibility of continuing an impaired pregnancy. They also consider such selection to be incompatible with a desirable ideal that parents "unconditionally welcome" their children, whatever they might be like, and obscures the fact that even able-bodied children may deviate from parental expectations. In this chapter, Asch and Wasserman argue that although selecting to have certain kinds of children might seem to empower parents, it can also serve to undermine the status of entire communities.

26

CONSCIENTIOUS REFUSAL AND ACCESS TO ABORTION AND CONTRACEPTION

Carolyn McLeod and Chloë FitzGerald

Conscientious refusal in health care refers to refusals by health care professionals to provide (or not to provide) certain health care services. The most widely cited examples involve physicians and nurses who refuse to perform or assist with the performance of an abortion and pharmacists who refuse to dispense contraceptives. The topic of conscientious refusal in bioethics is closely tied to debates about access to abortion and contraception and about how we conceive of the role of health care professionals and their obligations to their patients.

Abortion and contraception raise issues of conscience among health care professionals because strong religious or moral beliefs that concern the legitimacy of these services are common. Prime examples are beliefs about the status of fetuses and embryos, women's reproductive freedom, and the purpose of procreation. There are opposing views on these issues that can polarize societies, despite the fact that abortion and contraception are legally available in most of the developed world and often covered by state-funded health provision.

Although conscientious refusals *to* provide abortions or contraception are more well known, conscientious refusals *not to* provide these services have also occurred. In other words, some health care professionals insist on offering abortion or contraceptive services even when they are prohibited, because not doing so violates their conscience. James Childress mentions the example of physicians who secretly provided information on contraception to couples in Connecticut when there was still an anti-contraceptive law in vigor, an action he calls "evasive noncompliance" (Childress 1985, 68–9; see also Harris 2012). Which professionals make conscientious refusals on an issue depends to some extent on the legal status quo. In the current situation, where abortion and contraception are typically legal and form part of the standard services provided by health care professionals, conscientious refusals that concern abortion or contraception will be refusals to provide (rather than not provide) services. We focus predominantly on these refusals.

In the first section, we provide more details on the nature of conscientious refusal in health care and discuss how refusal impinges on access to abortion and contraception. We approach the considerable, while qualified, support for this phenomenon by bioethicists in the second section. We express worries in the third section about certain aspects of this support and the view of conscience on which much of it is based. Finally, the fourth section explores the implications of alternative conceptions of conscience—those that we have each proposed elsewhere—for the bioethics education of health care professionals. Our focus here is on education about patient access to abortion and contraception. Our general position on conscientious refusal, which informs our discussion throughout, is that accommodation for conscience in health care can be appropriate. But such a policy must be grounded in a more nuanced view about conscience than what we tend to see in the bioethics literature; and it must take seriously the political nature of conscientious refusals and their likely impact on women's access to abortion and contraception.

Conscientious Refusal: The Phenomenon and Its Impact

The phenomenon of conscientious refusal by health care professionals is complicated by the variety of kinds of services that the refusals can target and by how the phenomenon differs from paradigm cases of conscientious objection. We cover these issues first and then turn to what is known about the impact of conscientious refusals on access by patients to abortion and contraceptive services.

Depending on the kind of professional involved (doctor, nurse, or pharmacist), conscientious refusal that concerns abortion or contraception can be a refusal to do the following: Perform an abortion; prescribe or dispense contraception, emergency or otherwise; prescribe or dispense contraception to a particular group (e.g., unmarried women); refer a patient to another professional for abortion or contraceptive services; provide information on abortion or contraception; train to perform abortions and related procedures; stock contraception (i.e., in one's pharmacy); or simply participate in any way in the provision of these services. Conscientious refusal can therefore target a range of services, from providing patients with a particular service to offering them information about it.

However, conscientious refusal is directed not only at a certain health care service (or set of services), but also at the expectation that the relevant professional will provide the required service. This expectation comes from professional norms or policies, or from legal rules. Normally, the objector does not refuse a direct order by an authority to meet the relevant expectation; and in this way, conscientious objection in health care differs from the tradition of conscientious objection by pacifists to comply with the military draft. What many objectors in health care refuse to do is accede to a request by a patient, who may hold an expectation of care, but who neither issues an order nor has authority over the objector. As a result, relevant authorities (e.g., the health care professional's college or professional association) will not know about an objector's refusal unless the patient complains about it or the objector makes her objection public. To be sure, some conscientious objectors in health care are like pacifist objectors in that they refuse to comply with a direct order by an authority (e.g., an order by a physician to a nurse); however, many enjoy too much autonomy in their practice for that to be true.

Conscientious refusals in health care can go unnoticed not only by authorities, but also by patients themselves, particularly if health care professionals are not clear about why they will not fulfill patients' requests. Thus, because of how very private they can be, the frequency of conscientious refusals in health care is unknown. However, their impact on others can be substantial. Unlike a citizen refusing the military draft whose action has at most a statistical effect on the numbers fighting for a nation, a conscientious refusal in health care typically has direct effects on patients, some of which can be severe (e.g., unwanted pregnancy). Moreover, when conscientious refusals in health care target abortion or contraceptive services, women are disproportionately affected.

Although the numbers of conscientious refusals by health professionals are difficult to measure, they seem to be significant enough to create serious obstacles to access to abortion or contraception in some places. In the United States, for example, the political and legal prominence of the issue (many health care professionals in the U.S. have a legal right to conscientious refusal; Charo 2007; Downie 2012; Dykes 2002) and the media attention it attracts (Dale 2004; Editorial 2007; Stein 2006, 2008, 2012) suggest that the frequency of conscientious refusals is quite high. The issue is growing in political importance in other countries, including Canada (Downie and Nassar 2008; Rodgers and Downie 2006), the U.K. (Deans 2013; Laurance 2007), Spain (Sánchez Esparza 2012), South Africa (van Bogaert 2002), and Italy (Palma 2012). There have been reports in some of these countries of serious restrictions, even "black-outs," to abortion access because of conscientious refusals. (See Cannold 1994 for an example from Australia.) The potential for conscientious refusals to limit access to abortion severely is a reality in some parts of the world.

Conscientious refusal in health care is intimately tied to the political and moral debate about abortion, especially in the U.S. There, the right of health care professionals to issue such refusals was not a topic of serious debate until the Supreme Court decriminalized certain kinds of abortion in *Roe v. Wade* (Stein 2012). Nonetheless, some bioethicists approach the issue as though it had little to no connection to the politics of abortion. We criticize this tendency in the next section.

Support for Conscientious Refusal in Health Care

There is broad support in the bioethics literature for the claim that health care professionals have a right (or at least should be permitted) to refuse conscientiously to provide services; however, this support is not unqualified. In this section, we outline the different qualifications that bioethicists defend to this right. We also discuss the method that some of them use to defend their moderate endorsement of conscientious refusals.

The majority of bioethicists who have commented on conscientious refusal take a moderate stance: That is, one that permits refusal but at the same time restricts it. The limitations on refusal that bioethicists defend concern the kinds of refusals that health care professionals can make, when they can make them (e.g., not in emergencies), and possibly how they do so (Benjamin 1995; Blustein 1993; Brock 2008; Card 2011; Charo 2007; Childress 1997; Deans 2013; Fenton and Lomasky 2005; LaFollette and LaFollette 2007; Lynch 2008; McLeod 2010; Meyers and Woods 2007; Wicclair 2000, 2011). Julian Savulescu is somewhat unusual in his extreme view that health care professionals (he focuses on physicians) have no right to conscientious objection, although they could permissibly make objections that do not compromise "the quality, efficiency, or equitable delivery of a service" (2006: 296; see also Kelleher 2010 and Kolers 2014). According to Savulescu (2006: 296), physicians are responsible for providing all "legal and beneficial care," and their conscience should not interfere with them doing so.

Different limitations on what is permitted distinguish different versions of the moderate position on conscientious refusal in health care. The following is a non-exhaustive list of moderate views that appear in the literature. A conscientious refusal is permissible if and only if:

- The objector is willing to make a timely referral to a professional who will perform the relevant service (Cantor and Baum 2004; Charo 2007).
- The objector is able to show that her objection is genuine—that it stems from a sincerely held moral or religious belief (Benjamin 1995; Lynch 2008; Meyers and Woods 1996).
- The refusal respects the "core values" of the profession (Deans 2013; Wicclair 2000, 2011).
- The objector has registered her refusal with her licensing board, which is an institution that should be charged with ensuring that patients get the services they need (Lynch 2008).
- The objector works in an area in which the patient could easily get the service somewhere else close by (Fenton and Lomasky 2005).

Most authors also argue that to be morally permissible, a conscientious refusal cannot be explicitly discriminate against a minority social group (e.g., be racist), nor can it occur in an emergency situation.

Most of the above restrictions do not preclude health care professionals from refusing in many contexts to perform abortions or to prescribe or dispense contraception. More generally, many bioethicists have taken positions that, while qualified, do not prevent them from endorsing or allowing much conscientious refusal in health care. Overall, support among bioethicists for conscientious refusal is considerable. We point this out, not because we believe that conscientious refusal should be banned necessarily, but because we worry about the implications that such support has for women's freedom to access abortion or contraception. As noted above, conscientious refusals can have a substantial negative impact on women's ability to obtain these services.

Granted, support from bioethicists tends to be weaker for pharmacists who object to emergency contraception (EC), compared with physicians who refuse to perform abortions. Pharmacists who object to EC often do so because they believe that EC is an abortifacient and is, as a consequence, morally wrong. Such refusals by pharmacists are typically grounded in empirical beliefs about the mechanisms of action of EC that are questionable at best, which helps to explain why bioethicists have little sympathy for them. In general, refusals to prescribe EC are heavily criticized in the literature (e.g., Card 2011; Greenberger and Vogelstein 2005; Kelleher 2010).

In defending moderate positions on conscientious refusal, bioethicists often employ extreme examples unrelated to abortion and contraception that most of us, regardless of our views on abortion, would agree are highly morally desirable or morally undesirable. Bioethicists use the former type—the morally desirable refusal—to help motivate the view that conscience is worth protecting among health care professionals. For instance, if a physician who was working under the Nazi regime in Germany conscientiously refused to be involved in the killing of Jews, he would reveal the kind of conscience most of us would want to protect in health care (McLeod 2008: 37).

Bioethicists use cases at the opposite extreme—that is, refusals that almost anyone would consider morally abhorrent—to show that limits on conscientious refusal in health care are essential, even when the refusals are based on sincere moral convictions. Mark Wicclair (2000: 216) invents the example of a physician who has a deeply held moral belief that pain is a sign of a moral flaw and therefore should be endured. This physician conscientiously refuses to prescribe medication for pain. Dan Brock (2008: 190) imagines a white physician who sincerely believes that racial mixing is morally wrong and thus conscientiously refuses to treat black patients. Both of these examples are of conscientious refusals that are clearly unacceptable. Because of cases like them, conscientious refusal, or protection for it, cannot be unlimited in health care.

It is worthwhile considering extreme examples of conscientious refusal that are removed from the debate over access to abortion and contraception; they can allow one to develop a universal analysis of conscientious refusal and can also provide clues about the moral dimensions of refusals to provide abortion and contraceptive services. However, too much focus on these cases and not enough on those that involve abortion, contraception, or the like (e.g., sterilization) is problematic for two reasons. First, it leaves us with theories that do not say enough about whether or when the latter are morally justified, given what is special about *them*: For instance, the significant impact they can have on women's reproductive freedom. Second, it simply misrepresents the phenomenon of conscientious refusal in health care (at least within the U.S.), which arose in the midst of heated debate about abortion and is still embedded to some degree in this political context. Conscientious refusal is tied—in health care, not in the military—generally speaking with right-wing political agendas and opposition to them, particularly agendas that favor the traditional family and women's place within it. Portraying the phenomenon as though it either did not have this connection or was politically neutral is misleading.

Further Criticisms of the Literature

We see at least two additional problems with the literature on conscientious refusal: It is often too one-sided, focusing more on the potential harm to conscientious objectors if forced to violate their conscience than on the consequences for patients if they do not have access to treatment; and much of the literature is grounded in a view about conscience that is unpersuasive. Let us discuss each of these issues in turn.

McLeod (2010) highlights an instance of the first problem when she argues that bioethicists have failed to think clearly about the negative consequences women (or girls) are likely to face when conscientious objectors deny them access to EC. In her view, these consequences amount to more than mere inconvenience, which is how some bioethicists assess them (e.g., Fenton and Lomasky 2005). It is more likely that women will be harmed rather than merely inconvenienced by a conscientious refusal of EC, according to McLeod, even when they could get the drug at another pharmacy close by. She explains how in circumstances where the drug is widely available, conscientious refusals to provide EC can still interfere with women's interests: More specifically with "their autonomy in obtaining EC . . . their moral identity (as a good or fine person), and [their] sense of security" (i.e., security in knowing that their society respects their ability to decide what happens to their own bodies) (2010: 19, 20). Women's reproductive autonomy is at stake because a refusal can be so emotionally difficult that a woman stops trying to get EC and decides to take her chances with getting pregnant (see also Kelleher 2010: 302). Such outcomes are dependent, according to McLeod, on the socio-political context in which conscientious objections to EC occur. Currently this context is one in which negative social stereotypes influence what it means for women to request EC and for someone to deny such requests on moral grounds. The relevant stereotypes include "that women who are sexually promiscuous are of low character—they are 'sluts' or 'whores'—and [that] women, more so than men, who have unprotected sex are 'irresponsible' or 'careless'" (McLeod 2010: 18, citing Stubblefield 1996).

Because of this oppressive social context, women tend already to be vulnerable when they seek EC. Their social position puts them at serious risk of harm when pharmacists or other health care professionals refuse them access to EC. Even if a woman who has this experience manages to continue her search for the drug and obtain it from another pharmacy, the refusal at the first pharmacy can be damaging to her (e.g., to her bodily security). Moreover, regardless of how the refusal is made, it can be harmful. The pharmacist could be as kind and caring as possible when stating his moral objection and yet still make the woman feel horrible, in part because one can only do so much to deflect the negative social meanings of one's actions.

Overall, McLeod's argument reminds us that bioethicists need to probe in detail what the effects of conscientious objections to abortion and contraception are on women *within* the societies in which they live: That is, societies that are sexist, racist, and in other ways morally non-ideal. If McLeod is correct about what these consequences are like, then the feminist struggle to ensure that women have access to abortion and contraception continues even where these services are legal *and* readily available, so long as there is some conscientious refusal.

The second problem we see with the literature on conscientious refusal is that it tends to rely on a particular understanding of conscience and why conscience is worth protecting that is flawed. What McLeod calls the "dominant view" of conscience in bioethics is explicitly defended by Martin Benjamin, Jeffrey Blustein, James Childress, and Mark Wicclair (McLeod 2012: 161–81; Benjamin 1995; Blustein 1993; Childress 1979, 1997; Wicclair 2000, 2006). These authors associate the value of conscience (or of listening to one's conscience) with having moral integrity, and in turn, define moral integrity in terms of psychological unity, or more specifically, unity between one's moral principles and commitments and one's actions. The violation of integrity, so understood, is harmful, according to this view.

We see three problems with the conception of conscience just described:

1. It prioritizes the preservation of psychological unity over the development of an individual's moral values.
2. It provides no incentive for an agent to rethink her moral values, encouraging a view of conscience as fixed.
3. It focuses exclusively on the explicit attitudes of conscientious objectors, neglecting the implicit attitudes that can also influence their behavior and thus lead them to violate their conscience.

The first concern lies with what the dominant view takes to be wrong with denying professionals the right to conscientious refusal. The idea is that if a health care professional cannot abide by her conscience, she loses psychological unity (i.e., integrity). And this is bad for two reasons: Unity is part of what constitutes a good life (Blustein 1993; Benjamin 1995: 470); and desire to repair "inner division" is an admirable characteristic of persons (Blustein 1993: 297).

However, it is not clear that the function and value of conscience lie in protecting psychological unity. Obeying one's conscience and going against the grain of social norms under considerable social pressure can make people feel less, rather than more, psychologically unified. McLeod describes an example (based on the real case of Lois Jenson) of a woman who listens to her conscience telling her to stand up for herself and press charges in the face of debilitating sexual harassment at work. Because the woman receives little support in her endeavor and instead faces a worsening situation and mounting social pressure, she begins to doubt that she has done the right thing in listening to her conscience. She loses confidence in her perspective and starts to loathe herself. In sum, she loses rather than gains psychological unity as a result of listening to her conscience (McLeod 2012).

McLeod's feminist relational perspective on conscience and consequent consideration of scenarios in which the protagonist is part of an oppressed group help to highlight the disunity that conscience can bring. However, the point can be made even if we limit ourselves to more traditional examples of powerful men in positions of privilege. Literature, film, and popular myth are replete with examples of heroes who struggle with their conscience. Moreover, obeying conscience is often depicted in these narratives as a process that makes one feel *less* psychologically unified. For instance, the Thomas More of the 1966 film, *A Man for All Seasons*, remains true to his religious and moral values and refuses to swear the oath required by law because it challenges the Pope's power; yet he doubts and struggles with himself in the process, particularly in the face of the suffering his decision inflicts on those dear to him. Granted, he might enjoy some psychological unity when he finally faces execution for his beliefs, at which point he appears to be at peace with himself. But even assuming that is true, obtaining such unity was not More's aim in following his conscience, nor does it capture what we value most in his actions. Rather, we appreciate the fact that he struggles to work out what he values and to do the right thing by his own lights. On this view, conscience is valuable precisely because it prevents us from blindly following whatever the social norms of the day dictate and encourages us to make our own moral choices (McLeod 2012; FitzGerald 2014).

A second and related problem with the dominant view about conscience in bioethics is that its insistence on psychological unity does not encourage rethinking the values that one upholds through one's conscience; instead it tends to present conscience as the reinforcement of a fixed set of values. For example, Mark Wicclair (2000: 214) refers to the "core ethical values" involved in conscience that are "integral" to a person's "self-conception or identity," as if these values did not change over time. Although Wicclair and other proponents of the dominant view do not explicitly say that conscience involves a fixed set of values, we suspect that this idea is lurking behind their conceptions of conscience and it is evident in the way that they discuss examples. There is rarely mention of the possibility of an individual's conscience developing and changing, nor of cases where the voice of one's conscience is in fact a recalcitrant emotion stemming from past values that one has disowned. For instance, a theatre-goer raised in a strict Puritan household may experience pangs of guilt when going to the theatre as an adult, even if he completely rejects the Puritan values of his upbringing (example originally from John Rawls 1972: 482; employed in the context of recalcitrant emotions by Brady 2007: 274). Psychologically complex cases such as these highlight the dangers of conceiving of conscience as the reinforcement of fixed values.

The notion that the values of conscience are fixed goes hand-in-hand with the idea that conscience protects psychological unity. Once one has a set of values that are unified, whatever those values might be, conscience will continue to reinforce them in order to preserve psychological unity, if that is the correct function of conscience. But there is no incentive here for the agent to change her values or rethink her conscience. This outcome is deeply problematic because there may be values influencing a person's conscience that she no longer endorses and perhaps has never endorsed.

The final problem is that the prevailing view ignores implicit attitudes, which may influence objectors' explicit attitudes about the services they find offensive. There is a wealth of empirical evidence showing that much of our behavior is influenced by implicit attitudes that are not under our direct rational control and that may even conflict with our explicit attitudes (Jost et al. 2009; Nosek and Riskind 2012). The Harvard Implicit Association Test (IAT) is widely used by social psychologists to measure implicit attitudes. Subjects are asked to match negatively and positively valenced words with, for example, black faces and white faces, at such a speed that conscious reflection is not involved in the task. Most white subjects and many black subjects who are tested connect negatively valenced words with black faces more quickly than they do with white faces. This is taken as an indication of an implicit, non-conscious association between negative evaluations and black people, amounting to a pro-white bias. Most who are found to exemplify an implicit pro-white bias hold explicit anti-racist views and are thus horrified to learn about their implicit attitudes. Biases related to a variety of factors, such as gender, socio-economic status, ethnicity, age, nationality, and sexual orientation have been tested in populations from all over the world and their widespread presence confirmed (Jost et al. 2009).

Importantly, these biases have been shown to influence behavior outside the laboratory (Jost et al. 2009; Nosek and Riskind 2012). Researchers have recently investigated implicit biases among health care professionals and shown how they affect patient care. A landmark study of this kind indicated a negative correlation between the level of implicit pro-white bias exhibited by white physicians and the probability that they would recommend an effective treatment option (thrombolysis) to a black patient (Green et al. 2007). Another study showed that clinicians with higher levels of implicit pro-white bias, compared with those with lower levels, delivered a poorer quality of care and clinical communication to black patients (Cooper et al. 2012). (For further studies, see Sabin and Greenwald 2012; von Hippel et al. 2008.) The results of this research are disturbing because they prove that even if a physician is explicitly and sincerely committed to being non-prejudiced towards her patients, she may still harbor implicit biases and give poor treatment to marginalized patients as a result.

Underlying the dominant view of conscience is the problematic assumption that only explicit beliefs influence behavior and are thus relevant to conscience. This view presents conscience as a mode of consciousness that examines whether past or future behavior accords with an individual's moral values, yet only mentions actions that an agent plans explicitly (Benjamin 1995; Blustein 1993; Childress 1979, 1997; Wicclair 2000, 2006). However, we know that implicit attitudes also influence behavior, behavior that can contravene an agent's values without her awareness. We know, for example, that some physicians unwittingly go against values they cherish by treating black patients differently from white patients.

Consider that a conscientious objector to abortion or contraception could genuinely believe that he objects to the service for non-sexist reasons; but he actually harbors implicit biases against women that influence his desire to object. Some feminists have worried that sexism lies behind some conscientious objection (e.g., Anderson 2005). The data on implicit bias operating under the radar of conscious thought makes this a more likely phenomenon. Of course, just because beliefs are explicit does not mean that they are a better justification for conscientious objection; but an objector is at least able to cite the explicit beliefs that lead him to object and to hold them up to scrutiny. The worry is that implicit attitudes of which he is unaware (and would not endorse if he were aware of them) could be influencing a health care professional's decision to conscientiously object. We argue that important work on implicit attitudes and their contribution to decisions and behavior needs to be acknowledged and integrated into a realistic conception of conscience.

In this section, we have made two broad claims. First, the support by bioethicists for conscientious refusal in health care tends to focus too much on the potential harm to objectors and fails to appreciate the seriousness of the consequences these refusals may have for patients, particularly when they concern female patients' access to abortion and contraception. The remedy for this problem is fairly obvious: Bioethicists need to consider the socio-political context in which refusals take place and supplement their theorizing with data from the terrain that reveal the effects refusals have on access to abortion and contraception. Second, there are three main flaws in the dominant view of conscience that informs much of the discussion in bioethics about the moral permissibility of conscientious refusals. In the final section, we briefly discuss the implications for health professional education of a revised conception of conscience—one that we believe is immune to the three worries we have raised with the dominant view.

Promoting a "Well-Functioning Conscience" Through Health Professional Education

Given the impact that conscientious refusal has on access to abortion and contraception, it is reasonable to ask health care professionals for something in return for the right to conscientiously refuse services. In our view, this something should be participation in educational workshops that encourage the development of "a well-functioning conscience" (a concept we explain below) and promote understanding of the ethics of abortion, contraception, and conscientious refusal.

Our discussion in the previous section indicated that there is more involved in having a well-functioning conscience than the bioethics literature suggests. On our view, a well-functioning conscience is one that effectively flags occasions where an individual is behaving, has behaved, or is about to behave in a way that goes against her moral commitments, whether this behavior is the result of an explicitly planned action or of implicit attitudes (FitzGerald 2014). People with a well-functioning conscience have an awareness of their implicit biases and work to mitigate or avoid manifesting them, especially biases that conflict with their explicit moral or religious views. They will also revise their explicit attitudes when given good reason to do so and in response to inconsistencies internal to them and between them and their behavior. Such individuals will not maintain psychological unity at all costs and thus their conscience is not fixed; rather, it is open to revision based on what the individual endorses. The work of cultivating such a conscience is best done with the help and input of others rather than in isolation (FitzGerald 2014; McLeod 2012). Others can help us to see when implicit attitudes shape our behavior, when we have good reason to revise our commitments, and when our commitments and behavior are inconsistent. At least some of this work could be done with colleagues in a workshop setting and simply through encouraging professionals to reflect on their behavior.

On our view, health care professionals whose conscience is well-functioning with respect to the issues of abortion and contraception should have some understanding of how conscientious refusals to provide these services can affect women. This will involve having some sense of why these services are important to women who seek them out.

Assuming this view is correct, ethics education for health professionals that covers abortion and contraception could help health care professionals improve the functioning of their conscience. This is not to say that those health care professionals who conscientiously object to abortion or contraception necessarily have badly functioning consciences, only to argue that any right to have one's conscience protected should be accompanied by a duty to ensure the cultivation of a well-functioning conscience.

In terms of training health care professionals to develop a well- (or better-) functioning conscience with respect to abortion and contraception, educators could employ the existing method of reflective practice. Reflective practice encourages health professionals to reflect critically on their professional experience and learn from this reflection; it helps them to integrate professional values with their personal beliefs; and it promotes self-awareness (Mann et al. 2007: 596). The practice involves teaching methods such as small group discussions, keeping private journals or portfolios, and developing a relationship with a mentor, which are all well suited to approaching sensitive and delicate topics. In one educational intervention, organizers held workshops for medical students that involved role-plays on conscientious refusal in reproductive health care. Students' responses indicated that the workshops were helpful for them, allowing them time to reflect on their own views, become more comfortable discussing them, and consider how to communicate a refusal to a patient (Lupi et al. 2009).

To target the specific threat that implicit attitudes pose to the well-functioning of a health professional's conscience, workshops designed to raise awareness of the dangers of implicit bias could be combined with reflective practice methods. Jeff Stone and Gordon Moskowitz (2011) provide recommendations on how to create such workshops. Organizers could invite health professionals to test their own implicit biases with tools such as the IAT, although the tests should be carried out in a supportive environment and the results should remain strictly confidential. The IAT in particular should be seen as a teaching tool rather than an exam that one must pass. Workshops could include methods of identifying implicit biases, along with advice on how to mitigate these biases or avoid their manifestation. Of course, great care should be taken with the way in which advice is proffered because there is a danger of provoking hostile and counterproductive reactions. Which techniques are most likely to be successful at reducing the manifestation of implicit bias remains a somewhat open question; empirical research in this area is at a very early stage and caution is needed. For instance, there is mixed evidence on whether intentional control has positive or negative effects on the manifestation of implicit stereotypes (Payne and Stewart 2008: 1333). However, indirect methods of control seem more effective, and there is evidence that the following in particular may be helpful: Focusing on one's past failures in the area of bias/discrimination before an encounter and thus activating the goal of "being egalitarian" (Moskowitz and Li 2011); holding in mind counter-stereotypical exemplars, such as a successful black person (Blair 2002: 248–9); and mentally rehearsing "implementation intentions," tied to specific environmental cues, such as "When I see a black person, I will think 'successful'" (Payne and Stewart 2008).

There is some indication that health professionals would welcome learning more about implicit attitudes. In the study cited in the previous section in which physicians with pro-white implicit bias tended to suggest thrombolysis less often as a treatment for black patients, 75 percent of the participants said that taking the IAT is a worthwhile experience for physicians, and 76 percent agreed with the statement that learning more about unconscious biases could improve the quality of their patient care (Green et al.

2007: 1235). This evidence shows at least that health professionals would not necessarily be hostile to learning about the influence that implicit attitudes may have on their practice.

Concluding Remarks

In summary, conscientious refusal in health care is closely connected to political and moral debates over abortion and contraception. It can, and in some places does, have a significant impact on access to these services. The majority of bioethicists support the ability of health professionals to conscientiously refuse to provide abortion or contraceptive services within certain limits; most of them restrict permissible refusals to those that are not based on discriminatory beliefs, that do not occur in an emergency situation, and that satisfy other criteria as well. Such views tend not to preclude much conscientious refusal, however. On the whole, the bioethics literature is quite supportive of conscientious refusal in health care.

We have objected to the bioethics literature on conscientious refusal because, in general, it focuses too much on harm to health care professionals and too little on harm to patients, and because much of it employs a conception of conscience that is problematic. Although we agree that health care professionals should probably be able to make conscientious refusals in some circumstances, we also think that they should be duty-bound to cultivate a well-functioning conscience. We have outlined a revised conception of conscience that explains what a well-functioning conscience would look like and that has implications for the ethics education of health care professionals. Our recommendations for education included using reflective practice that is centered on the specific topics of abortion, contraception, and conscientious refusal, and that encourages health care professionals to maintain or develop a well-functioning conscience. Specific training in implicit attitudes is also vital, in our opinion, to ensure that these professionals are aware of the danger of behaving in ways that are contrary to their explicit beliefs.

Related Topics

Chapter 28, "Regulating Reproduction: A Bioethical Approach," Isabel Karpin

References

A Man for All Seasons (1966) [film] Directed by Fred Zinnemann, UK: Colombia Pictures.

Anderson, E. (2005) "So You Want to Live in a Free Society? Common Property, Common Carriers, and the Case of the Conscientious Objecting Pharmacist," *Left2Right*, August 2. Available at: http://left2right.typepad.com/main/2005/08/so_you_want_to_.html (accessed June 2011).

Benjamin, M. (1995) "Conscience," in W.T. Reich (ed.) *Encyclopedia of Bioethics*, 2nd edition, London: Macmillan, volume I, pp. 469–72.

Blair, I. (2002) "The Malleability of Automatic Stereotypes and Prejudice," *Personality and Social Psychology Review* 3: 242–61.

Blustein, J. (1993) "Doing What the Patient Orders: Maintaining Integrity in the Doctor–Patient Relationships," *Bioethics* 7 (4): 289–314.

Brady, M. (2007) "Recalcitrant Emotions and Visual Illusions," *American Philosophical Quarterly* 44 (3): 273–84.

Brock, D. (2008) "Conscientious Refusal by Physicians and Pharmacists: Who Is Obligated to do What and Why?" *Theoretical Medicine and Bioethics* 29: 187–200.

Cannold, L. (1994) "Consequence for Patients of Health Care Professionals' Conscientious Actions: The Ban on Abortions in South Australia," *Journal of Medical Ethics* 20: 80–6.

Cantor, J. and Baum, K. (2004) "The Limits of Conscientious Objection: May Pharmacists Refuse to Fill Prescriptions for Emergency Contraception?" *New England Journal of Medicine* 351 (19): 2008–12.

Card, R. (2011) "Conscientious Objection, Emergency Contraception, and Public Policy," *Journal of Medicine and Philosophy* 36: 53–68.

Charo, A. (2007) "Health Care Provider Refusals to Treat, Prescribe, Refer or Inform: Professionalism and Conscience," *American Constitution Society*, White Paper Series.

Childress, J. (1979) "Appeals to Conscience," *Ethics* 89: 315–35.

Childress, J. (1985) "Civil Disobedience, Conscientious Objection, and Evasive Noncompliance: A Framework for the Analysis and Assessment of Illegal Actions in Health Care," *Journal of Medicine and Philosophy* 10 (1): 63–84.

Childress, J. (1997) "Conscience and Conscientious Actions in the Context of MCOs," *Kennedy Institute of Ethics Journal* 7: 403–41.

Cooper, L., Roter, D., Carson, K., Beach, M., Sabin, J., Greenwald, A. and Inui, T. (2012) "The Associations of Clinicians' Implicit Attitudes about Race with Medical Visit Communication and Patient Ratings of Interpersonal Care," *American Journal of Public Health* 102 (5): 979–88.

Dale, S.S. (2004) "Can a Pharmacist Refuse to Dispense Birth Control?" *Time Magazine*, May 30. Available at: http://content.time.com/time/magazine/article/0,9171,644153,00.html (accessed September 2013).

Deans, Z. (2013) "Conscientious Objection in Pharmacy Practice in Great Britain," *Bioethics* 27: 48–57.

Downie, J. (2012) "Resistance Is Essential: Relational Responses to Recent Law and Policy Initiatives Involving Reproduction," in J. Downie and J. Lewellyn (eds.) *Being Relational: Reflections on Relational Theory and Health Law*, Vancouver: University of British Columbia Press, pp. 209–29.

Downie, J. and Lewellyn, J. (eds.) (2012) *Being Relational: Reflections on Relational Theory and Health Law*, Vancouver: University of British Columbia Press.

Downie, J. and McLeod, C. (eds.) (2014) "Let Conscience be Their Guide? Conscientious Refusals in Health Care," Special Issue of *Bioethics* 28 (1): ii–iv, 1–48.

Downie, J. and Nassar, C. (2008) "Barriers to Access to Abortion Through a Legal Lens," *Health Law Journal* 15: 143–73.

Dykes, B. (2002) "Proposed Rights of Conscience Legislation: Expanding to Include Pharmacists and Other Health Care Providers," *Georgia Law Review* 36.

Editorial. (2007) "Doctors Who Fail Their Patients," *The New York Times*, February 13. Available at: http://www.nytimes.com/2007/02/13/opinion/13tue3.html?_r=0 (accessed September 2013).

Fenton, E. and Lomasky, L. (2005) "Dispensing with Liberty: Conscientious Refusal and the 'Morning-After-Pill,'" *Journal of Medicine and Philosophy* 30: 579–92.

FitzGerald, C. (2014) "A Neglected Aspect of Conscience: Awareness of Implicit Attitudes," Special Issue of *Bioethics* 28 (1): 24–32.

Green, A., Carney, D., Pallin, D., Ngo, L., Raymond, K., Iezzoni, L. and Banaji, M. (2007) "Implicit Bias Among Physicians and Its Prediction of Thrombolysis Decisions for Black and White Patients," *Journal of General Internal Medicine* 22: 1231–8.

Greenberger, M. and Vogelstein, R. (2005) "Pharmacist Refusals: A Threat to Women's Health," *Science* 308: 1557–8.

Harris, L.H. (2012) "Recognizing Conscience in Abortion Provision," *New England Journal of Medicine* 367: 981–3.

Jost, J., Rudman, L., Blair, I., Carney, D., Dasgupta, N., Glaser, J. and Hardin, C. (2009) "The Existence of Implicit Bias Is Beyond Reasonable Doubt: A Refutation of Ideological and Methodological Objections and Executive Summary of Ten Studies That No Manager Should Ignore," *Research in Organizational Behavior* 29: 39–69.

Kelleher, J.P. (2010) "Emergency Contraception and Conscientious Refusal," *Journal of Applied Philosophy* 27 (3): 290–304.

Kolers, A. (2014) "Am I My Profession's Keeper?" Special Issue of *Bioethics* 28 (1): 1–7.

LaFollette, E. and LaFollette, H. (2007) "Private Conscience, Public Acts," *Journal of Medical Ethics* 33: 249–54.

Laurance, J. (2007) "Abortion Crisis as Doctors Refuse to Perform Surgery," *The Independent* April 16. Available at: http://www.independent.co.uk/news/uk/health_medical/article2452408.ece (accessed December 2010).

Lupi, C., Estes, C., Broome, M. and Schreiber, N. (2009) "Conscientious Refusal in Reproductive Medicine: An Educational Intervention," *American Journal of Obstetrics and Gynaecology* 201 (5): 502.e1–502.e7.

Lynch, H.F. (2008) *Conflicts of Conscience in Health Care: An Institutional Compromise*, Cambridge, MA: MIT Press.

Mann, K., Gordon, J. and MacLeod, A. (2007) "Reflection and Reflective Practice in Health Professions Education: A Systematic Review," *Advances in Health Sciences Education* 14: 595–621.

McLeod, C. (2008) "Referral in the Wake of Conscientious Objection to Abortion," *Hypatia* 23(4): 30–47.

McLeod, C. (2010) "Harm or Mere Inconvenience? Denying Women Emergency Contraception," *Hypatia* 25 (1): 11–30.

McLeod, C. (2012) "Taking a Feminist Relational Perspective on Conscience," in J. Downie and J. Lewellyn (eds.) *Being Relational: Reflections on Relational Theory and Health Law*, Vancouver: University of British Columbia Press, pp. 161–81.

Meyers, C. and Woods, R. (1996) "An Obligation to Provide Abortion Services: What Happens When Physicians Refuse?" *Journal of Medical Ethics* 22: 115–20.

Meyers, C. and Woods, R. (2007) "Conscientious Objection? Yes, but Make Sure it is Genuine," *American Journal of Bioethics* 7 (6): 19–20.

Moskowitz, G. and Li, P. (2011) "Egalitarian Goals Trigger Stereotype Inhibition: A Proactive Form of Stereotype Control," *Journal of Experimental Social Psychology* 47: 103–16.

Nosek, B. and Riskind, R. (2012) "Policy Implications of Implicit Social Cognition," *Social Issues and Policy Review* 6 (1): 113–47.

Palma, A. (2012) "Aborto, in Italia l'80% dei medici è obiettore di coscienza" [Blog]. Available at: http://www.fanpage.it/aborto-in-italia-l-80-dei-medici-e-obiettore-di-coscienza/#ixzz24AFpu7An (accessed June 2012).

Payne, B. and Stewart, B. (2008) "Bringing Automatic Stereotyping Under Control: Implementation Intentions as Efficient Means of Thought Control," *Personality and Social Psychology Bulletin* 34 (10): 1332–45.

Rawls, J. (1972) *A Theory of Justice*, Oxford: Clarendon Press.

Rodgers, S. and Downie, J. (2006) "Abortion: Ensuring Access," *Canadian Medical Association Journal* 175 (1): 9.

Sabin, J. and Greenwald, A. (2012) "The Influence of Implicit Bias on Treatment Recommendations for 4 Common Pediatric Conditions: Pain, Urinary Tract Infection, Attention Deficit Hyperactivity Disorder, and Asthma," *American Journal of Public Health* 102 (5): 988–95.

Sánchez Esparza, M. (2012) "Médicos de atención primaria podrán objetar en los casos de aborto." Available at: http://www.elmundo.es/elmundo/2012/03/05/andalucia_malaga/1330973795.html (accessed June 2012).

Savulescu, J. (2006) "Conscientious Objection in Medicine," *British Medical Journal* 332: 294–7.

Stein, R. (2006) "Medical Practices Blend Health and Faith," *Washington Post*, August 31. Available at: http://www.washingtonpost.com/wp-dyn/content/article/2006/08/30/AR2006083003290.html (accessed September 2013).

Stein, R. (2008) "Rule Shields Health Workers Who Withhold Care Based on Beliefs," *Washington Post* December 19. Available at: http://www.washingtonpost.com/wp-dyn/content/article/2008/12/18/AR2008121801556.html?sub=AR (accessed September 2013).

Stein, R. (2012) "Birth Control: Latest Collision between Individual Conscience and Society," *NPR Health News*, February 16. Available at: http://www.npr.org/blogs/health/2012/02/16/146921508/birth-control-latest-collision-between-individual-conscience-and-society (accessed September 2013).

Stone, J. and Moskowitz, G. (2011) "Non-conscious Bias in Medical Decision-Making: What Can be Done to Reduce It?" *Medical Education* 45: 768–76.

Stubblefield, A. (1996) "Contraceptive Risk-Taking and Norms of Chastity," *Journal of Social Philosophy* 27 (3): 81–100.

van Bogaert, L. (2002) "The Limits of Conscientious Objection to Abortion in the Developing World," *Developing World Bioethics* 2 (2): 131–43.

von Hippel, W., Brener, L. and von Hippel, C. (2008) "Implicit Prejudice Toward Injecting Drug Users Predicts Intentions to Change Jobs Among Drug and Alcohol Nurses," *Psychological Science* 19: 7–11.

Wicclair, M. (2000) "Conscientious Objection in Medicine," *Bioethics* 14: 205–27.

Wicclair, M. (2006) "Pharmacies, Pharmacists, and Conscientious Objection," *Kennedy Institute of Ethics Journal* 16 (3): 225–50.

Wicclair, M. (2011) *Conscientious Objection in Health Care: An Ethical Analysis*, Cambridge: Cambridge University Press.

Further Reading

Card, R. (2011) "Conscientious Objection, Emergency Contraception, and Public Policy," *Journal of Medicine and Philosophy* 36: 53–68 (an argument against conscientious refusal by pharmacists in the case of emergency contraception).

Childress, J. (1979) "Appeals to Conscience," *Ethics* 89: 315–35 (a classic contemporary defence of appeals to conscience).

Lynch, H.F. (2008) *Conflicts of Conscience in Health Care: An Institutional Compromise*, Cambridge, MA: MIT Press (a detailed treatment of an institutional solution to conscientious refusal in health care).

Wicclair, M. (2011) *Conscientious Objection in Health Care: An Ethical Analysis*, Cambridge: Cambridge University (an extended argument for moderate support of conscientious refusal in health care).

27
HUMAN EMBRYOS FOR REPRODUCTION AND RESEARCH

Françoise Baylis

Introduction

Ex utero (i.e., extracorporeal) human embryos created by *in vitro* fertilization (IVF) are now widely used for reproductive and research purposes. Individuals or couples who are infertile or who are at risk of having a child with a genetic disorder can use IVF, with or without third-party gametes, to create embryos for reproductive use. In addition, individuals and same-sex couples who are not infertile, but who want a genetic link to their child, can avail themselves of this reproductive technology.

Typically, more IVF embryos are created per cycle than can reasonably be transferred in the cycle in which they were created. While practice differs between IVF clinics, in many countries the current norm is to transfer no more than three IVF embryos per cycle (unless there are sound clinical reasons to increase this to four or five), and increasingly there is a move towards single embryo transfer (which is now legislated in some jurisdictions). IVF embryos not transferred in the cycle in which they were created can be discarded; donated or sold for reproductive, teaching, or research use by others; or cryopreserved (hereafter, frozen) for later own reproductive use (provided they are deemed suitable for transfer). If, at some later date, these frozen IVF embryos are no longer wanted by the prospective social parent(s) (i.e., those who planned to care for the child(ren) born of IVF and embryo transfer), then they can be transferred to a third-party for their reproductive use; an IVF clinic to improve assisted human reproduction or to provide instruction in assisted human reproduction; or a research team to pursue basic science or clinical research. Not all human embryos used for research purposes are IVF embryos in excess of reproductive need. In some jurisdictions it is legal to create human embryos expressly for research purposes, using IVF or other technologies.

A brief review of some of the ethical issues associated with the reproductive and research uses of human embryos follows, but first, some (very) basic biology and terminology. In science, the term "human embryo" refers to the developing human organism from day 14 after fertilization is complete until day 56. Prior to 14 days, the developing human organism is, according to some, a pre-embryo. When a human egg is fertilized by human sperm a new cell, called a zygote, is created. The zygote contains genetic information from the egg and sperm providers. As this cell continues to divide it becomes a morula, then a blastocyst, and only once implantation is complete (approximately 14 days after fertilization) is the developing human organism technically a human embryo. More commonly, however, in guidelines, regulations, and laws, the term human embryo refers to the developing human organism from the completion of fertilization (i.e., the appearance of the two cell zygote) until eight weeks' gestational age (i.e., 56 days). Potentially, however, human embryos need not be created by fertilization. For example, they could be created by parthenogenesis, somatic cell nuclear transfer (hereafter, cloning), single-cell embryo biopsy, and the reprogramming of somatic nuclei. In what follows, the term human embryo is used to describe the developing human organism from the time it is created (whether by fertilization or some other means) until it becomes a fetus at eight weeks' gestational age.

The Moral Status of the Human Embryo

In the years surrounding the 1978 birth of Louise Brown (the first human born using IVF technology), debate on the ethics of this technology focused primarily on the moral (and legal) status of the developing human embryo, including the right to life. In many respects, this early debate mirrored the abortion debate insofar as one's view on abortion typically informed one's view on the moral status of the IVF embryo, despite there being important differences in developmental stage (embryo versus fetus) and location (outside or inside the woman's body) (Robertson 1986). Particular attention was given to religious claims about ensoulment, philosophical claims about potentiality and personhood, and biological claims about human development.

For some, the developing human embryo "from the moment of conception" has the same moral status as all other humans (be they infants, children, or adults). This view is defended in particular by the Catholic Church. In the 1987 *Instruction on Respect for Human Life in its Origin and on the Dignity of Procreation (Donum Vitae)* the Church reaffirmed its view that "[h]uman life must be absolutely respected and protected from the moment of conception" (Congregation for the Doctrine of the Faith 1987). From a secular perspective, similar arguments have been advanced on the basis of human origin and potentiality. The human embryo is undeniably of the species *Homo sapiens* and it has the potential to become what everyone recognizes as a human person with full moral status—provided the embryo is of "good quality" and placed in a physiologically receptive uterus. Proponents of this view believe that with the completion of fertilization there is protectable human life. Many scientists, however, suggest that fertilization is "only incidental to the beginning of life" as there are other processes from which humans could potentially develop, including parthenogenesis and nuclear transfer, and that "potentiality for life must therefore reside in the unfertilized egg and all of its precursors" (Edwards 1974: 13).

For others, the developing human embryo is just human material; it is a collection of cells, similar to skin, blood, bone marrow, and other bodily tissues; it has no moral status. Rather (in)famously, Helga Kuhse and Peter Singer (1990) have compared the early human embryo to a lettuce. Proponents of this view insist that species membership (i.e., genetic humanity) is neither necessary nor sufficient for moral status. Personhood is a sufficient condition for moral status, but not all humans are persons, and not all persons are humans. Persons are beings to whom we have moral obligations; they are beings endowed with rights, dignity, and value. Sentience (the capacity to feel pain), rationality (the powers of reason), and relationality (being part of a particular social and biological community) are among the criteria that have been proposed for assigning moral status (Warren 1998; Strong 1997).

Between these extremes (of full moral status for human embryos on the one hand and near complete disregard for human embryos on the other) are those who believe, for different reasons, that the developing human embryo has special moral status, but not the same moral status as a full-fledged person. The proponents of this view maintain that the human embryo is deserving of "profound respect" but that such respect does not preclude the use of human embryos for reproductive and research purposes when the anticipated benefits outweigh the harms of embryo death and destruction (Ethics Advisory Board 1979a). The United States National Institutes of Health Human Embryo Research Panel, for example, concluded that "the preimplantation embryo warrants serious moral consideration but not the same as that due infants or children" (National Institutes of Health 1994: 50). In support of this view, the Panel noted "[t]he very high natural mortality, the absence of developmental individuation, the lack of even the possibility of sentience and most other qualities considered relevant to personhood" (National Institutes of Health 1994: 50). Others, however, insist that the hoped-for benefits in scientific knowledge and human health do not justify the wholesale destruction of human embryos. They note that a majority of the human embryos used for reproductive purposes will not survive, and typically all of the human embryos used for research purposes either will be destroyed during the course of experimentation, or will be destroyed thereafter owing to prohibitions on the transfer of human embryos that have been the subject of experimentation so as to avoid harm to future offspring.

Against this backdrop, and in an effort to side-step the intractable debate about the moral status of the developing human embryo, some have suggested that human organisms created through the reprogramming of somatic nuclei, parthenogenesis, cloning, and altered nuclear transfer would be different in kind and moral status from human embryos created by joining egg and sperm and thus could be used for research without any moral qualms (for a summary overview, see Baylis 2008; Green 2007). Others contest such claims. They insist that human origin and potentiality, not the means of creation, determine moral status.

An important feature of the contemporary debate on the moral status of the developing human embryo is the unwavering attention to the physical/material properties of the embryo as if there were biological facts about the embryo amenable to discovery that would authoritatively resolve the moral status debate. This is not so, however, as the debate is ultimately about values not facts.

Reproductive Use of Human Embryos: Beyond the Moral Status Debate

With the development of IVF technology and *ex utero* access to the developing human embryo concerns about procreative liberty (and marital privacy), potential harms to embryos manipulated outside of the body, informed choice, equitable access to reproductive technologies, resource allocation, slippery slopes, and impact on the family were added to early concerns about the moral status of the human embryo (Ethics Advisory Board 1979b). Concerns about procreative liberty focused on the right to reproduce and found a family. Concerns about potential harms to embryos focused on the risk of congenital defects as a direct result of *ex utero* manipulation, and on the potential for long-term physical and psychological harms to children born of IVF and embryo transfer.

Concerns about informed choice focused on the obligation to disclose the potential harms of IVF and embryo transfer to improve reproductive decision-making, and on the importance of ensuring voluntariness. Concerns about access focused on discrimination, typically on the basis of marital status and sexual orientation, as originally IVF and embryo transfer were limited to lawfully married couples. Concerns about resource allocation—a thorny issue in countries with government-funded health care systems—focused on whether to include IVF and embryo transfer in the basket of services paid for by the state, given competing health care priorities. Concerns about slippery slopes focused on the possibilities of surrogacy (hereafter, contract pregnancy); undesirable genetic interventions (e.g., cloning to produce children or for biomedical research), altering the cellular and genetic composition of embryos, and creating part-human hybrids and chimeras; and the commercialization of reproductive materials (e.g., gametes and embryos). Finally, initial concerns about impact on the family highlighted the splintering of parental roles. At that time, it was understood that as many as five individuals could have a parental role *vis-à-vis* a child born of IVF and embryo transfer—a biological mother and a biological father who each make a genetic contribution, an additional biological mother who provides a gestational service, and two social parents who together plan to care for the child. Today, there is the prospect of further splintering as many families have more than two social (and sometimes legal) parents and as two women may be involved in providing the genetic contribution, using mitochondrial replacement technology—the woman who provides the nuclear DNA (removed from an egg with "unhealthy" mitochondrial DNA), and the woman who provides the enucleated egg containing the "healthy" mitochondrial DNA.

From a practice and policy perspective, some of the ethical issues identified above are more or less settled in some jurisdictions. In other jurisdictions, these issues remain contentious and ethical debate continues. In addition, as the range of assisted human reproductive technologies has expanded beyond IVF and embryo transfer to include pre-implantation genetic diagnosis (PGD) (and, more recently, comprehensive chromosome screening, embryo and oocyte (hereafter, egg) freezing, *in vitro* maturation of eggs, and (pending) mitochondrial replacement technology), so too the range of contentious ethical issues has expanded.

For example, concerns about PGD (a technique used to diagnose a range of chromosomal and single gene traits in the eight-cell IVF embryo prior to transfer) focus on how we choose our children—most commonly, what kind of children we choose not to have, or not to have again (Glover 2007; Scott 2007). Initially, this technology was available to "select against" human embryos at significant risk for incurable, early onset, sex-linked, seriously disabling traits. Now, it is used to "select against" less serious early and late onset disorders. One example in the category of late onset disorders is heritable breast and ovarian cancer associated with two abnormal genes: BRCA1 and BRCA2 (Krahn 2009). Critics of the use of PGD to identify embryos "affected" with late onset disorders compared with early onset disorders insist that these embryos could become people with rich lives if they were transferred to a uterus, successfully implanted and were born. By the time their condition manifested, treatments (even cures) might be available. These same critics argue that the ever expanding use of PGD reinforces the false belief that embryos are fungible (i.e., completely replaceable/interchangeable with nothing lost in choosing between one embryo and another). The fact is, however, that different people would be born of so-called "healthy" and so-called "affected" embryos and the difference would not be reducible to the presence or absence of one undesirable trait. Critics of PGD also argue that use of this technology not only expresses disvalue for persons with disabilities, but ultimately could result in diminished support for persons with the disabilities targeted by PGD (Parens and Asch 2000).

From another perspective, if one chooses to avail oneself of PGD and there are embryos identified as "affected" it would be foolish (if not morally wrong) to transfer these "affected" embryos, regardless of the severity of the diagnosed condition or the age of onset. And yet there are some, who would "select for" what others might consider "affected" embryos. Deaf parents, for example, may want a child who will also be a member of the Deaf Community. PGD to "select for" human embryos with desired traits has also been used to select for HLA compatibility (when parents want a child who will become a donor for a sibling in need of a cell transplant— i.e., savior sibling) and could be used for social sex-selection (Wilkinson 2010).

Concerns about embryo freezing initially focused on potential harms to the offspring and on decisional authority and control over frozen embryos. With time and clinical experience, concerns about potential harms to children born of frozen–thawed embryos have diminished, though there are still conflicting reports on the potential harms of embryo freezing. As regards the relevant decision-making, particular attention has been given to the "who," "what," and "when" of informed choice. Who should decide whether embryos are frozen? Who should decide whether frozen embryos are discarded or donated/sold for reproductive, teaching, or research use? What information should be available to those who will make this decision? And, when should the decision about the eventual disposition of unused frozen embryos be made—before embryos are created, before they are frozen, when they are no longer needed for their original reproductive purpose, or when they are to be "handed over" to another? And, in relation to this point in time, if an option other than discarding frozen embryos is chosen, when and if so, how often, should there be the option to renew or withdraw consent?

In answer to the first of these questions, IVF clinics typically allow the prospective social parent(s) to decide whether to freeze good quality embryos for later use. Possible objectives in choosing embryo freezing include: reducing multiple gestations, avoiding embryo destruction, reducing costs, and preserving future options. Some clinics, however, until quite recently would only allow this if there were more than two good quality embryos to freeze. If there were only one or two such embryos, then embryo freezing was not available, but donation for human embryonic stem cell (hESC) and other research was an option (Haimes and Taylor 2009). In answer to the second of these questions, there are those who insist that the gamete providers (i.e., the sperm and egg providers) should be the ones to determine the disposition of any frozen embryos created using their genetic material. This perspective is ethically non-controversial when the gamete providers and the prospective social parents are the same people. When third-party gametes are used, however, the situation is more complicated as the prospective social parents (who are prospective embryo providers) may not be authorized to consent to the research use of embryos created with someone else's genetic material. Consider, for example, a situation in which a woman donated her eggs to create embryos for an infertile heterosexual couple to have a child using the sperm of the male partner. When that couple has finished their reproductive project, what should happen to any remaining frozen embryos? While it is clear that the sperm provider (who is one of the prospective social parents) should be involved in decision-making regarding the disposition of these embryos, the roles of the egg provider and the prospective social mother are contested. What if, for example, the egg provider consented to the use of her eggs to create an embryo to assist an infertile couple, but expressly objected to embryo research (Schaefer et al. 2012)? In some jurisdictions (e.g., Canada), only the gamete providers have dispositional authority over frozen embryos. In other jurisdictions (e.g., the United States), the gamete providers typically have no control over embryos created using their gametes; the prospective social parents have sole dispositional authority over frozen embryos.

With egg freezing, dispositional authority is not (yet) a contested ethical issue, but it may become one should there be large quantities of abandoned eggs in storage. Initially, egg freezing was offered to women with cancer prior to chemotherapy or radiotherapy. Now, it is also widely offered to women as insurance against ovarian insufficiency when pregnancy is delayed because of educational pursuits, career goals, or later age of establishing committed relationships. It is anticipated that so-called "social egg freezing" will amount to an expensive and unnecessary form of insurance as many of the women who will have frozen large numbers of eggs for their future reproductive use will become pregnant without using their frozen–thawed eggs (Darnovsky 2008). Should there be large quantities of unused, unwanted eggs in storage, these could become a valuable resource for embryo research.

On the horizon is mitochondrial replacement technology using pronuclear transfer or maternal spindle transfer to avoid the transmission of disease-linked mitochondrial DNA (mtDNA). Typically, babies are made from the sperm of one man and the egg of one woman. But, some women's eggs include unhealthy mtDNA. If these women reproduce using their own eggs, their children could be affected with a mitochondrial disease and this could result in serious health problems, including neurodegenerative disease, stroke-like episodes, blindness, and muscular dystrophy. The plan to avoid the vertical transmission of mtDNA mutations involves replacing disease-linked mtDNA with healthy donor mtDNA to create children with three genetic parents: the man who contributes nuclear DNA; the woman who contributes nuclear DNA; and the woman who contributes healthy mtDNA. In addition to concerns about the further splintering of parentage (noted above), concerns with this technology focus on the potential harms to the eggs providers and the increased risk of coercion and exploitation, the potential short- and long-term harms to offspring and their progeny, the move to embrace germline genetic modification, and the opportunity costs associated with the technology which ultimately will benefit very few (Baylis 2013).

Research Use of Human Embryos: Beyond the Moral Status Debate

In 1998, James Thomson and colleagues reported on the successful derivation of hESCs. This research, with the attendant promise of future treatments for everything from Alzheimer's, to burns, to cancers, and so on reenergized the debate on the moral status of the developing human embryo. It also introduced new ethical concerns focused on the source of eggs and embryos for research, the potential harms to the providers of eggs and embryos, the need for regulatory and research ethics oversight, and the ethics of volitional evolution (i.e., willful control of inheritable genetic traits through research involving cloning, human admixed embryos, and mitochondrial replacement, all with a view to changing the genetic inheritance of future generations).

Should human embryo research be permitted? This question has been answered in the affirmative in countries that permit (and in some cases fund) both fertility treatments involving IVF (which is the fruit of early and ongoing embryo research as new methods are developed, applied, and perfected) and hESC research in pursuit of clinical applications in regenerative medicine. Indeed, tolerance for, if not active endorsement of, these practices continues to shape the ethical debate. Ethical questions of pivotal importance include: What embryo research should be permitted? And, which embryos should be used for research?

What embryo research should be permitted? The proponents of human embryo research typically agree that such research should not exceed 14 days after fertilization. The 14-day limit on human embryo research was proposed by the Ethics Advisory Board of the United States Department of Health, Education, and Welfare (1979a). Writing in support of research involving IVF and embryo transfer, the Ethics Advisory Board recommended that human embryos not "be sustained *in vitro* beyond the stage normally associated with the completion of implantation (14 days after fertilization)" (1979a: 107). Underlying this recommendation was the belief that moral status could only be conferred on individuals, and that until implantation was complete the developing human organism might or might not be an individual, as both twinning and recombination were possible. With twinning, two genetically identical individuals could be created from one embryo. With recombination, two genetically different twin embryos could fuse together to create a chimera, or one twin embryo could envelop (wrap around) the other twin embryo (which ceases development during gestation) to create what is called a fetus *in fetu*.

Five years after this recommendation, in 1984, the Committee of Inquiry into Human Fertilisation and Embryology (the Warnock Committee) in the United Kingdom also recommended a 14-day limit on human embryo research, using the formation of the primitive streak (the precursor to brain development) as the "reference point" for individuality (a presumed necessary condition for moral status). At the time, most authorities placed this developmental process at about 15 days after fertilization, and on this basis the Warnock Committee endorsed a precautionary 14-day limit on human embryo research (Department of Health & Social Security 1984). That same year, the Committee to Consider the Social, Ethical and Legal Issues Arising from In Vitro Fertilization in Victoria, Australia (the Waller Committee) also endorsed a 14-day limit on human embryo research (Victoria 1984). Some Australian scholars, however, advocated a different (later) time limit. Kuhse and Singer (1990), for example, suggested a 28-day limit. On their view, sentience (the capacity to feel pleasure or pain) determines moral status and prior to 28 days the embryo is not sentient and so does not have moral status.

The 14-day limit is now widely entrenched in legislation and research ethics guidelines around the world. In important respects, however, this limit (from the time it was first proposed to this day) is mostly irrelevant because researchers typically do not have the ability to maintain an *ex utero* human embryo beyond approximately six days (Edwards 1974), at which time the embryo (at the blastocyst stage) hatches. Once this happens, the embryo needs to implant and get access to a blood supply. If the embryo is in a petri dish (not a uterus) it will attempt to "implant" on the bottom of the dish and it will fail to develop. So, from a practical perspective, the 14-day limit at most serves a political purpose. In anticipation of new science, however, it has been suggested that if it were possible to maintain a human embryo in culture up to and beyond 14 days, there should be national (or perhaps international) oversight committees that determine the time limit for specific embryo research projects based on research objectives and potential clinical value. Instead of an arbitrary 14-day limit for all embryo research, some such research would be limited to a few days (perhaps as little as 3 or 5 days), whereas other human embryo research could be permitted beyond 14 days. For example, it might be permissible to do cancer research until day 21 of embryonic development (beginning of closure of the neural tube).

In addition to specifying the length of time during which human embryo research is permitted, countries that regulate human embryo research typically also specify the scope of permissible research. The most liberal of the regulated regimes is the United Kingdom. In 1990, the *Human Fertilization and Embryology Act* (1990) was introduced. Schedule 2 of the Act identified the following research activities as "necessary and desirable":

(a) promoting advances in the treatment of infertility,
(b) increasing knowledge about the causes of congenital disease,
(c) increasing knowledge about the causes of miscarriages,
(d) developing more effective techniques of contraception, or
(e) developing methods for detecting the presence of gene or chromosome abnormalities in embryos before implantation.

Ten years later, this list was expanded in recognition of the potential of regenerative medicine (following the first successful derivation of hESCs). In January 2001, the *Human Fertilization and Embryology (Research Purposes) Regulations* were passed to specifically expand allowable embryo research beyond reproductive purposes. Currently, the *Human Fertilization and Embryology Act* (2008) (Schedule 2) permits the following research:

(a) increasing knowledge about serious disease or other serious medical conditions,
(b) developing treatments for serious disease or other serious medical conditions,
(c) increasing knowledge about the causes of any congenital disease or congenital medical condition that does not fall within paragraph (a),
(d) promoting advances in the treatment of infertility,
(e) increasing knowledge about the causes of miscarriage,
(f) developing more effective techniques of contraception,
(g) developing methods for detecting the presence of gene, chromosome or mitochondrion abnormalities in embryos before implantation, or
(h) increasing knowledge about the development of embryos.

In reviewing this list of legally permitted research, one might wonder "what research is excluded"? The "not-so-facetious" answer would be "nothing that could not somehow be described (or re-described) as relevant to health care." Why then expand the list of permitted embryo research instead of eliminate the list altogether? Some speculate that this approach better fits with the overarching goal of having a permissive regime with the appearance of robust national oversight.

Which embryos should be used for research? In the early days of human embryo research for reproductive purposes, it was suggested that non-viable embryos—embryos with no potential for ongoing growth and development because of a genetic or metabolic disorder—were morally equivalent to other human somatic cells and could be used for research (Baylis 1990). This idea was revisited in the late 1990s and early 2000s in debates about hESC research, at which time it was suggested that organismically dead embryos (embryos with irreversible cessation of cell division), and "pseudo-embryos" (embryos created by altered nuclear transfer to ensure that certain essential elements of embryogenesis are lacking) were non-viable and thus could be used for research (President's Council on Bioethics 2005). These specific proposals did not gain much traction. Meanwhile, researchers around the world continue to use embryos classified as "poor quality" on the basis of appearance or progress, as well as embryos identified as genetically "affected" through the use of PGD, for hESC research (Ehrich et al. 2010).

Another proposed distinction is between "spare" embryos (embryos originally created for reproduction, that are no longer wanted for this purpose) and "research" embryos (embryos specifically created for research purposes). In some countries only "spare" embryos—an ethically contentious category—can be used for research. Typically, this means that only women and couples undergoing fertility treatment who have embryos in storage and have completed their reproductive project can provide embryos to research. Beyond this, in some instances, embryos that are abandoned (as when the women or couples neglect to pay their storage fees and are lost to follow-up) can be made available for research. In other countries it is permissible to create human embryos specifically for research. So doing is ethically contentious, however, because of the need to access eggs from fertility patients or healthy volunteers. Women normally produce one egg a month. To increase the number of eggs potentially available for treatment or research, hormones are administered to women to stimulate the production of multiple eggs. These eggs are then removed by a needle inserted through the vagina.

Technologically assisted egg production is widely recognized as an onerous, invasive, and potentially harmful activity (Schaefer et al. 2012). The primary physical risk of hormonal stimulation is ovarian hyperstimulation syndrome. This may only result in abdominal bloating and mild abdominal pain, but in rare instances it can produce life-threatening complications including hemorrhage from ovarian rupture and thromboembolism. There have also been anecdotal reports of ovarian cancer, breast cancer, and colon cancer that suggest an increased risk of these cancers among those who undergo hormonal stimulation. In addition to the physical risks of hormonal stimulation, there are the physical risks of egg retrieval including bleeding, infection and adverse responses to the anesthesia. Other surgical risks include acute ovarian trauma, infection, infertility, vaginal bleeding, and lacerations.

It has been suggested that if the egg providers are fertility patients, they have presumably consented to the potential harms of ovarian stimulation and egg retrieval in pursuit of their own reproductive project and, as such, there are no potential physical harms specifically attributable to their decision to provide some of their eggs for research. This is inaccurate, however. Fertility patients who provide eggs for research and who do not become pregnant in their treatment cycle may have to undergo additional cycles of hormonal stimulation and egg retrieval to produce more eggs—eggs that would otherwise have been available to them (as either frozen eggs or embryos). In this situation, egg providers who are fertility patients would experience additional physical harms. In the alternative scenario, if the egg providers are healthy volunteers, then clearly the potential physical harms of hormonal stimulation and egg retrieval are solely a function of the decision to become an egg provider. It is one thing for infertile women to assume the potential harms of egg production in the hope of having a child using IVF, but quite another to encourage healthy volunteers to expose themselves to these potential harms for no potential benefit to themselves. From this perspective, restricting embryo research to "spare" embryos protects women (both healthy volunteers and fertility patients) from potential physical harms.

In those jurisdictions where human embryo research is limited to "spare" embryos, a further distinction can be drawn between fresh and frozen embryos. By definition, "spare" embryos are embryos "in excess of reproductive need." Following Carolyn McLeod and Françoise Baylis (2007), this category includes fresh embryos that are unsuitable for transfer and thus unsuitable for freezing (for example, embryos classified as "poor quality" as well as "affected PGD" embryos); and frozen embryos that are surplus to fertility treatment. As it is in the best interest of women pursuing fertility treatment to freeze their good quality fresh embryos for future reproductive use, good quality fresh embryos that are suitable for freezing are not "in excess of reproductive need" (unless it is known that there will be no subsequent embryo transfer cycle using frozen–thawed embryos). Others reject this distinction. In their view, "spare" embryos are any and all embryos not transferred in the cycle in which they were created, including good quality fresh embryos suitable for freezing. Interest in defining "spare" embryos in this way was originally motivated by a desire to have access to these embryos for hESC research, in the belief these embryos were superior to frozen embryos. Notwithstanding efforts to popularize this definition of spare embryos, the fact is that IVF clinic staff and embryo research staff appear "more 'comfortable' with donation of frozen, not fresh, embryos to hESC research" (Ehrich et al. 2010: 2206) and so the debate about whether fresh embryos count as "spare" embryos is, in some sense, moot.

Providing eggs for hESC research. While some jurisdictions limit human embryo research to "spare" embryos, other jurisdictions permit the creation of embryos specifically for research purposes. Typically, where creating human embryos for research is permitted, so too are payments, cash or in-kind (e.g., reduced IVF fees), to provide eggs to create embryos. These could be cash payments to healthy volunteers, or in-kind payments to women undergoing fertility treatment. Well known and controversial is the Newcastle "egg sharing for research" scheme (NSER) funded by the United Kingdom's Medical Research Council (Haimes 2013). With this scheme, IVF patients were eligible to receive a £1,500 reduction in fees for one IVF cycle (at a cost of £3,000 to £3,700) if they agreed to provide 50 percent of their fresh eggs for nuclear transfer research.

With the buying and selling of eggs, the ethical debate is about commodification, commercialization, and exploitation on the one hand, and rights, freedom of choice, and dignity on the other (Widdows 2009; Baylis and McLeod 2007). Some jurisdictions, such as the United Kingdom, Canada, Australia, New Zealand, and Israel prohibit payment for eggs (whether for reproduction or research) on the grounds that such payment is likely to induce financially disadvantaged women to assume serious risks they would not otherwise assume. These (and other) countries allow egg donation, however, and they generally permit compensation for out-of-pocket expenses incurred as a direct result of donation.

Other jurisdictions, most notably the United States, distinguish between eggs for reproduction and eggs for research. Some states (e.g., Massachusetts and California), allow payment for eggs for reproduction, but not for research. Other states (e.g., New York), allow payment for eggs irrespective of intended use. Those who support commercial trade in human eggs argue that women should be compensated fairly for egg production whether the eggs are for reproduction or for research. It should not be the case that women who undergo ovarian hyperstimulation and egg retrieval procedures to produce eggs for reproductive purposes are paid, while those who undergo the very same procedures with the same attendant risks to produce eggs for research purposes are not (Spar 2007). As well, it should not be the case that researchers may benefit financially from embryo research while those who provide the essential research material and services are prohibited from doing so. On this view, if there is exploitation, it is in expecting women to undergo hormonal stimulation and egg retrieval without fair compensation.

But what is fair compensation and what is unfair inducement? In the United Kingdom, patients undergoing ovarian stimulation and egg retrieval for their own reproductive project can provide eggs for research in exchange for a £1,500 reduction in treatment fees. Is this "egg sharing for research" scheme fair compensation? The market price in the United States for human eggs for reproduction is supposed to be around US$5,000 per cycle, as recommended by the Ethics Committee of the American Society for Reproductive Medicine and this has been used as a reference point for compensation for eggs for research. Meanwhile, there are advertisements soliciting elite egg donors from college students at Ivy League schools in the United States for as much as US$100,000 per cycle (Subrahmanyam 2008), and reports of student egg providers in Romania receiving as little as €600–800 per cycle (Zeiger 2013).What then is fair compensation for women in the United Kingdom or the United States who sell their eggs for research use? And, in the context of globalized trade in human eggs, what is fair compensation for women in middle income or poor countries who provide the same "services," for the same "product," with the same attendant risks?

Notwithstanding efforts to increase the number of eggs available for embryo research through various compensation/payment schemes, human eggs for research remain in short supply relative to the increasing demand. In 2007, in a further effort to address the problem of supply and demand, the Human Fertilisation and Embryology Authority—the national regulatory body responsible for licensing embryo research in the United Kingdom—granted several licenses for stem cell research involving the creation of cytoplasmic hybrid embryos—embryos created by inserting a human nucleus into a non-human enucleated egg. Shortly thereafter, in 2008, the United Kingdom passed legislation specifically permitting the creation of human admixed embryos as defined in Section 4A(6) of the *Human Fertilisation and Embryology Act* (2008).

For various reasons, the proposed use of enucleated animal eggs to create research embryos has had no impact on the problem of supply and demand. This problem may be time limited, however, given increasing enthusiasm for social egg freezing, at least in North America. Not all of the eggs being frozen will be used for reproduction, as many of the women with eggs in storage likely will become pregnant without using assisted human reproduction. And, of those who do reproduce using their frozen–thawed eggs, many likely will have considerably more frozen eggs than they will use. This means that, *de facto*, we are in the process of creating human egg banks, thereby obviating the need to create part-human cytoplasmic hybrid embryos for research purposes.

Conclusion

The promises and perils of human embryo manipulation, whether for reproduction or for research, are considerable. But this need not be so. With more informed debate and discussion that critically engages the moral imagination, we should be able to direct the reproductive and research use of embryos in ways that will serve the interests of human kind. This is not to suggest that consensus or even harmonization is possible. It is to say that in the context of global health and global science we need to critically examine the range of ethical issues remaining attentive to the broader, global implications of national policies and practices.

Related Topics

Chapter 28, "Regulating Reproduction: A Bioethical Approach," Isabel Karpin
Chapter 32, "Reproductive Testing for Disability," Adrienne Asch and David Wasserman

References

Baylis, F. (1990) "The Ethics of Ex Utero Research on Spare 'Nonviable' IVF Human Embryos," *Bioethics* 4 (4): 311–29.

Baylis, F. (2008) "Animal Eggs for Stem Cell Research: A Path Not Worth Taking," *American Journal of Bioethics* 8 (12): 18–32.

Baylis, F. (2013) "The Ethics of Creating Children with Three Genetic Parents," *Reproductive BioMedicine Online* 26: 531–4.

Baylis, F. and McLeod, C. (2007) "The Stem Cell Debate Continues: The Buying and Selling of Eggs for Research," *Journal of Medical Ethics* 33 (12): 726–31.

Congregation for the Doctrine of the Faith (1987) *Instruction on Respect for Human Life in its Origin and on the Dignity of Procreation Replies to Certain Questions of the Day*. Available at: http://www.vatican.va/roman_curia/congregations/cfaith/documents/rc_con_cfaith_doc_19870222_respect-for-human-life_en.html (accessed July 21, 2014).

Darnovsky, M. (2008) "Eggs on Ice: New Profit Center for the Baby Business," *Biopolitical Times* [Online]. Available at: http://www.biopoliticaltimes.org/article.php?id=4239 (accessed July 21, 2014).

Department of Health & Social Security (1984) *Report of the Committee of Inquiry into Human Fertilisation and Embryology*, London: Her Majesty's Stationery Office. Available at: http://www.hfea.gov.uk/docs/Warnock_Report_of_the_Committee_of_Inquiry_into_Human_Fertilisation_and_Embryology_1984.pdf (accessed July 21, 2014).

Edwards, R. (1974) "Fertilization of Human Eggs In Vitro: Morals, Ethics and the Law," *The Quarterly Review of Biology* 49: 3–26.

Ehrich, K., Williams, C. and Farsides, B. (2008) "The Embryo as Moral Work Object: PGD/IVF Staff Views and Experiences," *Sociology of Health and Illness* 30: 772–87.

Ehrich, K., Williams, C. and Farsides, B. (2010) "Fresh or Frozen? Classifying 'Spare' Embryos for Donation to Human Embryonic Stem Cell Research," *Social Science and Medicine* 71: 2204–11.

Ethics Advisory Board (1979a) *Report and Conclusions: HEW Support of Research Involving Human In Vitro Fertilization and Embryo Transfer*, Washington, DC: U.S. Department of Health, Education, and Welfare.

Ethics Advisory Board (1979b) *Appendix: HEW Support of Research Involving Human In Vitro Fertilization and Embryo Transfer*, Washington, DC: U.S. Department of Health, Education, and Welfare.

Glover, J. (2007) *Choosing our Children*, Oxford and New York: Oxford University Press.

Green, R.M. (2007) "Can We Develop Ethically Universal Embryonic Stem-Cell Lines?" *Nature Reviews Genetics* 8 (6): 480–5.

Haimes, E. (2013) "Juggling on a Rollercoaster? Gains, Loss and Uncertainties in IVF Patients' Accounts of Volunteering for a U.K. 'Egg Sharing for Research' Scheme," *Social Science in Medicine* 86: 45–51.

Haimes, E. and Taylor, K. (2009) "Fresh Embryo Donation for Human Embryonic Stem Cell (hESC) Research: The Experiences and Values of IVF Couples Asked to be Embryo Donors," *Human Reproduction* 24: 2142–50.

Human Fertilisation and Embryology Act (1990) c. 37, Schedule 2. United Kingdom. Available at: http://www.legislation.gov.uk/ukpga/1990/37/pdfs/ukpga_19900037_en.pdf (accessed July 21, 2014).

Human Fertilisation and Embryology Act (2008) c. 22, Schedule 2. United Kingdom. Available at: http://www.legislation.gov.uk/ukpga/2008/22/schedule/2 (accessed July 21, 2014).

Krahn, T. (2009) "Preimplantation Genetic Diagnosis: Does Age of Onset Matter (Anymore)?" *Medicine, Health Care and Philosophy* 12 (2): 187–202.

Kuhse, H. and Singer, P. (1990) *Embryo Experimentation*, New York: Cambridge University Press.

McLeod, C. and Baylis, F. (2007) "Donating Fresh Versus Frozen Embryos to Stem Cell Research: In Whose Interests?" *Bioethics* 21: 465–77.

National Institutes of Health (1994) *Report of the Human Embryo Research Panel*. Vol. 1. Maryland: National Institutes of Health. Available at: http://bioethics.georgetown.edu/pcbe/reports/past_commissions/human_embryo_vol_1.pdf (accessed July 21, 2014).

Parens, E. and Asch, A. (2000) "The Disability Rights Critique of Prenatal Genetic Testing: Reflections and Recommendations," in Parens, E. and Asch, A. (eds.) *Prenatal Testing and Disability Rights*, Washington, DC: Georgetown University Press, pp. 3–43.

President's Council on Bioethics (2005) *Alternative Sources of Human Pluripotent Stem Cells: A White Paper*. Washington DC. Available at: http://bioethics.georgetown.edu/pcbe/reports/white_paper/alternative_sources_white_paper.pdf (accessed July 21, 2014).

Robertson, J. A. (1986) "Extracorporeal Embryos and the Abortion Debate," *Journal of Contemporary Health Law Policy* 2: 53–70.

Schaefer, G.O., Sinaii, N. and Grady, C. (2012) "Informing Egg Donors of the Potential for Embryonic Research: A Survey of Consent Forms from U.S. In Vitro Fertilization Clinics," *Fertility and Sterility* 97: 427–33.

Scott, R. (2007) *Choosing Between Possible Lives: Law and Ethics of Prenatal and Preimplantation Genetic Diagnosis*, Portland, OR: Hart Publishing.

Spar, D. (2007) "The Egg Trade: Making Sense of the Market for Human Oocytes," *New England Journal of Medicine* 356: 1289–91.

Strong, C. (1997) "The Moral Status of Preembryos, Embryos, Fetuses, and Infants," *Journal of Medicine and Philosophy* 22: 457–78.

Subrahmanyam, D. (2008) "Ivy League Egg Donor Wanted," *Yale News* April 23. Available at: http://yaledailynews.com/blog/2008/04/23/ivy-league-egg-donor-wanted/ (accessed July 21, 2014).

Victoria. Committee to Consider the Social, Ethical and Legal Issues Arising from In Vitro Fertilization (1984) Available at: http://nla.gov.au/nla.party-783771 (accessed July 21, 2014).

Warren, M.A. (1998) *Moral Status: Obligations to Persons and Other Living Things*, Oxford: Oxford University Press.

Widdows, H. (2009) "Border Disputes Across Bodies: Exploitation in Trafficking for Prostitution and Egg Sale for Stem Cell Research," *International Journal of Feminist Approaches to Bioethics* 2: 5–24.

Wilkinson, S. (2010) *Choosing Tomorrow's Children: The Ethics of Selective Reproduction*, Oxford: Clarendon Press.

Zeiger, A. (2013) "Israelis Held in Romanian Ova Trafficking Case," *The Times of Israel*. February 19. Available at: http://www.timesofisrael.com/israelis-held-in-romanian-ova-trafficking-case/ (accessed July 21, 2014).

28
REGULATING REPRODUCTION
A Bioethical Approach

Isabel Karpin

Introduction

Over the last 10 years, across the globe, there has been a steady increase in the use of assisted reproductive technologies (ARTs). The European Society of Human Reproduction and Embryology (ESHRE) reports the highest uptake in Belgium, Denmark, Finland, Iceland, Norway, Slovenia, and Sweden where more than 3.0 percent of all babies born in 2010 were conceived by ARTs (ESHRE 2010). In Australia the figure from 2008 data is as high as 3.3 percent of Australian babies, having risen by 10 percent per year over the previous five years (Wang et al. 2010: viii). In the U.K. the Human Fertilisation and Embryology Authority (HFEA) reports that, in 2010, 2 percent of babies were born using *in vitro* fertilization (IVF) procedures (HFEA 2013: 39). The figure is lower in the U.S. (approximately 1 percent) (ESHRE 2010), however the number is still significant given the high cost of this developing technology and the comparative lack of public health funding for these procedures in the U.S. It is not surprising, then, that many countries have introduced laws dealing with ARTs and IVF that attempt to impose limits on their use.

The regulation of reproductive technology, and human reproduction more broadly, raises significant bioethical concerns. This chapter focuses primarily on the ramifications of regulating reproduction on women's freedom of choice and autonomy, but also briefly considers the impact on alternate familial relationships. It is uncontroversial that laws about reproduction have a greater effect on women because, more often than not, a woman's body is central to the reproductive process. Indeed, this has been recognized in Canada in the *Assisted Human Reproduction Act* (2004) (AHRA) which has, as one of its overarching principles: "2(*c*) while all persons are affected by these technologies, women more than men are directly and significantly affected by their application and the health and well-being of women must be protected in the application of these technologies." Further, advances in reproductive technology challenge the way in which human reproduction is conventionally conceived. New family forms such as those constituted by same-sex parents, those formed through egg or sperm donation, or those created through careful genetic testing and selection shift assumptions about what kinds of families are both possible and desirable. With this in mind, the aim of this chapter is to map out a bioethics of reproductive regulation from a feminist and postmodern philosophical perspective.

The Laws

Together with laws governing access to abortion and regulating the behavior of pregnant women, new laws that seek to regulate ART are key to any analysis of the bioethical issues raised by the regulation of reproduction. To this end, this chapter will draw on legal examples of reproductive regulation from the U.K., Canada, Australia, and the U.S. The U.K. has comprehensive national legislation governing all aspects of reproductive technology and embryo research (*Human Fertilisation and Embryology Act* 1990 (HFE)) and a national authority—the HFEA—charged with licensing and monitoring all activities covered by the legislation. Canada, too, has national ART legislation—the AHRA—however, a number of its central provisions were found unconstitutional in 2010 and its effectiveness has been significantly reduced. In Australia there is a mixture of highly regulated, unregulated, and self-regulated jurisdictions among the several states and territories (*Human Reproductive Technology Act* WA (1991); *Assisted Reproductive Treatment Act* VIC (2008); *Assisted Reproductive Technology Act* NSW (2007); *Assisted Reproductive Treatment Act* SA (1988)) as well as national laws (the *Prohibition of Human Cloning for Reproduction Act* (2002) and the *Research Involving Human Embryos Act* (2002)) and national ethical guidelines with which clinics must comply in order to achieve accreditation (*National Health and Medical Research Council Ethical Guidelines on the use of Assisted Reproductive Technology in Clinical Practice and Research* (2007) (NHMRC ART Guidelines)). The U.S. is one notable country that has left the area of ARTs largely unregulated.

In the jurisdictions covered here, laws dealing with reproduction are typically of two types: Those that prohibit certain practices outright, and those that permit certain practices under specific conditions. In the U.K., Australia, and Canada, for example, sex selection of embryos is allowed under limited circumstances; namely, where there is a sex-linked disorder that is being screened (Sched 2 S1ZA, HFE (1990) U.K.; s11, NHMRC ART Guidelines (2007) Aus.; s5(1)(e) AHRA (2004) Can.). However, all three of these jurisdictions prohibit outright the creation of cloned, hybrid, or chimeric (containing cells from human and non-human sources) embryos for human reproduction. These are common legislative concerns in many countries across the globe. Paradoxically, however, laws that seek to prospectively prohibit the reproduction of a class of entirely speculative beings grant them a concrete reality through the act of prohibition itself. In light of this, and related developments, it is necessary to ask: What role should law play in the area of reproduction?

The Role of Law

Technologies that enable cloning, same-sex reproduction, or multiple biological parentage (three or more genetic parents) can produce entities that would radically destabilize conventional accounts of reproduction. Canadian law professor Roxanne Mykitiuk and I have argued that, in the early days of ARTs, regulatory responses to these reproductive technologies attempted to counter their destabilizing effects by imposing limits that reinforced traditional notions of "natural" reproduction. For instance, the potential impact of new reproductive technologies was moderated in some jurisdictions by legal requirements that assisted reproduction only take place between a man and a woman within a heterosexual relationship and "that the product of that technologically enhanced reproduction has a blood/genetic line that only traces back to two progenitors" (Karpin and Mykitiuk 2006: 196).

More recently, however, law has played a role in creating the conditions for a new radically transformed understanding of the "natural." For example, some jurisdictions have introduced legal recognition of same-sex parents (Millbank 2006a, 2006b, 2008; McCandless and Sheldon 2010). In those jurisdictions this not only attributes legal legitimacy to this parenting form but goes some way to establishing same-sex parenting as a new "natural." Similarly, recent moves in the U.K. to allow the creation of embryos with more than two progenitors under s3ZA(5) of the HFE Act (1990) will begin to challenge the orthodoxy of dyadic genetic parenting (Sample 2013). In March 2013, the U.K. HFEA recommended the government consider allowing mitochondria replacement for women with mitochondria disease. This would have the effect of creating embryos using reproductive material from three people and thus merging three partial sets of DNA (HFEA 2013).

Thus the category of what is natural is not fixed and law can play a role in its revision. What is allowed and disallowed under law becomes a key marker for what is natural and unnatural and this has implications for what is perceived as ethical. We might ask: Is this an appropriate role for the law?

Feminist postmodern legal thinkers argue that law contributes to a provisional and changing understanding of bodies (Murphy and Ó Cuinn 2013; Fox et al. 2010; Fineman 2000). They contend that law, in conjunction with other discourses, actively *creates* the meaning attributed to these bodies rather than merely performing a regulatory role. Thus in the case of reproduction, entities such as eggs, sperm, fetuses, and embryos are given meaning through the convergence of cultural, biotechnological, legal, and other discourses. This account contrasts with more conventional views that regard law as a mechanism only, protecting individuals from potential harm by placing appropriate limits on that which is already discovered, created, or imagined.

Mary Ford argues that, typically, "law defines and approaches its subjects in a way that presupposes the liberal, modernist model of selfhood" (Ford 2009: 32)—that is, a bounded autonomous individual. In this more traditional view, law is charged with upholding individual liberty and equality by protecting independence and autonomy. For feminist legal thinkers, these individualistic ideals are problematic because they deemphasize, and thus devalue, the importance of the relationships and context that give these bodies their shape and meaning. This is borne out in the context of the regulation of the reproductive body. Traditionally, law is concerned with defending the individual against unauthorized incursion and controlling the boundaries of the self. However, pregnancy, in its very essence, confounds and crosses boundaries, complicating the concept of individual identity. Thus, a great deal of legal and regulatory work aims to define the boundaries of the pregnant female body to give effect to the liberal individual subject of law. Much of that work involves drawing a line around where the individuality of the woman stops and that of the fetus or, more recently, the embryo, begins.

Instead of rejecting these ideals outright, Jennifer Nedelsky has offered a critical reconceptualization of autonomy and selfhood. Nedelsky's "relational autonomy":

> acknowledges both the ways in which we are profoundly shaped by, indeed significantly constituted by the relationships of which we are a part (whether personal, cultural, national or global) and at the same time captures the way in which we genuinely are autonomous beings who are not *determined* by these relationships.
>
> (Nedelsky 2011: 167)

The remainder of this chapter examines the *legal* creation of reproductive bodies at key moments in the recent history of biotechnology to consider how variants of this relational approach might offer viable alternatives to the individualist model.

Displacing the Female Body

While laws vary across different nations, in Australia, the U.K., Canada, and most parts of the U.S., a fetus does not acquire legal personhood status until it is "born alive." The key constitutive moment then, when legal personhood is said to accrue to a fetus, is when it exists independently from the gestating woman. It is at this point that a distinct rights bearing individual can be identified (Savell 2006). Nevertheless, in many jurisdictions the fetus is viewed as a potential person afforded a special status in law. Sonia Harris-Short has noted that in the English context, for example, "both the *HFE* Act 1990 and the *Abortion Act* 1967 are premised on the principle that the embryo/foetus, as a potential person, has a special status . . . worthy of protection" (Harris-Short 2009: 65). This seeming contradiction illustrates the ongoing struggle within law to find a way to account for fetal value. The debate often polarizes between those who wish to attribute individuality to the fetus at varying stages of development and those who wish to deny it any value until it is born. Neither of these positions, however, adequately deals with, nor attempts to document, the way in which women themselves value their pregnancies.

In the late 1980s and early 1990s, for example, the characterization of the fetus as on the cusp of individuation played out in courtrooms and legislatures across the U.S. There were a series of so-called "protective incarcerations" of pregnant, drug-addicted women. Some received forced medical treatments, including court-ordered cesarean sections. Women who gave birth to babies testing positive for drugs were also prosecuted for harm allegedly caused *in utero*. These interventions were initiated in the wake of a moral panic about "crack babies" that revealed, as Dorothy Roberts documents, systemic racism against poor African American women (Roberts 1991: 1420–1, n6–8; see also Paltrow 1992) and very little scientific grounding (Okie 2009). In one particularly notable case a prosecutor charged a woman with supplying an illegal substance to her child via her own blood after the child was born but in the seconds before the umbilical cord was cut (*Jennifer Clarice Johnson v State of Florida* (1991) 578 So. 2d 419 (5th Dis., Ct of Appeals)).

Feminist lawyers have spoken against these cases, insisting that they inappropriately attribute personhood to the unborn fetus and they deny that same status to the woman whose addiction disorder is used against her. Despite these arguments, prosecutions continue in states like Alabama (Calhoun 2012) and there have been numerous unsuccessful attempts to establish personhood rights for the fetus in states such as Mississippi, North Dakota, Montana, and Oklahoma (Calhoun 2012). In response, Lynn Paltrow, executive director of the National Advocates for Pregnant Women, has said "there is no way to treat fertilized eggs, embryos and fetuses as separate constitutional persons without subtracting pregnant women from the community of constitutional persons" (Calhoun 2012: 4). This analysis sums up the dilemma of a system that is based on individualism. The only options within the individualist model are either to attribute individual status to both the woman and her fetus, thus creating a potentially antagonistic relationship, or to deny any value to the fetus. But, what happens when the pregnant woman wants to assert both her own right to selfhood, and that of her fetus? The story of Australian woman, Brodie Donegan, who lost her 32-week pregnancy when she was hit by a negligently driven car, offers an interesting demonstration of this problem. The woman driving the car was found guilty of causing grievous bodily harm to Donegan, which included the loss of her pregnancy, however there was no legal claim that could be made on behalf of the fetus itself because it never took a breath and thus never attained legal personhood status. Donegan states:

> The current law allows the foetus/baby to be listed in the mother's injuries. But the offence is against the mother. The baby's existence is not recognised separately to the mother until he/she takes a breath.
>
> My problem with this law is that . . . she was not my injury. She was my baby. I felt her move; I'd [. . .] been to check ups, ultrasounds, and had pictures of her. I had bought clothes for her, set up a room for her, and carried her for 8 months.
> (Donegan 2013)

Donegan, who is pro-choice, has subsequently attempted to propose a new law—*Zoe's Law 2*—that would enable a separate charge of grievous bodily harm to be introduced on behalf of the fetus, but only under limited circumstances. Most importantly, *Zoe's Law 2* would specifically exclude any claim for harm caused by a mother or "medical professionals during the course of a procedure, treatment or assisting a pregnant woman" (Donegan 2013).

This law is currently before the New South Wales state parliament but it has raised significant concern among pro-choice activists who are apprehensive that allowing this change in status for fetuses, even in these limited circumstances, would be just the beginning of a slide towards attributing individual legal personhood to them more broadly. The concern is that this would then be used to trump the autonomous rights of the gestating woman. Law academic Hannah Robert suffered a similar pregnancy loss when her car was hit by a 4WD when she was eight months pregnant. Robert opposes the law because, she argues, the fetus "is a life completely contained within a legal person (the mother), [and] any interests or rights it could have can only be advanced through the consent of the mother" (Robert 2013). She suggests instead "a specific offence addressing conduct that ends the life of a foetus without the mother's consent."

The idea of the fetus as a separate entity is, however, evident in laws that seek to establish a concept of fetal viability to limit reproductive choice for women. Fetal viability describes a developmental stage when it might be possible for a fetus to survive outside the womb. In the context of American abortion law, for example, in the watershed case *Roe v. Wade* ((1973) 410 U.S. 113) the fetus was deemed to have attained a limited form of legal subjectivity or personhood at the point of viability, which was said to occur in the third trimester. In that case states could have regulated to limit abortion in the third trimester of pregnancy except where necessary to preserve the life of the mother. However, in the later case of *Casey v Planned Parenthood* ((1992) 112 S.Ct. 2791) the rigid trimester system was abandoned and instead the court ruled that state laws must not place an undue burden on a woman seeking an abortion up to the point of viability. Justice Sandra Day O'Connor noted in that case that viability might arise earlier than the third trimester if, for example, technology is used to enhance fetal respiratory capacity. Thus, the effect of "viability" has been to artificially construct a moment when the fetus attains individuality in law. In these moments, law rather than the woman gives birth to the individual.

This emphasis placed on identifying the point at which an individual is formed distorts our understanding of what is really at stake in the attribution of legal personhood. If we come back to the pregnant woman, we can see that her bodily boundaries are intermingled with the developing fetus and the potential new person. Postmodern feminists embrace an account of the body as never fully individuated, never fully separated from the other (Shildrick 1997; Haraway 1991). How then might a feminist postmodern *legal* bioethics reframe the pregnant woman? First, it would seek to craft laws that were able to accommodate and celebrate fluid boundaries. For example, the relational view of autonomy outlined above requires the development of laws that respond to female agency, and which are formed through a non-traditional understanding of selfhood. Rather than relying on a bounded, individual self, such laws would permit a more complex and embodied account of the self constituted within a matrix of relationships to other persons, as well as things, societal institutions, practices, and beliefs (Nedelsky 2011; Downie and Llewellyn 2011).

Drawing on the work of feminist philosopher Luce Irigaray (1985), in the early 1990s I proposed a relational strategy that reconfigured the pregnant woman in law as not-one-but-not-two (Karpin 1992). The conceptualization of the pregnant woman as not-one-but-not-two aimed to retain the primacy of the woman's selfhood while not subscribing to individualist models that demand either that the woman and her fetus are equal and, therefore, potential protagonists, or that the fetus has no value to the woman until it is born. Both Brodie Donegan's law reform and Hannah Robert's alternative proposal attempt to articulate this form of relational identity. Significantly, neither wants to describe the fetus as entirely distinct and separate from the mother. Under Donegan's form of the law, the mother is exempted from claims for harm she may have caused to the fetus. Presumably this exemption rests on an understanding that the mother's embodied, life-giving relationship to the fetus is unique and must be protected. However, because this is not made explicit, Donegan's law reform appears to attribute separate legal personhood to the fetus. As Robert notes, "[o]nce the foetus is defined as a legal person, the law has a direct relationship with it, and the mother's consent becomes irrelevant" (Robert 2013). Robert's proposal, however, offers a law where the identity and selfhood of the fetus is contingent upon its relationship to the woman and thus is to be preferred if applying a relational model.

Given developments in ARTs, it is worth asking: Can this relational conceptualization of reproduction be extended to cover embryos formed outside the body of a woman?

The Pre-Gestated Embryo

In IVF practice an embryo is created outside the body of a woman by fertilizing a human egg with a human sperm in a petrie dish. The fertilized ovum is usually grown to blastocyst stage and then either transferred to the woman's uterus in the hopes of achieving a pregnancy, or stored for future reproductive use. Cryopreservation, or the freezing of embryos, became a significant part of IVF with the shift from natural cycle IVF (involving collecting and fertilizing the single egg that a woman releases during her monthly cycle) to stimulated IVF (involving suppression of the natural cycle and the introduction of a follicle-stimulating hormone to increase the number of eggs produced from one cycle). In some cases not all frozen embryos are used and these remain in storage pending a disposition decision.

Laws controlling the development and use of these embryos created outside the female body typically concern how they may be "made," who may make them, for what purpose, how long they may be stored, the manner of their disposal and destruction, and the genetic conditions for which they may be tested (see, for example, HFE 1990).

One key way in which law has had a direct impact is through the process of definition. For example, defining a "cluster of cells" as an "embryo" because it meets a set of artificially imposed conditions, constitutes a transformative moment. As a newly defined embryo, these bundled cells attract a clutch of values, expectations, and narrative trajectories.

In the Australian context the legal definition of an embryo has been through a number of iterations. The latest definition has arguably opened a space for scientific experimentation on fertilized cells that did not previously exist. An embryo is now defined in the *Australian Prohibition of Human Cloning for Reproduction Act* (2002) (PHCRA) as:

> a discrete entity that has arisen from either: (a) the first mitotic division when fertilization of a human oocyte by a human sperm is complete; or (b) any other process that initiates organized development of a biological entity with a human nuclear genome or altered human nuclear genome that has the potential to develop up to, or beyond, the stage at which the primitive streak appears; and has not yet reached 8 weeks of development since the first mitotic division.
>
> (PHCRA s8)

Thus, fertilized cells before the first mitotic cell division are not defined as embryos and therefore are not subject to the same research limitations (Lockhart Committee 2005: xv, 174). This distinction was justified on the grounds that the first mitotic cell division inaugurated a unique genetic entity (Lockhart Committee 2005: xv). By privileging genetic identity, however, an account of selfhood as synonymous with DNA is given the force of law while the necessity for female gestation to create the individual is obscured. In other words, the embryo takes on an individual identity that cannot be sustained.

Feminists who wish to destabilize the existing legal characterization of these embryos as entities in and of themselves, disconnected from the female body that is otherwise necessary for their development, have found ways of critically re-describing the process (Franklin 2001; Fox 2000; Ford 2009; Thomson 1997; Morgan and Michaels 1999). For example, I have coined the phrase "pre-gestated embryos" in order to reintroduce the erased female body, and the necessity of gestation for individual personhood to be established. By simply altering the language we can expose the law's constitutive role and highlight the possibility of an alternative account that insists that embryos exist only within a matrix of relatedness.

A relational account of autonomy would regard embryos as constituted through their relationship with the woman who created them and who might gestate them in the future. This is reflected in a recent study exploring women's feelings about their frozen embryos in which a number of women described their own, often highly embodied, relationship to their frozen embryos (Millbank et al. 2012). For some of these women the pre-gestated embryo did not possess a separate identity, but was an extension of the relational and familial network of which the woman who created it was a part.

What Next? Cell-Based Reproductive Ubiquity

In 2007 a group of scientists reported that they had successfully cloned a mouse embryo using adult skin cells (Li et al. 2007). The development occurred using a cell reprogramming method that induces pluripotency in adult stem cells (iPS cells). In other words, it returns the adult cells to an immature state, similar to that of an embryonic stem cell, enabling them to differentiate into all cell types—muscle, bone, blood, nervous system, and many more. There are some indications that the pluripotency of these cells may well be as potent as the human embryonic stem cell (hES cell) (Kang et al. 2009). It is not surprising then that Professor Bob Williamson was prompted by this research to ask: "if every cell in the body has the potential to become an embryo, do people who are opposed to embryonic stem cell research believe that every skin cell deserves the respect that is accorded to an embryo made in the usual way?"(Cronin 2007).

Apart from the obvious potential future uses of iPS cells to create whole human beings, there is another use that is much closer to reality and has already been foreshadowed by its legal prohibition in the U.K.: The creation of artificial gametes. Advances in stem cell technology in the U.K. have shown the capacity to produce what appears to be mature human sperm from hES cells (Nayernia et al. 2006a, 2006b). Because the cell reprogramming method of iPS looks increasingly likely to mimic most if not all the capacities of an hES cell, it seems likely that this technology could also be used to create gametes (West et al. 2013).

Thus we have a situation where it might be possible to use a sperm generated from a skin cell of a man to fertilize an egg (either natural or artificially generated). While this may seem a distant fantasy, the U.K. legislature has been sufficiently concerned to explicitly prohibit the use of artificial gametes in assisted reproduction. Clause 3ZA of the HFE Act defines "permitted embryo," "permitted sperm," and "permitted eggs." Paragraph 29 of the *Explanatory Notes* to the 2008 HFE Amendment Act states "Permitted eggs are defined as eggs produced by or extracted from the ovaries of a woman and permitted sperm as sperm produced by or extracted from the testes of a man."

If it becomes safe to use artificial gametes, some of the most significant applications will be for women rendered infertile from cancer treatment who could create new eggs from her skin cells; the capacity of two men (and possibly two women) to have a child that is genetically related to both parties; and, as Emily Jackson points out, the capacity to create "a child [with] only one genetic parent whose natural gametes could be used to fertilize their artificially derived gametes" (Jackson 2008).

While views may differ about the value and research uses of the human embryo, the development of induced pluripotent stem cells has focused legal inquiry on a new moral/ethical and legal question: If pluripotency theoretically elevates the skin cell to a point of reproductive capacity where it may generate any cell type in the body, then what limits should be placed on the future uses of such cells? More importantly, who will be authorized to make decisions governing use of these cells? Is it the tissue donor's choice, or the law that determines whether or not for instance an individual can use his or her own skin cell to develop an entire human embryo? And where is the reproductive body of the woman in all of this? These questions will be central to the ongoing debate in this area of law and bioethics and in the last part of this chapter I begin to map out some possible responses.

Conclusion

In modern biomedicine, human reproduction has taken on a multitude of forms across a multitude of bodies. As we have seen, the emergence of new technologies of fetal viability, embryo creation, and cryopreservation have led to various attempts to regulate the fetal and embryonic form as if it were a distinct individual. In addition, law has played a key role in determining what is, and what is not, an acceptable form of reproduction. The prohibition against the use of cloned embryos for reproduction is more often understood as a curtailment of scientific ambition rather than of women's reproductive freedom but, in fact, it is also a law that determines the kind of embryos/fetuses that women can gestate. Typically, however, respect for the autonomy of the individual woman has meant that legal regulation of the embryo is curtailed at the point at which the embryo is transferred to the woman's womb. However, regulatory capacity revives, as we have seen, at the point where some kind of fetal viability is proclaimed even while *in utero*. It seems inevitable that as technology develops, the period of maternal or female agency over the embryo/fetus will become narrower and notions of embryonic and fetal identity broadened.

The gradual removal of female embodiment from the center of reproductive regulatory regimes, and the concomitant foregrounding of the fetal and embryonic form, has made regulations that limit reproductive freedoms seem more palatable. This is because they are crafted so they do not look like laws about women's bodies. Recent clinical innovations that highlight the reproductive potential of every cell in the body pose a unique challenge for law. Who, if anyone, should determine how these technologies are developed? The legislative response in the U.K. to the possibility of the creation of artificial gametes suggests women will be further diminished as decisional agents rather than, as might have been the alternate approach, given enhanced reproductive choice and opportunity.

In this context, more work is required to consider alternate ways of constituting the reproductive body in law. Nedelsky's concept of the relational self is a useful architecture around which to construct rights, duties, and responsibilities. By using the idea of relational autonomy we can develop laws that foreground female agency at the same time as they acknowledge that we exist as part of a matrix of relations and familial possibilities (Karpin 2012: 143). If such a model were legally endorsed then technologies such as human cloning, embryos formed through genetic manipulation technologies, embryos formed from iPS cells, and other innovative interventions would not be prohibited if shown to be otherwise safe. Instead, they would form part of a range of potential reproductive options for women and their families. In earlier work, cultural theorist David Ellison and I suggested that in the future women might "choose radically novel family arrangements that will find their origins in (among others) human clones, female sperm and male eggs" (Karpin and Ellison 2009: 33). A legal bioethics of reproduction that utilizes a relational feminist and postmodern approach to regulating would insist that this is a central and appropriate role for female decisional agency.

Related Topics

Chapter 21, "Autonomy," Catriona Mackenzie
Chapter 27, "Human Embryos for Reproduction and Research," Françoise Baylis
Chapter 30, "Reproductive Travel and Tourism," G.K.D. Crozier

References

Calhoun, A. (2012) "The Criminalization of Bad Mothers," *New York Times* April 25.

Cronin, D. (2007) "Cell Research Creates New Ethical Concerns," *Canberra Times*, November 22.

Donegan, B. (2013) "Busting the Myths around Zoe's Law," SBS Comments. Available at: http://www.sbs.com.au/news/article/2013/09/22/comment-busting-myths-around-zoes-law (accessed September 23, 2013).

Downie, J. and Llewellyn, J. (eds.) (2011) *Being Relational: Reflections on Relational Theory and Health Law*, Vancouver: UBC Press.

European Society of Human Reproduction and Embryology (ESHRE) (2010) *ART Fact Sheet*. Available at http://www.eshre.eu/Guidelines-and-Legal/ART-fact-sheet.aspx (accessed September 27, 2013).

Fineman, M.A. (2000) "Cracking the Foundational Myths: Independence, Autonomy and Self-Sufficiency," *Journal of Gender, Social Policy and the Law* 8: 13–31.

Ford, M. (2009) "Nothing and Not-Nothing: Law's Ambivalent Response to Transformation and Transgression at the Beginning of Life," in S.W. Smith and R. Deazley (eds.) *The Legal Medical and Cultural Regulation of the Body*, Farnham, Surrey: Ashgate Publishing Group, pp. 21–44.

Fox, M. (2000) "Pre-persons, Commodities or Cyborgs: The Legal Construction and Representation of the Embryo," *Health Care Analysis* 8 (2): 171–88.

Fox, M. et al. (2010) "Embryonic Hopes: Controversy, Alliance, and Reproductive Entities in Law and the Social Sciences," *Social and Legal Studies* 19 (4): 497–517.

Franklin, S. (2001) "Biologization Revisited: Kinship Theory in the Context of the New Biologies," in S.F. Franklin and S. McKinnon (eds.) *Relative Values: Reconfiguring Kinship Studies*, Durham and London: Duke University Press.

Haraway, D. (1991) *Simians, Cyborgs and Women: The Reinvention of Nature*, New York: Routledge.

Harris-Short, S. (2009) "Regulating Reproduction: Frozen Embryos, Consent, Welfare and the Equality Myth," in S.W. Smith and R. Deazley (eds.) *The Legal Medical and Cultural Regulation of the Body*, Farnham, Surrey: Ashgate Publishing Group, pp. 47–75.

Human Fertilisation and Embryology Authority (HFEA) (2011) *Fertility Treatment in 2011 Trends and Figures*, London.

Human Fertilisation and Embryology Authority (HFEA) (2013) *Mitochondria Replacement Consultation: Advice to Government*, March, London.

Irigaray, L. (1985) *This Sex Which Is Not One*, Ithaca New York: Cornell University Press.

Jackson, E. (2008) "Degendering Reproduction?" *Medical Law Review* 16: 346–68.

Kang, L., Wang, J., Zhang, K. and Gao, S. (2009) "iPS Cells Can Support Full-Term Development of Tetraploid Blastocyst-Complemented Embryos," *Cell Stem Cell* 5: 135–8.

Karpin, I. (1992) "Legislating the Female Body: Reproductive Technology and the Reconstructed Woman," *Columbia Journal of Gender and Law* 3 (1): 325–49.

Karpin, I. (2012) "The Legal and Relational Identity of the 'Not-Yet' Generation," *Law Innovation and Technology* 4 (2): 122–43.

Karpin, I. and Ellison, D. (2010) "Reproduction Without Women: *Frankenstein* and the Prohibition Against Human Modification," in C. Kevin (ed.) *Feminism and the Body, Interdisciplinary Perspectives*, Cambridge: Cambridge Scholars Publishing, pp. 29–48.

Karpin, I. and Mykitiuk, R. (2006) "Regulating Inheritable Genetic Modification or Policing the Fertile Scientific Imagination a Feminist Response," in J. Basko, G. O'Sullivan and R. Ankeny (eds.), *The Ethics of Inheritable Genetic Modification: A Dividing Line*, New York: Cambridge University Press, pp. 193–222.

Li, J., Greco, V., Guasch, G., Fuchs, E. and Mombaerts, P. (2007) "Mice Cloned from Skin Cell," *Proceedings of the National Academy of Sciences of the United States of America* 104 (8): 2738–43.

Lockhart Committee (2005) *Legislation Review: Prohibition of Human Cloning Act 2002 and Research Involving Human Embryos Act 2002*, Legislation Review Committee Reports: Commonwealth of Australia.

McCandless, J. and Sheldon, S. (2010) "The Human Fertilisation and Embryology Act (2008) and the Tenacity of the Sexual Family," *Modern Law Review*, 73 (2): 175–207.

Millbank, J. (2006a) "The Recognition of Lesbian and Gay Families in Australian Law: Part 1 Couples," *Federal Law Review* 34 (1): 1–44.

Millbank, J. (2006b) "The Recognition of Lesbian and Gay Families in Australian Law: Part 2 Children," *Federal Law Review* 34 (2): 205–260.

Millbank, J. (2008) "Unlikely Fissures and Uneasy Resonances: Lesbian Co-Mothers, Surrogate Parenthood And Fathers' Rights," *Feminist Legal Studies* 16 (2) 141–67.

Millbank, J., Stuhmcke, A., Karpin, I. and Chandler, E. (2012) *Enhancing Reproductive Opportunity: A Study of Decision-Making Concerning Stored Embryos*, Sydney: UTS.

Morgan, L. and Michaels, M. (eds.) (1999) *Fetal Subjects Feminist Positions*, Philadelphia: University of Pennsylvania Press.

Murphy, T. and Ó Cuinn, G. (2013) "Taking Technology Seriously: STS as Human Rights Method," in M.L. Flear, A.-M. Farrell, T.K. Hervey and T. Murphy (eds.) *European Law and New Health Technologies*, Oxford: Oxford University Press.

Nayernia, K., Lee, J.H., Drusenheimer, N., Nolte, J., Wulf, G., Dressel, R. et al. (2006a) "Derivation of Male Germ Cells from Bone Marrow Stem Cells," *Laboratory Investigation* 86: 654–63.

Nayernia, K., Nolte, J., Michaelmann, H.W., Lee, J.H., Rathsack, K., Drusenheimer, N. et al. (2006b) "In vitro-differentiated Embryonic Stem Cells Give Rise to Male Gametes That Can Generate Offspring Mice," *Developmental Cell* 11: 125–32.

Nedelsky, J. (2011) *Law's Relations: A Relational Theory of Self, Autonomy and Law*, Oxford: Oxford University Press.

Okie, S. (2009) "The Epidemic That Wasn't," *New York Times* January 27.

Paltrow, L.M. (1992) "Criminal Prosecution of Pregnant Women: National Update and Overview," *Reproductive Freedom Project of the Australian Civil Liberties Union*, New York: Civil Liberties Union.

Roberts, D.E. (1991) "Punishing Drug Addicts Who Have Babies: Women of Color, Equality and the Right to Privacy," *Harvard Law Review* 104: 1419–82.

Robert, H. (2013) "Why Losing My Daughter Means I Don't Support Zoe's Law," *The Conversation*. Available at: https://theconversation.com/why-losing-my-daughter-means-i-dont-support-zoes-law-19985 (accessed December 6, 2013).

Sample, I. (2013) "Britain Ponders 'Three-Person Embryos' to Combat Genetic Disease," *The Guardian* 20 March.

Savell, K. (2006) "Is the 'Born Alive' Rule Outdated and Indefensible?" *Sydney Law Review* 28: 625–64.

Shildrick, M. (1997) *Leaky Bodies and Boundaries: Feminism, Postmodernism and (Bio)Ethics*, New York: Routledge.

Thomson, M. (1997) "Legislating for the Monstrous: Access to Reproductive Services and the Monstrous Feminism," *Social and Legal Studies* 6 (3): 401–24.

Wang, Y., Chambers, G. and Sullivan, E. (2010) "Assisted Reproductive Technology in Australia and New Zealand 2008," *Assisted Reproduction Technology Series* No. 14, Cat. No. PER 49, Canberra: AIHW.

West, F.D., Ozcan, S., Shirazi, R., Soleimanpour-Lichaei, H.R., Dinc, G., Hodges, D.H. et al. (2013) "In Vitro-Derived Gametes from Stem Cells," *Seminars in Reproductive Medicine* 31 (1): 33–8.

29

CHILDREN, PARENTS, AND RESPONSIBILITY FOR CHILDREN'S HEALTH

Amy Mullin

We typically take children's health concerns very seriously, and severely blame those who contribute to children's ill health through negligence or abuse. But what are the grounds for holding people responsible for avoiding bad outcomes or aiming at good ones when it comes to children's health? Who should be held responsible—and for what? I argue that parents are among those to be held responsible, *but* expecting parents to maximize children's health is too high a standard *and* other individuals and groups share responsibility with parents. Different examples of how children's health can be affected will draw attention more to the responsibilities of some rather than others. As a result, this essay will survey five different contexts affecting children's health: Infant feeding, obesity, exposure to tobacco smoke, parental resistance to medical treatment, and emotional maltreatment.

Identifying Social Parents

In this essay I discuss only responsibility for children's health after they are born, and focus on responsibility that individuals and groups have for the health of children in their own society. I will not explore circumstances in pregnancy that affect the health of children.

It is relatively uncontroversial to say that parents have significant responsibility for children's health, but we need to be clearer about who counts as a parent, and why parents are responsible. It is important to distinguish between biological, legal, and social parents. A social parent is an adult who interacts regularly with a child over an extended time period with many of those interactions concerning the child's health, safety, and overall development. A social parent assumes significant responsibility for a child's well-being and development, and is recognized by others as having it. Social parents have accepted, if not always voluntarily assumed, responsibilities for care in a context in which "parental rights and obligations are attached to socially constructed roles" (Brake 2010: 151). Social parents may relinquish their responsibility when options such as adoption and foster parenting are available. Should parental roles unfairly distribute the work of caring for children, they could be critiqued for injustice, but until roles are transformed, social parents have assumed that work.

Social parents may discharge some of their responsibility by arranging for others to meet a child's needs, but nevertheless know a child well and interact regularly with him or her. A child's legal parent may fail to fulfill the role of social parent, culpably so if other social parents do not pick up the slack, and many biological parents will never know or engage with their genetic or gestational children. By contrast, extended kin, stepparents, and some long-term paid caregivers, often without the legal status of parent, may serve as a child's social parent.

Responsibility for Children's Health

If social parents assume significant responsibility for a child's health, what does that entail? Who else shares responsibility? To what standard of health are they required to aspire? Few would argue that parents are solely responsible. Medical professionals, occasional caregivers, teachers, social workers, youth program leaders, those who design and market products that affect children's health, and the state all plausibly share responsibility to keep children healthy. Some acquire responsibility in virtue of their roles or when their activities can predictably be expected to affect children's health. Some acquire a duty of rescue by becoming aware of a child in crisis. The state bears some responsibility for meeting the needs of its members.

Both the state and members of the community other than a child's parents are widely recognized to have a range of legitimate concerns that extend beyond children's interests. The state's legitimate concerns include the interests of adult citizens, non-citizen residents, and needy members of the international community. Other individuals and groups may be legitimately concerned with their own projects, health, and the flourishing of other adults they care about. Given the need to balance interests, it is implausible to expect those with responsibility for children's health, including their social parents, to strive always to maximize children's health and wellbeing.

We nonetheless frequently encounter references to the "best interests" of children in policy and legal contexts. The United Nations Convention on the Rights of the Child dictates: "In all actions concerning children, whether undertaken by public or private social welfare institutions, courts of law, administrative authorities or legislative bodies, the best interests of the child shall be a primary consideration" (UN General Assembly 1989: article 3.1). Parents are assigned primary responsibility for children's care and it is expected that "the best interests of the child will be their basic concern" (UN General Assembly 1989: article 18.1), while article 24 of the convention outlines children's right to the "highest attainable standard of health." This could mean that parents would be obliged to make significant sacrifices to make generally healthy children better off.

In contrast to policy documents, philosophers who discuss children's interests find the requirement to maximize those interests vague, since children have as yet no stable sense of what makes for the best life for them. It is also too strict, as individuals with responsibility for children's health have other morally acceptable priorities. Søren Holm raises both objections: "There is no way family decision-making can make the best interest of the child paramount in real life. The interest of other family members must almost always play a role and there is furthermore in many cases no clear answer as to what the best interest of the child is" (Holm 2008: 22). A more plausible approach holds parents and others accountable for aiming to provide children with minimally decent care. For example, David Archard writes: "The state should . . . always be seen as a 'positive' guarantor that every child within its jurisdiction enjoys a minimally decent upbringing" (Archard 2004: 215).

What constitutes minimally decent care? The capability approach, developed by Martha Nussbaum (2006) and Amartya Sen (1985), is a useful way to think about this question. On this approach, justice requires us to aim at universal access to important capabilities. The resources people need to develop and sustain capabilities differ depending on their traits (what some need to be mobile will differ from others, depending on their ability to walk) and social context (for some access to clean water might require long journeys). A capability approach to identifying minimally decent care is preferable to one that identifies a minimal bundle of resources children require because of the former's recognition of the impact of individual differences and social circumstances on the ability to realize important capabilities even when supplied with similar resources. The capability approach also reminds us that justice for children requires not only resources, but also people to interact with them in ways that develop their basic capabilities.

Lists of basic capabilities can be controversial, but not as controversial as accounts of the best life. Some capabilities such as the ability to survive and be healthy, the capacity to engage in various social relationships, and the ability to move about in and have some control over one's material environment, will be relatively uncontroversial. Minimally decent care will be care that strives to develop children's basic capabilities.

Theoretical Frameworks Explaining Responsibility for Health

What theoretical framework best explains parental responsibilities? The main contenders are claims about children's rights, and claims about the need to respond to dependency and vulnerability with care. Appeals to rights may be grounded in protection of choices (agency rights) or interests (welfare rights). Rights put limits on acceptable interactions others can have with a rights holder. Advocates of children's rights typically argue that: "children move gradually from having their rights primarily protect their interests to having their rights primarily protect their choices" (Brennan 2002: 62). For most advocates of children's rights, rights are ultimately grounded in what promotes one's most significant interests (Brennan 2002: 63; Brighouse 2002: 40; see also Archard 2004). On a rights-based approach, minimally decent care would be care that promotes children's most significant interests (for instance by developing their basic capabilities).

Children's interests in care will not be served by giving them rights only insofar as they are capable of making informed choices. Children who will predictably die before maturity and those who will not become autonomous will not have their interests respected if rights are grounded solely in potential for autonomy, or self-direction. Any rights-based approach should reflect a broader account of capacities worthy of moral respect (including the ability to enter into morally valuable relationships) (see Mullin 2011).

Rights-based approaches need not ground parents' responsibilities for children's health solely in children's significant interests, as children are not the only ones affected by their poor health. Children are societies' means of sustaining themselves over time. The social contributions children can make when they mature gives another reason for the state to ensure that parents assume some responsibility for children's health.

The second major theoretical approach focuses on obligations to respond to dependency (a need to rely extensively on others for survival and flourishing) and vulnerability (susceptibility to physical and emotional harm) with care. Children have significant and unavoidable dependency and are vulnerable because of their relatively fragile physicality and need for support to develop capacities important to their future. Physically or emotionally damaging interactions that affect children not only cause temporary suffering and suspension of ability to engage in activities (as with adults). They also prevent children from developing basic capacities.

Martha Fineman (2010) and Eva Kittay (1999) emphasize the importance of recognizing vulnerability and unavoidable dependency, including that of children. Since children share vulnerability and dependency with others, including often their parents, this puts limits on requiring those with responsibility for their care to make children's interests paramount. No one should be expected to compromise their own basic needs, or the basic needs of others in their care, to maximize children's interests.

To understand the obligation to respond to dependency and vulnerability with care, we must define "care": "Care may be said to include everything we do directly to help others to meet their basic needs, develop or sustain their basic capabilities, and alleviate or avoid pain and suffering, in an attentive, responsive and respectful manner" (Engster 2005: 55). Everyone inevitably experiences periods of both vulnerability and dependency and so all of us are indebted to others' care for our health and our lives. Societies are not sustainable without extensive provision of care. Given the care that all have received and may urgently need in the future, and the stake members of a society share in its sustainability, both basic fairness and the moral value of belonging to a caring society make *prima facie* calls upon all who may meet dependency and vulnerability with care to do so. This is particularly true for care of children whose future prospects are affected dramatically by its lack.

Primary responsibility for children's health falls upon parents who have assumed that responsibility in a social context. However, unmet needs and broader social causes of poor health make claims upon all with ability to respond—even if only by supporting state mechanisms to afford children a social safety net. Robert Goodin (1985: 779) argues that responsibility to meet vulnerable people's needs includes responsibility to assist those allocated primary responsibility, to set up collective mechanisms to respond to need, and to monitor the failures of others to meet their primary responsibility. Daniel Engster, in addition, draws our attention to the importance of ensuring that social allocation of responsibilities to care is not unjust (Engster 2005: 66).

Care ethics insists on the importance of thinking about both those who receive and those who provide care, with the latter's interests putting limits on any maximizing claims about those of the former. It recognizes social interests in raising children to be productive members of society, and avoids a narrow (economic) construal of productivity. A society will only be sustainable if its children develop capacities to serve as providers of care, and recognize a responsibility to do so.

Rights-based approaches that recognize the importance of significant interests and care ethics approaches both attribute direct moral status to children. This means children are held morally considerable in their own right: "If an entity has moral status, then we may not treat it in just any way we please, we are morally obliged to give weight in our deliberations to its needs, interests or well-being" (Warren 1997: 3). Both approaches assign responsibility to other actors to meet children's most significant interests.

Children's rights to care will differ considerably from more prototypical rights to limit others' interference with the rights holder. Some theorists worry that emphasis on children's rights will therefore encourage children and parents to have the wrong kind of attitude toward what needs to be a supportive and emotionally close relationship, by pitting children (or at least their advocates) against parents and demanding that parents do not interfere with their children (O'Neill 1989). However, children's rights are not primarily rights to freedom from interference, and insistence on their rights may be strategically important as a way to emphasize children's moral status: Appeals to rights remind us of "the independent standing of the child, and the centrality of her interests in determining policy" (Brighouse 2002: 36). Care ethics can additionally draw attention to injustices in the allocation of responsibilities for children's care, both in terms of the burdens on children's parents (especially mothers), and the inequities that result for children when the only resources available to meet their needs are those possessed by their families. The two approaches, in the versions sketched above, are not fundamentally incompatible.

Examples Highlighting Shared Responsibility for Children's Health

The remainder of this essay will present five instances in which parents have some, but not all responsibility for children's health, and discuss how that responsibility must be shared with others, including the state. The first draws attention to the gendered nature of some aspects of responsibility for children's health, and the importance of context for balancing the interests of mothers and children.

Infant Feeding

Infant feeding, before children can eat solid foods, can involve either breastfeeding or formula. There are clear health advantages to breastfeeding, but the extent of the advantage depends on the ability of families to access high-quality alternatives. When formula is affordable and clean water is easily available, the main health advantages are lowering the risk of gastrointestinal and ear infections (Wolf 2006). There are many claims about other health benefits from breastfeeding, such as reducing childhood obesity, but evidence is not always compelling, with small sample sizes and no adjustment for other factors that may lead to differences, or signs of only modest benefits (Armstrong and Reilly 2002: 2003). When alternatives to breastfeeding do not compromise children's ability to lead minimally decent lives, it is important to recall that a standard of maximizing children's health is too high, particularly when breastfeeding involves significant burdens on the mother.

By contrast, in situations where formula is of low quality, or clean water is not reliably available, health advantages are huge: "suboptimum breastfeeding, especially non-exclusive breastfeeding in the first 6 months of life, results in 1.4 million deaths and 10 percent of disease burden in children younger than 5 years" (Black et al. 2008: 243). In countries where more impoverished families live, only 47–57 percent of infants under two months old, and far fewer older children, are exclusively breastfed (Black et al. 2008: 250). Yet studies of infants in low-income countries show that breastfeeding significantly reduces child death and disease (Black et al. 2008: 250). This points to the clear difference social context makes in determining the relative merits of different approaches to infant feeding—and to the need to regulate claims about safety of infant formula to reflect that context. The extent of maternal responsibility to breastfeed, since based on provision of minimally decent care, will depend upon the safety and quality of available alternatives. Either when social context makes infant formula unavailable or unreliable or when a child's particular health needs make formula feeding a poor alternative (as when infants cannot tolerate formula, or risk very significant negative outcomes from gastrointestinal infections), breastfeeding may be important to protect children's basic capabilities.

Because only women can breastfeed, they bear the burdens associated with it—burdens that may be psychological (attitudes towards the display of breasts, or sexuality and breastfeeding, as outlined in Kukla (2006)), but can also include prolonged pain and discomfort in breastfeeding (cracked and bleeding nipples, blistering, exhaustion, and infections like mastitis). In a study (based on a small sample), several women found breastfeeding more painful than labor and childbirth (Kelleher 2006: 2731). Breastfeeding women have increased nutritional needs, and may need to monitor their diet and refuse medications in order not to compromise their breast milk. Problems with breastfeeding and decisions not to breastfeed often involve guilt, shame, and feelings of failure in a context in which public health messages emphasize the superiority of breastfeeding over formula feeding (Kukla 2006). Given the range of potential burdens on women, more balanced public health messages about infant feeding choices should be encouraged.

Evidence is clear that mothers with working conditions less favorable to breastfeeding (no or short paid maternity leave, little opportunity to take breaks to pump, no facility for keeping pumped milk) are less likely to initiate or continue breastfeeding (Kelly and Watt 2005). As a result children whose mothers are in lower socioeconomic classes are far less likely to be breastfed. Justice requires measures to ensure that breastfeeding is accommodated and supported (for instance, with the ability to pump at work, and public provision of medical advice for breastfeeding women who forego regular medication) whenever it is important to providing minimally decent care. Societies that share in funding the potentially increased health costs associated with formula feeding (such as more infections in infants) have reasons beyond a commitment to protecting children's basic capabilities to support breastfeeding. However, support for breastfeeding should not make women who cannot or choose not to breastfeed feel that they have failed their infants. When breastfeeding is undertaken even though not required for minimally decent care, an increase in the share of childcare done by parents who are not breastfeeding would help compensate for the increased burden of mothers who do.

Obesity

Undernutrition is the cause of extensive death and disease in children: "Maternal and child undernutrition is the underlying cause of 3.5 million deaths, 35 percent of the disease burden in children under 5 years and 11 percent of global DALYs [that is, disability-adjusted life years]" (Black et al. 2008: 243). Parents are not typically blamed for undernutrition (supposing they live in impoverished conditions). Undernutrition instead raises questions about the responsibility of states to allocate more fairly the resources available within them, and of other states (and individuals) to provide international assistance. There are effective interventions available to remedy undernutrition, such as access to a larger supply of food and provision of missing micronutrients (Bhutta et al. 2008: 417). By contrast, child obesity raises questions about parental responsibility.

Child obesity affects more than one-fifth of children in developed countries, with considerable impact on future health (increased risk of cancer, cardiovascular problems, and diabetes) and current health (physical and psycho-social) (Lotz 2004). Public health authorities are often reluctant to intervene directly with family practices around food intake and exercise, because this would require fairly extensive interference with parental liberty, although interventions would be justified by risk of harm to children's health that undermines their development of basic capabilities. Instead public health interventions are typically indirect, such as education campaigns, or campaigns to provide information about nutrition or limit portion size in restaurants.

Mianna Lotz recommends direct intervention in the form of mandatory obesity programs—parents would have to get medical advice and monitoring, supply nutritious food, limit high-fat and high-sugar foods, and get children to exercise (Lotz 2004: 291). However, this may require parents to change their own patterns of eating and physical exercise; nutritious food can take more time to prepare than higher calorie alternatives (and be more expensive/less available); and parents of older children may have limited ability to control what their children eat and how often they exercise. To achieve short-term reductions in children's weight, families must change their lifestyles considerably, including reducing sedentary activities such as watching television and using computers. To be sustainable, these changes likely need to be supplemented by broader societal changes in what are often termed "obesogenic" societies (including limiting the significant exposure children have to advertising of foods high in fat and sugar, reducing portion sizes in restaurants, and making more low-cost opportunities for physical activity available). Moreover, few direct interventions in family practices have been proven to be effective in sustaining long-term weight loss in children. Holm argues that there are "no known interventions targeted at individuals and families that lead to long-term sustainable reductions in obesity" (Holm 2008: 23). Clearly we cannot support invasive interventions in the absence of evidence they are effective.

Despite Lotz's careful use of the term "parents," most public health and media coverage of obesity tends to differentially blame mothers, who are often culturally expected to buy and prepare food and monitor children's behavior (Maher et al. 2010: 240). This not only excludes fathers from sharing responsibility, but also ignores the significant contribution that socioeconomic class makes to obesity, with lower socioeconomic class correlating to increased obesity (Bell et al. 2009). It also ignores the extent to which older children share responsibility when they both make choices about what they eat and how often they exercise, and can understand the impact of their choices.

Parents have some responsibility for children's obesity, because they influence children's food intake, physical activity, and sedentary habits. There is some as yet preliminary evidence that a preventive approach may be effective, given that different parental feeding styles are associated differentially with obesity. The style least associated with obesity involves parents making healthy foods available but not controlling what children eat, to encourage children's development of self-control and attentiveness to internal cues of hunger (Golan and Crow 2004: 43; Patrick et al. 2005). However, if parents are to make healthy options available and let children choose, this may increase time and costs associated with meal preparation. Some new interventions include parent counseling, with emotional support for parents working to reduce their children's weight, and acknowledgment of difficulty in changing children's behavior, but there are as yet little data on their effectiveness (Golan and Crow 2004: 46). Treatment programs have to date not been proven to be effective long term.

In addition to lack of evidence about their effectiveness, we have another reason to be concerned about mandatory imposition of obesity programs. Obesity is higher in children from lower socioeconomic backgrounds and therefore poorer families are more likely to be expected to participate in mandatory programs to combat obesity than families with more resources. Mandatory participation would add stress and public oversight to lives that are already subject to high stress and greater monitoring than wealthier families. Instead I recommend further research and public education with respect to evidence-based claims about approaches to feeding children, and support for parents who choose to seek interventions. In addition, public health campaigns should continue to support broader societal changes with respect to easy availability and advertising of high-fat and high-sugar foods, and call for better access for lower-income families to free and inexpensive forms of enjoyable physical recreation.

Exposure to Tobacco Smoke

As with obesity, there is a clear social gradient with respect to children's exposure to tobacco smoke, since people from lower socioeconomic positions are more likely both to smoke and to have their health negatively affected by smoking (Graham 2004: 104). Many advocate legislation against exposing children to secondhand smoke, because of the demonstrated negative health effects and importance of protecting children from harm (Brennan and White 2007: 105). Few may be willing to devote significant state resources to entering homes to detect parental smoking, or willing to countenance extensive interference with family privacy. However, making it illegal to smoke in enclosed spaces (homes, cars, or public spaces) could lead to significant moral pressure for smokers to reduce children's exposure to tobacco. Alternatively or additionally, states could increase taxes on cigarettes, since demand is sensitive to price. Meredith Minkler notes that "A 10% increase in the price of cigarettes, for example, has been shown to decrease teen smoking by 14%, and it is projected that a $2 per pack tax would decrease adolescent tobacco use by almost 46%" (Minkler 1999: 129).

Monique Jonas and Simon Thornley argue that when significantly harmful effects of a parental practice are widely established, interference with parental liberty and privacy is warranted on the basis of children's interests (Jonas and Thornley 2011: 130). One could further argue there are social interests in ensuring that children's health is not diminished to the point that they require substantial care and will be less likely to make constructive contributions to their societies. Jonas and Thornley claim that smoking in enclosed spaces around children meets the following criteria for prohibiting a parental practice: It is clearly identifiable; strong evidence suggests it typically leads to significant harm; it is avoidable without great difficulty (since parental smoking could take place outside enclosed spaces they share with their children); it does not have significant benefits; harm reduction is not easily attainable by other means; there will be no troubling consequences (Jonas and Thornley 2011: 136–8).

There is significant evidence that children's regular exposure to tobacco smoke harms their health to the extent of compromising provision of minimally decent care (especially increasing children's susceptibility to respiratory illness), and the studies are high quality, with large sample sizes conducted in different settings (Jonas and Thornley 2011: 138). However, Jonas and Thornley's claim that there are no potentially troubling consequences to prohibition of parental smoking is unwarranted. If parental smoking around children is prohibited, it is foreseeable that children may be left unsupervised and/or parents may become more stressed, and so any such prohibition would need to be accompanied by some limited public provision of paid childcare, particularly when parents are in the process of ceasing or decreasing their smoking.

It is reasonable to assume that people are generally aware of the negative effects of smoking, and an educative approach (that includes limits on tobacco advertising) has not been sufficient to stop parents and others from smoking around children. While less coercive approaches should be tried (including public funding for smoking cessation programs for smokers from lower socioeconomic classes or financial incentives for people willing both to stop smoking and having their success monitored), legislation that prohibits parental smoking around children in enclosed spaces may be called for. Any such legislation should generally not be accompanied by intrusive practices with respect to family privacy within the home. One exception would be children whose health status is such that their basic capabilities are threatened by even occasionally being in enclosed spaces with smoking parents. With the exception of these cases, any legislation would serve primarily as a clear statement of social values with respect to protection of children's health, and a way to limit children's exposure to smoking in situations that are already open to public observation.

Parental Resistance to Children Receiving Medical Treatment

Parents have legitimate interests in having intimate relationships with the children they rear, and the importance of privacy to the realization of intimacy requires a certain freedom from state or social interference with childrearing arrangements (Brighouse and Swift 2006). However, as Harry Brighouse and Adam Swift note, freedom from interference should apply only when parents are doing an adequate job (Brighouse and Swift 2006: 97), in other words, providing minimally decent care. It should not extend to resistance to medical treatment for children's serious health problems that lead to children's death or limit their basic capabilities.

In the U.S., for many years religious exemption clauses allowed religious parents "to withhold preventive and diagnostic measures from and to refuse medical care for their sick children," and most states permitted religious defenses to criminal charges of medical neglect of children (Hughes 2004: 253). In 1996, federal requirements that states have such exemptions (to be eligible to receive federal grants to deal with child abuse) were withdrawn. As a result, and due to increased attention to very difficult deaths of children whose parents believed that all healing should be spiritual (Hughes 2004), many states repealed these exemptions. It is hard to disagree with Richard Hughes' conclusion that the "duty to care is more compelling than a subjective right of religious liberty" (Hughes 2004: 265).

James Dwyer similarly argues that children should be afforded the same respect as other persons incompetent to make health care decisions, and their interests in being treated medically for significant health problems should outweigh parents' religious liberty (Dwyer 2000: 177). By contrast, Susan Dudley focuses on parents whose views about medical treatment differ from many health care professionals for cultural reasons (Dudley 2003). She recommends a balanced approach to court cases concerning children whose parents' beliefs about appropriate medical care clash with the medical establishment. She urges courts to acknowledge the complexity of the issues involved including the potential injustice of giving greater autonomy to parents whose disputes concern religion than those whose disagreements with contemporary medical practice concern culture. She recommends that courts identify the costs and benefits of different options for treating children's health problems and recognize the possibility that medical decisions may be in error (Dudley 2003: 1295).

Dudley's encouragement of dialogue between medical professionals and patients' families is to be supported, and her reminder that medical professionals can err in their judgments is salutary. However, parents' pursuit of alternative medical treatment cannot be supported when children's basic capabilities are at serious risk and there is substantial evidence that one option will be much better for a child than the other. When the stakes are not high (with respect to provision of minimally decent care), or when the stakes are high but the balance of evidence does not strongly support one option, then it is appropriate to let parents choose. Agents of the state, such as judges, should assess not only the scale of consequences of making one choice versus another but also the presence (or lack) of expert consensus with respect to medical care.

Emotional Maltreatment

Children's emotional health was for years considered secondary to physical health, but is now widely recognized as significant. A World Health Organization Commission outlines the "importance of early child development, including not only physical and cognitive or linguistic development but also, crucially, social and emotional development" for health (Marmot et al. 2008: 1662). Children's emotional maltreatment is a better predictor of long-term negative outcomes for children than physical abuse (Glaser 2002: 698). But how should emotional maltreatment be understood?

To identify emotional maltreatment one must identify children's basic emotional needs and how parents meet them. Children need to feel safe by having parents comfort them when they are upset. When this need is unmet, they find it hard to trust anyone or develop empathy (Davidov and Grusec 2006). Children also need to experience positive emotions such as warmth and interest in relationships with their parents. These emotionally positive interactions correlate with children's developing a conscience and being accepted by others (Grusec and Davidov 2007, 301). Without them, children's basic capacity to have relationships with others is threatened. Emotional maltreatment may therefore be understood as patterns of interactions between parents and children that do not provide comfort in response to distress and do not include warmth and interest. Maltreatment may be due to various causes, including parental indifference or hostility, parents' mental health needs, and misunderstanding of children's emotional needs. When children are emotionally maltreated, their basic capabilities are threatened.

Social parents are primarily responsible for meeting children's emotional needs, but other members of society, and the state, have important subsidiary responsibilities to ensure children receive minimally decent care, as is typically well recognized when it comes to physical abuse or neglect. Public responsibilities include improving education about children's emotional needs (this could be introduced as part of health curricula in public schools), improved detection of emotional maltreatment, support for parents who need assistance in meeting the emotional needs of children, and supplying alternative forms of care when parents are unwilling or unable to meet those needs.

Given the power and responsibility of the state, its interventions should not reflect discriminatory views about who is likely to abuse or neglect children. For instance, in the U.S. there is evidence that "racism may affect child welfare decision making, leading to disproportionate scrutiny and reporting" (McRoy 2004: 483) Given that over half of children are in foster care because their caregivers have substance abuse problems, it is also important for the state to develop better substance abuse and treatment plans (McRoy 2004: 479). Finally, once there is greater public awareness of the nature of children's emotional needs, it will be important for all adults to recognize a responsibility to report suspicions of emotional maltreatment—with the understanding that suspicions will be investigated, and may lead to better education of parents, or treatment and support, rather than only removal of children from their homes.

Conclusion

Parents, particularly mothers, are sometimes assigned too much responsibility for children's health and expected to aim at too high a standard. Parents share responsibility with the state, and with other individuals and groups, including those who are in a position to detect that children's basic emotional needs are not being met, and those who can effect changes in policy that affect children's lives. Public policies should aim to ensure that children receive care that develops their basic capabilities. Since these policies include those that distribute social resources in ways that impact on children's health, citizens who choose government representatives, as well as the state representatives themselves, all bear a share of the responsibility for protecting children's health.

Related Topics

Chapter 32, "Reproductive Testing for Disability," Adrienne Asch and David Wasserman
Chapter 34, "Family Caregivers, Long-Term Care, and Global Justice," Lisa Eckenwiler

References

Archard, D. (2004) *Children: Rights and Childhood*, 2nd edition, London: Routledge.

Armstrong, J. and Reilly, J. (2002) "Breastfeeding and Lowering the Risk of Childhood Obesity," *Lancet* 359: 2003–4.

Bell, K., McNaughton, D. and Salmon, A. (2009) "Medicine, Morality and Mothering: Public Health Discourses on Foetal Alcohol Exposure, Smoking around Children and Childhood Overnutrition," *Critical Public Health* 19 (2): 155–70.

Bhutta, Z., Ahmed, T., Black, R., Cousnes, S., Dewey, K., Giugliani, E. et al. (2008) "What Works? Interventions for Maternal and Child Undernutrition and Survival," *Lancet* 371: 417–40.

Black, R., Allen, L., Bhutta, Z., Caufield, L., de Onis, M., Ezzati, M. et al. (2008) "Maternal and Child Undernutrition: Global and Regional Exposures and Health Consequences," *Lancet* 371: 243–60.

Brake, E. (2010) "Willing Parents: A Voluntarist Account of Parental Role Obligations," in D. Archard and D. Benatar (eds.) *Procreation and Parenthood*, Oxford: Oxford University Press, pp. 151–77.

Brennan, S. (2002) "Children's Choices or Children's Interests: Which Do Their Rights Protect?" in C.M. MacLeod and D. Archard (eds.) *The Moral and Political Status of Children*, Oxford: Oxford University Press, pp. 53–69.

Brennan, S. and White, A. (2007) "Responsibility and Children's Rights: The Case for Restricting Parental Smoking," in S. Brennan and R. Noggle (eds.) *Taking Responsibility for Children*, Waterloo, ON: Wilfrid Laurier Press, pp. 97–111.

Brighouse, H. (2002) "What Rights (if Any) Do Children Have?" in C.M. MacLeod and D. Archard (eds.) *The Moral and Political Status of Children*, Oxford: Oxford University Press, pp. 31–52.

Brighouse, H. and A. Swift (2006) "Parents Rights and the Value of the Family," *Ethics* 117 (1): 80–108.

Davidov, M. and Grusec, J. (2006) "Untangling the Links of Parental Responsiveness to Distress and Warmth to Child Outcomes," *Child Development* 77: 44–58.

Dudley, S. (2003) "Medical Treatment for Asian Immigrant Children: Does Mother Know Best?" *Georgetown Law Review* 92: 1287–307.

Dwyer, J. (2000) "Spiritual Treatment Exemptions to Child Medical Neglect Laws: What We Outsiders Should Think," *Notre Dame Law Review* 76: 147–77.

Engster, D. (2005) "Rethinking Care Theory: The Practice of Caring and the Obligation to Care," *Hypatia* 20 (3): 50–74.

Fineman, M. (2010) "The Vulnerable Subject and the Responsive State," *Emory Law Journal* 60: 251–75.

Glaser, D. (2002) "Emotional Abuse and Neglect," *Child Abuse and Neglect* 26: 697–714.

Golan, M and Crow, S. (2004) "Parents Are Key Players in the Prevention and Treatment of Weight-Related Problems," *Nutrition Reviews* 62 (1): 39–50.
Goodin, R. (1985) "Vulnerabilities and Responsibilities: An Ethical Defense of the Welfare State," *The American Political Science Review* 79 (3): 775–87.
Graham, H. (2004) "Social Determinants and Their Unequal Distribution: Clarifying Policy Understandings," *The Milbank Quarterly* 82 (1): 101–24.
Grusec, J. and Davidov, M. (2007), "Socialization in the Family: The Roles of Parents" in J. Grusec and D. Hastings (eds.) *Handbook of Socialization: Theory and Research*, New York: Guilford Press, pp. 284–308.
Holm, S. (2008) "Parental Responsibility and Obesity in Children," *Public Health Ethics* 1 (1): 21–9.
Hughes, R. (2004) "The Death of Children by Faith-Based Medical Neglect," *Journal of Law and Religion* 20: 247–65.
Jonas, M. and Thornley, S. (2011) "Smoky Rooms and Fuzzy Harms: How Should the Law Respond to Harmful Parental Practices?" *Public Health Ethics* 4 (2): 129–42.
Kelleher, C. (2006) "The Physical Challenges of Early Breastfeeding," *Social Science and Medicine* 63: 2727–38.
Kelly, Y. and Watt, R. (2005) "Breast-Feeding Initiation and Exclusive Duration at 6 Months by Social Class: Results of the Millennium Cohort Study," *Public Health Nutrition* 8 (4): 417–21.
Kittay, E. (1999) *Love's Labor: Essays on Women, Equality and Dependency*, New York: Routledge.
Kukla, R. (2006) "Ethics and Ideology in Breastfeeding Advocacy Campaigns," *Hypatia* 21 (1): 157–80.
Lotz, M. (2004) "Childhood Obesity and the Question of Parental Liberty," *Journal of Social Philosophy* 35 (2): 288–303.
Maher, J., Fraser, S. and Wright, J. (2010), "Framing the Mother: Childhood Obesity, Maternal Responsibility and Care," *Journal of Gender Studies* 19 (3): 233–47.
Marmot, M. and Field, S., Bell, R., Houweling, T. and Taylor, S. (2008) "Closing the Gap in a Generation: Health Equity through Action on the Social Determinants of Health," *Lancet* 372: 1661–9.
McRoy, R. (2004) "Expedited Permanency: Implications for African-American Children and Families," *Virginia Journal of Social Policy and Law* 12 (3): 475–89.
Minkler, M. (1999) "Personal Responsibility for Health? A Review of the Arguments and the Evidence at Century's End," *Health Education Behavior* 26: 121–41.
Mullin, A. (2011), "Children and the Argument from 'Marginal' Cases," *Ethical Theory and Moral Practice* 14: 291–305.
Nussbaum, M. (2006) *Frontiers of Justice: Disability, Nationality, Species Membership*, Cambridge: Cambridge University Press.
O'Neill, O. (1989) "Children's Rights and Children's Lives," in O. O'Neill (ed.) *Constructions of Reason*, Cambridge: Cambridge University Press, pp. 445–63.
Patrick, H., Nicklas, T., Hughes, S. and Morales, M. (2005) "The Benefits of Authoritative Feeding Style: Caregiver Feeding Styles and Children's Food Consumption Patterns," *Appetite* 44: 243–9.
Sen, A. (1985) *Commodities and Capabilities*, Oxford: Oxford University Press.
UN General Assembly (1989) *Convention on the Rights of the Child*, United Nations, Treaty Series. Available at: http://www.unhcr.org/refworld/docid/3ae6b38f0.html (accessed July 18, 2012).
Warren, A. (1997) *Moral Status: Obligations to Persons and Other Living Things*, Oxford: Oxford University Press.
Wolf, J. (2006), "What Feminists Can Do for Breastfeeding and What Breastfeeding Can Do for Feminists," *Signs: Journal of Women in Culture and Society* 31 (2): 397–424.

Further Reading

Brake, E. and Millum, J. (2012) "Parenthood and Procreation," *Stanford Encyclopedia of Philosophy*. Available at: http://plato.stanford.edu/entries/parenthood/ (accessed May 28, 2012).
Nettle, D. (2010) "Why Are There Social Gradients in Preventative Health Behavior? A Perspective from Behavioral Ecology," *PLoS ONE* 5 (10): e13371.

30
REPRODUCTIVE TRAVEL AND TOURISM

G.K.D. Crozier

Technological advancements in medicine, communications, and travel have had a significant impact on how people address their medical and reproductive health needs (Reed 2008). Increasingly, patients are crossing national borders to seek reproductive goods and services, including those requiring human bodily resources such as gametes (eggs and sperm) or the services of a surrogate mother. This phenomenon—referred to here as "reproductive travel"—raises a host of ethical issues, many of which resist easy solutions. Although these ethical issues overlap considerably with those raised by surrogacy (paid and unpaid), ova harvesting, medical tourism, and other topics discussed in this volume, this essay will focus primarily on those issues that are unique to the phenomenon of reproductive travel. Specifically, I focus on tensions between reproductive autonomy of individuals and the duties of nations, the racial and gendered dimensions of reproductive travel, and the exploitation and constraints on consent of women who are paid to provide reproductive bodily resources (ova and surrogacy services, specifically).

The case of Diane Blood is widely discussed as the first high-profile contemporary case of reproductive travel. In 1995, Mrs Blood's husband died after contracting bacterial meningitis and falling into a coma. Since Mr and Mrs Blood had been trying to reproduce before he fell ill, Mrs Blood wanted to use her husband's semen to have a child with him posthumously. This was not permitted in her native United Kingdom because there was no written record of Mr Blood's consent. However, Mrs. Blood succeeded in achieving her reproductive objective by traveling to nearby Belgium, where legislation permitted the use of her deceased husband's sperm (Deech 2003). On two separate occasions, Mrs Blood was successfully impregnated using *in vitro* fertilization (IVF) and embryos created with her ova and her husband's spermatozoa, and she gave birth to two sons three years apart.

From the time of this highly publicized case, reproductive travel has become an increasingly widespread phenomenon. The accessibility of information and communication via the Internet and the ease of international travel have changed how people look for solutions to challenges they encounter in all aspects of their lives. This is no less true in the domain of reproductive medicine (Chung 2006; Korn 2012). Patients are able to locate and communicate with physicians overseas, clinics are able to advertise to foreign customers, and support groups and information forums have emerged online to connect patients with each other in order to share insights and resources regarding their experiences.

Throughout this essay, the term "reproductive travel" is used to refer to all cases where people cross national borders in order to obtain reproductive medical goods and services. This practice (or a subset of it) has variously been referred to as "reproductive tourism," "gamete travel," and "fertility tourism," among other terms. My preference for "reproductive travel" reflects the following observations: The term "tourism" potentially trivializes the activity which, for many patients, involves no recreational activities and a certain level of emotional and physical distress; the practice need not involve any medical procedures on the people who are traveling or paying for the services (for example, when prospective parents seek a surrogate mother); travel may not involve the manipulation of gametes; and fertility is not the goal in some cases of reproductive travel. Rather, the common factor here is that some kind of medical care involving reproductive health experts is required, and the activity involves the crossing of national borders by some party—whether by patients, prospective parents, gamete providers, or medical specialists.

Various practices fall under the category of reproductive travel. The attention of academia and the press has focused mainly on travel whose objective is to enhance fertility and facilitate procreation, such as travel for IVF, either with or without the gametes or surrogacy services of third parties. But it is not inconsequential that medical procedures unrelated to increasing fertility might also be involved, such as contraception, abortions, and related phenomena such as gender reassignment, female genital cutting, prostatectomies, or hysterectomies.

Motivations for Reproductive Travel

One useful way to understand the growing phenomenon of reproductive travel is to consider the various (sometimes overlapping) motivations of those who participate in it: (1) Cost, (2) limited domestic availability of goods or services, (3) avoidance of domestic legislation designed to protect the participants, and (4) avoidance of domestic legislation designed to promote social values (Crozier and Baylis 2010).

(1) One of the central motivations for reproductive travel is *cost*. Medical procedures can vary greatly in their cost among countries, and procedures relating to reproductive health are no exception. Prospective parents in wealthier countries can save thousands of dollars by obtaining medical procedures abroad, such as IVF and other medical fertility enhancing procedures, or even human gametes or surrogacy services. Countries such as Thailand and India are actively competing for a share of this lucrative market in medical travel in general, including reproductive travel. Some clinics even advertise romantic getaway packages where clients can bundle inexpensive fertility treatments with vacations in romantic locations.

(2) *Limited domestic availability* of reproductive goods and services is another factor that can drive patients abroad. Long waiting lists for gametes or IVF, for example, may be deemed unsupportable by couples for whom each additional year of waiting decreases their chances of successfully achieving a pregnancy. This category of reproductive travel also houses some of the most controversial cases—those cases motivated by domestic restrictions on payment for human reproductive resources, such as gametes or surrogacy services. Many countries limit the amount of money that can be paid to sperm and ova providers and to surrogates; frequently, payment is restricted to only what would be considered necessary to compensate the provider for time, lost wages, and expenses. This has led to shortages in human reproductive

resources in these countries (Levine 2011), and it has motivated a growing industry in reproductive travel for the purchase of gametes and paid surrogacy in countries where the regulations regarding compensation for human reproductive resources are more permissive, such as Thailand and India.

(3) In some cases, people seek to circumvent domestic regulations that are in place to *protect the health or wellbeing* of those people who would be directly involved in the procedure—prospective parents, future children, and people providing human reproductive resources. The case of Diane Blood also falls into this category, since the procedure was denied in the U.K. on the basis of consent—it is deemed in the best interests of U.K. citizens that their prior written consent must be secured if their bodily resources are to be used for posthumous reproduction.

Also falling under this category are cases of reproductive travel motivated by the desire to circumvent policies prohibiting risky procedures. For example, IVF resulting in post-menopausal pregnancy, or in higher-order multiples such as triplets or quadruplets, is unavailable in many countries because the risk to the health of the mother and offspring is deemed to be too high. By traveling abroad to countries with less restrictive policies, patients are able to obtain these procedures—sometimes resulting in high costs to their own healthcare systems at a later stage. In one recent high-profile case, a 62-year-old woman gave birth to twins after traveling to India for assisted reproductive procedures that were denied to her in Canada on account of her advanced age (Baylis and Crozier 2009).

Along similar lines, many countries do not permit gamete providers to remain anonymous on the grounds that this is contrary to the interests of the resulting offspring. For example, Denmark has become a popular destination for Europeans seeking sperm in part because, unlike some of its neighboring countries, such as Sweden, it permits providers to remain anonymous.

(4) Reproductive travel has proven to be particularly controversial in cases where legal restrictions rooted in *social or religious values* drive people abroad for goods and services related to reproductive health and fertility. Travel for contraception and abortion, although not widely discussed in the context of the reproductive travel industry, which tends to focus on people whose goal is procreation, is a perfect example of this kind of case phenomenon. Many countries reflect the social/religious values of their citizens by restricting access to contraception or abortion, either by banning it outright or by rendering it a scarce resource. One response to this is for women to travel to nearby countries with less stringent regulations. For instance, in response to the ban on abortion in Ireland, Irish women in need of abortion frequently travel to Britain for this service (Department of Health 2012; McDonald 2012). One response has been the "abortion boat" run by Women on Waves, a non-profit founded by Dutch gynecologist Rebecca Gomberts. By keeping the ship in international waters where the more permissive Dutch laws are in effect on the vessel, this group is able to offer abortion services to women who live in countries that prohibit these treatments.

(*The Week* Staff 2012)

The desire to select the sex of prospective offspring is yet another reason for reproductive travel based on social values. While the selection of certain embryos for implantation during IVF on the basis of sex is not permitted in many countries for ethical or demographic reasons, some prospective parents are willing to travel abroad for this service. Thailand, in particular, has become a popular destination for reproductive travel in part because its clinics may offer sex selection services (Whittaker 2009).

Some countries have developed legislation regarding assisted reproduction that is grounded in a particular conception of the characteristics of an "acceptable family." For example, same-sex couples or unmarried people are not permitted access to IVF or other fertility procedures in Italy since it introduced strict regulations in 2004 limiting these procedures to heterosexual married couples. For people wishing to have "non-traditional families" in countries with strict socio-religious restrictions regarding fertility assistance, travel abroad can be a compelling alternative.

Reproductive Autonomy and the State

One focal point of discussions regarding the ethics of reproductive travel has been the tensions arising between the reproductive rights claimed by individual citizens and the objectives of the countries in which they live. Advocates of assisted reproductive technologies (ARTs) have long cited reproductive autonomy as the central benefit of these interventions. For example, although IVF is currently accepted as "normal," if not common practice, this was not always the case. In the 1970s and 1980s, critics argued that IVF was too medically risky for the "test tube babies" that would be born this way, and they also worried about the sociological ramifications of this practice for the very definition of "family"—a concept that has always been highly normatively charged. In response to these arguments, R.G. Edwards (1974) defended IVF on the basis of infertile couples' right to procreate. Similarly, advocates of reproductive travel frequently refer to the reproductive autonomy of prospective travelers as one of the strongest reasons for supporting the existence and viability of these markets.

Guido Pennings (2004) is widely cited for his arguments favoring reproductive travel as a means for balancing the reproductive autonomy of citizens with the duty of a government to adopt legislation that reflects the socio-religious views of its populace—or at least those values that are shared by the majority of the citizens of that state. National governments, Pennings argues, have a responsibility to adopt legislation that reflects the values of the majority of the people in that country, even if this means that its legislation will be inconsistent with the values of minority groups. For example, countries where predominant socio-religious mores strongly favor traditional notions of "family" will restrict access to fertility treatments—for instance, Italy's laws deny treatments to unmarried persons or same-sex couples (Boggio 2005), and Iran forbids any treatments using third-party gametes (Inhorn 2011). These laws hold despite the fact that all the countries' citizens do not universally share the values underlying them. Given the availability of reproductive travel, however, this fact need not effectively curtail the reproductive autonomy of those denied access to fertility treatments in their home countries if they can meet their needs by going abroad. Thus, Pennings favors reproductive travel as a way of ensuring the reproductive autonomy of minority groups in various nations as well as the rule of the majority.

However, reproductive tourism is unlikely to satisfactorily resolve the tension between reproductive autonomy and the rule of law. Crucially, it is not the case that anyone who wants access to these reproductive goods and services can simply travel abroad to obtain them—access to reproductive travel remains the purview of relatively wealthy and otherwise socially privileged citizens. This poses a challenge for nations with deep (constitutional or otherwise) commitments to equitable access to medical care for all citizens (Boggio 2005), and it runs the risk of creating a class of global elites who have increased access to medical care at the expense of the poor (Martin 2009; Sengupta 2011). Additionally, the availability (even if only in principle) of reproductive travel gives the travelers' countries more leeway to pass even more restrictive laws within their borders, potentially constraining reproductive autonomy even further for citizens unable to travel abroad (Storrow 2010). Furthermore, if a country opts to push certain ART procedures abroad because they are deemed to have bad consequences, this potentially undermines the very rationale behind restricting them domestically (Storrow 2010). For these reasons, reproductive travel seems not to serve as a very effective "safety valve" (as Pennings refers to it) for easing the challenges posed by countries with diverse populations. Some authors have preferred the term "reproductive exile" to "reproductive travel" since the vast majority of these travelers would obtain treatment at home if it were possible, but instead they are forced to go abroad due to various constraints that restrict their access to key reproductive goods and services (Matorras 2005; Inhorn and Patrizio 2009).

Various measures have been suggested for minimizing reproductive travel, including punishments for physicians or clinics that inform patients about reproductive travel or facilitate this practice; suggested punishments include fines, license revocations, and even imprisonment (Heng 2006; Shanks 2010). Punishments for reproductive travelers have also been explored as a means to curtail the industry; Turkey, for example, has recently introduced legislation whereby women who go abroad for fertility treatments involving third-party gametes may be imprisoned for up to three years on their return (Shanks 2010; Van Hoof and Pennings 2011). The threat to states may be even more severe in the case of the destination countries for reproductive travelers. If competition among these countries for a share in this market becomes particularly fierce, destination countries may be tempted to enact increasingly permissive legislations regarding reproductive medical goods and services, regardless of their risks or their ethical implications. This would effectively result in what has been referred to as a "race to the bottom" (Millns 2002; Carbone and Gottheim 2006).

The health and future welfare of prospective children must also be given careful consideration in this discussion. Just as in the early debates concerning IVF, prospective parents are not the only relevant parties, even within their own families. For instance, many nations have taken measures to ensure that children born from third-party gametes have access to information about their genetic parents. By traveling abroad, parents from these countries are able to obtain anonymous gametes, with potential negative effects for the children who will be born (Blyth and Farrand 2005). There are additional risks for babies born of foreign surrogates regarding legal parenthood and citizenship, and there have been cases where commissioning parents have been unable to bring the offspring home with them (Parks 2010). Until and unless both the source and destination countries guarantee legal rights regarding parenthood and citizenship of children, offspring produced through reproductive travel are in an insecure position and the ethics of the practice will remain problematic.

Feminism, Gender, Race, and Global Justice

There are many reasons for which feminist analysis should figure prominently in bioethical investigations of reproductive travel. Questions involving sexual orientation and women's choices are among the most ethically salient features of reproductive travel, and these are questions for which feminist scholarship has developed a specific set of conceptual tools. Feminist scholarship challenges the traditional distinction by which decisions made within the family are considered private matters, whereas decisions made outside the family are considered public, and thereby subject to evaluation in terms of equity and justice. Although reproductive travel is often the result of a deeply personal decision made by prospective parent(s) to expand their family, this intimate act has broad political implications—both within the travelers' own countries and internationally. The kinds of choices made by the people involved in the various aspects of this phenomenon—parents, ova providers and surrogates, clinicians, etc.—manifest patterns that reveal the systematic social constraints in which they find themselves. These social pressures may not be apparent to the individual people in question, but they may nevertheless be visible on analysis of groups of individuals, all of whom share particular characteristics (social status, nationality, gender, etc.) and life decisions (Young 2007; Donchin 2010).

For example, on the one hand it would ostensibly seem that the availability of reproductive travel widens the options available to women—making it possible for them to conceive without a male spouse, presenting greater opportunities for having children later in life, or when they suffer from other fertility challenges. On the other hand, in a society (as are most) where women are significantly valued for their reproductive capabilities, the increasing availability of ART in general means that women can be expected to experience greater social pressure to have children and to engage in social reproduction—for example, to have children when they might otherwise be pleased to remain childless, to engage in post-menopausal reproduction despite the costs and health risks, or to carry to term pregnancies involving multiple embryos.

Reproductive travel involving surrogacy and third-party ova requires the intimate use of another woman's body. Contrasted with sperm collection, the procedures by which ova are harvested involve multiple injections to administer hormones and a transvaginal needle to extract the ova—this is painful and invasive for the provider, and it carries medical risks such as ovarian hyper-stimulation syndrome, which can be fatal. Surrogacy itself brings obvious risks of physical discomforts and dangers, but in a transnational setting, much of the surrogacy that takes place is "gestational surrogacy" whereby surrogates carry offspring from the embryos of other women. This is preferred because it permits commissioning parents greater control over the genetic makeup of the offspring (including degree of relatedness or ethnic/physical characteristics) and also because it reduces the emotional connection a surrogate might feel towards the baby. Surrogates are encouraged to care for the developing fetus like they would their own children, but to perceive the status of the relationship they hold to that child as inferior to the bonds of genetic or contractual parenthood.

Frequently, when prospective parents are purchasing gametes to create a child, a significant consideration is the phenotypic characteristics or ethnic-cultural background of the gamete provider. For example, although Spanish legislation guarantees the anonymity of gamete providers, measures are taken to match providers and recipients across multiple phenotypic features, including coloring, height, weight, and even blood group. This serves to not only mask ART by creating the façade of a "natural" family, which renders the practice more "socially acceptable," it is also based on an outdated view of European countries as ethnically homogeneous societies (Bergmann 2011).

Within the Indian market, women who are lighter skinned or Brahmin can receive higher compensation for their ova than darker skinned women (Pande 2010). Similarly, there is a strong market within Northern Europe for ova from women of former eastern-block countries, such as Romania, because their fair coloring is in high demand and because of the low price of their ova due to the generally low levels of prosperity common among former citizens of the USSR (Storrow 2005; Ferrari Morris 2007). Indeed, there are even clinics that import Eastern European women for their reproductive resources because the premium on their genetic predisposition for fair coloring is so high and their relative wages are so low (Sarojini et al. 2011).

Choices of prospective parents regarding where to travel and with whom to contract are frequently influenced by preferences that are rooted in global injustices. Without significant inequalities between countries and their citizens underwriting the price differential and the availability of human bodily resources (surrogacy and ova), for instance, the phenomenon of reproductive travel might not be so widespread (Ikemoto 2009).

With respect to domestic ova and surrogacy provisioning, many Organization for Economic Cooperation and Development (OECD) countries limit the compensation that can be offered to women to an amount sufficient to cover the costs involved, including time and expenses, even though restricting compensation can have a negative effect on the supply of female reproductive resources (Levine 2011; Smith 2012). There is concern in these countries that commoditization of these resources will undermine existing altruistic systems wherein these human bodily resources are perceived as gifts given freely, and altruistic gifting is preferred on the grounds that it minimizes the exploitation of those who provide these resources (Martin 2010; Crozier and Martin 2012). A central concern is that, if more money were offered than merely that which would serve as compensation for expenses incurred, people might be enticed to sell their bodily resources for profit, which would disproportionately attract providers from less privileged socio-economic groups. Arguably, a system wherein the wealthy effectively procure organs or reproductive resources from the poor in a non-reciprocal manner is exploitative of providers. The term "exploitative" typically refers to arrangements wherein one party is at a significant disadvantage relative to the other such that this results in them putting forth a disproportionately large share of the effort or other costs into an arrangement in exchange for a disproportionately small share of the benefit.

But, if a domestic market in ova or surrogacy would be exploitative, then this exploitation would likely be exacerbated when extended transnationally since the socio-economic discrepancies between commissioning parents and potential ova and surrogacy providers would tend to be increased substantially. In the reproductive travel market, women from whom these reproductive goods and services are procured are typically from countries with emerging or developing economies, and are more socio-economically vulnerable than commissioning parents. This raises concerns over coercion, exploitation, and justice—an acute concern in light of the relatively poor reproductive health care often otherwise available to women in these countries (Sengupta 2011; Jaiswal 2012). (For illuminating discussions of exploitation in the context of domestic and transnational surrogacy, see Wertheimer (1999) and Panitch (2013), respectively.)

Certainly both the commissioning parents and the surrogates gain something particularly valuable to them in the exchange—the former gain children and the latter gain money that is significant to their families. This wage is significant, and in India, for example, it is sometimes in excess of five times the average annual wage. These funds are used to eliminate debts, to start businesses, to pay for education and (sometimes life-saving) medical care for family members, and to achieve other ends that are both of huge value to them and otherwise unobtainable (Bhatia 2012). However, the conditions under which gestational surrogates and ova providers enter into the contracts are of concern. There are documented cases wherein consent has been hampered by misleading and outright fraudulent recruitment tactics on behalf of brokers and by the providers' relatively impoverished education levels and access to information about the industry (Sarojini et al. 2011). Arguably, however, even if the conditions of the contract are completely transparent, poor women in countries with emerging and developing economies are unable to properly consent to these contracts precisely because the background conditions of their poverty provide them with no viable alternatives, and this undermines the legitimacy of their consent—they are effectively coerced into entering into a contract that they might otherwise resist (Panich 2013).

Furthermore, the working conditions of gestational surrogates working in the reproductive travel industry can be quite striking. Indian surrogates, for example, are subjected to stringent screening prior to, and monitoring throughout, the pregnancy. Often, surrogates are housed in group homes with limited contact with their own families; their diets and activities are closely controlled; and they relinquish the ability to make medical decisions related to their pregnancies, including difficult choices regarding selective termination (which is often medically recommended in the case of triplets or other higher-order multiples) (Pande 2010). Indeed, part of what makes Indian surrogacy services so attractive to many customers is that commissioning parents are able to assert a great deal of control over the conditions of the pregnancy and birth relative to what would be possible if the surrogates were hired domestically or from the U.S., for example; and the reason Indian surrogates accept these conditions is because they are unable to bargain for more favorable contracts.

What, then, can be done? The contracts can be exploitative of surrogates and ova providers, yet increasing the wages risks (it has been argued) hampered consent by increasing the coercive factor of the offer (Panitch 2013). Some advocate quashing the practice of transnational surrogacy and ova sales by criminalizing it, or by increasing the supply of domestic providers by increasing their payments (PS 2012), or by promoting national networks such that countries can be self-sufficient in their use of these female reproductive resources (Martin 2010). Others suggest that, given that this market is likely to persist, legislation introducing some minimum standards of care to ensure the informed consent and the safety of participants and resulting children is required—for example, in the form of regional trade agreements (Chung 2006; Ferrari Morris 2007) or global measures similar to the Hague Adoption Convention (Storrow 2005; Martin 2009). Beyond this, some suggest letting the free market dictate the details of contracts in order to maximize the reproductive autonomy of commissioning parents, while others suggest basic requirements for surrogacy contracts, minimizing the share taken by brokers and middle-men, measures to improve the bargaining power and benefits received by providers of surrogacy and ova (Sarojini et al. 2011; Jaiswal 2012; Panitch 2013), and strengthening the social connections between surrogates and commissioning parents (Donchin 2010; Parks 2010).

Conclusion

This essay represents a brief introduction to some of the ethical issues raised by reproductive travel. I have, as much as possible, avoided focusing too much on ethical issues that overlap considerably with other areas of bioethics—many of which are discussed elsewhere in this book. Insofar as reproductive travel deals with the movement of patients across national borders (often from nations with more prosperous economies to nations with less prosperous ones), the chapter on Medical Tourism will be relevant to this one (see Chapter 8 in this volume). Because some reproductive travel involves payment for human reproductive resources such as gametes and surrogacy, there is much to be learned from discussions of commoditization of human biological resources, including organ sales and the sale of tissue for research purposes. Furthermore, there is overlap between this area and bioethical investigations of research conducted on test subjects in developing countries; similar to markets in reproductive travel, there are significant risks of exploiting the test subjects and their communities unless they derive sufficient benefits from the exchange—and it is no simple matter how to define "sufficient benefits." Although I have tried to minimize discussion of those issues that are likely to overlap significantly with topics in other chapters of this book, I encourage readers to investigate these issues if they wish to have a fuller appreciation of the complex ethical dimensions of reproductive travel.

Related Topics

Chapter 8, "Medical Tourism," I. Glenn Cohen
Chapter 28, "Regulating Reproduction: A Bioethical Approach," Isabel Karpin

References

Baylis, F. and Crozier, G.K.D. (2009) "Postmenopausal Reproduction: In Whose Interests?" *Journal of Obstetrics and Gynaecology Canada* 31 (5): 457–8.

Bergmann, S. (2011) "Fertility Tourism: Circumventive Routes That Enable Access to Reproductive Technologies and Substances," *Signs* 36 (2): 280–9.

Bhatia, S. (2012) "Women Line Up to Rent Out Wombs: There May Be Ethical Concerns, But Poor Villagers Are Earning Enough Money to Transform Lives," *Sunday Telegraph* June 9.

Blyth, E. and Farrand, A. (2005) "Reproductive Tourism: A Price Worth Paying for Reproductive Autonomy?" *Critical Social Policy* 25: 91–114.

Boggio, A. (2005) "Italy Enacts New Law on Medically Assisted Reproduction," *Human Reproduction* 20 (5): 1153–7.

Carbone, J. and Gottheim, P. (2006) "Markets, Subsidies, Regulation, and Trust: Building Ethical Understandings into the Market for Fertility Services," *The Journal for Gender, Race and Justice* 9 (1): 521–3.

Chung, L.H. (2006) "Free Trade in Human Reproductive Cells: A Solution to Procreative Tourism and the Unregulated Internet," *Minnesota Journal of International Law* 15 (1): 263–96.

Crozier, G.K.D. and Baylis, F. (2010) "The Ethical Physician Encounters International Medical Travel," *Journal of Medical Ethics* 36 (6): 297–301.

Crozier, G.K.D. and Martin, D. (2012) "How to Address the Ethics of Reproductive Travel to Developing Countries: A Comparison and National Self-Sufficiency and Regulated Market Approaches," *Developing World Bioethics* 12 (1): 45–54.

Deech, R. (2003) "Reproductive Tourism in Europe: Infertility and Human Rights," *Global Governance* 9 (4): 425–32.

Department of Health (2012) "Abortion Statistics, England and Wales: 2011," *GOV.UK* May 29. Available at: http://www.gov.uk/government/uploads/system/uploads/attachment_data/file/200529/Abortion_statistics__England_and_Wales_2011.pdf (accessed July 23, 2014).

Donchin, A. (2010) "Reproductive Tourism and the Quest for Global Gender Justice," *Bioethics* 24 (7): 323–32.

Edwards, R. (1974) "Fertilization of Human Eggs In Vitro: Moral, Ethics and the Law," *The Quarterly Review of Biology* 49: 3–26.

Ferrari Morris, E. (2007) "Reproductive Tourism and the Role of the European Union," *Chinese Journal of International Law* 8 (2): 701–13.

Heng, B.C. (2006) "'Reproductive Tourism': Should Locally Registered Fertility Doctors Be Held Accountable for Channelling Patients to Foreign Medical Establishments?" *Human Reproduction* 21 (3): 840–2.

Ikemoto, L.C. (2009) Reproductive Tourism: Equality Concerns in the Global Market for Fertility Services," *Law and Inequality* 27: 277–309.
Inhorn, M. (2011) "Globalization and Gametes: Reproductive 'Tourism,' Islamic Bioethics, and Middle Eastern Modernity," *Anthropology and Medicine* 18 (1): 87–103.
Inhorn, M. and Patrizio, P. (2009) "Rethinking Reproductive 'Tourism' as Reproductive 'Exile,'" *Fertility and Sterility* 92 (3): 904–5.
Jaiswal, S. (2012) "Commercial Surrogacy in India: An Ethical Assessment of Existing Legal Scenario from the Perspective of Women's Autonomy and Reproductive Rights," *Gender, Technology and Development* 16 (1): 1–28.
Korn, P. (2012) "Surrogacy Gives Birth to Industry," *Portland Tribune* June 21.
Levine, A.D. (2011) "The Oversight and Practice of Oocyte Donation in the United States, United Kingdom and Canada," *HEC Forum* 23: 15–30.
Martin, D. (2010) "Medical Travel and the Sale of Human Biological Materials: Suggestions for Ethical Policy Development," *Global Social Policy* 10: 377–95.
Martin, L.J. (2009) "Reproductive Tourism in the Age of Globalization," *Globalizations* 6 (2): 249–63.
Matorras, R. (2005) "Reproductive Exile Versus Reproductive Tourism," *Human Reproduction* 20 (12): 3571. Available at: humrep.oxfordjournals.org/content/20/12/3571.1.full.pdf (accessed July 23, 2014).
McDonald, H. (2012) "Hundreds of Irish Women Forced to Come to Britain for Abortions," *The Guardian* November 16. Available at: http://www.guardian.co.uk/world/2012/nov/16/ireland-abortion-women-forced-abroad (accessed July 23, 2014).
Millns, S. (2002) "Reproducing Inequalities: Assisted Conception and the Challenge of Legal Pluralism," *Journal of Social Welfare and Family Law* 24 (1): 19–36.
Pande, A. (2010) "Commercial Surrogacy in India: Manufacturing a Perfect Worker-Mother," *Signs* 35 (4): 969–92.
Panich, V. (2013) "Surrogate Tourism and Reproductive Rights," *Hypatia* 28 (2): 274–89.
Parks, J.A. (2010) "Care Ethics and the Global Practice of Commercial Surrogacy," *Bioethics* 24 (7): 333–40.
Pennings, G. (2004) "Legal Harmonization and Reproductive Tourism in Europe," *Human Reproduction* 19: 2689–94.
PS (2012) "Calls for Increased Compensation for Egg Donors," *The Copenhagen Post* December 3.
Reed, C.M. (2008) "Medical Tourism," *Medical Clinics of North America* 92: 1433–46.
Sarojini, N., Marwah, V. and Shenoi, A. (2011) "Globalisation of Birth Markets: A Case Study of Assisted Reproductive Technologies in India," *Globalization and Health* 7: 27. http://www.globalizationandhealth.com/content/7/1/27 (accessed July 23, 2014).
Sengupta, A. (2011) "Medical Tourism: A Reverse Subsidy for the Elite," *Signs* 36 (2): 312–19.
Shanks, P. (2010) "Struggling to Control Fertility Tourism," *Biopolitical Times* April 17. http://www.biopoliticaltimes.org/article.php?id=5156 (accessed July 23, 2014).
Smith, R. (2012) "Fertility Treatment Waiting Times Halve after Increased Payments to Donors," *The Telegraph (UK)* November 26.
Storrow, R.F. (2005) "Quests for Conception: Fertility Tourists, Globalization and Feminist Legal Theory," *Hastings Law Journal* 57: 295–330.
Storrow, R. F. (2010) "Travel into the Future of Reproductive Technology," *UMKC Law Review* 79 (2): 295–307.
The Week Staff (2012) "'Women on Waves': A Guide to the Dutch 'Abortion Ship,'" *The Week* October 4. Available at: theweek.com/article/index/234374/women-on-waves-a-guide-to-the-dutch-abortion-ship (accessed July 23, 2014).
Van Hoof, W. and Pennings, G. (2011) "Extraterritoriality for Cross-Border Reproductive Care: Should States Act Against Citizens Travelling Abroad for Illegal Infertility Treatment?" *Reproductive BioMedicine Online* 23 (5): 546–54.
Wertheimer, A. (1999) *Exploitation*, Princeton: Princeton University Press.
Whittaker, A. (2009) "Global Technologies and Transnational Reproduction in Thailand," *Asian Studies Review* 33 (3): 319–32.
Young, I. (2007) *Global Challenges: War, Self-Determination and Responsibility for Justice*, Malden, MA: Polity Press.

31
POPULATION GROWTH AND DECLINE
Issues of Justice

Margaret P. Battin

Let's start with what is supposed to be the solution to population issues, but is actually part of the problem. That's the figure at the end of many of the classic population projections, the so-called "leveling off" point at which population growth will cease to be a threat to the globe. The question is whether "leveling off" is a realistic prediction or an unsupported and dangerous fantasy, and if it's the latter what we can do to transform it into the former with a reasonable degree of justice.

"Levelling Off"

The "leveling-off" assumption relies on projections concerning what has been known as the demographic transition, a pattern of four distinct stages that a society is said to go through in moving from an undeveloped, agrarian economy to an industrialized, developed one. In the first stage of the demographic transition, that characterizing premodern, undeveloped, non-industrial, agrarian economies, birth rates are high, but so are death rates: In the absence of modern medicine and many other factors, life is hard, infant mortality is high, maternal mortality in childbirth is also high, and the average lifespan is short. Thus population size remains comparatively stable: There are many births, but many early deaths. In the second stage, the introduction of immunization programs, clean water supplies, antibiotics, and other developments from the technologically advanced nations leads to a sharp drop in death rates, but traditional social patterns continue to favor high birth rates. With high birth rates and low death rates, the population soars. With increasing development, however, a third stage begins: As women are increasingly educated, as infant mortality drops and families find they do not need many children born to ensure that a few survive, as social insurance systems mean that parents do not need to rely on their children for support in their old age, and as additional children no longer mean an additional source of labor in tasks like wood gathering, water hauling, and farm work but instead begin to represent a liability in schooling costs, clothing costs, entertainment, and supervision in an urban environment, birth rates begin to decline; thus population growth rates slow. In the fourth stage, which characterizes industrialized nations like those of Europe and North America, both birth and death rates are low—births are fewer but lifespans longer—and population size "levels off" or stabilizes.

Paul Ehrlich raised a global alarm with the publication of *The Population Bomb* in 1968, pointing out that the global population was increasing at an unsupportable rate. Indeed, it doubled from 3 billion in 1959 to 6 billion in 1999; the 7 billion mark was reached just a dozen years later, the 8 billion mark forecast for 2025. But various projections showed the global total leveling off at some 9, or 10, or as high as 12 billion at the middle of the twenty-first century or the beginning of the twenty-second. Whenever growth leveled off, it was widely assumed, the population problem would then be solved.

Indeed, in many countries fertility rates have dropped dramatically. Some have had sub-replacement fertility rates, and fertility rates in others—Japan, Germany, and Lithuania, for example—have dropped so low as to cause population decline. Indeed, some observers believe the population problem will be reversed: "In 2050," claim Noriyuki Takayama and Martin Werding (2011: cover blurb), "world population growth is predicted to come almost to a halt. Shortly thereafter it may well start to shrink."

"Leveling off," or even global population decrease, may seem to be an attractive picture. But are the measures designed to achieve leveling off, or even population decline, just? Many questions of justice arise. For instance, leveling off assumes that every woman, on average, will have at most 2.1 children—so for any woman who has three children, there must be another woman who has only one; and for every woman who has four, there must be another who remains childless altogether. Are the various forms of population "control" even workable solutions? Are alternative strategies, like enhancing development, fairer as a way to achieve population stabilization? By inquiring into the seemingly pie-in-the-sky assumption about eventual leveling off, we can unearth some of the most troubling issues about population and justice.

Most nations now have family-planning programs, though these vary tremendously in character, methods, and effectiveness; some are governmental, some are conducted by non-governmental organizations; and some rely entirely on local private groups. They vary in nearly every aspect of their existence: Funding, level of education, services provided or denied, and rhetoric used. Yet despite their enormous variety, virtually all of these family-planning programs face several basic ethical dilemmas about the strategies they employ.

Issues of Justice in the Early Programs of Population Control

Concern with runaway population growth erupted in the mid-1960s, as the development of public health measures, preventative measures, effective therapies, and other modern medical techniques meant that death rates (especially among infants and young children) began to fall while birth rates remained high. India and then China, each home to about a fifth of the world's population, were among the first to respond, and their population-control programs—India's male sterilization program and China's one-child policy—exhibit some of the most vivid questions of justice.

Incentives and Disincentives

Perhaps most notorious for its use of problematic incentives was India's vigorously pursued population-control policy of 1975–6. Though this may well be a myth and no documentation of the practice is apparently available, Indian officials were widely believed to offer a transistor radio to any man who would consent to a vasectomy on the spot. Financial incentives were offered to local officials who could persuade villagers to accept sterilization, often at the mobile "vasectomy camps" created around the country. At the same time, disincentives were also used to secure compliance: Fines, denial of benefits, denial of medical treatment for government officers, denial of governmental quarters for civil servants, denial of accommodations in housing projects for the public, and disqualification for most government scholarships.

China's one-child program, initiated in 1979 and imposed in the early 1980s, also used a wide range of incentives (better jobs, better housing, better pay) for couples with one child only, together with disincentives (fines, demotions, penalties, forcible abortions and sterilizations, even house-burnings) to discourage those having more than the permitted number of children. Incentives and disincentives to influence reproductive behavior have been used in many other societies: The Nazis used bronze, silver, and gold medals to reinforce large family size for Aryan (but not Jewish) women: Four, six, and eight children, respectively; Ceauşescu's Romania used a variety of harsh disincentives and penalties for abortion or failure to have an adequate number of children, set at five; and Singapore's 1983 combination pronatalist/antinatalist program provided a wide array of benefits and preferences to encourage educated women to have large families, but also used incentive payments for sterilization to decrease fertility among uneducated women.

Both incentives and disincentives can violate fundamental principles of autonomy if they undermine someone's ability to rationally deliberate or are coercive in some way. Basic principles of reproductive liberty require informed, voluntary choice about matters relevant to procreation, and the voluntariness of such choices can quite easily be infringed. India's notorious transistor radios, even if fictional, compromise voluntary choice in two ways: Not only might they have been too attractive to resist for poor villagers, but the way in which they were allegedly offered would have undercut the possibility of reflective deliberation for a man as well as the possibility of consultation with his wife.

Contraception Mandates versus Family Size Ceilings

India's vasectomy program emphasized promoting contraception, targeting larger families; China's program, however, promulgated a family size limit, coupled with the supply and surveillance of contraception to maintain this limit. While in practice contraception mandates and family size ceilings are often intertwined, they are conceptually different. Contraception mandates may alter the decisional structure of childbearing choices but still recognize individual preferences in choices about family size; family size limits impose a ceiling but allow the couple to determine how to prevent childbearing. Contraception mandates seem particularly problematic when the contraceptive poses health risks to the user, involves unacceptable side effects, or, as in sterilization, is irreversible. Family size limits are problematic where they are very severe (as in a one-child policy), are inequitably imposed, or are not necessitated by a country's demographic situation. Contraceptive mandates tend to impose burdens of restricted childbearing on just some individuals; in contrast, family size limits affect everyone and in this sense are more just, but they typically function by punishing violators after the fact, even those where pregnancy is unintended, and in this different sense appear unjust.

But both contraceptive mandates and family size limits may be viewed as just in other ways. Under its one-child policy, China effectively mandated contraceptive use, used fertility surveillance, and limited birth permits, but it in principle imposed these mandates on *all* women. Simultaneously, its family size ceiling has been comparatively egalitarian: One child for all couples (with the exception of two in some rural provinces and no ceiling for the tiny populations of the non-Han ethnic areas), not, say, five children for Party members and no children for non-members. This policy came to be seen by the populace as a demographic necessity and therefore understandable and normal (Nie 2005; Nie and Wyman 2005), and thus, it can be claimed, not unjustly imposed. Although officially still in force, the one-child policy is now beginning to erode, as well-to-do couples sometimes elect to pay large fines for having additional children; it is also being deliberately relaxed as China considers ways to move away from the one-child policy to a more stable, long-term population management plan compatible with "leveling off." In 2013 it announced a further incremental reform in the one-child policy that would allow couples to have two children if just one of the parents was an only child, and further relaxations can be expected in the future.

Targeting

Even in countries with less acute population problems, issues of justice may arise in family-planning programs. For example, programs may target groups segregated by income, ethnicity, or race that are perceived to be at higher risk of excess childbearing. Even if targeted contraceptive programs do not violate canons of voluntary choice, they may be unjust because they approach people identified primarily as members of specific, often stereotyped subgroups (e.g., black inner-city teenagers), making assumptions about the members of a subgroup that are not true of all individuals in it. Access to programs can be discriminatory both in terms of whom it excludes and whom it targets. Other issues include adherence to veiled family size limitations: Target ceilings entertained by program officials or governments, but not known to recipients of family-planning services or available for public discussion. And family-planning programs may also violate informed consent by withholding information, such as risks, reversibility, and side effects of the contraceptives involved.

Population Stabilization Over Time

The issue of "leveling off" involves not just how high population growth can climb or how far it can decline, but what population size can be sustained over time. Since population control measures—disincentives, incentives, mandates, etc.—work at the individual level —just one reproductively capable couple at a time—they cannot guarantee long-term results. Population stabilization, thus, requires ongoing, long-term, indeed permanent attention; there is no "end point" at which population problems are definitively solved.

Declines in fertility in developed and many developing countries have lulled many thinkers into concluding that there is no real problem. However, population futures are not easy to predict (Caldwell 2004; Demeny 2004). As John Bongaarts pointed out, fertility measures in many developed countries may be temporarily depressed by a rise in the mean age of childbearing: As women procreate in later ages, a drop in total fertility may turn out to be only a postponement, corresponding to increases in apparent fertility rates when social patterns of postponement end and the timing of childbearing stabilizes or shifts back to earlier ages (Bongaarts 2002, 2008). Societal framing may also play a role in reproductive behavior: For example, with the most recent relaxation of China's one-child policy, some couples reported that although they would now be permitted a second child, they still planned to remain at one: Such preferences are clearly subject to societal expectations and the behavior of other couples in the same age cohort. Thus the sense that the population "explosion" is over may be misinformed in several ways: It does not account for population pressures in the still-developing world; it over-interprets its own current "birth dearth" (Vallin 2002); and it overlooks the vicissitudes of family size preferences within populations.

Some observers have been concerned that "population entrapment" in societies now experiencing high growth rates would mean failed societal infrastructures as the population outstrips their capacity, something most likely in the least developed nations with most rapid population growth and greatest population momentum. In these countries, it was argued, the demographic transition may not take place after all, leading to famine, war, and overall die-back—that is, human death or non-reproduction on a widespread scale, whether from starvation, water and resource depletion, global pollution or climate change, or other population-size related causes. However, enshrined in the strategies explicitly favored in the U.N. Millennium Development Goals, economic development has been a strategy actively pursued as a means of population growth control. Goals associated with it have included increased education for both women and children, especially female children; lowering infant mortality rates, enhancing the status of women, the creation of jobs for women, etc. These measures have been supplemented by greater involvement of the wealthy nations in matters like infectious disease control, especially in malaria and HIV/AIDS, leading to reduced mortality. Personal incomes in many developing nations have increased; so has the gross domestic product of many countries. Yet economic development brings with it dramatic increases in rates of consumption: Diets consisting of more fats and meats (less efficient foodstuffs than grains), more extensive energy uses, more uses of consumer and industrial products that pollute or exhaust environmental resources. The specter here is sometimes pictured as more than a billion inhabitants of China (a fifth of the world's population), all having just one child, maybe two, but, like the inhabitants of the United States, all wanting refrigerators and automobiles. For "lean" developing countries, emulating Western economic models may also mean emulating "fat" Western domestic models as well, with low family size but huge uses of resources. Not only is economic development typically uneven in its benefits for individuals, but in the absence of other alterations in human behavior, it risks increasing, rather than decreasing, strains on the earth's carrying capacity. Thus economic development is hardly a panacea to population stabilization, and without other limitations offers a problematic and in many ways patently unjust solution to population problems.

The Malthusian Warning: An Issue of Justice

Part of what raises these issues of justice was voiced, though perhaps less noticed from an ethical point of view, by Thomas Malthus in his classic 1798 work on population. Malthus warned that human beings, like other species, may reproduce at a rate that outstrips the carrying capacity of the site they inhabit and so doom themselves to destruction. Malthus posited that the growth of the human population tends to be exponential, but their food resources are ultimately limited by the productive capacity of the land. When a species exceeds the carrying capacity of its site, it "crashes" or dies back, either partially or completely. Widespread starvation, epidemics of disease exacerbated by the poor nutritional status of the population, pathological or aggressive behavior aggravated by overcrowding, and other factors lead to dramatic, involuntary population loss. "Die-backs" were to be expected, in Malthus's view, the foreseeable consequence of humans' inability to restrain themselves in matters of procreation.

Of course, Malthus lived in an era in which, although infant mortality was high and death rates in general high, people had few reliable methods of controlling procreation. There was abstinence and withdrawal; and while various forms of condoms had been used at much earlier times in history, the latex condom, the contraceptive pill, and safe methods of sterilization were yet to be developed. With these and other medical developments, however, it has become much more possible to control reproductive outcomes. Early population-control programs relied heavily on permanent sterilization, either male or female; newer family-planning programs have stressed reversible contraception, including condoms, oral contraceptives (the Pill), depot injectables (Depo-Provera and related forms), transdermal patches, intrauterine devices (IUDs), subdermal implants (Norplant and Implanon, its single-rod successor), and other forms of fertility regulation, using contraception both to delay the onset of childbearing and yield greater spacing between children as ways of decreasing total family size.

Thanks both to development and to family planning programs, population growth rates have declined substantially in many parts of the world. But slowed growth is still growth and, due to population momentum as large numbers of young people reach reproductive age, especially in the developing world, total global population is still increasing. Population projections for the year 2050 have ranged from the U.N. low of 7.78 billion (likely to be surpassed by the time this chapter is published), to the 2012 estimates of 9.4 billion (U.S. Census Bureau) or 9.6 billion (U.N. Population Division), to a high-variant estimate of almost 11 billion if fertility rates are just half a child higher per woman than the medium estimate. What is often overlooked is the narrowness of this margin: At just half a child higher per woman on average, population growth would continue to climb and keep climbing indefinitely until, presumably, either some form of global behavior change occurred or there were catastrophic die-backs.

Population Control and Its Critics

Religious Critics

Among religious groups, two have conspicuously opposed population limitation, Catholicism and Islam, though in somewhat different ways.

Drawing on earlier roots but articulated in response to the development of the Pill, Catholic teaching, which permits sex only within marriage, insists that the marital act must be both "unitive" and "procreative"—that every act of sexual activity must be open to the transmission of new life (Paul VI 1968). The use of all forms of "artificial" contraception is forbidden, as is sterilization. Catholics may licitly use only "natural family planning," that is, only rhythm methods which rely on abstinence during the woman's fertile period. The teaching in *Humanae Vitae* (it is a teaching, not doctrine, and is not articulated as infallible) has heavily influenced public policy in Latin America, the Philippines, and elsewhere, where family-planning programs, abortion, sterilization, and the distribution of contraception have been prohibited, underfunded, or in other ways impeded by governments. In the U.S. and much of Western Europe it has been largely ignored: Catholic women practice contraception at about the same rate as non-Catholic women. Yet Catholic opposition to population control has played a major role in both international and domestic policy in two ways: It has at times influenced governments to discontinue funding for family-planning programs and has blocked contraceptive coverage by the insurers of employees at Catholic institutions at home; this has been said by many to be unjust. Nevertheless, Catholic teaching also directs attention to issues of unequal distribution of resources and disparate levels of development as a way of understanding how economic injustice can contribute to population pressures.

Islam has traditionally strongly emphasized the importance of procreation. It too has been concerned about the permissibility of "artificial" contraception, though it clearly accepts the Holy Prophet's endorsement of *azl*, male withdrawal during intercourse. Some authorities allow modern contraception; some prohibit it; and some adopt a position of conditional acceptance, permitting it, for instance, only with the wife's consent or if a diaphragm or IUD is fitted by a woman physician. Spermicides and oral contraceptives or other hormonal methods are considered permissible only if it can be shown that they do not harm the woman.

Both Catholicism and Islam are undergoing considerable evolution in response to population issues. Although Catholicism still prohibits all "artificial" contraception and sterilization, it places increasing emphasis on responsible planning of family size, especially through the use of the rhythm method of timed abstinence and contemporary fertility-awareness based methods. Some Islamic countries, like Iran, Tunisia, Turkey, Bangladesh, and Indonesia, have had very successful family-planning programs, with dramatic drops in average family size. Others, particularly in the Middle East, have begun to introduce family-planning programs that seek to introduce concepts of condom use and responsible family-size planning to men, rather than women, on the assumption that this is more in accord with basic Islamic religious teachings and with the realities of reproductive choice in male-dominated societies.

Feminist Critics

Meanwhile, feminist critics, among them Betsy Hartmann, have examined the nature and methods of programs designed to control population growth (Hartmann 1995 [1987]). Controlling population growth means controlling people, they have argued, and it means especially controlling women. Population programs have typically targeted "acceptors"—women who can be pressured into accepting contraception or sterilization—and have paid little or no attention to women's subordinate situations in patriarchal societies, their precarious economic circumstances, their lack of education and familiarity with modern medicine, their compromised nutritional status, and their desperate need of other health care (Dixon-Mueller 1993; Women's Global Network for Reproductive Rights, multiple newsletters). For instance, some programs encouraged the implantation of various kinds of long-acting contraceptives, especially the IUD and the subdermal implant, without regard to side effects and with no provisions for removal of the device should the woman experience side effects or wish to have a child: Once it was in, there was nowhere to go to get it removed. Contraceptive testing, feminist critics have also claimed (though this is not documented), sometimes lacked informed consent or used placebo controls (some women got dummy pills, risking a pregnancy they did not want). Other contraceptive testing has been conducted, the feminist critique continues, with drugs whose long-term effects are not known, like the antifertility vaccines, or modalities easily abused, like quinacrine sterilization. Compounding the damage, feminists have argued, population-control programs seem to have committed a conceptual error as well: These programs appear to *blame* poor, uneducated women in the third world for unrestrained, "excess" fertility, as if problems of global population growth, including environmental degradation and immigration pressures on wealthy nations, were exclusively their fault.

Another target of continuing criticism has been China's effectively imposed one-child policy, condemned by feminists and others for its policies of required contraception, forced abortion, and mandatory sterilization (Gu et al. 2007). In addition, in a cultural tradition with pronounced son preference, China has seen widespread selective sex-based abortion, concealment and abandonment of female children, and in some cases, female infanticide, all contributing to a stark imbalance in male : female gender ratios. Feminist critics of China's policy have focused largely on individual abuses; supporters focus largely on apparent social consent and dramatic economic gains.

Cornucopian Critics

A third school of researchers, usually dubbed the cornucopians, has attempted to show that supposed limits on population growth are not well founded and hence that population control is not needed. Julian Simon was particularly vocal among this group, pointing out there is no agreement on the actual "carrying capacity" of the globe and insisting that human ingenuity can be counted upon to develop new food production techniques and new ways of exploiting and conserving resources (Simon 1981). It is sometimes also said that Malthus's pessimistic predictions were wrong, since they were followed by the Green Revolution, a vast expansion of agricultural productivity increasing the carrying capacity of the earth.

Many cornucopian researchers have focused on specific areas such as agriculture, fisheries, fresh water, fuels, air quality, and so on to try to demonstrate that substantial increases in global population can still be accommodated. But, as critics point out, even if it were possible to produce food for 1,000 billion people, this does not mean that it is possible to dispose of the domestic and industrial wastes of 1,000 billion people and their engines; and even if there were adequate agricultural water supplies, there may not be sufficient resources for fertilizer. The Green Revolution has been a one-time event, critics point out, and cannot be counted on for indefinite expansion. Cornucopianism is limited by the weakest essential link.

Critiques of Population Programs Per Se

Although more than half a century has passed since the initial concern with global population arose in the 1960s with Paul Ehrlich's talk of "population explosion," and as public perceptions in the developed world to some degree shifted away from these issues, several further lines of criticism have emerged in very recent years. In one, a handful of contemporary critics are combining religious, feminist, cornucopian, and other concerns into a much more severe critique of population control. The claim is that the population-control movement itself over the past half-century was or has become both practically and morally problematic. For example, Matthew Connelly launches a "withering" critique of "a humanitarian movement gone terribly awry" (Connelly 2008: back cover). Stephen Mosher identifies policies he takes to have been "wrong-headed" and counterproductive, saying that it is "too late to simply call off the dogs of population control" where fertility is below replacement; he argues that the "entire edifice of institutions, policies, and programs" which form the "population control juggernaut" should be scrapped, along with the "nasty theory" that there are "*too many people*" (Mosher 2008: 256–7; 3). The Christian Right is said to see international population policy as "a horror story of devastation and destruction visited upon women and the 'natural family'" (Buss and Herman 2003: 63); the Christian Right movement has consistently opposed population-control programs.

The arguments of many of these critics share an underlying commitment to value-of-life and family-values principles, a mistrust of government and of targeted programs, and the view that population increase is necessary for economic growth; but they also exhibit a tendency to exaggeration, to fail to see issues of unwanted fertility and its particular impact on poor women, to confuse a decline in growth rates with an absolute decline in total population, and to fail to consider what would have happened to global population had family-planning programs not been instituted in the first place. They also fail to recognize what may be the consequences of politically motivated declines in foreign aid for family planning, which dropped precipitously from $723 million in 1955 to $442 million in 2004 before easing up again to $648.5 million in 2010, and the implications that may have both for future fertility rates and for the precarious situation of women in severe economic or personal straits facing an unwanted pregnancy. These critics develop an almost paranoid view of "population controllers," according to which they have over the past half century, as Mosher puts it, "perpetrated a gigantic, costly and inhumane fraud upon the human race, defrauding the people of the developing countries of their progeny and the people of the developed world of their pocketbooks" (Mosher 2008: ix).

At the same time, continuing a theme first developed by Zero Population Growth (founded by Paul Ehlich in 1968) and strengthened by Negative Population Growth (founded in 1972), those who are primarily concerned with the practical implications of increasing global population and consumption, both for social issues like immigration and aging but particularly for environmental sustainability, assert that the globe is already seriously overpopulated and that we must reduce the global numbers if it is to survive. Negative Population Growth (NPG) makes the case for fewer people, encouraging:

> every country in the entire world, to put into effect national programs with the goals of first achieving a negative rate of population growth, then eventually stabilizing population size at a far lower level than today's—a size that would be sustainable indefinitely in a sound and healthy environment.
>
> (Grant 2006: iv)

Optimal Population Size: Fewer with More, or More with Less?

Dire predictions about overpopulation, unsustainable patterns of consumption, future generations, and the threat of die-back and crash presuppose a set of theoretical reflections concerning justice most vigorously pursued in philosophy by Derek Parfit (Parfit 1984), and in related versions in social-choice theory by Blackorby and collaborators (Blackorby et al. 2005). Although Parfit's concern is presented in a philosophically sophisticated form, the question he poses is simple: Which is to be preferred, when speaking of populations, a situation which yields the highest average level of welfare, or that which yields the greatest aggregate total of welfare? Put in another way, which is to be preferred, a situation in which there are fewer people though their quality of life is high, or one in which there is just as much happiness altogether, but more people with a lower quality of life? Such questions of course raise issues, like those framed by Amartya Sen and Martha Nussbaum (Sen 1992; Nussbaum 1999; Nussbaum and Glover 1995), about how human wellbeing should be measured and what factors "quality of life" assessments should consider, such as adequate nutrition and housing; freedom from exploitation, abuse, or grinding labor; adequate health, including reproductive health; personal autonomy and leisure; and whatever else contributes to human happiness and flourishing. But the central theoretical problem is about numbers: When we think about population size in general, should there be fewer people better off, or more people, but worse off? After all, the sum total of welfare or happiness in the world might be the same.

Translated into the context of the actual world, with wide gaps between rich nations and very rich population subgroups within them, and desperately poor nations with populations enduring chronic hunger or starvation, the problem might look like this: Is it better to have a world in which a small population lives as the global rich now do, with ample houses, automobiles, and the generous use of resources? Or, as a matter of justice, is it better to have more people, even if they must live at the subsistence levels of the global poor? Then, there could be many, many more people who have life, with just the same use of resources. Take any two people in absolute poverty: Would it be better if there were just one of them, poor, but not on the edge of starvation? Instead of any five in absolute poverty, one who was rich? Or instead of one comfortable, well nourished, well equipped person, three who are poor, but surviving? There is no easy answer to these questions, but they are central to issues of justice in population theory and policy.

In the eyes of Alan Weisman, a *global* one-child policy is our last, best hope for a future on earth—presumably a policy to be instituted *now*, and only relaxed as the global population declines enough and it is possible to stabilize the population at an acceptable level indefinitely. There would be procedural questions of justice about how a policy would be developed and enforced, whether it should be attentive to the special claims of population groups that had been the victims of genocide or natural disaster, and whether "credits" from women who did not want or could not have even one child could be "traded" to other women who wanted more. A global one-child policy—one child per woman—would be at least prima facie just when applied equally to the entire human population. It is, however, difficult to imagine how such a policy could realistically be imposed on a global scale anytime in the near future, so enormous would be the enforcement structures required and so great the limitations of reproductive freedom it would involve.

A Thought Experiment about a Solution to the Population Problem

I think there is at least a partial solution (Battin 1995, 1996, 1997). What if, instead of continuing reproductive patterns in which fertile individuals either accept pregnancy as the consequence of sexual intercourse, decide whether and how to practice contraception, or resort to abortion if unwanted pregnancy occurs, the default mode of human biology were such that conceiving or fathering a child required a *positive* decision, followed by deliberate action intended to allow pregnancy to occur? This shift already occurs with long-acting reversible contraception, or LARC—like the IUD and the subdermal implant—which maintains a condition in which a woman is not open to pregnancy unless she has the contraceptive neutralized or removed.

Let us thus entertain a conjecture: What if *everybody*, both male and female, used long-acting, reversible, "automatic" contraception, LARC, such that sustaining or contributing to pregnancy required a positive choice, rather than a negative choice to prevent it? This conjecture is morally tolerable only with two essential guarantees: No-targeting universality, and no-questions-asked reversibility. The two principal technologies now available for women are not perfect, and such technologies are not yet available for men, though research on long-term contraception for men progresses in many countries, especially India and China (Turok 2007; Male Contraception Information Project, ongoing). We can nevertheless imagine the further development of safe, reliable, and reversible contraceptive technologies, free of substantial side effects, nuisance, or risks, for all reproductively fertile human beings.

This thought experiment is not advanced as a practical proposal, and it sidesteps the question of how it might come to be that way. If it were framed as a proposal, half the discussion would focus on how to get from here to there, and on what sorts of (repressive) measures would be required to make it be the case that everyone used "automatic" contraception. That's not the interesting part. What's interesting is the question of what it would be like *if* we were already there—if long-acting reversible contraceptive were simply routinely and uncontroversially used by everybody—except when they wanted to have a child. That's the interesting question: What would the world be like?

This thought experiment poses a powerful challenge, eliciting a picture that seems far preferable to our current difficulties with unwanted and unintended fertility. If *everyone* routinely used automatic contraception, then all childbearing would require a simultaneous choice by both male and female to try to conceive a child. This would be to make family planning as fully voluntary as possible: Both parents must want the children they have, though they may have as many as they want. Nevertheless, since people will *accept having* more children than they would *choose to have*, reversing the default would give people of all backgrounds and educational and wealth levels everywhere in the world the freedom to make their own decisions about the size of their families—but it would still lower fertility. It would virtually eliminate all unintended or unwanted pregnancy—most teen pregnancy; most pregnancy following incest, rape, mass rape, and other sexual violence; most ill-timed pregnancy in serious maternal illness; and, of course, most call for abortion, even as it also reduced population growth rates. This change might not solve all population problems, and would not bring as dramatic a decline as Weisman's hypothetical global one-child policy, but it would reduce greatly growth without infringing reproductive rights. After all, an estimated 40 percent of pregnancies worldwide are unintended, as are almost 50 percent in the U.S.

The alternative, it might be feared, would be some variant of China's imposition of severe birth limits. Whether imposed birth ceilings in other countries would be as comparatively egalitarian as China's originally were and whether they would involve as great a degree of apparent popular assent is hard to predict; but the likelihood is that stark population control policies could be enforced in far more biased ways in other countries if the perception of population "emergency" resurfaces. China's policy has involved dramatic infringements of reproductive liberties in some cases; other nations, still more threatened by population pressures, might move to enforce population control—especially of disfavored minorities—in more ruthless ways.

The third alternative is no population control. It is potentially starker and more cruel since it risks widespread crash and die-back. The neo-Malthusian advocacy of population control is to some degree rejected by religious, feminist, and cornucopian thinkers, but the wholesale rejection of attention to population size at all may invite still worse consequences, though it often seems to be the direction in which we are headed.

At the same time, population "emergencies" in the other direction could also occur, whether sharply declining birthrates or major die-offs, including both slow processes like declining fertility due to environmental toxins and rapid catastrophes like high-mortality infectious-disease pandemics, or global nuclear or biological warfare. Population policy in many countries has emphasized permanent methods of fertility discontinuation—starting with India's emphasis on vasectomies for men and many other countries' reliance on tubal ligation or quinacrine cauterization for women. Voluntary sterilization has been the single most popular method in both the U.S. and the U.K. But these permanent methods are typically difficult and expensive to reverse, so they cannot be favored if it is uncertain whether population growth or population decline is the more serious risk.

Thus the universal use of long-acting *reversible* contraception, envisioned in this thought experiment, has a dramatic advantage in the contexts of both population growth and population decline: With it, childbearing rates can be expected to decline, but childbearing can also be resumed in the event not only of a personal tragedy like losing a child, but if some form of negative population emergency occurs. The thought-experiment presented here concerning long-acting, always-reversible, "automatic" contraception, in continuous use for both men and women except when they actively choose to have a child, can, I believe, go a long way toward showing us a route between two undesirable alternatives, uncontrolled population growth and catastrophic population decline, a route that can survive close ethical scrutiny in that it serves both essential objectives but at the same time protects individual reproductive rights.

Related Topics

Chapter 10, "Moral Responsibility for Addressing Climate Change," Madison Powers

Chapter 26, "Conscientious Refusal and Access to Abortion and Contraception," Carolyn McLeod and Chloë FitzGerald

Chapter 28, "Regulating Reproduction: A Bioethical Approach," Isabel Karpin

Bibliography

Avery, D.T. (1995) *Saving the Planet with Pesticides and Plastic: The Environmental Triumph of High-Yield Farming*, Indianapolis, IN: Hudson Institute.

Bandarage, A. (1997) *Women, Population and Global Crisis*, London: Zed Books.

Battin, M.P. (1995) Editorial: A Better Approach to Adolescent Pregnancy. *Social Science & Medicine* 41 (9): 1203–5.

Battin, M.P. (1996) Roundtable on Focus Article, "Adolescent Pregnancy: When it is a Problem, What is the Solution?" *Reproductive Health Matters* 8 (November): 110–12.

Battin, M.P. (1997) Sex and Consequences: World Population Growth versus Reproductive Rights," *Philosophic Exchange* 27: 17–31.

Blackorby, C., Bosssert, W. and Donaldson, D. (2005) *Population Issues in Social Choice Theory, Welfare Economics, and Ethics*, Cambridge and New York: Cambridge University Press.

Bongaarts, J. (2002) The End of the Fertility Transition in the Developed World, *Population and Development Review* 28 (3): 419–43.

Bongaarts, J. (2008) Fertility Transitions in Developing Countries: Progress or Stagnation? *Studies in Family Planning* 39 (2): 105–10.

Brown, L.R. (1997) *State of the World 1997: A Worldwatch Institute Report on Progress Toward a Sustainable Society*, New York and London: W.W. Norton.
Buss, D. and Herman, D. (2003) *Globalizing Family Values: The Christian Right in International Politics*, Minneapolis, MN and London: University of Minnesota Press.
Caldwell, J.C. (2004) Demographic Theory: A Long View. *Population and Development Review* 30 (2): 297–316.
Campbell, M.M. (1998) Schools of Thought: An Analysis of Interest Groups Influential in International Population Policy. *Population and Environment* 19 (6): 487–512.
Campbell, M., Nalan-Sahin-Hodoglugil, N. and Potts, M. (2006) Barriers to Fertility Regulation: A Review of the Literature, *Studies in Family Planning* 37 (2): 87–98.
Cleland, J. (2008) Fatal Misconception or Fatal Misinterpretation? Review of Matthew Connelly, *Fatal Misconception, Population and Development Review* 34 (3).
Cohen, J.E. (1995) *How Many People Can the Earth Support?* New York and London: W.W. Norton.
Connelly, M. (2008) *Fatal Misconception: The Struggle to Control World Population*, Cambridge, MA and London: The Belknap Press of Harvard University Press.
Demeny, P. (2004) Population Futures for the Next Three Hundred Years: Soft Landing or Surprises to Come? *Population and Development Review* 30 (3): 507–17.
Dixon-Mueller, R. (1993) *Population Policy & Women's Rights: Transforming Reproductive Choice*, Westport, CT and London: Praeger.
Ehrlich, P.R. (1968) *The Population Bomb*, New York: Ballantine Books.
Ehrlich, P.R. and Ehrlich, A.H. (1990) *The Population Explosion*, New York: Simon and Schuster.
Gee, E.M. and Gutman, G.M. (eds.) (2002) *The Overselling of Population Aging: Apocalyptic Demography, Intergenerational Challenges, and Social Policy*, Don Mills, Ontario: Oxford University Press.
Goldberg, M. (2009) *The Means of Reproduction: Sex, Power, and the Future of the World*, New York: Penguin,
Gore, A. (1992) *Earth in the Balance: Ecology and the Human Spirit*, New York: Houghton Mifflin.
Grant, L. (ed.) (2006) *The Case for Fewer People: The NPG Forum Papers*, Santa Ana, CA: Seven Locks Press.
Greenhalgh, S. and Winckler, E.A. (2005) *Governing China's Population: From Leninist to Neoliberal Biopolitics*, Stanford, CA: Stanford University Press.
Gu Baochang, Wang Feng, Guo Zhigang and Zhang Erli (2007) China's Local and National Fertility Policies at the End of the Twentieth Century, *Population and Development Review* 33 (1): 129–47.
Hartmann, B. (1995) [1987] *Reproductive Rights & Wrongs: The Global Politics of Population Control*. Boston, MA: South End Press.
Kennedy, P. (1993) *Preparing for the Twenty-First Century*, New York: HarperCollins Publishers.
Male Contraception Information Project (ongoing) E. Lissner (ed.). Available at: www.malecontraceptives.org (accessed July 28, 2014).
Malthus, T.R. (1960) [1798] *An Essay on the Principle of Population, as it Affects the Future Improvement of Society* (complete 1st ed. and partial 7th ed. (1872), reprinted in *On Population*, G. Himmelfarb (ed.)), New York: Modern Library.
Mosher, S.W. (2008) *Population Control: Real Costs, Illusory Benefits*, New Brunswick, NJ and London: Transaction Publishers.
Nie, J.-B.(2005) *Behind the Silence: Chinese Voices on Abortion*, Lanham, MD: Rowman & Littlefield.
Nie, Y. and Wyman, R.J. (2005) The One-Child Policy in Shanghai: Acceptance and Internalization, *Population and Development Review* 31 (2): 313–36.
Noonan, J.T., Jr (1986) *Contraception: A History of Its Treatment by the Catholic Theologians and Canonists* (enlarged edition). Cambridge and London: Belknap/Harvard University Press.
Nussbaum, M.C. (1999) *Sex and Social Justice*, New York: Oxford University Press.
Nussbaum, M. and Glover, J. (eds.) (1995) *Women, Culture, and Development: A Study of Capabilities*, Oxford: Clarendon Press.
Obono, O. (2003) Cultural Diversity and Population Policy in Nigeria, *Population and Development Review* 29 (1): 103–11.
Parfit, D. (1984) *Reasons and Persons*, Oxford: Clarendon Press.
Paul VI, Pope. 1968. *Humanae Vitae*. Encyclical Letter of His Holiness Paul VI on the regulation of birth, 25 July 1968. Available at: http://www.vatican.va/holy_father/paul_vi/encyclicals/documents/hf_p-vi_enc_25071968_humanae-vitae_en.html (accessed June 9, 2008).
Potts, M. (2008) Review of *Fatal Misconception, Population and Development Review* 34 (3).
Sen, A. (1992) *Inequality Reexamined*, Cambridge: Harvard University Press.

Sen, G., Germain, A. and Chen, L.C. (eds.) (1994) *Population Policies Reconsidered: Health, Empowerment, and Rights*. Harvard Series on Population and International Health. Cambridge, MA: Harvard School of Public Health and International Women's Health Coalition, distributed by Harvard University Press.

Simon, J.L. (1981) *The Ultimate Resource*, Princeton, NJ: Princeton University Press.

Takayama, N. and Werding, M. (2011) *Fertility and Public Policy: How to Reverse the Trend of Declining Birth Rates*, Cambridge, MA and London: The MIT Press.

Takeshita, C. (2012) *The Global Biopolitics of the IUD: How Science Constructs Contraceptive Users and Women's Bodies*, Cambridge, MA and London: The MIT Press.

Turok, D. (2007) The Quest for Better Contraception: Future Methods, *Obstetrics and Gynecology Clinics of North America* 34: 137–66.

U.N. Population Division (2007) *World Population Prospects: The 2006 Revision*. Available at: http://www.un.org/esa/population/publications/wpp2006/English.pdf (accessed June 9, 2008).

U.S. Census Bureau, World Population Information and Population Clocks. Available at: http://www.census.gov/ipc/www/idb/worldpopinfo.html (accessed June 9, 2008).

Vallin, J. (2002) The End of the Demographic Transition: Relief or Concern? *Population and Development Review* 28 (1): 105–20.

Weiner, M. and Teitelbaum, M.S. (2001) *Political Demography, Demographic Engineering*, New York and Oxford: Berghahn Books.

Weisman, A. (2013) *Countdown: Our Last, Best Hope for a Future on Earth?* New York, Boston and London: Little, Brown and Co.

Worldwatch Institute (2014) *State of the World 2014: Governing for Sustainability*. Washington, DC: Island Press.

Women's Global Network for Reproductive Rights (WGNRR), Amsterdam. Multiple newsletters. Available at: http://www.wgnrr.org/ (accessed July 28, 2014).

Zeng, Y. (2007) Options for Fertility Policy Transition in China, *Population and Development Review* 33 (2): 215–46.

32
REPRODUCTIVE TESTING FOR DISABILITY

Adrienne Asch and David Wasserman

Two developments in the 1970s and 1980s led to a striking contrast in public attitudes and policies toward having children with disabilities. On the one hand, the more routine character of prenatal genetic testing (and the availability of legal abortions) made it increasingly common, and perhaps expected, for parents to abort fetuses found to have "serious" disabilities. The termination rate for fetuses with one of the most common and easily detected conditions, Down syndrome, was estimated to be at or over 90 percent (e.g., Shaffer et al. 2006). On the other hand, those two decades saw the emergence of a strong disability rights movement and the reconceptualization of disability as a social phenomenon, the interaction of a physical or mental condition with an exclusionary environment. Informed by this social model, the disability rights movement played a major role in the passage of landmark disability discrimination laws in the United States in 1973 and 1990. As the abortion of fetuses with disabilities became routine, children and adults with disabilities became more visible and better integrated into educational and social activities. It was not long before proponents of the latter development observed a deep tension with the former.

As early as the mid-1980s, some scholars in bioethics and disability studies questioned the practice of prenatal selection against disability and the assumptions about disability informing it. In particular, they expressed concern about its ready acceptance by clinicians and the limited opportunity afforded prospective parents to reflect on its use. They argued that the speed at which testing became the standard of care for reproductive medicine, and the frequency with which positive results led to abortion, reflected and perpetuated harmful stereotypes about disability. This critique was independent of, and cut across, the abortion debate: It was not based on the moral status of the embryo or fetus, and many, though by no means all, of its proponents were pro-choice. Few sought special legal restrictions on disability-based termination.

These concerns have gained a greater hearing as it has become easier and less expensive to test early embryos and fetuses for an increasing number of health conditions. Selecting for sex and other "non-medical" traits has long been controversial, criticized by most bioethicists and reproductive professionals. In the past decade, some of these critics have recognized that selecting against disability also requires close examination. Routine disability testing is now coming under scrutiny from the media, healthcare professions, social sciences, philosophy, religion, and law. The issue of disability as a basis for selection became even more prominent with a recent controversy over selection *for* disability, a controversy provoked by a highly publicized case in which a deaf couple sought to have deaf children (Mundy 2007).

A variety of concerns have been raised about the practice of disability selection and the exercise of selectivity by prospective parents: That decisions to test and terminate for disability are typically made without adequate information or opportunity for reflection (Asch 1989, 1999; Press and Browner 1997; Fine and Asch 1982; Asch and Wasserman 2009); that professional sponsorship of such testing demeans people with disabilities by assuming the lesser value or greater burden of disabled lives (Saxton 1998); and that the use of such testing by prospective parents to select against disability conflicts with the most attractive ideal of the parent–child relationship (Asch 2000; Asch and Wasserman 2005). These critiques differ in emphasis and in their reliance on normative and empirical claims. But all hold that routine prenatal selection against disability is incompatible, in theory or practice, with the social equality of people with disabilities and with their full inclusion in society (Reinders 2000; Asch 2003).

Many bioethicists and philosophers deny or downplay this conflict, arguing that prenatal selection against disability is compatible with full social inclusion. Some argue that the conflict can be avoided by distinguishing negative attitudes toward disability from negative attitudes toward people with disabilities (Buchanan et al. 2000; Steinbock 2000; Baily 2000; Nelson 2000). If that distinction is recognized, then prenatal selection should not be offensive; if that distinction is rejected, then it will also be offensive to prevent or treat disability. Some defenders of selection contend as well that the decision of individual couples to select against disability need not reflect a general view that it is undesirable or burdensome to have a child with a disability (Nelson 2000; Kittay and Kittay 2000). Finally, some defenders claim that the harms and costs of creating children with severe disabilities outweigh any damage to the inclusion of, or offense to, existing people with disabilities (Buchanan et al. 2000; Murphy 2011).

In the remainder of this chapter, we will consider the variety of concerns that have been raised about disability—those that are widely shared, and those that are held by only some critics. We begin by discussing the different ways disability is defined and conceptualized, because they provide a context for understanding the different critiques of prenatal testing.

What Is a Disability? What Are Its Causes?

Many different characteristics are considered disabilities. Paraplegia, deafness, blindness, diabetes, autism, epilepsy, depression, and HIV have all been classified as "disabilities." The term covers such diverse conditions as the congenital absence or adventitious loss of a limb or a sensory function, progressive neurological conditions like multiple sclerosis, chronic diseases like diabetes or arteriosclerosis, the inability or limited ability to perform such cognitive functions as remembering faces or calculating sums, and psychiatric disorders like schizophrenia and bipolar disorder. There seems to be little about the functional or experiential states of people with these various conditions to justify a common concept; indeed, there is at least as much variation among "disabled" people with respect to their experiences and bodily states as there is among people who lack disabilities.

Two common features stand out in most official definitions of disability, such as those in the World Health Organization, the *U.K. Disability Discrimination Act*, and the *Americans with Disabilities Act*. There must be (1) an impairment (or a perceived impairment) and

(2) some personal or social limitation associated with that impairment. The notion of a limitation encompasses restrictions on such "basic" actions as moving one's arms or legs (Nordenfelt 1997); on daily activities such as dressing and toileting; and on social activities, such as working. The classification of a physical or mental variation as an impairment may be statistical, based on the average in some reference groups; it may be biological, based on explicit or implicit theories of human functioning; or it may be normative, based on some understanding of what is good for human beings (Tremain 2006). Most often, it probably involves some combination of these.

The most controversial aspect of the definition of disability is the relationship between the two elements—between the impairment and limitation. At one extreme are definitions that imply, or are read to imply, that impairments are the sole causes of limitation. At the other extreme are definitions that appear to treat the physical and social environment as the sole cause of disability. Between these extremes are definitions that regard the impairment and environment as interacting to cause limitation. Thus, for example, an individual with a mobility impairment is limited in getting around by the interaction of his inability to move his legs and the lack of ramps and wide doors in the buildings he frequents.

These different understandings of the relationship of impairment to limitation inform two contrasting approaches to disability, often described as opposing models: The medical and social. The *medical model* understands a disability as both a physical or mental impairment and as the personal and social consequences of that impairment. It regards the limitations faced by people with disabilities as resulting primarily or solely from their impairments. In contrast, the *social model* understands disability as a social process or condition: The exclusion of people with certain physical and mental characteristics from important domains of social life. The exclusion is manifested not only by shunning and confinement, but also by a built environment and organized social activity that do not accommodate people with disabilities.

Two versions of the social model are embraced by disability scholars and activists. The minority group model sees people with disabilities as a "discrete and insular" group facing stigmatization and exclusion. The disadvantages they face arise from the discrimination they suffer, like racial, ethnic, or sexual minorities. The human variation model sees many of the challenges faced by disabled people as arising less from their exclusion as a stigmatized group than from a mismatch between their characteristics and society's institutions. These two versions of the social model differ in emphasis, but their goals overlap, since discrimination has led to, and been expressed in the failure of society to accommodate the variations presented by people with disabilities. If one goal of social policy is to remove discrimination and its enduring disadvantages, another is to encompass the full range of human variation in the design of the physical environment and social practices.

In their extreme forms, the medical and social models serve to chart the space of possible relationships between impairment and limitation more than to reflect the actual views of individuals, groups, or institutions. The medical model is rarely defended, but often adopted unreflectively by health care professionals, bioethicists, and philosophers who fail to appreciate the disabling effects of environmental and social factors.

The medical and social models suggest (although they do not strictly imply) different views about the impact of disability on wellbeing, and different views about how disability is relevant to reproductive decisions, medical interventions, and social policy. Those who accept a social model of disability regard the association between disability and wellbeing as highly contingent, mediated by a variety of environmental and social factors. They also tend to favor conceptions of wellbeing that do not give central importance to the exercise of the standard array of physical and mental functions. These two views are formally independent—one could regard the adverse impact of disability on wellbeing as substantial, but largely due to social causes; conversely, one could regard the adverse impact of disability as comparatively minor, yet largely attributable to the impairment itself.

The attribution of disadvantage to social causes may matter less for assessing prenatal selection. Even if the disadvantages associated with diagnosable impairments are primarily or solely attributable to social factors, there may be little that prospective parents can do to mitigate those disadvantages. What may be more important to their decision to test or terminate is the impact those disadvantages have on the overall wellbeing of the future child and its family. Critics of prenatal selection maintain that the adverse impact is greatly exaggerated by health professionals and mainstream bioethicists. Their disagreement is reflected in conflicting assessments of life with disabilities found in the bioethics and public policy literature on the one hand, and disability scholarship on the other.

Routine Termination for Disability Is Based on Unfounded Assumptions and Misinformation about the Difficulties of Disabilities for Children, Parents, and Families

Clearly, many health professionals, bioethicists, and laypeople believe that being born with a disability is almost always damaging and often disastrous for the child, her parents, and her siblings. Parents must give up other important life goals; non-disabled children are neglected as parents focus on the needs of the child with the disability; mothers especially must forsake or curtail other interests to "cope with" their child; resources of time and money are often strained to or past the breaking point (Wertz and Fletcher 1993; Botkin 1995). Despite parental commitment and increased social acceptance, life with a disability is almost always of lesser quality than life without one (Purdy 1995; Buchanan et al. 2000; Brock 2005; Green 2008). Research suggests that some of these views are shared by prospective parents who accept prenatal testing (Gottfreðsdóttir et al. 2009b).

But are these assumptions warranted? Chronic illness and disability are not equivalent to acute illness or sudden injury, in which an active disease process or unexpected change in physical function disrupts life's routines. Most people with conditions such as spina bifida, achondroplasia, Down syndrome, and many other mobility and sensory impairments perceive themselves as healthy, not sick, and describe their conditions as givens of their lives—the equipment with which they meet the world. The same is true for people with chronic conditions such as cystic fibrosis, diabetes, hemophilia, and muscular dystrophy. These conditions include intermittent flare-ups requiring medical care and adjustments in daily living, but they do not render the person as unhealthy as most of the public—and members of the health profession—often imagine.

Like everyone else, people with disabilities are enmeshed in the details of everyday life. They are thinking about a traffic jam, a disagreement with a friend, which movie to attend, or which team will win the World Series—not just about their diagnosis. Having a disability can intrude into a person's consciousness if events bring it to the fore: For example, if two lift-equipped buses in a row fail to stop for a man using a wheelchair; if the theater ticket agent insults a patron with Down syndrome by refusing to take money for her ticket; or if a hearing-impaired person misses a train connection because he did not know that a track change had been announced.

Many proponents of prenatal testing and termination insist that critics ignore the fact that some conditions for which tests are available can be lethal in early childhood (Tay-Sachs), and can impair cognitive, physical, and sensory capacities to an extreme degree (Trisomy 13 or 18)—making it unclear how the child could have rewarding interactions in any environment. We acknowledge that given our knowledge of these conditions in 2013, medicine, education, and environmental design have not yet improved the potential for children with these conditions to have lives that most parents could conceive as satisfying. Nonetheless, the vast majority of diagnosable impairments are neither lethal in early childhood nor so capacity limiting. The availability of tests for such rare conditions hardly supports selection against all significant disabilities; it merely reinforces the case that prospective parents should make testing decisions based on a careful assessment of information about specific impairments and on how a child's particular condition will influence their family goals.

Most research on the wellbeing of people with disabilities relies on self-reports, and those reports do not confirm the grim views of third parties. Most people with disabilities report a quality of life similar to people without disabilities (Saigal et al. 1996; Albrecht and Devlieger 1999; Gill 2000; Goering 2008). However, the interpretation of self-reported wellbeing is complex and disputed (Menzel et al. 2002; Schwartz et al. 2007; Barnes 2009), and it raises the question about the extent to which appraisals of wellbeing should rely solely on subjective self-appraisal. This is not, or not entirely, an empirical question; it depends on the conception of wellbeing we regard as most appropriate in the context of procreation, where the individual in question is not (yet) capable of self-appraisal, desire formation, or the experiences of pleasure and pain.

There is a need for more empirical research, using a variety of methods, on the impact of children's disabilities on families. Existing studies of families paint a more complex picture than that found in most medical and bioethical literature. Many studies do find that parents of children with significant disabilities face considerable stress and hardship at various stages in their children's lives. Thus, Gerstein et al. (2009) note that "a wealth of research continues to suggest that families of children with ID [intellectual disabilities] face increased stressors . . .. Indeed, levels of stress have been found to be higher in parents of children with ID than in their typically developing counterparts." Eisenhower et al. (2009) find that mothers of children with developmental delays have poorer physical health outcomes, as well as the poorer mental health outcomes already shown in extensive research. The challenges may be especially great for parents of adult children with psychiatric disabilities, where "a body of research suggests that older parents of adults with serious mental illness experience on average, higher levels of burden and elevated health and mental health symptoms" (Aschbrenner et al. 2010).

Yet there is also considerable research, including some of the studies just cited, suggesting that these negative findings need to be qualified in several ways. First, the findings are not uniform. Some studies find that families of children with significant disabilities fare on average about as well as other families (Ferguson 2001; Walker et al. 1987). Some find that the additional challenges facing parents of children with disabilities are largely attributable to external factors like a lack of support services, or to pre-existing family, social, or economic circumstances (Hatton et al. 2010). And some find that although families with disabled children face additional challenges, they experience equal or distinct rewards. This is true even for parents of adult children with serious psychiatric disabilities, "while later stages of the life course may involve unprecedented difficulties, they may also present unique opportunities for positive parenting experiences, including personal growth and a greater awareness of family strengths" (Aschbrenner et al. 2010).

A 2002 review of the existing research on families of disabled children noted that evidence of positive outcomes may have been overlooked because of the prevailing emphasis on negative ones. "If we ask negatively phrased questions, we are not very likely to get positive answers . . ." (Hastings and Taunt 2002: 117). Taking up this challenge five years later, Blacher and Baker (2007: 343) found that "the expression of common benefits across families with and without disability, despite differences in negative impact . . . tempers the exclusively negative perspective that has characterized earlier literature on family and disability."

Prospective parents with disabilities have the personal experience enabling them to reject the exaggerated assumptions about disability held by many people without disabilities. They are often harshly confronted with those assumptions in deciding to have their own children. And yet, having experienced a variety of challenges related to their disabilities, from frequent hospitalization to pervasive stigma, they have a wide range of responses to testing and termination (Skotko 2005; Gottfreðsdóttir et al. 2009b). Some refuse testing, some use it only for preparation, some test and terminate, much like their non-disabled counterparts, and some choose not to reproduce (Kelly 2009; Boardman 2013; Walsh-Gallagher et al. 2012).

Yet even if we reject exaggerated assumptions about the hardships of disability, and attribute many or most to an exclusionary environment, the question remains of whether to regard disabilities, or the underlying impairments, as conditions it is better to live without. In their discussion of prenatal testing for disability in 2000, Parens and Asch noted that the most "contentious" issues in evaluating critiques of routine testing stem from the question of how much the disadvantage in having an "impairment" or being a person with a disability is socially constructed, and how much it is "intrinsic" to the condition itself, independent of any social environment (Parens and Asch 2000: 24). Should a disabling trait, an impairment, be differentiated from any other characteristic that a person will exhibit? Genetics professionals, bioethicists, and prospective parents all recognize that most normal variations will predispose an individual to some valuable experiences and make others harder to come by. Parents and others generally appreciate the pleasures of both the "mellow" and the "energetic" child, although they may later comment on how mellow children may stay close to home, may miss out on certain opportunities to discover new experiences and people; conversely, the energetic child may get into scrapes by barging into new territory and getting to know new people, without paying attention to cues that her more reserved brother might notice as reasons to stay away.

Most people who recognize the social contribution to disability and the flourishing of many disabled people, would still deny that impairments are merely "neutral" variations like mellowness. They hold that, on balance, in any imaginable world, an impairment is something it is better not to have. Why does this conclusion seem obvious, and should it? Even if further exploration reinforces the prevailing view, this question deserves to be taken seriously, and explored both conceptually and empirically.

Many (though not all) people with a wide range of disabilities articulate life's benefits from their non-species-typical modes of being in the world. Even if we reject or qualify these claims after fuller investigation, it would be important to find out what lies behind them, to endeavor to understand why these people with disabilities perceive their conditions as valuable. Hearing their voices would at least give pause to philosophers who "know" that disabilities preclude most reasonable life plans, make life harder overall, and must be treated as different from all other human variations that parents and society should expect to incorporate.

We ourselves find it plausible to regard disabilities, like many other characteristics and variations, as neither wholly positive nor wholly negative; rather, in some circumstances a disability, like a personality type, height, or the place one lives will promote some experiences and preclude others (Asch and Wasserman 2010). The question that needs further exploration is why disability, but not female sex, minority race, or rural residence, should be presumed to have a detrimental effect on wellbeing rather than being treated as one of many factors that contribute in complex ways to how well a life goes overall.

The Process and Content of Prenatal Health Care Should be Modified to Provide More Opportunity for Reflection and More Accurate Information about Living with a Disability

In one sense, prenatal testing and selective termination increase reproductive options. Before ultrasound, and chromosomal and genetic testing, women and couples faced an unconditional decision about whether or not to continue a pregnancy. Since the introduction of those technologies, that decision can be based on an increasing amount of medical detail about the fetus or embryo—even before implantation.

This increase in options may not, however, lead to an increase in reproductive autonomy if women are misinformed about the nature of the tests, and subjected to pressure to test and terminate in the face of "positive" results. Research over the past 15 years raises serious questions about whether consent to prenatal testing and selective abortion can be regarded as truly informed and voluntary.

It should not be surprising that many reproductive health professionals share the general views of non-disabled people about the overwhelming burdens of raising children with disabilities. Whether or not the mere offer of a prenatal test is itself directive (Clarke 1992; Wachbroit and Wasserman 1995), conveying the expectation that a prospective parent will terminate if the result is positive may make it more difficult for prospective parents to continue a pregnancy, especially if the result is accompanied by one-sided information about disability. Several studies suggest that when reproductive health professionals do talk to their patients about the reasons for prenatal testing and termination, they tend to focus narrowly on the medical issues associated with disability (Lippman and Wilfond 1992; Wertz 2000; Skotko 2005; Klein 2011). They emphasize "the array of potential medical complications and physical limitations that may occur in children with the condition" (Lippman and Wilfond 1992: 936). A 2011 literature review concluded that a high proportion of reproductive clinicians held extremely negative attitudes towards life with a disability, which they conveyed to their patients (Klein 2011). Other research suggests that such negative information has a significant impact on decisions about whether to terminate in the face of positive test results.

As reproductive testing becomes routine and comprehensive, issues of informed consent become more acute. In 1997, Press and Browner reported that women were being presented with prenatal testing as part of routine prenatal care, as "just another blood test." Many were not told that the test concerned fetal health, not their own health; nor were they told that the results would not help them or their doctor to manage their pregnancy or to improve the health of their fetus. The option of abortion after positive results was rarely mentioned. A 2009 study suggests a continuing failure to explain the implications of prenatal testing to pregnant women: "Approximately one half of the women surveyed who underwent both ultrasound and biochemical screening did not foresee that they might ultimately be confronted with the need to make the decision about whether or not to terminate the pregnancy" (Seror and Ville 2009). The introduction of non-invasive tests may further discourage reflection and discussion on the implications of testing. In a 2009 study, a woman explained her decision in these terms: "I just thought, well this is something you do when you are pregnant" (Gottfreðsdóttir et al. 2009a: 716). The frequent absence of clear communication and discussion should trouble conscientious health professionals, because it means that pregnant women are being led to obtain information they may not want to have, and to make decisions they may not want to make.

The solution does not lie in providing clinical detail about each of the conditions tested for. The sheer number of conditions that can now or soon be tested for, and the diagnostic and predictive limitations of many of those tests, make a comprehensive consent process virtually impossible. What is needed is not more detail, but a broader focus. It is important for clinicians to learn about the knowledge, attitudes, and values of pregnant women concerning reproductive testing, termination, and raising a child with a disability. And prospective parents must be able to obtain information about a subject they may know very little about, that is, what it is like to raise children with disabilities. This may also be a subject on which they are not expecting to reflect in a clinical setting. It would be helpful for reproductive health professionals to shift the focus from the clinical severity of the diagnosed condition to the expectations of the prospective parents in having a child: "What are you looking for in your experience of child-rearing and how do you think a child's motor, cognitive, emotional, or sensory impairment might affect that experience?" If prospective parents have a chance to reflect on and respond to such questions, professionals may be in a much better position to discuss their concerns about the effect of impairments on parental goals and experiences (The Boston Women's Health Book Collective 2008).

In 2008, the U.S. Congress took a major step in making that information available to pregnant women by enacting, with wide bipartisan support, the *Prenatally and Postnatally Diagnosed Conditions Awareness Act* (known as the *Kennedy–Brownback Act*). The Act requires the federal government to arrange for the collection and dissemination of evidence-based, up-to-date information about the conditions subject to diagnosis. This information encompasses "the range of outcomes for individuals living with the diagnosed condition, including physical, developmental, educational, and psychosocial outcomes." Such information should provide a powerful corrective to the "bad news" typically delivered to pregnant women whose fetuses are diagnosed with the tested conditions. The Act may have an even greater impact on prenatal decision-making if it helps reframe how those women and their partners view their choices after positive test results (Asch and Wasserman 2009). Information on the range of outcomes for individuals living with the diagnosed condition may help pregnant women and their partners see their decision as one about parenting a child who will have a disabling trait, not about preventing disability.

The Act, however, has a built-in limitation: It mandates better information only for women who have already been tested and received positive results, not for women deciding whether to obtain testing. The information the Act collects may come too late in the process to be fully effective in reframing prenatal decision making. A woman who has already been led to regard such testing as a routine part of reproductive health care may have difficulty in seeing the testing as a prelude to a decision about what kind of child she is willing to parent. She might not want to make that decision, and, if she had understood the test's purpose before consenting to it, she might have refused to put herself in a position where she had to make such a choice.

Education about disability must begin much earlier, and for a much broader population of individuals contemplating having children, reproductive health professionals, and the general public. In order for this information to be meaningfully integrated into the decision-making of prospective parents, the processes by which prenatal testing is now offered them may have to be restructured. It will be a formidable challenge to incorporate the offer and provision of this information into an increasingly complex and congested informed-consent process.

The Practice of Prenatal Testing Is in Tension with the Social Equality of People with Disabilities, But Can Be Reformed in Ways that May Reduce this Tension

Unlike the difficult, complex, often confused decisions of individuals and couples, which need not "send a message" to others regarding the lives of disabled persons, official policies and practices can indeed send a message of inferiority. This would be obvious for race or sex. Imagine a state-funded research program to identify genetic variants associated with dark complexion or African ancestry, designed to enable prospective parents to terminate fetuses with those variants. Such research would rightly be denounced as eugenic and racist. The fact that there is no popular concern over similar research programs to promote selection against disability suggests that—even if there are important differences between disability and race as minority characteristics—the expressive significance of such practices and policies has been overlooked. Whether or not they identified with or celebrated their disabilities, people with disabilities might reasonably be troubled by state or professional sponsorship of programs that treated the birth of people with conditions like theirs as a highly undesirable outcome.

Two approaches have been proposed for weakening the expressive force of the connection between prenatal testing and selection against disability. First, prenatal testing can be used more frequently to arrange appropriate medical and social services for children expected to have disabilities. Although the dominant use of prenatal genomic testing is, and will remain, to decide about pregnancy termination or embryo selection, its clinical utility is not limited to those decisions. An early diagnosis of intellectual or developmental disabilities can significantly benefit prospective parents who intend to have the child regardless of the diagnosis. There is a growing recognition that prenatal diagnosis of these conditions can spare parents a painful and expensive diagnostic odyssey after birth. It can also facilitate early intervention, which can be helpful, even critical, in achieving better outcomes for some of the diagnosable conditions (Makela et al. 2009; Lopez-Rangel et al. 2008). Moreover, even when testing only yields probabilities, it may help identify environmental factors that increase risk or exacerbate symptoms. Thus, prenatal testing can be used to promote early intervention, heightened vigilance, improved treatment, and greater continuity of care. The professional and societal expectation that some parents will choose to bear children with diagnosed impairments, as well as the specific arrangements reflecting that expectation, may well reduce the proportion of women and couples choosing to terminate after such a diagnosis (Le Dref et al. 2013).

A second, more controversial measure would be to allow prenatal testing for any genetically detectable condition or trait, whether or not it was associated with disease or disability. By permitting reproductive testing for any condition or trait, policy makers and professionals could support reproductive choice without singling out disability as a basis for selective embryo implantation or pregnancy termination (Asch 2003; Wasserman 2003; Gavaghan 2007). Such a policy would avoid the heightened stigmatization likely to result from the line-drawing, now widely advocated (Botkin 1995; Wertz 2000), to limit testing to more "serious" or "severe" disabilities. The more restricted the list of conditions subject to testing, the more stigmatizing testing will be for people living with those conditions.

The comparative virtue of this approach—of permitting any and all available testing—is that it would give no official or privileged role to disabilities in the determination of whether to offer testing or termination. Perhaps it would make little practical difference. Most prospective parents might well test only for disabilities (which would limit the costs of unrestricted testing), because they shared prevailing attitudes toward disability, and because there may be fewer reliable tests for characteristics besides sex and disability. But this is not all that matters in gauging the expressive significance of a prenatal testing regime. A policy that gave no special status to disabilities, that did not treat them as providing a presumptively stronger basis for selection than any other trait or variation, would emphatically disavow the exceptionalism about disability that has dominated prenatal testing since its inception. It would "send the message" that disability did not give prospective parents a privileged reason to screen out embryos or terminate a pregnancy, that disabilities were just some among the myriad variations that might be relevant to some prospective parents in deciding whether to bring a child into the world. At the same time, an unrestricted testing policy might well encourage a consumerist approach toward parenting; it might appear to endorse the treatment of embryos and fetuses, if not children, as commodities. To choose a policy of unrestricted testing is to treat this as a lesser evil than the heightened stigmatization of those disabilities subject to testing under a more restrictive policy.

An unrestricted policy would also permit selection *for* disability, a controversial issue in the recent bioethics literature. Most criticism of such selection concerns the welfare of the children chosen or its impact on aggregate wellbeing. Despite their skepticism about standard objections to creating children with disabilities, many disability advocates are reluctant to endorse their deliberate creation. Sometimes, the skepticism reflects doubts about "disability neutrality"—the view that there is nothing worse in having a disability than in lacking it (Asch and Wasserman 2010). But it may also reflect misgivings about the selection of a child based on any detectable trait—disability, sex, skin or eye color (Asch and Wasserman 2005; see next section).

Even if we adopt policies responsive to expressivist concerns about routine selection against disability, difficult questions remain. Can our society maintain a commitment to moral and political equality for people who are born with undiagnosable disabilities, or who acquire them later in life, while geneticists, reproductive health professionals, and bioethicists urge that families not knowingly bring to term fetuses who will have similar disabling traits? What grounds does a society have to demand that a teacher, employer, or business owner make provisions for someone with characteristics that the same teacher, employer, or businessperson was urged to treat as inimical to membership in her family? On the other hand, how do we respond to arguments that prospective parents should avoid creating children they expect to be significantly worse off, for medical or social reasons, than some minimum level, thereby increasing inequality (Wilkinson 2010) or imposing further costs (for cost estimates, see Stabile and Allin 2012)? Or does a society lack the moral authority to criticize any procreative choice until it achieves a level of justice most societies fall far below?

Prenatal Selectivity Is Incompatible with the Most Attractive Ideal of the Parent–Child Relationship

One version of the disability critique—put forward by Asch (1989, 2000) and most fully developed by Asch and Wasserman (2005)—emphasizes an ideal of the parent–child relationship that is relevant to prospective parents. It distinguishes between the decision to not become a parent at this time (whether for the first time or not) and the decision to not become the parent of a particular child or kind of child—one with a diagnosable impairment. Although put forward earlier than many critiques of sex and other "non-medically" based selection, this objection is similar to some of these in drawing on a notion of parental acceptance (Wertz and Fletcher 1993; Sandel 2007; Herissone-Kelly 2007).[1]

This critique has two parts. First, it maintains that prenatal selectivity is problematic in basing the decision to form a parent–child relationship on a single attribute of the future child—the diagnosable impairment. Selecting against disability involves a paradigmatic form of stigmatization—reducing the complex whole the future child would become to that single, disvalued part. Prenatal testing invites stigmatization because it makes that single part so salient. This does not imply that all parental decisions to terminate must be misinformed and stigma-driven; merely that stigmatization is a significant danger for prospective parents in the context of prenatal testing, a danger that reproductive health professionals and practices often exacerbate.

But even if the decision to terminate on the basis of a diagnosed impairment is not misinformed or driven by stigma, it involves a problematic exercise of selectivity. Choosing a future child of the basis of any trait—whether positive or negative—arguably falls short of what Asch and Wasserman call an ideal of "unconditional welcome." This ideal is the counterpart for prospective parents of the ideal of unconditional love or commitment for actual parents. Prospective parents can hardly be expected to make an unconditional commitment toward an early-term fetus, let alone towards any or all of the embryos in an *in vitro* fertilization array. The ideal of unconditional welcome urges them to *anticipate* the commitment they would make on becoming parents by not conditioning their willingness to bear and raise a child on the expected presence or absence of virtually any trait (see also Herissone-Kelly 2007, 2009). Asch and Wasserman argue that this posture distinguishes prospective parents from prospective friends and lovers, who may and should exercise selectivity in choosing to form their intimate relationships. It also suggests a role for prospective parents continuous with that of actual parents, whose attachment to their children is expected to be even less dependent on the loss or acquisition of important traits than the attachment to a friend or lover.

Unlike Sandel (2007), Asch and Wasserman do not rely on the notion that children are "gifts." They simply argue that prospective parents should recognize that their children, disabled or not, may differ greatly from their expectations in a host of ways. They should recognize that they exercise only limited control over who their children become, and should validate and foster their children's unique characteristics. If disability is understood as more similar to than different from other attributes in its impact on a child's and family's life, then a child's disability can be incorporated into the parent's appreciation of the child. Just as parents must accommodate a non-disabled child's interest in some favored family pursuits and aversions to others, so should prospective parents be willing to accommodate the different tastes and capacities of children with disabilities. This critique rejects the claim, made most cogently by Mary Ann Baily (2000), that the very fact that any child can pose unexpected challenges gives prospective parents a reason to "improve their odds." Asch and Wasserman counter that the attempt to do so by prenatal testing exaggerates the singular challenges of disability, mistakenly assuming that it is additive, and creates a false sense of security.

This version of the disability critique eschews parental selection *for* disability for the same reasons that it rejects selection *against* disability. Parents should recognize that disability is only one of a child's attributes, and that possessing or not possessing a disability does not in itself guarantee a child's potential for having a satisfying relationship with her parents or a rewarding and productive life outside the family. An impairment is just one source of possible affinity with parents who share it, just as it is only one source of possible lack of affinity with parents who lack it. In neither case should it be a basis for prenatal selection.

Thus, the ideal of unconditional welcome draws support from two insights. The first concerns parental attitudes that promote a child's sense of being loved and valued as a unique individual; the second concerns the limited role that any single trait, where an impairment like blindness or Down syndrome, or personality traits like extroversion or impatience, play a part in defining that individual. This hardly means that parents should accept any expression or manifestation of a trait in their child rather than attempt to control or modulate its expression. They should thoughtfully guide the development of any child, disabled or not.

This critique is not threatened by the claim (Nelson 2000) that the decision to terminate any pregnancy, for any reason, can be formally expressed as a refusal to bear a child with a particular trait—e.g., "our first/second/nth child." Why, Nelson, asks, is it objectionable to abort on the basis of an impairment, but not a "trait" such as being the fourth conceived? First, "traits" like the latter are not stigmatized—parents rarely decline to add an nth additional child based on birth-order stigma. Second, whether or not such relational characteristics qualify as traits—a question we leave to others—the decision not to have one's nth child is a decision not to enter a parent–child relationship with an additional human being. In declining to assume the role, one can hardly be held to an ideal specific to it.

Nor is this critique in tension with the social model, which understands disability as a relational characteristic (Kukla and Wayne 2011). It is doubtful that most health professionals and prospective parents involved in routine prenatal testing *see* diagnosed disabilities in relational terms, as conditions that are disadvantageous because of an unaccommodating environment. For those who do—for example, those who are successfully raising a disabled child but decline to have another child with the same disability because of realistically estimated costs—the critique would apply with lesser force, and the departure from the ideal of unconditional welcome would be less significant. In the extreme case of prospective parents living under a regime that killed those with significant disabilities, the critique would not apply at all.

A final concern is that the ideal of unconditional welcome is too narrow (Ruddick 2000) or too demanding—particularly on women (Gedge 2011). Ruddick argues that it is only one, i.e., the "maternal" model, of three reasonable models of parenthood. It is not clearly superior to two others: The "familial"—where decisions about a child are based on its role in, and likely impact on the family as a whole; and the "projectivist" model, where decisions are based on whether the traits of a child are compatible with the goals or projects of its prospective parents. Asch and Wasserman (2005) argue that the familial model is rarely incompatible with unconditional welcome, which is an ideal both for parents and families. The perceived incompatibility, they argue, arises largely from exaggerated or unsupported beliefs about the adverse impact of children with significant disabilities on other family members. The projectivist model is indeed incompatible with our ideal, but it is arguably too inflexible and self-oriented, failing to recognize the limitations in treating the creation and rearing of a child as an individual "project." It is important to recognize that a projectivist parent may be thwarted by a non-disabled child who turns out to be able but not willing to participate in valued family activities; who simply eschews the parents' values and projects. Parents must be willing to support their children in their own pursuits, however little they resemble those of the parents, as long as those pursuits are respectful to others and not self-destructive. A child is not a "creation" like an artwork, but a separate person who may or may not express the values or vision of its creators.

There are at least two responses to the demandingness objection. The first, more general one, is that unconditional welcome is offered as an ideal, one to which prospective parents should aspire even if they will inevitably fall short (Wasserman and Asch 2007a, 2007b). For example, a couple may decide with deep misgivings not to have a child very likely to predecease them, or at risk of unemployment and institutionalization in surviving them. Such a decision may be unduly pessimistic, but if made with serious reflection and careful research, it is hardly one for which the couple should be criticized. The more specific worry, that the burden of welcoming will fall disproportionately on the mother, seems realistic as a practical concern but not as an objection. A moral ideal should not be rejected because of the likelihood that it would be abused or distorted by a sexist society.

In earlier writing, we extended Sara Ruddick's (1995) conception of the work of mothers (or parents) to include not only protection, nurturance, education, and socialization, but also fostering an appreciation of the child as a unique individual, however much her characteristics diverge from those of her parents. Although we believe that such appreciation is a critical part of good parenting, it has not been seriously discussed in the literature—with the notable exception of Rosalind McDougall's (2007, 2009) account of "acceptingness" as a core virtue for parents and prospective parents. We believe the parental role of appreciation, and the virtue of acceptingness, deserve further discussion, in the context of a broader examination of the goals of parenthood.

Related Topics

Chapter 17, "Ethical Issues in Genetic Research," Dena S. Davis
Chapter 29, "Children, Parents, and Responsibility for Children's Health," Amy Mullin
Chapter 39, "Medicalization, 'Normal Function,' and the Definition of Health," Rebecca Kukla

Note

1 It is striking that few opponents of sex selection extend their critique to selection against disability. Indeed, most would permit selection in the case of sex-linked disorders. Herissone-Kelly (2009) is one of the few to offer a critique general enough to encompass selection against disability.

References

Albrecht, G.L. and Devlieger, G. (1999) "The Disability Paradox: High Quality of Life Against the Odds," *Social Science & Medicine* 48: 977–88.

Asch, A. (1989) "Reproductive Technology and Disability," in S. Cohen and N. Taub (eds.) *Reproductive Laws for the 1990s*, Clifton, NJ: Humana Press, pp. 69–124.

Asch, A. (1999) "Prenatal Diagnosis and Selective Abortion: A Challenge to Practice and Policy," *American Journal of Public Health* 89 (11): 1649–57.

Asch, A. (2000) "Why I Haven't Changed My Mind about Prenatal Diagnosis: Reflections and Refinements," in E. Parens and A. Asch (eds.) *Prenatal Testing and Disability Rights*, Washington, DC: Georgetown University Press, pp. 234–58.

Asch, A. (2003) "Disability, Equality and Prenatal Testing: Contradictory or Compatible?" *Florida State University Law Review* 30 (2): 315–42.

Asch, A. and Wasserman, D. (2005) "Where Is the Sin in Synecdoche: Prenatal Testing and the Parent–Child Relationship," in D. Wasserman, R. Wachbroit and J. Bickenbach (eds.) *Quality of Life and Human Difference: Genetic Testing, Health Care, and Disability*, New York: Cambridge University Press, pp. 172–216.

Asch, A. and Wasserman, D. (2009) "Informed Consent and Prenatal Testing: The Kennedy-Brownback Act," *Virtual Mentor* 11 (9): 721–4.

Asch, A. and Wasserman, D. (2010) "Making Embryos Healthy or Making Healthy Embryos: How Much of a Difference Between Prenatal Treatment and Selection?" in J. Nisker, K.A. Aschbrenner, J.S. Greenberg, S.A. Allen and M.M. Seltzer (2010) "Subjective Burden and Personal Gains Among Older Parents of Adults with Serious Mental Illness," *Psychiatric Services* (Washington, DC) 61 (6): 605–11.

Baily, M.A. (2000) "Why I had Amniocentesis," in E. Parens and A. Asch (eds.) *Prenatal Testing and Disability Rights*, Washington, DC: Georgetown University Press, pp. 64–71.

Barnes, E. (2009) "Disability, Minority, and Difference," *Journal of Applied Philosophy* 26 (4): 337–55.

Blacher, J. and Baker, B.J. (2007) "Positive Impact of Intellectual Disabilities on Families," *American Journal on Mental Retardation*, 112: 330–480.

Boardman, F.K. (2013) "Knowledge Is Power? The Role of Experiential Knowledge in Genetically 'Risky' Reproductive Decisions," *Sociology of Health & Illness* 36: 137–50.

Botkin, J.R. (1995) "Fetal Privacy and Confidentiality," *Hastings Center Report* 25 (5): 32–9.

Brock, D.W. (2005) "Preventing Genetically Transmitted Disabilities while Respecting Persons with Disabilities," in D. Wasserman, R. Wachbroit and J. Bickenbach (eds.) *Quality of Life and Human Difference: Genetic Testing, Health Care, and Disability*, New York: Cambridge University Press, pp. 67–100.

Buchanan, A., Brock, D.W., Daniels, N. and Wikler, D. (2000) *From Chance to Choice: Genetics & Justice*, New York: Cambridge University Press.

Clarke, A. (1992) "Is Non-directive Genetic Counseling Possible?" *Obstetrical & Gynecological Survey* 47 (5): 304–5.

Eisenhower, A.S., Baker, B.L. and Blacher, J. (2009) "Children's Delayed Development and Behavior Problems: Impact on Mothers' Perceived Physical Health Across Early Childhood," *Social Science & Medicine* 68 (1): 89–99.

Ferguson, P. (2001) "Mapping the Family: Disability Studies and the Exploration of Parental Response to Disability," in G. Albrecht, K. Seelman and M. Bury (eds.) *Handbook of Disability Studies*, Thousand Oaks, CA: Sage Publications, pp. 373–96.

Fine, M. and Asch, A. (1982) "The Question of Disability: No Easy Answers for the Women's Movement, *Reproductive Rights Newsletter* 4 (3): 19–20.

Gavaghan, C. (2007) "Right Problem, Wrong Solution: A Pro-choice Response to 'Expressivist' Concerns about Preimplantation Genetic Diagnosis," *Cambridge Quarterly of Healthcare Ethics* 16 (1): 20–34.

Gedge, E. (2011) "Reproductive Choice and the Ideals of Parenting," *International Journal of Feminist Approaches to Bioethics* 4 (2): 32–47.

Gerstein, E.D., Crnic, K.A., Blacher, J. and Baker, B.L. (2009) "Resilience and the Course of Daily Parenting Stress in Families of Young Children with Intellectual Disabilities," *Journal of Intellectual Disability Research*, 53 (12): 981–97.

Gill, C.J. (2000) "Health Professionals, Disability, and Assisted Suicide: An Examination of Empirical Evidence," *Psychology, Public Policy, and Law* 6 (2): 526–45.

Goering, S. (2008) "'You Say You're Happy, but . . .': Contested Quality of Life Judgments in Bioethics and Disability Studies," *Journal of Bioethical Inquiry* 5 (2/3): 125–35.

Gottfreðsdóttir, H., Björnsdóttir, K. and Sandall, J. (2009a) "This Is Just What You Do When You Are Pregnant: A Qualitative Study of Prospective Parents in Iceland Who Accept Nuchal Translucency Screening," *Midwifery* 25 (6): 711–20.

Gottfreðsdóttir, H., Björnsdóttir, K. and Sandall, J. (2009b) "How Do Prospective Parents Who Decline Prenatal Screening Account for Their Decision? A Qualitative Study," *Social Science & Medicine* 69 (2): 274–7.

Green, R. (2008) *Babies by Design: The Ethics of Genetic Choice*, New Haven, CT: Yale University Press.

Hastings, R.P. and Taunt, H.M. (2002) "Positive Perceptions in Families of Children with Disabilities," *American Journal on Mental Retardation* 107: 116–27.

Hatton, C., Emerson, E., Graham, H., Blacher, J. and Llewellyn, G. (2010) "Changes in Family Composition and Marital Status in Families with a Young Child with Cognitive Delay," *Journal of Applied Research in Intellectual Disabilities* 23: 14–26.

Herissone-Kelly, P. (2007) "The 'Parental Love' Objection to Nonmedical Sex Selection: Deepening the Argument," *Cambridge Quarterly of Healthcare Ethics* 16 (4): 446.

Herissone-Kelly, P. (2009) "Two Varieties of 'Better-For' Judgements," in M.A. Roberts and D.T. Wasserman (2009) *Harming Future Persons: Ethics, Genetics and the Nonidentity Problem*, Dordrecht: Springer, 249–63.

Kelly, S.E. (2009) "Choosing Not to Choose: Reproductive Responses of Parents of Children with Genetic Conditions or Impairments," *Sociology of Health & Illness* 31: 81–97.

Kittay, E.F. and Kittay, L. (2000) "On the Expressivity and Ethics of Selective Abortion for Disability: Conversations with My Son," in E. Parens and A. Asch (eds.) *Prenatal Testing and Disability Rights*, Washington, DC: Georgetown University Press, pp. 165–95.

Klein, D.A. (2011) "Medical Disparagement of the Disability Experience: Empirical Evidence for the 'Expressivist Objection,'" *AJOB Primary Research* 2: 8–20.

Kukla, R. and Wayne, K. (2011) "Pregnancy, Birth, and Medicine", in E.N. Zalta (ed.) *The Stanford Encyclopedia of Philosophy* (Spring 2011 edition). Available at: http://plato.stanford.edu/archives/spr2011/entries/ethics-pregnancy/ (accessed July 29, 2014).

Le Dref, G., Grollemund, B., Danion-Grilliat, A. and Weber, J.C. (2013) "Towards a New Procreation Ethic: The Exemplary Instance of Cleft Lip and Palate," *Medicine, Health Care and Philosophy* 16: 365–75.

Lippman, A. and Wilfond, B.S. (1992) "Twice-Told Tales: Stories about Genetic Disorders," *American Journal of Human Genetics* 51: 936–7.

Lopez-Rangel, E., Mickelson, E.C.R. and Lewis, M.E.S. (2008) "The Value of a Genetic Diagnosis for Individuals with Intellectual Disabilities: Optimising Healthcare and Function Across the Lifespan," *British Journal of Developmental Disabilities* 54: 69–82.

Makela, N.L., Birch, P.H., Friedman, J.M. and Marra, C.A. (2009) "Parental Perceived Value of a Diagnosis for Intellectual Disability (ID): A Qualitative Comparison of Families with and without a Diagnosis for Their Child's ID," *American Journal of Medical Genetics* A 149A: 2393–402.

McDougall, R. (2007) "Parental Virtue: A New Way of Thinking about the Morality of Reproductive Actions," *Bioethics* 21: 181–90.

McDougall, R. (2009) "Impairment, Flourishing and the Moral Nature of Parenthood," in K. Brownlee and A. Cureton (eds.) *Disability and Disadvantage*, Oxford: Oxford University Press, pp. 352–68.

Menzel, P., Dolan, P., Richardson, J. and Olsen, J.A. (2002) "The Role of Adaptation to Disability and Disease in Health State Valuation: A Preliminary Normative Analysis," *Social Science & Medicine* 55 (12): 2149–58.

Mundy, L. (2007) *Everything Conceivable: How Assisted Reproduction Is Changing Men, Women, and the World*, New York: Alfred A. Knopf, 319–20.

Murphy, T.F. (2011) "When Choosing the Traits of Children Is Hurtful to Others," *Journal of Medical Ethics* 37 (2): 105–8.

Nelson, J. (2000) "The Meaning of the Act: Reflections on the Expressive Force of Reproductive Decision Making and Politics," in E. Parens and A. Asch (eds.) *Prenatal Testing and Disability Rights*, Washington, DC: Georgetown University Press, pp. 196–213.

Nordenfelt, L. (1997) "The Importance of a Disability/Handicap Distinction," *Journal of Medicine and Philosophy* 22: 607–22.

Parens, E. and Asch, A. (2000) "Introduction," in *Prenatal Testing and Disability Rights*, Washington, DC: Georgetown University Press.

Prenatally and Postnatally Diagnosed Conditions Awareness Act (2008) S.1810: 110–374.

Press, N. and Browner, C.H. (1997) "Why Women Say Yes to Prenatal Diagnosis," *Social Science & Medicine* 45: 979–89.

Purdy, L. (1995) "Loving Future People," in J. Callahan (ed.) *Reproduction, Ethics and the Law*, Bloomington, IN: Indiana University Press, pp. 300–27.

Reinders, H.S. (2000) *The Future of the Disabled in Liberal Society: An Ethical Analysis*, Notre Dame, IN: University of Notre Dame Press.

Ruddick, S. (1995) *Maternal Thinking: Toward a Politics of Peace*, Boston, MA: Beacon Press.

Ruddick, W. (2000) "Ways to Limit Prenatal Testing," in E. Parens and A. Asch, (eds.) *Prenatal Testing and Disability Rights*, Washington DC: Georgetown University Press, pp. 95–107.

Saigal, S., Feeny, D., Rosenbaum, P., Furlong, W., Burrows, E. and Stoskopf, B. (1996) "Self-perceived Health Status and Health-Related Quality of Life of Extremely Low-Birth-Weight Infants at Adolescence," *Journal of the American Medical Association* 276: 453–9.

Sandel, M.J. (2007) *The Case Against Perfection*, Cambridge, MA: The Belknap Press of Harvard University Press.

Saxton, M. (1998) "Disability Rights and Selective Abortion," in R. Solinger (ed.) *Abortion Wars: A Half Century of Struggle, 1950–2000*, Berkeley, CA: University of California Press, pp. 374–94.

Schwartz, C.E., Andresen, E.M., Nosek, M.A. and Krahn, G.L. (2007) "Response Shift Theory: Important Implications for Measuring Quality of Life in People With Disability," *Archives of Physical Medicine and Rehabilitation* 88 (4), 529–36.

Seror, V. and Ville, Y. (2009) "Prenatal Screening for Down Syndrome: Women's Involvement in Decision-Making and Their Attitudes to Screening," *Prenatal Diagnosis* 29 (2): 120–8.

Shaffer, B.L., Caughey, A.B. and Norton, M.E. (2006) "Variation in the Decision to Terminate Pregnancy in the Setting of Fetal Aneuploidy, *Prenatal Diagnosis* 26 (8): 667–71.

Skotko, B.G. (2005) "Prenatally Diagnosed Down Syndrome: Mothers Who Continued Their Pregnancies Evaluate Their Health Care Providers," *American Journal of Obstetrics & Gynecology* 192: 670–7.

Stabile, M. and Allin, S. (2012) "The Economic Costs of Childhood Disability," *The Future of Children* 22 (1): 65–96.

Steinbock, B. (2000) "Disability, Prenatal Testing, and Selective Abortion," in E. Parens and A. Asch (eds.) *Prenatal Testing and Disability Rights*, Washington, DC: Georgetown University Press, pp. 108–23.

The Boston Women's Health Book Collective (2008) "Prenatal Testing," in *Our Bodies, Ourselves: Pregnancy and Birth*, New York: Touchstone Book/Simon & Schuster, pp. 109–27.

Tremain, S. (2006) "Reproductive Freedom, Self-Regulation, and the Government of Impairment in Utero," *Hypatia* 21 (1): 35–53.

Wachbroit, R. and Wasserman, D. (1995) "Patient Autonomy and Value Neutrality in Nondirective Genetic Counseling," *Stanford Journal of Law and Social Policy* 6 (2): 103–11.

Walker, L.S., Ford, M.B. and Donald, W.D. (1987) "Cystic Fibrosis and Family Stress: Effects of Age and Severity of Illness," *Pediatrics* 79: 239–46.

Walsh-Gallagher, D., Sinclair, M. and Mc Conkey, R. (2012) "The Ambiguity of Disabled Women's Experiences of Pregnancy, Childbirth and Motherhood: A Phenomenological Understanding," *Midwifery* 28 (2): 156–62.

Wasserman, D. (2003) "A Choice of Evils in Prenatal Testing," *Florida Law Review* 30 (2): 295–313.

Wasserman, D. and Asch, A. (2007a) "A Response to Mahowald and Nelson," *Cambridge Quarterly of Healthcare Ethics* 16 (4): 468–75.

Wasserman, D. and Asch, A. (2007b) "Reply to Nelson," *Cambridge Quarterly of Healthcare Ethics* 16 (4): 478–82.

Wertz, D.C. (2000) "Drawing Lines: Notes for Policymakers," in E. Parens and A. Asch (eds.) *Prenatal Testing and Disability Rights*, Washington, DC: Georgetown University Press, pp. 261–87.

Wertz, D.C. and Fletcher, J.C. (1993) "A Critique of Some Feminist Challenges to Prenatal Diagnosis," *Journal of Women's Health* 2 (2): 173–88.

Wilkinson, S. (2010) *Choosing Tomorrow's Children: The Ethics of Selective Reproduction*, New York: Oxford University Press.

Part VII

END-OF-LIFE AND LONG-TERM CARE

This section highlights two sets of related issues: First, the ethical issues posed by chronic illness and our individual, familial, and social responses to it; second, the traditional bioethical problems of defining death, forgoing life-sustaining treatments, and active euthanasia. In keeping with the overall orientation of this volume, justice issues are presented front and center whenever appropriate.

We begin with Bruce Jennings' chapter on the challenges of Alzheimer's disease, a chronic and degenerative brain disorder that gradually erodes memory and effaces the patient's capacity for self-control as well as their sense of personal identity and selfhood. Whereas a popular conception of Alzheimer's tends to focus exclusively on the burdens to self, caregivers, and society, Jennings proposes an alternative approach, based upon capability theories, which emphasizes the patient's remaining capacities for human flourishing. And in place of a dominant philosophy of caring that emphasizes merely physical comforts, discomforts, and protection against harm, he advocates for a more person-centered approach that attempts to salvage and support whatever remains of the patient's identity, sense of agency, and previously held values.

In a world in which more and more people will live longer due to the successes of contemporary medicine and public health, more and more people will suffer from diseases like Alzheimer's, cancer, and other chronic, debilitating conditions. Who will provide care for all these people? The traditional response has been the provision of care within large, extended families, but in developed countries today family caregivers are often squeezed between the demands of looking after loved ones, young and old, and by the demands of outside jobs that support their families. A widespread solution to this problem has been to hire caregivers driven from their home countries by poverty and lack of opportunity. At the level of social policy, this migration of caregivers from poor to developed countries represents a troubling brain drain, especially with regard to the thousands of physicians and nurses trained at great expense in their home countries. By actively soliciting such health care workers to attend to the needs of patients and families in developed countries, well-off nations play an active role in undermining the provision of health services to some of the most needy people on earth. This is clearly an injustice of the first order that demands worldwide recognition of the problem and concerted efforts to stem the tide of the brain drain.

On a more personal level, what do the families of patients in developed states owe to those who undertake the hardships of leaving their home countries to care for their loved ones in private households, nursing homes, and hospitals? Lisa Eckenweiler fills a large gap in the existing bioethical literature by confronting this question directly as a problem of justice. She concludes that those who utilize the services of these migrant care providers owe them recognition, solidarity, and "preventive foresight" in anticipating looming problems on both the personal and policy levels.

Whether we die from a chronic, debilitating disease like Alzheimer's, or from accident or old age, we all die. But what is death anyway, and how do we know that a human being has died? Traditionally, before the advent of mechanical ventilators and the modern intensive care unit, this question was not particularly difficult to answer. A person was dead when their breathing and heartbeat had permanently stopped, period. But the development of technologies to keep the heart beating and blood flowing by mechanical means, coupled with the advent of organ transplantation, called for a serious rethinking of the very nature of death and the criteria and clinical tests for determining that someone has died. A conception of death as "whole brain death" involving the destruction of the entire brain—including both the brain stem and the neocortex—quickly emerged as the accepted standard in both medicine and law, but recent developments in intensive care medicine have called this longstanding consensus into question. Winston Chiong provides a helpful history of this long-running controversy, and offers his own philosophical and policy solution that rejects standard approaches based on a quest for a set of air tight necessary and sufficient conditions for death. Instead, Chiong proposes a more flexible account that would view death as a "cluster concept" composed of a variety of human functions that normally go together but that can be disaggregated in some circumstances that call for nuanced policy judgments based upon the nature of the decision at hand, such as transplantation, the continuation of treatment, or burial.

A focal point in bioethical debates about the definition of death and the ethics for forgoing life-sustaining treatments has been the permanent vegetative state (PVS). In this condition, the patient's higher brain functions and capacity for conscious awareness have been permanently destroyed by cardiac arrest or traumatic brain injury, but the brain stem remains intact, thus leaving the patient in a state of "wakeful unresponsiveness." Some advocates of a "higher brain" conception of death claim that patients who are permanently vegetative should be considered dead, and several of the salient cases in the ethics and law of forgoing treatment have centered on such patients (e.g., Quinlan, Cruzan, Schiavo). If the moral and legal valence of PVS were insufficiently controversial, we now have evidence from functional neuroimaging tests (fMRI) that many patients formerly diagnosed as persistently or permanently vegetative actually exhibit some degree of motor, spatial, and linguistic neural activities. In other words, such patients are actually conscious to some degree ("minimally conscious"), and up to 40 percent of patients diagnosed as in PVS by standard behavioral measures may have been misdiagnosed according to these new techniques. Joseph Fins underscores the clinical and ethical complexities of such developments emanating from the neuroscience laboratory and charts their implications for clinical ethics.

The ethics of forgoing life-sustaining treatments, always controversial, has become even more heated with the advent of the disability critique of bioethical orthodoxy. The standard bioethical approach to forgoing such treatments has consisted of two steps: First, discern what the patient wants or would have wanted; second, in the absence of such subjective information, choose so as to advance the patient's best interests.

Advocates for individuals who are disabled often claim that what might seem at first glance to be an autonomous wish to die might instead be a not fully autonomous response to negative social judgments, and that the quality of life of these individuals, judged from their own perspective, might be much higher than physicians might think. Although they concede that some versions of this disability critique might be exaggerated and problematically paternalistic, Leslie Frances and Anita Silvers maintain that our standard bioethical assumptions bearing on decisions to die need to be rethought in light of the circumstances of the disabled within societies that often marginalize their voice and denigrate their quality of life.

Beyond the ethics of treatment refusal and termination, there are the far more controversial practices of physician-assisted dying and active euthanasia—i.e., assisting patients' attempts to terminate their own lives (e.g., by prescribing a lethal dose) or actively killing patients unable to accomplish death on their own. Whether or not one ultimately approves or disapproves of such practices, there is at least a strong autonomy-based moral and legal argument for them: viz., death is sought by virtue of the patient's own choice. Even more controversial, then, are cases of active euthanasia without any appeal to the patient's wishes or values. Here death is sought on the sole ground of mercy, to end a patient's suffering. And within this category by far the most controversial cases involve newborn children freighted with lethal and painful conditions. Focusing on the Dutch "Groningen Protocol" for regulating infanticide for children, Marian Verkerk and Hilde Lindemann explore the darker side of the neonatal intensive care unit that now salvages many children who would have mercifully died in previous decades, but now live on only to experience unbearable suffering.

33

ALZHEIMER'S DISEASE

Quality of Life and the Goals of Care

Bruce Jennings

Introduction

There are approximately one hundred forms of dementing illness, but Alzheimer's disease (AD) is the most prevalent type, accounting for over 60 percent of all cases. The risk of symptomatic AD increases with age. Today it affects an estimated 5.4 million people in the U.S. and 432,000 in the U.K. Worldwide, the prevalence of all forms of dementia is over 24 million people. In 2050 there will be an estimated 11–16 million people with AD in the U.S., and the cost of their care will exceed $1.1 trillion (Alzheimer's Association 2012: 13–21; Nuffield Council on Bioethics 2009: 4–6).

AD is a progressive and degenerative brain disorder that gradually undermines cognitive function and emotional control. The disease lends itself to the mapping of various stages of impairment and dysfunction, although the manifestation of behavioral symptoms varies significantly among individuals. In addition to the loss of short-term memory and disorientation in relation to everyday activities, AD also progressively manifests changes in the individual's personality; the onset of psychiatric conditions such as depression, paranoia, hallucinations; the erosion of executive functions regarding such things as personal hygiene, apparel, and social etiquette; and loss of self-control in the presence of strong feelings such as anger, frustration, or fear. Fine motor function, judgment, and physical response time may also be affected during the course of the disease.

In bioethics and moral philosophy, neither the ethics of dementia care, nor indeed more generally the ethics of cognitive impairment and chronic long-term care, have been a central focus of research or analysis (Nussbaum 2006; Kittay 1999; Kittay and Carlson 2010). This is surprising given the social impact of AD. Even today there are relatively few extended treatments of the ethical aspects of AD and dementia (Post 1995; Agich 2003; Hughes and Baldwin 2006; Hughes et al. 2006; Nuffield Council on Bioethics 2009). In the broader culture, the background presence of dementia is evident, but it is not often openly or seriously discussed; it remains shrouded in fear, shame, and taboo. Alzheimer's leads us to think about a condition that is profoundly at odds with a culture enamored with open horizons, independence, youth, physical vitality, and cognitive acuity.

Broadly defined, the ethical challenge of AD is twofold. It puts self-identity, personhood, and the value of continued living in question. And it puts what we owe to one another in question. Careful thinking about AD forces one to confront the *imperative for care*—that is, to face up to our common human need, fragility, vulnerability, and dependency on others. It is also presents the ethical challenge of the *imperative to care*—to face up to moral responsibility or obligation in recognizing and responding to the needful vulnerability of others, despite the involuntary limits—or in any case, the "transformation"—that giving care to someone with AD brings about in one's life and future.

If the message of impairment that goes with AD is that our bodies and our brains are vulnerable, the message of care is that we are also fragile in ourselves and our minds (MacIntyre 1999). We cannot flourish humanly solely on our own, or on our own terms. We cannot *be* alone because we cannot subsist without being cared about and cared for. Moreover, we cannot *become* alone because we cannot realize our human potential without caring for, being cared about, and, especially, without caring with. Human flourishing happens in the space of interrelationships of mutual accommodation with others.

Care as a Structure of Meaning

AD creates circumstances in which particular decisions involve ethical dilemmas and require the application of general principles and values in order to resolve them. However, AD care is not simply a series of individual treatment or care decisions. It is a pattern of decisions, treatment plans, and caregiving practices that take on a certain shape and tend in a certain direction over a long period of time. Therefore, what a bioethics perspective can bring to Alzheimer's is not simply well formulated moral rules or principles, but in addition a careful understanding of the appropriate metaphors, resonance, sensibility, and moral imagination required by the challenge of AD. The bioethics of dementia requires careful attention to the task of interpretation so that beneath the surface, or between the lines, of the memory loss, confusion, disorientation and the other symptoms of AD, can be seen a remaining person who is experiencing a life of a certain quality and still capable of a certain kind and degree of communication and relationship with others.

Considered as a pattern of interaction, Alzheimer's care must be discerning and interpretative, and it must also be intentional and directed toward certain ethical and humane goals. The structure of long-term relationships between persons living with AD and those who care for and protect them has an impact on the quality of life and experience of the individual. That structure of interactions forms a kind of social environment or ecology, which, like the physical and architectural environment of the patient with AD, has a direct influence on the person's impairment and its manifestation and consequences. A social and physical environment can greatly reinforce and exacerbate the impairment caused by the progressive neurological damage and loss of function; a particular pattern and place of caregiving can be a disabling condition in the context of AD. By the same token, the environment within which care is given can be an enabling and sustaining influence. The social dimension of AD care may not be enough to overcome the neuro-physical and chemical aspects of the disease, for which at the moment there is no effective cure or medical treatment. However with the right goals, resources, and techniques, social care can stave off the loss of personhood and meaningful living for a considerable period of time (Kitwood 1993, 1997; Kitwood and Breden 1992; Killick and Allan 2001; Jennings 2010). Stated somewhat differently, if the brain cannot be restored through cure, that does not mean that the mind cannot be preserved and healed for a time through care. As Steven Sabat and Rom Harré argue:

> . . . if [in dementia] there is a loss of the capacity to present an appropriate self, in many cases the fundamental cause is to be found not in the neurofibrillary tangles and senile plaques in the brains of sufferers, but in the character of the social interactions and their interpretation that follow in the wake of the symptoms.
>
> (Sabat and Harré 1992: 460)

Alzheimer's creates the need for the conservation of mind and self in the face of the deterioration and disintegration of the brain (Harré 1998; Harré and Gillett 1994). So in an important sense AD care is a form of reminding. It is reminding in the ordinary sense of recalling to mind something that has been forgotten; in AD care a person's memory of past abilities and experiences can be nurtured and used therapeutically, and the loss of short-term memory and behavioral control can (to some extent) be mitigated and compensated for.

Alzheimer's care is reminding in another sense of reconstructing the subject, the person. It is a rediscovering and refashioning of relationality and specific modes of communicating and interacting with others (Killick and Allan 2001). Reminding is changing the environment and the external support system that surrounds the person so that *different* abilities do not become *the absence of* abilities. Reminding, as the play on words suggests, is remembering who and where one is, most fundamentally, as a human person (a "subject" who still has the ability to act as distinct from an "object" who is merely acted upon by others); and how one must be treated by family and society. The tragedy of AD is not only that it alters brain function and changes what people do; the deeper tragedy occurs when and if the long-term care and health care systems allow—or even cause—those changes to "objectify" persons, reducing them to the status of mere objects and not subjects, and treat them only in terms of their impaired body and altered behavior, rather than working with them to re-mind themselves and to be re-membered among those with whom they are living.

The Imagined Reality of Alzheimer's

Alzheimer's has an objective, scientific and physical reality, a social reality, and what might be called an imagined reality. The imagined reality consists of paradigms, icons, and images concerning dementia. These are the lenses and filters through which we most habitually perceive and create assumptions, attitudes, and reactions to AD. Among the most important facets of this imagined reality are beliefs that have to do with the loss of mind, self, and personhood due to the neurological impairment AD involves and with the lack of continuity of self-identity over time. Work in bioethics should critically reexamine this imagined reality and the social construction of AD.

In the face of AD, family members (and other caregivers) have to fashion new patterns and new structures of meaning for themselves. This is shown clearly in the literature of various memoirs, autobiographical accounts, and "pathographies" of AD (Bayley 1999; Bernlef 1988; DeBaggio 2002, 2003; Cooney 2003; Davidson 1997; McGowin 2003; Mitchell 2002). At least in the early stages of dementia, individuals with AD who are aware of their own symptoms and changes must do this, too. Still sensitive to the cues and reactions of others around them, persons living with dementia may assimilate and take such patterns of response into their own work of reminding and healing. They also carry with them into the course of their disease expectations about dementia previously drawn from the culture and perhaps their own experience with a parent or loved one. They, like others with disability, will have to refashion such expectations to preserve their self-identity and esteem from the negative interpretation that encroaches upon them (Davidson 1997; Bayley 1999).

There are three aspects of the imagined reality of AD and the conventional patterns of response to it that should be examined carefully before the issues of quality of life and the goals of care can be addressed. Careful analysis and reflection may lead us to reject or drastically modify each of these factors in the imagined reality of AD.

The first aspect is the assumption that the impairment of brain must of necessity erase the ability to make meaning, what can be called *communicative ability*, and thereby erode one's membership in the human moral community, a membership status that involves being understood by yourself and others as a subject rather than an object. The absence of amyloid plaques and neurological tangles does not guarantee, in and of itself, a normal self; similarly the presence of these abnormalities in the brain need not, in and of itself, preclude the continued exercise of communicative ability or erase one's status as a person or subject.

The second widely held view that should be examined critically is the notion that quality of life for persons with moderate to severe cognitive and behavioral impairments from dementia involves primarily security, comfort, and the fulfillment of immediate, experiential interests. This is the hedonic (comfort and safety) notion of quality of life. An alternative conception of quality of life, to be discussed below, holds that the preservation and restoration of capacities for human flourishing and self-realization, appropriate within the context of AD, are the ethically warranted goals of care.

And, third, the notion that the proper stance of the family (or others with the legal and moral authority to make decisions on behalf of the patient with AD) *vis-à-vis* a person with moderate to severe dementia is one of "guardianship," the purpose of which is to protect the best interests of the person with dementia as defined by their hedonic and experiential quality of life. An alternative conception, which I refer to as "trusteeship," is that the ethically (and legally) appropriate standard for caregivers entrusts them with pursuing the conditions necessary for the preservation of capacity and personhood of the individual receiving care.

Quality of Life

The phrase, "quality of life," is almost always controversial. The basic idea behind the concept of quality of life is that some characteristics of the person and his or her surrounding environment are better than others from the point of view of the human good or human flourishing (Nehamas 1998; Nussbaum and Sen 1993). Yet, despite its difficulty and frequent lack of clarity, the concept of quality of life seems to be an indispensable one. It is especially pertinent to the situation and care of persons with dementia and is very commonly brought up in this context. Therefore, a consideration of the various meanings the concept of quality of life has and the controversies surrounding it are central to a consideration of the goals of dementia care.

What are we talking about when we invoke a person's "quality of life"? There are two common notions that are often conflated and should be clearly distinguished, especially when dementia is the focus of discussion; the first is useful, the second pernicious.

Quality of Life as a Goal of Care

One common meaning of quality of life defines it as a goal of care. The moral point of our dealings with another (whether the situation be health care or some other form of relationship) is to sustain and improve the quality of life. In this sense, quality of life becomes a benchmark to guide human activity and a norm of assessment and evaluation. But notice that the evaluation here is directed primarily at the caregiver and the caregiving process, not at the recipient of care, who partakes of the quality of life achieved but is not judged by it. Moreover, quality of life can be thought of as an interaction between the person and his or her surrounding circumstances, including other people. Thus understood as a goal or outcome of care, an improved quality of life may be a change (for the better) in the person's symptoms or perceptions; or it may be a change in the person's relationship with his or her environment. Medical cure, symptom relief, psychological happiness, or social empowerment may all be goals of care as comprehended by the concept of quality of life.

Quality of Life as the Moral Worth of a Life

The term quality of life is sometimes also used to refer to the moral worth or value of a person and his or her life. Pushed to its logical extreme, this understanding of the quality of life takes us to the infamous Nazi concept of "life unworthy of life" (*lebensunwertes Leben*), which was used to rationalize everything from active euthanasia of those with disabilities to the genocidal death camps (Lifton 1986; Cohen 1983). To say that a person has no quality of life or a very low quality of life is to say that prolonging this person's life has no moral significance, either to the person himself or to society.

In my own view, it is a mistake to use quality of life as a measure of the moral worth of human beings. The notion of the moral worth of a life is logically quite distinct from the notion of quality of life. An account of moral worth is based on an underlying account of humanness or the human person; an account, that is, of what it is to be human. The concept of quality of life, however, is based on an account of a person's inherent capacities and external circumstances. Quality of life may legitimately reveal what is required in order to *become (more fully) human*, but it cannot completely define the value of *being human*.

Let us now consider the main philosophical theories of quality of life. In the history of philosophy there are many such accounts. Most of the theories that are pertinent to dementia and dementia care fall into two categories (Brock 1993; McCormick 1978; Parfit 1984: 493–502; Scanlon 1993): Hedonic theories and capability theories.

Hedonic Theories

These accounts identify quality of life with the individual's awareness, consciousness, or experience. Happiness or pleasure, however those terms are precisely to be defined, are the *sine qua non* of quality of life. This allows for considerable individual variation in assessing good quality of life because different things make different people happy, but it also allows for some kind of common metric (at least on the negative side) because there are seemingly universal negative states of pain or suffering or unhappiness that all (normal) persons avoid.

An interesting question is whether the kind of happiness (or pleasure) that makes for a good quality of life is a direct, unmediated sensation, or instead a more complex psychic state that results from some act of self-interpretation. If it is the former, then it would seem to follow that a person locked in a cell with an electrode implanted in a pleasure center of the brain would be experiencing the highest quality of life. That conclusion must be mistaken and counts against the theory. However, if the pleasure or happiness the theory requires involves some form of cognitive mediation and secondary interpretation, then persons who have serious cognitive deficits will be automatically judged to have a poor quality of life by definition, and that view seems unduly biased against non-intellectual goods in life.

Capability Theories

This type of philosophical theory attempts to base our understanding of the good life on an account of those functions, capacities, and excellences that are most fully and constitutively human. To the extent that we attain and master those capacities, and to the extent that we avoid those conditions that would stunt or undermine those capacities, we flourish as human beings. Theories of this type also usually have a developmental component built into them, for those most fully human capacities are ones that are not mastered at birth or automatically expressed by instinct, but must be developed and nurtured by education, interaction with others, and practice over the course of a lifetime. To the extent, then, that the individual continues to grow and develop throughout his or her life, quality of life on the capability view is enhanced by that growth.

Accounts of these important capacities differ among philosophers, but as a generalization we can say that they usually emphasize the following elements: (1) The human capacity to take part fully in social relationships of intimacy, friendship, and cooperation; (2) the capacity to use reason and to develop and follow a life plan of self-fulfillment and self-realization; (3) the capacity for independence and self-reliance; and (4) the human need for an appropriate social and cultural environment that provides the individual with various types of resources necessary to meet both basic and secondary needs (Nussbaum 2011).

In mainstream medical and legal approaches to AD care, the most commonly adopted philosophical perspective is the hedonic (Cantor 2005). It may seem that only this type of theory is compatible with the radically diminished cognitive capacity in dementia, but this may be a serious conceptual bias. The relative strengths and weaknesses of these two types of philosophical theory have not been explicitly discussed in the medical literature, and the hedonic approach has been adopted without sufficient critical analysis.

There is nothing in the capability theory of quality of life that necessarily makes it inapplicable to the situation of AD. When applying capability theory to this context, for example, the question becomes how to supplement and perpetuate those capacities that we value as expressive of our humanity. When one of the bodily (neurologic) preconditions for the exercise of these capacities is damaged, caregivers could try to find a social, environmental functional equivalent for it. If a speech disorder manifests itself in a person's dementia, caregivers could try to compensate with resources for nonverbal communication, for it is in the communication itself that important ethical goals of dementia care—such as respect for the person and the preservation of agency and capability—are met, not in the particular medium of communication (Killick and Allan 2001). If short-term memory loss is a problem, environmental cues, interior renovations, and the like could be used to facilitate a daily round of social relationships that do not require a robust memory.

Although capability theories often stress high-level cognitive skills in their accounts of quality of life, relational and communicative factors that remain present in dementia, virtually until its end stage, can easily be shifted to the center of attention. Making sense together, remembering a distant past and self, making judgments and expressing evaluations, even though non-verbally through emotional responses and bodily, kinetic gestures—these are some of the constituent elements or capabilities of a quality life, whatever the degree of one's other abilities at short-term memory processing and reasoning.

Those without the impairments of dementia do these and other things in many different ways with an audience of others or with an audience of various "selves" or perspectives within their own minds. Those with the impairments of dementia do them differently, more tenuously, and need different kinds of audiences and help, but they do them, sometimes for a remarkably long time into the progress of the disease. Life lived with and in spite of dementia, then, even well into its later stages, can be appreciated and understood by drawing on conceptions of human agency and flourishing; and it need not be assessed only in the most directly sensate, hedonic terms (Albert and Logsdon 2000; Burgener 1998; Lawton 1995; Russell 1996).

The Goals of Care and the Obligations of Caregivers

AD involves memory impairment, cognitive impairment, loss of emotional and behavioral control, and loss of "executive function," or the person's sense of what conduct is socially appropriate. Consequently, caregiving often involves restraining or deflecting the willful behavior of the affected person, sometimes by physical and coercive means. Who then should superintend the person with dementia? What norms of conduct should govern dementia care and the exercise of power and authority it involves so that protective measures do not become abusive and excessive? The ethical boundaries within which dementia caregivers operate are related to one's views on the goals of care and the quality of life that should be preserved for the person.

There are two contrasting frameworks within which ethics and the law have tried to address these issues. The first is the *guardian model*; the second is what may be called the *trustee model* (Jennings 2001).

The guardian model is concerned primarily with the health, safety, comfort, and hedonic quality of life of the incompetent person. The trustee model is more broadly concerned with sustaining and preserving the person's capacities and abilities in ways appropriate to the developmental course of the disease. The guardianship model is grounded on a duty of protection. The trustee model, by contrast, is principally grounded on a duty to promote, preserve, and sustain the agency and the dignity of the person being cared for. Its aim is environmental adaptation in order to accommodate ongoing impairments to agency and to preserve remaining capacities for agency by the person living with AD.

How well does the model of guardianship fit the circumstances of AD? The guardian model is close to the everyday look and feel of Alzheimer care in homes and families, where most persons with mild to moderate AD still reside. It is even closer to the attitude toward caregiving prevalent in nursing homes. However, the guardian model has some problems and limitations when applied to the circumstances of risky behavior in AD care.

One problem is the tendency of the guardian model to treat decision-making capacity as an all or nothing proposition. A guardian is not appointed at all unless a person is determined to be legally incompetent, and once that is done the guardian assumes the entire decision-making function and is not bound by the person's current preferences. (A person without competence is considered to be a person whose "preferences"—if he or she can be said to have preferences at all—do not legally matter.) The directing goal of the guardian's decision-making is the best interests of the ward. In clinical settings matters are not usually so formal and legalistic, but it is not uncommon for the patient to fade into invisibility as a person if a determination of incapacity is made. Unfortunately, this is particularly likely in the case of persons with AD, even in its early stages.

In the field of bioethics, the all or nothing approach of the guardian model is not endorsed as the best practice of surrogate decision-making (Buchanan and Brock 1990). On the contrary, decision-making capacity is understood as constituting a spectrum of ability; the patient may be significantly involved in some decisions where he or she has a definite preference and excluded or overridden in others. This style of caregiving, which fits the trustee model more closely than the guardian model, is done not primarily for reasons of expedience, tranquility, and humane patient control, but for the explicitly ethical goals of preserving agency and respecting the person being cared for.

In the early stages of AD's long course of decline, patients are situated on the margins of decision-making capacity and personal judgment, not clearly in the realm of either autonomy or incompetence. Here caregiving involves small coercions, the little skirmishes through which the management of risky or inappropriate behavior is conducted. The decisions of a person with AD in its early stages are shaky, fallible, and debatable. Clearly, this is a matter of degree, for this kind of fallibility characterizes the situation of all of us some of the time. But during early AD the tension escalates, and conflicts between the person with early AD and family and caregivers inevitably arise.

In the ethics of AD care we must therefore consider the complex dynamics of justified "paternalism" in the context of marginal capacity. Paternalism has been defined as any case where one person acts to diminish another person's freedom or violates their rights (e.g., to be informed), to the end that the other person's good may be secured (Kleinig 1984; De Marneffe 2006; Conly 2012; Coons and Weber 2013). Paternalism thus is often an issue for ethical analysis in health and long-term care settings. Many philosophers have argued that paternalism can be justified under certain conditions. Feinberg (1986), for example, considers the proportionality between the importance of the liberty lost and that of the harm to the self that is prevented. G. Dworkin (1988, 2010) emphasizes the future-oriented nature of the person's interests being served by the paternalistic intervention. Paternalism is justified now if it serves greater freedom or autonomy later and if the person whose freedom was limited can ultimately acknowledge that benefit.

Such arguments are generally persuasive, but they do not perfectly fit the situation of controlling behavior in early AD. For one thing, analyses of paternalism of this kind do not shed much light on the problem of assessing relative risk; instead, they tend to assume that as a starting point. This is a flaw in the guardian model generally. Once relative risk has been assessed, and the risk has been found to be immediate and serious, then the duties to protect the incompetent against harm to self and the duties of promoting a loved one's best interests clearly apply. But in mild dementia the risk assessment stage is difficult. If we look at risk narrowly, then forgoing all kinds of activities is almost always the most reasonable thing to do. As one's capacities erode, one constricts one's repertoire of behavior accordingly, like closing concentric circles. But if we take the psycho-social costs of restricting freedom and curtailing activity seriously, then excessive caution may not be in the best interest of the person with dementia. Such overly cautious guardianship may indeed prove harmful to the ward. Even at the level of physical health and wellbeing, such a course of caretaking for persons with AD leads to an earlier sedentary existence, more rapid loss of cognitive skills, and increased morbidity and mortality. This is one instance in which the goals of guardianship (understood as protection against harm) and trusteeship (understood as sustaining agency and capacity) are most clearly at odds.

Most of the inappropriate or dangerous behavior that patients with early AD wish to engage in grows out of their desire to sustain some part of themselves that they, perhaps inchoately, feel is being lost. This interpretation of early stage AD behavior is attested to in both first person and family member memoirs of the experience of the disease (DeBaggio 2001; Davidson 1997) and in more social scientific and clinical observational accounts (Kitwood 1997). If this is the case, then we take too narrow a view of the moral reality of the situation presented by dementia when we focus exclusively on coercion and the limitation of behavior. Curtailing behavior is only an early step in a morally justified response to the problem. What persons living with early and mid-stage AD need is more than protective restraint; they need help in effecting a transition from one set of behavioral skills to another. They need an environment (both physical and human) that provides them with alternative ways of sustaining their sense of self other than those past activities that have now become inappropriate or dangerous. Here a sheer clash of wills is *not* always inevitable, and there is room for accommodation and adjustment.

Persons with AD can be led to move the focus of their attention and intention from one object to another and from one activity to another. Cooking is not the only way to validate your identity as someone who cares for her family, and driving is not the only way to sustain your sense of independence and self-reliance. Creativity in caregiving is required to find viable and acceptable substitutes; finding a morally desirable outcome is sometimes difficult, but it is not impossible. Often some minor risk is not the principal evil to be avoided; the devastating ripple effects of continuous conflicts and clashes of will can be much more destructive.

In the care and superintendence of persons with AD, the trustee model emphasizes the preservation and restoration of capacities for human communicative relations and an honoring of the identity of the person with dementia as the principal goals of care. Work in the bioethics of Alzheimer's care should assist the broader health care system in reconceptualizing the concept of best interests so that it is not exclusively defined by the hedonic conception of quality of life and its preoccupation with security, comfort, and the fulfillment of immediate, experiential interests. The focus of trusteeship is the person, the subject, the self as an active being in the world of meaning and relationships with others. Trustees view progressive dementia not so much as a declining state in which capacity, agency, and personhood are lost, but as a state of transitions and transformations. Without romanticizing the devastating aspects of AD, trustees stress difference rather than loss, and look for whatever value and meaning can be found in those states of being and capacities for agency that do remain available to the self prior to the end stage of the disease (Burgener 1998).

The goal of trusteeship is to sustain the person's human flourishing and quality of life in ways suggested by capability theory. For trusteeship, providing comfort, pleasant sensation, and experience is not enough. The challenge is to create a caregiving environment or social ecology, containing the necessary caregiving skills and practices that meet the goals of preserving the communicative and relational capacity of the individual with dementia, and acknowledging that this individual remains someone to whom respect, dignity, and care, not just custodial comfort and safety, are owed. The problems posed by the symptoms of AD are attributed to the pathology of the patient's brain, but that is not sufficient because these problems are often exacerbated by the care-taking environment and the (usually well-intentioned) behavior of the caregivers. An ethical response to AD requires that the caregiving system accommodate these symptoms in creative ways and that it compensate for them as much and for as long as possible.

Alzheimer's and End-of-Life Care

If the hedonic conception of quality of life is too narrow in the early and middle stages of dementia, it also gives the wrong kind of guidance in the late stages.

One aspect of end-of-life dementia care that has provoked an important debate in bioethics has to do with the use of advance medical directives, standards of surrogate decision-making, and the use of life-sustaining technologies such as artificial nutrition and hydration through the use of percutaneous endoscopic gastrostomy (PEG) feeding tubes (Finucane and Bynum 1996; Grant et al. 1998; Finucane et al. 1999; Rudberg et al. 2000; Gillick 2000; Post 2001). Individuals who have lost decision-making capacity must have medical treatment decisions made by a designated representative or surrogate, and the standard view in bioethics is that individuals' prior wishes and instructions, when they exist, should guide the surrogate in making these decisions. In other words, end-of-life treatment decisions should be made on the basis of the patient's advance directive or on the basis of what the surrogate decision-maker infers would be the patient's express preference if he or she were able to make the decision (the so-called substituted judgment standard).

The hedonic conception of quality of life casts substantial doubt on the currently prevailing ethical and legal approach to end-of-life care in dementia in cases where prolonging life through technological means, such as PEG tube feeding, may be hedonically acceptable as in the patient's best interests, but where it would be forgone if the patient's advance directive were followed. Challenging the standard view, Dresser and others (1986; Dresser and Robinson 1989) have argued that a contemporaneous best interest standard, rather than an advance directive or substituted judgment approach, should be used in decision-making about forgoing life-sustaining treatments. Best interests on this view should be defined by assessing the quality of life of the patient with advanced dementia in hedonic terms. Counter-arguments by R. Dworkin (1993), Post (1995), and Jaworska (1999), among others, appeal to interests and senses of personhood that go beyond hedonic quality of life as reasons why we should honor a person's advance directive or longstanding wishes and values. R. Dworkin, for instance, makes a distinction between what he calls "experiential interests" and "critical interests," the former being those things that a person experiences as enhancing their good and the latter those things that rationally, objectively do enhance a person's good whether he or she is aware of it or not. A person with dementia may have lost all experiential interest in her previous values, beliefs, and instructions—because she has forgotten them or can no longer understand what they mean—but it does not follow that her critical interests in these things has been lost, or that their significance for the person's quality of life has been erased. And it is on the basis of a person's critical interests that both quality of life and the obligations of caregivers toward the person must be assessed; experiential interests (or hedonic quality of life) alone are important, but ethically insufficient to be the determining factor in end-of-life treatment decisions.

Conclusion

If it does nothing else, critical work in bioethics on quality of life and the goals of care in AD should increase our awareness of new possibilities for family, professional, and community caring for persons with dementia. Bioethics should teach our society how to read dementia properly. In AD there is a kind of personhood that seems devoid of relationality and is therefore limited to the protection of comfort and safety, not because it really is, but only because we do not know how to interpret it.

Related Topics

Chapter 21, "Autonomy," Catriona Mackenzie
Chapter 22, "Capacity and Competence," Jessica Berg and Katherine Shaw Makielski
Chapter 34, "Family Caregivers, Long-Term Care, and Global Justice," Lisa Eckenwiler

References

Agich, G.J. (2003) *Dependence and Autonomy in Old Age: An Ethical Framework for Long-Term Care*, Cambridge: Cambridge University Press.

Albert, S.M. and Logsdon, R.G. (eds.) (2000) *Assessing Quality of Life in Alzheimer's Disease*, New York: Springer.

Alzheimer's Association (2012) "Alzheimer's Disease Facts and Figures," *Alzheimer's and Dementia: The Journal of the Alzheimer's Association* 8 (March): 131–68.

Bayley, J. (1999) *Elegy for Iris*, New York: St Martin's Press.

Bernlef, J. (1988) *Out of Mind*, London: Farber and Farber.

Brock, D.W. (1993) "Quality of Life Measures in Health Care and Medical Ethics," in M.C. Nussbaum and A. Sen (eds.) *The Quality of Life*, New York: Cambridge University Press, pp. 95–139.

Buchanan, A.E. and Brock, D.W. (1990) *Deciding for Others: The Ethics of Surrogate Decision Making*, Cambridge: Cambridge University Press.

Burgener, S.C. (1998) "Quality of Life in Late Stage Dementia," in L. Volicer and A. Hurley (eds.) *Hospice Care for Patients with Advanced Progressive Dementia*, New York: Springer, pp. 88–113.

Cantor, N.L. (2005) *Making Medical Decisions for the Profoundly Mentally Disabled*, Boston, MA: MIT Press.

Cohen, C. (1983) "'Quality of Life' and the Analogy with the Nazis," *Journal of Medicine and Philosophy* 8: 113–35.

Conly, S. (2012) *Against Autonomy: Justifying Coercive Paternalism*, Cambridge: Cambridge University Press.

Cooney, E. (2003) *Death in Slow Motion: My Mother's Descent into Alzheimer's*, New York: HarperCollins.

Coons, C. and Weber, M. (eds.) (2013) *Paternalism: Theory and Practice*, Cambridge: Cambridge University Press.

Davidson, A. (1997) *Alzheimer's, a Love Story: One Year in My Husband's Journey*, Secaucus, NJ: Carol Publishing Group.

DeBaggio, T. (2002) *Losing My Mind: An Intimate Look at Life with Alzheimer's*, New York: The Free Press.

DeBaggio, T. (2003) *When It Gets Dark: An Enlightened Reflection on Life with Alzheimer's*, New York: The Free Press.

De Marneffe, P. (2006) "Avoiding Paternalism," *Philosophy and Public Affairs* 34 (1): 68–94.

Dresser, R.S. (1986) "Life, Death and Incompetent Patients: Conceptual Infirmities and Hidden Values in the Law," *Arizona Law Review* 28: 373–405.

Dresser, R.S. and Robertson, J.A. (1989) "Quality of Life and Non-treatment Decisions for Incompetent Patients: A Critique of the Orthodox Approach," *Law, Medicine, and Health Care* 17: 234–44.

Dworkin, G. (1988) *The Theory and Practice of Autonomy*, Cambridge: Cambridge University Press.

Dworkin, G. (2010) "Paternalism," in E.N. Zalta (ed.) *The Stanford Encyclopedia of Philosophy* (summer 2010 edition). Available at: http://plato.stanford.edu/archives/sum2010/entries/paternalism (accessed August 2, 2014).

Dworkin, R. (1993) *Life's Dominion*, New York: Knopf.

Feinberg, J. (1986) *Harm to Self*, New York: Oxford University Press.

Finucane, T.E. and Bynum, J.P.W. (1996) "Use of Tube Feeding to Prevent Aspiration Pneumonia," *Lancet* 348: 1421.

Finucane, T.E., Christmas, C. and Travis, K. (1999) "Tube Feeding in Patients with Advanced Dementia: A Review of the Evidence," *Journal of the American Medical Association* 282: 1365–70.

Gillick, M.R. (2000) "Rethinking the Role of Tube Feeding in Patients with Advanced Dementia," *New England Journal of Medicine* 342: 206–10.

Grant, M.D., Rudberg, M.A. and Brody, J.A. (1998) "Gastrostomy Placement and Mortality Among Hospitalized Medicare Beneficiaries," *Journal of the American Medical Association* 279: 1973–4.

Harré, R. (1998) *The Singular Self*, Thousand Oaks, CA: Sage Publications.

Harré, R. and Gillett, G. (1994) *The Discursive Mind*, Thousand Oaks, CA: Sage Publications.

Hughes, J.C. and Baldwin, C. (2006) *Ethical Issues in Dementia Care: Making Difficult Decisions*, London: Jessica Kingsley Publishers.

Hughes, J.C., Louw, S.J. and Sabat, S.R. (eds.) (2006) *Dementia: Mind, Meaning, and the Person*, New York: Oxford University Press.

Jaworska, A. (1999) "Respecting the Margins of Agency: Alzheimer's Patients and the Capacity to Value," *Philosophy and Public Affairs* 28 (2): 105–38.

Jennings, B. (2001) "Freedom Fading: On Dementia, Best Interests, and Public Safety," *Georgia Law Review* 35 (2): 593–619.

Jennings, B. (2010) "Agency and Moral Relationship in Dementia," in Kittay, E.F. and Carlson, L. (eds.) *Cognitive Disability and Its Challenge to Moral Philosophy*, Malden, MA: Wiley-Blackwell, pp. 171–82.

Killick, J. and Allan, K. (2001) *Communication and the Care of People with Dementia*, Buckingham: Open University Press.

Kittay, E.F. (1999) *Love's Labor: Essays on Women, Equality, and Dependency*, New York: Routledge.

Kittay, E.F. and Carlson, L. (eds.) (2010) *Cognitive Disability and Its Challenge to Moral Philosophy*, Malden, MA: Wiley-Blackwell.

Kitwood, T. (1993) "Towards a Theory of Dementia Care: The Interpersonal Process," *Ageing and Society* 13: 51–67.

Kitwood, T. (1997) *Dementia Reconsidered*, Buckingham: Open University Press.

Kitwood, T. and Breden, K. (1992) "Towards a Theory of Dementia Care: Personhood and Well-Being," *Ageing and Society* 12 (3): 269–87.

Kleinig, J. (1984) *Paternalism*, Totowa, NJ: Roman and Allenheld.

Lawton, M.P. (1995) "Quality of Life in Alzheimer's Disease," *Alzheimer's Disease and Associated Disorders* 8 (Suppl. 3): 138–50.

Lifton, R.J. (1986) *The Nazi Doctors*, New York: Basic Books.

MacIntyre, A. (1999) *Dependent Rational Animals*, Chicago: Open Court Publishing Co.

McCormick, R. (1978) "The Quality of Life, the Sanctity of Life," *Hastings Center Report* (February): 30–6.

McGowin, D.F. (1993) *Living in the Labyrinth: A Personal Journey through the Maze of Alzheimer's*, New York: Delta Books.

Mitchell, M. (2002) *Dancing on Quicksand; a Gift of Friendship in the Age of Alzheimer's*, Boulder, CO: Johnson Books.

Nehamas, A. (1998) *The Art of Living*, Berkeley, CA: University of California Press.

Nuffield Council on Bioethics (2009) *Dementia: Ethical Issues*, Cambridge: Cambridge Publishers Ltd.

Nussbaum, M.C. (2006) *Frontiers of Justice*, Cambridge, MA: Harvard University Press.

Nussbaum, M.C. (2011) *Creating Capabilities: The Human Development Approach*, Cambridge, MA: Harvard University Press.

Nussbaum, M.C. and Sen, A. (eds.) (1993) *The Quality of Life*, New York: Cambridge University Press.

Parfit, D. (1984) *Reasons and Persons*, Oxford: Oxford University Press.

Post, S.G. (1995) *The Moral Challenge of Alzheimer Disease*, Baltimore, MD: The Johns Hopkins University Press.

Post, S.G. (2001) "Tube Feeding and Advanced Progressive Dementia," *Hastings Center Report* Jan–Feb: 36–42.

Rudberg, M.A., Egleston, B.L., Grant, M.D. and Brody, J.A. (2000) "Effectiveness of Feeding Tubes in Nursing Home Residents with Swallowing Disorders," *Parenteral and Enteral Nutrition* 24: 97–100.

Russell, C.K. (1996) "Passion and Heretics: Meaning in Life and Quality of Life of Persons with Dementia," *Journal of the American Geriatrics Society* 44: 1400–1.

Sabat, S.R. and Harré, R. (1992) "The Construction and Deconstruction of Self in Alzheimer's Disease," *Ageing and Society* 12: 443–61.

Scanlon, T.M. (1993) "Value, Desire, and Quality of Life," in M.C. Nussbaum and A. Sen (eds.) *The Quality of Life*, New York: Cambridge University Press, pp. 185–200.

34
FAMILY CAREGIVERS, LONG-TERM CARE, AND GLOBAL JUSTICE

Lisa Eckenwiler

One important explanation for the flow of health care workers across national borders is the growing demand and expectation in affluent countries, including Western welfare states, for affordable, quality long-term care services (OECD 2005: 10). This is one part of a global trend. Foreign-trained health care workers are increasingly likely to move from low-income countries with an inadequate number of care workers and high disease burdens to more prosperous and healthy parts of the world, especially North America, Western Europe, and the high-income countries in the Gulf and the Western Pacific (Polsky *et al.* 2007). This migration is skewing the distribution of the global health workforce and deepening health inequities, creating a global "crisis in health" (WHO 2006).

The most pressing question is what is owed to countries confronting health worker shortages and high disease burdens, particularly countries from which these care workers (and for that matter all nurses, physicians, pharmacists, etc.) migrate, after having been in many cases actively recruited. Still other crucial matters concern what is owed, by whom and why, to migrant care workers. We might consider governments in both destination and source countries, employers such as health care systems and institutions, and profit-making recruiters as primary moral agents here. And indeed, the responsibilities of some of these agents have been identified and enumerated in bi-lateral agreements, codes, guidelines, conventions, and other international instruments. These ethical interventions aim mostly at protecting health systems of source countries by enumerating principles for managing migration, but they also condemn deception and misrepresentation in recruitment practices, and call for employers and governments to treat migrant care workers with respect and to provide them with labor protections equal to those of citizens (Academy Health 2008; Commonwealth Health Ministers 2003; U.K. Department of Health 2004).

In this essay, I shall focus on the special moral agency of families in destination countries, and consider what they might owe care workers upon whom they rely to support their dependent, elderly family members in home and institutional care settings. Family caregivers are situated together with migrant care workers at the epicenter of shifting economic and care regimes, and find themselves forging cross-border relations as they care for and/or about elders in affluent countries. While most interventions aimed at addressing injustices in migrant health worker recruitment, migration, and employment have taken the shape of political-legal-institutional responses and calls for reform, I investigate the potential of practices (Kurasawa 2007), or particular forms of moral engagement, by family caregivers to advance the work of global justice.

I begin by describing the influx of migrant care workers into the U.S. long-term care labor sector. In this section I also identify and chart the ethical implications of a host of factors that compel care workers in low-income countries to cross borders for their own benefit and that of their families. Next I situate family caregivers within their social, economic, and political context and describe their plight as they try to care for loved ones while contributing to injustice in relying on workers from abroad. I show how both groups manage amidst structural injustice given their respective social and economic circumstances, and explain why family caregivers might have responsibilities to these workers, emphasizing their contribution to the identities of the dependent elderly and their loved ones, and even to the broader culture of destination countries. In the last section, I examine the potential for three practices of what I call "privileged responsibility"—recognition, solidarity, and preventive foresight—to advance the work of justice. Even as structural injustice persists in the transnational organization of long-term care and global health inequities fester (Eckenwiler 2012), my hope is to carve out a space for small steps that ordinary people might take, engaging their moral agency to mitigate moral damage and perhaps, even, promote justice for migrant care workers and people in source countries facing shortages.

Migrant Long-Term Care Workers in the U.S.

Long a low-wage, female, and so-called "minority" industry, long-term care has also become a transnational endeavor (Browne and Braun 2008). In the U.S., as in other privileged countries, a growing number of migrant care workers—mostly women—now find employment in the long-term care sector. An estimated 30 percent of foreign-educated registered nurses (RNs) work in long-term care, and approximately 48 percent of RNs working in home care specifically come from abroad (Martin et al. 2009). Among foreign-educated licensed practical nurses (LPNs), as many as 80 percent are employed in long-term care. A similar trend can be seen among direct care workers like nurses' aides and home health workers, the frontline of the paid long-term care workforce. Approximately 20 percent of direct care workers are born outside the U.S., most of them in low-income countries (Paraprofessional Health Institute 2011). Among home health aides, the foreign born and educated make up an estimated 24 percent. Although the data are difficult to come by, the top countries of origin for these workers are the Philippines, Jamaica, Haiti, India, Nigeria, and Ghana (Martin et al. 2009).

Demand for home health aides is rising especially quickly with the demographic shift toward a more elderly population and as the impacts of budget constraints unfold. Cuts to health and social service programs work partly by shifting from public to privatized service provision—most often provided at home and sometimes with cash transfers—that enable the elderly to purchase services "independently." These structural shifts are significant given that by 2040 the number of older adults using paid home care is expected to increase by three-quarters (Johnson et al. 2006). Home health and personal care aides have been identified as being among the fastest-growing occupational groups (U.S. Bureau of Labor Statistics 2007). Many of these workers are migrants.

Several factors align to facilitate the unprecedented flow of care workers across borders. Colonialism and longstanding interdependent relationships (Raghuram 2009: 30) have contributed to transnational health worker production and exchange. U.S. missionary and military involvement in the Philippines, along with targeted foreign policy strategies, began fueling the mobility of Filipino nurses over a century ago (Choy 2003). Similarly, the modern-day migration of Indian nurses can trace its roots back to the British Empire's Colonial Nursing Association (Rafferty 2005).

More recently, the re-structuring by international financial institutions of economies and public institutions in low and middle-income countries has generated job losses in many sectors, including health care. At the same time, some of these countries have come to organize their economies around the training and export of human resources, with the hope that remittances will help to reduce the burden of debt and poverty. In addition, efforts are underway to craft global trade policies (specifically the Global Agreement on Trade in Services, or GATS) to allow for the commodification and trading of care services on the global market (Connell 2010).

Selective immigration, especially for skilled workers in areas facing shortages, is an essential instrument of industrial policy under globalization (Ahmad 2005). Health and long-term care industry organizations in high-income countries, who regard international recruitment as a way to address shortages and reduce hiring costs and improve retention, often lobby to ease immigration requirements in order to gain access to nurses and other care workers (Buchan et al. 2003). A for-profit recruitment industry that services health care corporations has blossomed in this environment (Pittman et al. 2007).

Meanwhile, extremely poor working conditions and inadequate planning for demographic shifts in well-off countries have resulted in long-term care workforce shortages (Institute of Medicine 2008). A recent report argues that the unprecedented reliance on migrant care workers around the world is a symptom of the lack of comprehensive long-term care policy (International Organization for Migration 2010: 7). More generally, countries' "care regimes" can contribute to the flow of migrant workers. How governments structure provisions for the care of children, the ill and the elderly, including support for family caregivers, has implications for the demand for migrant workers. In countries with strong welfare states and provisions for care of the dependent, there appears to be less demand for such workers than in countries with weak welfare states (Michel 2010). I will say more on this below.

Transnational Identities, Autonomy, and Equity

What are the implications for migrant care workers' autonomy and prospects for equity? If we understand autonomy to mean something like being relatively free to choose one's actions and course in life from a decent set of options within a complex set of relations—familial, social, and economic—and equity to mean something like the absence of avoidable and unfair inequalities, the picture that emerges is complex.

Long-term care harbors some of the worst working conditions found anywhere. The people who are working in long-term care are frequently devalued, not treated with respect, and paid extremely low wages (Paraprofessional Health Institute 2010). These workers report high rates of job stress and low satisfaction, even when they say that they believe in the importance of their work (Castle et al. 2007). Direct care workers tend to fare the worst. Using the U.S. Census definition, approximately 15 percent are poor; two out of every five rely on public benefits such as food stamps and Medicaid. Many of them, especially home health aides, also lack benefits, including health insurance and sick leave. Nearly 30 percent go without health insurance. Perversely, however, nurses' aides and home health workers have higher than average rates of diabetes, asthma, and other chronic conditions, and have one of the highest rates of job-related injury among all occupations (U.S. Bureau of Labor Statistics 2009). They also often lack retirement benefits, which can, over time, place them in economically perilous conditions (Paraprofessional Health Institute 2011).

Threats to autonomy and equity for migrant care workers, in particular, come from several other sources. Women seeking employment in more affluent countries as maids, nannies, and nurses are now an integral part of the global and increasingly service-oriented economy (Dumont et al. 2007). Yet to the extent that their migration is fueled by gender norms and racial and cultural stereotypes that help to organize who does what work, and assign reduced meaning and value to various forms of work (Brush and Vasupuram 2006), it raises ethical concerns. At the same time would-be migrants from low- and middle-income countries are situated amidst nationalist rhetoric that supports neoliberal economic policies and encourages migration. One form encourages workers to organize their conduct around what is beneficial to states' economies (Ilcan et al. 2007). Another variety emphasizes "the active citizen," who allegedly maximizes quality of life by being not just a consumer, but also a participant in the global labor market (Schild 2007: 181). When it comes to migrant care workers, Filipinas, for example, are frequently stereotyped as caring, obedient, meticulous workers, or as "sacrificing heroines" (Schwenken 2008). These rhetorical strategies operate with a caring face, suggesting that labor migrants, especially women, will enjoy expanded opportunities for choice and prospects for equality. Yet by helping to create and nurture subjectivities that align with economic structures and modes of organizing labor, that, among other things, here serve to sustain restrictive gender roles and enforce expectations for individual (as opposed to social) responsibility for familial and national wellbeing, they constrain imaginations and opportunities for women and girls.

Most migrant laborers are subject to "flexibilization," Nancy Fraser's term for a "process of self-constitution that correlates with, arises, from, and resembles a mode of social organization" (Fraser 2009: 129). Its central features, on her account, are fluidity, provisionality, and a short-term temporal horizon. Transnational economic and other structures compel care workers to mobilize, when most say they would rather work in their home countries. Movement to care-related labor markets in the North may involve taking jobs below the education and skill level of care workers, a practice known as "down-skilling." There is also the rapid expansion of the "gray" economy, and the tendency under neoliberal economic policies to define more and more jobs as temporary and unskilled. Inequities may persist under such schemes, and choices may be constrained. Furthermore, although countries often incentivize immigration for some workers, they differentially incorporate migrants when it comes to immigration and citizenship status (Carens 2008). Care workers, especially the allegedly "unskilled," often lack citizenship in the countries where they are employed, and therefore, have a limited set of political rights and, even more than other long-term care workers, limited labor protections and access to health and social services (Bosniak 2009). Recent studies have found that the differential granting of rights to migrants through immigration policies has significant implications for the kinds of work they get, their "exit powers," and "voice" concerning their working conditions, and for their abilities to meet their goals (Shutes 2012).

More generally, like other migrants who describe feelings of dislocation, many nurses working abroad report a sense of "having a foot here, a foot there, and a foot nowhere" (DiCicco-Bloom 2004: 28). Many live in transnational families (Baldock 2000). To the extent that people are shaped by familial relationships and engagement in the communities and places from which we come, migration leads not just to a geographic but a "self-rupture" in many instances (Kittay unpublished). Indeed, these care workers, according to Kittay, experience a sort of "bi-placement" of identity, that is, of "never feeling oneself as fully here." These moral harms faced by individuals can at the same time threaten the relationships themselves; they may lead to the thinning of bonds, and the reinterpretation of status and standing (Miller 2009: 513).

Evidence suggests that migration can have adverse effects on health (Migrant Clinicians' Network). Undocumented, non-citizen care workers are especially vulnerable. They generally cannot seek work in institutional settings that offer employer-sponsored health insurance. While many care workers who are U.S. citizens do not have health insurance as part of their employment package, they might qualify for Medicaid. In contrast, all undocumented non-citizens were rendered ineligible for Medicaid by the 1996 *Illegal Immigration Reform and Immigrant Responsibility Act*. That group is also not positioned to purchase health insurance because its members do not have social security numbers or sufficient financial resources. Moreover, fears of deportation deter them from seeking care in public health clinics or emergency rooms. In short, although undocumented care workers are increasingly essential to social welfare in destination countries, they are often excluded from their benefits (Meghani and Eckenwiler 2009).

Migrant care workers can, of course, reap significant benefits by working abroad. There can be important gains for women in areas like self-trust and confidence, household decision-making and expenditures, as well as in spatial mobility and freedom from restrictive gender norms (McKay 2004). They may advance their respective migration projects, that is, achieve goals they have set for themselves, albeit under constrained conditions, whether this means contributing to wellbeing for their families and themselves at home, or ultimately gaining traction and stability in destination countries. Depending upon a range of factors, many care workers may well be vulnerable, yet become more autonomous and gain greater opportunity (Straehle 2013). Granting this potential, it nevertheless seems reasonable to conclude that migrants' overall prospects for autonomy and equality are at the very best highly uncertain (Abraham 2004).

Situating Families

The work of family caregivers—the vast majority of whom are women—is integral to the global health workforce. Around the world, family members are the primary providers of care, including long-term care for the elderly. At least 30 percent of adults in the U.S. are family caregivers, offering on average 200 hours of support per month, serving as a source of emotional support, coordinating care, accompanying the elderly to medical appointments, managing finances, and often delivering medical care (National Alliance for Caregiving and AARP 2009).

In spite of its integral contribution to social organization and cooperation, the care provided within families has long lacked social standing and respect in many places. Care labor is not typically seen as work, or in economic terms, as productive. Yet those who have tried to attach a dollar figure suggest that in the U.S. alone, the estimated worth of the long-term care work done by family members is somewhere over $375 billion and on the rise (AARP 2008).

The changing circumstances facing families in many affluent countries add to the challenges of ensuring adequate long-term care for elders in need of assistance. Families are having fewer children and are increasingly likely to be dispersed geographically. Meanwhile, opportunities for women in the paid labor force have expanded. In a shift from earlier eras, the majority of family caregivers in the U.S. and other high-income countries are employed in the paid labor force. The support of households, even in wealthy countries, increasingly demands the wages of two earners. This represents a departure from one of the pillars of the traditional, nationalist welfare state, the gendered division of labor involving male breadwinners and female homemakers.

At the same time, however, as many governments restructure to spend less on health and social needs, and health care institutions cut costs, a "care gap" has emerged that ultimately relies upon family caregivers to contribute additional energy and resources. Arguing on the basis of cost-effectiveness and consumer self-determination, choice, and benefit, many governments have begun to restructure their role in the provision of care and welfare services—especially home care and personal care assistance—and moved toward greater privatization and informalization (Shutes 2012). At the same time persistent efforts to cut health care costs have included shortened stays in hospital settings and early discharge of patients. These economic strategies have shifted responsibilities onto family members (Christopherson 2006).

In this context, U.S. employers offer little support. While this phenomenon holds true in many other countries, the U.S. has been described as having "the most family-hostile public policy in the developed world" (Williams and Boushey 2010: 1). Given the rigidity of many contemporary work schedules, family caregivers must conform and make do. Those in the paid labor force typically find themselves distracted, distressed, able to work fewer hours than they did before, and taking unpaid leaves. They often pass up opportunities for advancement. The reduction in work hours that some find necessary tends to translate into a loss of economic and other benefits. Finally, a growing body of research finds that family caregivers are at heightened risk for chronic, elevated stress and depression, poor physical health, and death (Godfrey and Warshaw 2009).

In all, family caregivers manage in the face of serious inequalities and constraints. Embedded in family ties and entangled within social and economic norms and institutional policies that are deficient from the perspective of care, the loved ones of the elderly who can do so increasingly rely on migrant workers to play a supporting role.

Injustice and Responsibility

The threats to autonomy and equity confronting family members and migrants amount to structural injustice. Structural injustice exists when social norms and economic structures and other social processes systematically thwart some people's prospects for self-development and self-determination as they simultaneously expand the prospects of others (Young 2006: 114). The examination above of the plight of family caregivers and migrant care workers reveals the extent to which both are situated amid social norms and economic structures, institutional rules, and patterns of interaction which expand opportunities for the well-to-do and contract them for the less well off.

When it comes to our focus here, relationships between family caregivers and migrants, there are glaring asymmetries in their experience of structural injustice. Family caregivers in the North indisputably struggle to varied degrees, depending upon their social and economic position. Yet they are far better situated than care workers who have migrated, given their elevated global economic position, wider range of options, and greater purchasing power. Indeed, the dense and radically asymmetrical relations of interdependence connecting them to migrant workers in long-term care ground responsibilities for family caregivers. There are several ways to think about this interdependence.

In the broadest terms, we might consider obligations of global justice as being grounded in our shared humanity. On a view that attempts to account for more specificity in our relationships, an agent's moral obligations encompass all those people upon whom her own activities depend, including the geographically distant (O'Neill 2000). Another view holds that we are related through shaping and sustaining the institutions and processes that generate global poverty, and that, in turn, helps to motivate migration (Pogge 2005: 33). Closely related is the "social connection model of responsibility" in which contributions to the structural processes that produce injustice generate responsibilities to remedy them (Young 2006: 103).

As citizens of a democracy, family caregivers elect leaders who help to establish the health, labor, and immigration policies that help mobilize care workers from poor countries. These same citizens support leaders who create and perpetuate the policies of international financial institutions, such as the World Bank and the International Monetary Fund (IMF) and trade organizations like the World Trade Organization. Then too, there are the demands and expectations of privileged people concerning long-term care. When it comes to family caregiving, these demands and expectations rest in part on certain social norms families support regarding care. As Joan Tronto points out, the pervasive tendency, particularly among white middle and upper class families, to understand caring as a matter involving the needs of their loved ones, and to act exclusively according to what appears to be best for them, can lead to moral hazards. In understanding caring in such private terms—as families are socially and economically compelled to do in the U.S.—they may not consider the implications for those who support them or for their kith and kin in less well-off parts of the world. Such myopia constitutes, in Tronto's (2006) words, "privileged irresponsibility."

Reflection on the relationships between source and destination countries, and between migrant and family caregivers, invites consideration of another way of thinking about grounding responsibilities. Specifically, the global interdependence that increasingly characterizes care work reveals the relational nature of our identities. Underpinning the relational conceptions of justice described above are relational conceptions of persons (and also of places). In other words, identities are established and maintained inter-subjectively, through dependency relations and interactions with family members, friends, and other social relationships. The care provided by migrant workers—nannies, nurses, home care aides, and others—has long been and now is an increasingly integral part of the identities of those who benefit from it. It sustains individuals who are beneficiaries of care and members of their families, expanding their opportunities by enabling them to have expanded access to health care services, or even having a walk around or eating regularly. Family caregivers might gain, for example, more time with their children, the chance for evening walks, or hours to work on valued projects. The presence of migrant care workers seems also, in a general sense, to shape the identities of citizens of an affluent country as participants in and beneficiaries of economic and labor policies that rely on low wage workers. We are responsible for addressing injustices such workers suffer, then, not (merely) because of our participation in processes that generate injustice, but also because of their intimate and crucial contribution—given under some measure of constraint—to who we are (Eckenwiler 2012). The scope of this argument expands to relationships even between people unknown to one another. It holds special force when there are particular, intimate relations involving migrants and families.

It is important to add here that adverse effects—whether to migrants, their families, or their countries' health systems—are not necessarily intended. Indeed, structural injustice often occurs as a result of our (individual and institutional) choices and actions as we try to advance our own interests, typically within accepted rules and parameters (Young 2006: 114). Despite the absence of any intention to harm, and despite the constraints they too confront, family caregivers in destination countries have special obligations to the migrant care workers upon whom they rely.

So what, then, might constitute privileged *responsibility*?

Practices of Privileged Responsibility

Governments, along with networking institutions like the World Health Organization have crafted instruments aimed at responding to injustices against transnational health care workers and source countries. According to Fuyuki Kurasawa (2007: 6), however, understanding global justice as emerging principally through prescriptive or legislative means overlooks "the social labour and modes of practice that supply the ethical and political soil within which the norms, institutions and procedures of global justice are rooted." It is important, in other words, to imagine the potential of personal interactions and practices to advance justice.

Kurasawa identifies five practices that advance the work of global justice: Bearing witness, forgiveness, giving aid, solidarity, and preventive foresight. Such practices may accompany or in some cases facilitate political, legal, economic, and institutional reform aimed at global justice. I consider three practices through which family members who rely upon migrant care workers, whether for home-based or institutional care, might contribute to the expansion of autonomy and equality for migrant care workers: Recognition, solidarity, and preventive foresight.

Recognition

Researchers have examined the ways that people, in profoundly intimate relations of care and dependence, create boundaries between themselves and workers. This "boundary work" involves constituting and re-constituting their own identities, constructing layered, yet porous boundaries that include *and* exclude intimate employees, especially the foreign (Lan 2003: 546). Ethically speaking, these interactive processes ultimately serve to undermine respect and perpetuate inequalities.

The practice of recognition can help to respond to the harm done through global social economic processes, privileged irresponsibility, and the tendency to perpetuate divisions between "us" and "them." Building upon the notion of respect for persons, recognition has been theorized as a moral capacity that can be expressed in several interrelated senses, including recognition of another as an autonomous individual deserving of equality; an individual's unique identity; persons as being members of and in association with particular communities or groups; and others' needs for relationships and belonging, both interpersonal and associative (Gould 2007a, 2008).

Recognition of nurses, nurse aides, and home care workers as persons, their structural position, of the inevitable asymmetries mediating all interactions, should serve as starting points here; and from there, recognition of the conditions under which they have migrated, under which they have taken a particular job, and of their goals for migration. Their expertise and experience warrant recognition, as does their capacity for decision-making authority on the job. Recognizing migrant care workers should include explicit acknowledgment that many live in transnational families and are parents, children, and partners of people living apart from them, and citizens of another society. It should include acknowledgement that they suffer from the fracturing of relationships, social exclusion, and perhaps a lack of belonging and stability (social, financial, legal) as a result of migration. It should include appreciation for their need to form new relationships, and to seek out certain services and forms of assistance. Also important is recognition of the fact that many migrants feel silenced under the most serious conditions of inequality and uncertainty, and may even hide concerns and abuse. Their unequal structural positions shape their subjective dispositions, undermining their agency. Family caregivers should support them in encouraging them to ask questions and express concerns. And crucially, family caregivers owe recognition of a care worker's contribution to the family and to the society in which she's employed, most likely as a low wage, highly vulnerable worker. A fourth dimension here is recognition of the places from which migrants come and those in which they provide care. I am using "place" broadly here to refer to source countries—the societies themselves—and their health care systems, as well as the workplace conditions in which migrant care workers find themselves.

Recognition manifests itself in many ways: Morally perceptive questions and acknowledgments, listening, offering fair compensation, and other forms of material support, supporting good working conditions, offering assistance in finding help to address harm and/or injustice, or helping to address it oneself.

Solidarity

For the most part, solidarity has been theorized as concerning relations among members of a particular group, region, or society. In particular, social solidarity traditionally understood focuses on community members who are vulnerable. Recent work on solidarity, though, attempts to expand it beyond its traditional sources of a national community. Carol Gould (2007b: 159), for example, conceptualizes it as an openness to cultivating relationships with a range of others who may not be one's compatriots or fellow group members, who are suffering.

Solidarity is often understood as involving fellow feeling, "feeling with" others or feelings of mutual concern. Yet affective ties, if they imply *affective affinity*, may not be the only or even a desirable basis for solidarity in societies characterized by pluralist moral values and social stratification. Iris Marion Young proposes a reconceptualization of the basis of solidarity that reckons with pluralism and asymmetries: It is not affect but rather the fact that people are situated differently yet still "dwell together . . . within a set of problems and [complex, causal] relationships of structural interdependence" (2000: 197). This grounds what she calls "differentiated solidarity."

Family caregivers seem ideally situated for differential solidarity with migrant care workers. Despite asymmetries, both confront disrespect and deepening injustices, and at the same time are told that their opportunities are expanding and they have ever-greater choice. Neoliberal economic policies have imperiled both, through cuts in public spending and shifting responsibilities for welfare increasingly onto families, especially women, who are responsible for both unpaid care labor and participation in the paid labor force, which for some, perversely, takes some away from their homes and families. The informalization and privatization of care is especially worrisome for migrant women given that it has thrust them into the kinds of work settings where they are most vulnerable.

Solidarity in this context should involve family caregivers advocating for more coherent and comprehensive coordination of care, labor, and migration policies. This would include attention to improved wages and working conditions for migrant care workers; immigration and other policies that improve social and economic status and more equitable access to social and political rights for all caregivers; adequate state support for working families and appreciation for the contribution of care work to the state, and not only as export; and finally, global health equity.

Preventive Foresight

"Preventive foresight" calls for cultivating a sense of responsibility by striving to anticipate and, to the extent possible, avoid injustice and crisis (Kurasawa 2007: 97). For starters, individuals and families with resources in wealthy countries might practice preventive forsesight. This would call for family members to plan ahead for long-term care needs and to think critically about their anticipated use of resources. They might ask themselves, for example: Is there a difference between our expectations for care and our needs? To what extent might these expectations or actual needs have harmful implications for care workers, as well as others in need of care abroad, such as their family members, communities, and the ill and dependent in source countries with health worker shortages? Could we plan and provide for long-term care needs in such a way that we might avoid or lessen participation in the perpetuation of injustice, even in the midst of a complex political and economic landscape that constrains our options?

Not only do families tend not to take the long view, but critics have observed that the future is strikingly absent from view in health policy, including long-term care policy planning (Graham 2010). Family caregivers, finally, should encourage policy makers to plan for the long term of long-term care, and more broadly, human health resource needs. In light of the issues raised here, thinking that goes beyond the confines of narrow nationalism is essential.

Conclusion

Long-term care raises questions regarding justice in health care resource allocation and workplace conditions, justice in families, global justice, as well as questions of justice that arise at the intersections of these areas. Here I have focused on one such question: What do family caregivers owe migrant workers who contribute to the care of their aging loved ones? I have argued that given their contribution (however indirectly and unwitting) to the injustices migrants suffer, their more privileged position, and crucially, the contribution made by these care workers to their identities, family members owe them recognition and solidarity, and for those who might but have not yet come, preventive foresight.

Related Topics

Chapter 5, "Immigration and Access to Health Care," Norman Daniels and Keren Ladin
Chapter 9, "Do Health Workers Have a Duty to Work in Underserved Areas?" Nir Eyal and Samia Hurst
Chapter 33, "Alzheimer's Disease: Quality of Life and the Goals of Care," Bruce Jennings

References

AARP (2008) *Valuing the Invaluable: The Economic Value of Family Caregiving, 2008 Update*, Washington, DC: AARP.

Abraham, B. (2004) "Women Nurses and the Notion of Their 'Empowerment,'" Discussion paper no. 88, Kerala Research Programme on Local Level Development, Thiruvananthapuram: Centre for Development Studies.

Academy Health (2008) *Voluntary Code of Ethical Conduct for the Recruitment of Foreign-Educated Nurses to the United States*, Washington, DC: Academy Health.

Ahmad, O. (2005) "Managing Medical Migration from Poor Countries," *British Medical Journal* 331: 43–5.

Baldock, C.V. (2000) "Migrants and Their Parents: Caregiving from a Distance," *Journal of Family Issues* 21: 205–24.

Bosniak, L. (2009) "Citizenship, Non-citizenship, and the Transnationalization of Domestic Work," in S. Benhabib and J. Resnik (eds.) *Migrations and Mobilities: Citizenship, Borders, and Gender*, New York: New York University Press.

Browne, C. and Braun, K. (2008) "Globalization, Women's Migration, and the Long-Term Care Workforce," *Gerontologist* 48: 16–24.

Brush, B. and Vaspurum, V. (2006) "Nurses, Nannies, and Caring Work: Importation, Visibility, and Marketability," *Nursing Inquiry* 13: 181–5.

Buchan, J., Parkin, T. and Sochalski, J. (2003) *International Nurse Mobility: Trends and Policy Implications*, Geneva: WHO.

Carens, J. (2008) "Live-In Domestics, Seasonal Workers, and Others Hard to Locate on the Map of Democracy," *Journal of Political Philosophy* 16: 371–96.

Castle, N.G., Engberg, J., Anderson, R. and Men, A. (2007) "Job Satisfaction of Nurse Aides in Nursing Homes: Intent to Leave and Turnover," *Gerontologist* 47: 193–204.

Choy, C. (2003) *Empire of Care: Nursing and Migration in Filipino American History*, Durham, NC: Duke University Press.

Christopherson, S. (2006) "Women and the Restructuring of Care Work: Cross National Variations and Trends in Ten OECD Countries," in M.K. Zimmerman, J.S. Litt and C.E. Bose (eds.) *Global Dimensions of Gender and Carework*, Stanford, CA: Stanford Social Sciences.

Commonwealth Health Ministers (2003) Commonwealth Code of Practice for the International Recruitment of Health Workers, adopted at the Pre-WHA Meeting of Commonwealth Health Minsters, Geneva, May 18.

Connell, J. (2010) *Migration and the Globalization of Health Care: The Health Worker Exodus*, Cheltenham, UK: Edward Elgar.

DiCicco-Bloom, B. (2004) "The Racial and Gendered Experiences of Immigrant Nurses from Kerala, India," *Journal of Transcultural Nursing* 15: 26–33.

Dumont, J.-C., Martin, J. P. and Spielvogel, G. (2007) "Women on the Move: The Neglected Gender Dimension of the Brain Drain," IZA Discussion Paper no. 2920, Bonn.

Eckenwiler, L. (2012) *Long-Term Care, Globalization, and Justice*, Baltimore, MD: The Johns Hopkins University Press.

Fraser, N. (2009) *Scales of Justice: Reimagining Political Space in a Globalizing World*, New York: Columbia University Press.

Godfrey, J. and Warshaw, G. (2009) "Toward Optimal Health: Considering the Enhanced Healthcare Needs of Women Caregivers," *Journal of Women's Health* 18: 1739–42.

Gould, C. (2007a) "Recognition, Empathy, and Solidarity," in G. Bertram, R. Celikates, C. Laudou and D. Lauer (eds.) *Socialite et Reconnaissance: Grammaires de l'Humain*, Paris: Editions L'Harmattan.

Gould, C. (2007b) "Transnational Solidarities," *Journal of Social Philosophy* 38: 148–64.

Gould, C. (2008) "Recognition in Redistribution: Care and Diversity in Global Justice," *The Southern Journal of Philosophy* 46: 91–103.

Graham, H. (2010) "Where Is the Future in Public Health?" *Milbank Quarterly* 88: 149–68.

Ilcan, S., Oliver, M. and O'Connor, D. (2007) "Spaces of Governance: Gender and Public Sector Restructuring in Canada," *Gender, Place, and Culture: A Journal of Feminist Geography* 14: 71–92.

Institute of Medicine (2008) *Retooling for An Aging America*, Washington, DC: National Academies.
International Organization for Migration (2010) *The Role of Migrant Care Workers in Ageing Societies: Report on Research Findings in the United Kingdom, Ireland, and the United States*, Geneva: IOM.
Johnson, R., Lo Sasso, A. and Wiener, J. (2006) *A Profile of Frail Older Americans and Their Caregivers*, Washington, DC: The Urban Institute.
Kittay, E. Unpublished manuscript. "The Body as the Place of Care."
Kurasawa, F. (2007) *The Work of Global Justice: Human Rights as Practices*, Cambridge: Cambridge University Press.
Lan, P. (2003) "Negotiating Social Boundaries and Private Zones: The Micropolitics of Employing Migrant Domestic Workers," *Social Problems* 50: 525–49.
Martin, S., Lowell, B.L., Gozdziak, E.M., Bump, M. and Breeding, M.E. (2009) *The Role of Migrant Care Workers in Aging Societies: Report on Research Findings in the United States*, Washington, DC: Institute for the Study of International Migration, Georgetown University.
McKay, D. (2004) "Performing Identities, Creating Cultures of Circulation: Filipina Migrants between Home and Abroad," Presented at Asian Studies Association of Australia, Canberra, June 29.
Meghani, Z. and Eckenwiler, L. (2009) "Care for the Caregivers: Transnational Justice and Undocumented Non-citizen Care Workers," *International Journal of Feminist Approaches to Bioethics* 2: 77–101.
Michel, S. (2010) "Filling the Gaps: Migrants and Care Work in Europe and North America," Paper presented at ESPA, Budapest.
Migrant Clinicians' Network. *Migrant Health Issues*. Available at: http://www.migrantclinician.org/issues/migrant-info/health-problems.html (accessed August 2, 2014).
Miller, S. (2009) "Moral Injury and Relational Harm: Analyzing Rape in Darfur," *Journal of Social Philosophy* 40: 504–23.
Ministers of Health for Pacific Island Countries (2007) *Pacific Code of Practice for Recruitment of Health Workers*, Port Vila, Vanuatu: WHO.
National Alliance for Caregiving and AARP (2009) Caregiving in the US. http://www.caregiving.org/data/Caregiving_in_the_US_2009_full_report.pdf (accessed August 20, 2014).
O'Neill, O. (2000) *Bounds of Justice*, Cambridge: Cambridge University Press.
OECD (Organisation for Economic Cooperation and Development) (2005) *Ensuring Quality Long-Term Care for Older People*, Paris: OECD.
Paraprofessional Health Institute (2010) *State Chart Book on Wages for Personal and Home Care Aides, 1999–2009*, Bronx, NY: PHI.
Paraprofessional Health Institute (2011) *Who Are Direct Care Workers?* Bronx, NY: PHI.
Pittman, P., Folsom, A., Bass, E. and Leonhardy, K. (2007) *U.S. Based International Nurse Recruitment: Structure and Practices of a Burgeoning Industry*, Washington, DC: Academy Health.
Pogge, T. (2005) "Real World Justice," *Journal of Ethics* 9: 29–53.
Polsky, D., Ross, S., Brush, B. and Sochalski, J. (2007) "Trends in Characteristics and Country of Origin among Foreign-Trained Nurses in the United States, 1990 and 2000," *American Journal of Public Health* 97: 895–9.
Rafferty, A. (2005) "The Seductions of History and the Nursing Diaspora," *Health and History* 7: 2–16.
Raghuram, P. (2009) "Caring about 'Brain Drain' Migration in a Postcolonial World," *Geoforum* 40: 25–33.
Schild, V. (2007) "Empowering 'Consumer-Citizens' or Governing Female Subjects? The Institutionalization of 'Self-Development' in the Chilean Social Policy Field," *Journal of Consumer Culture* 7: 179–203.
Schwenken, H. (2008) "Beautiful Victims and Sacrificing Heroines: Exploring the Role of Gender Knowledge in Migration Policies," *Signs* 33: 770–6.
Shutes, I. (2012) "The Employment of Migrant Workers in Long-Term Care: Dynamics of Choice and Control," *Journal of Social Policy* 41: 43–59.
Straehle, C. (2013) "Conditions of Care: Migration, Vulnerability, and Individual Autonomy," *International Journal of Feminist Approaches to Bioethics* 6 (2): 122–40.
Tronto, J. (2006) "Vicious Circles of Privatized Caring," in M. Hamington and D. Miller (eds.) *Socializing Care*, Lanham, MD: Rowman and Littlefield, pp. 3–26.
U.K. Department of Health (2004) *Code of Practice of the International Recruitment of Healthcare Professionals*, Leeds: U.K. Department of Health. Available at: http://webarchive.nationalarchives.gov.uk/20130107105354/http:/dh.gov.uk/prod_consum_dh/groups/dh_digitalassets/@dh/@en/documents/digitalasset/dh_4097734.pdf (accessed August 20, 2014).
U.S. Bureau of Labor Statistics (2007) "Occupational Employment Projections to 2016," *Monthly Labor Review* (November).

U.S. Bureau of Labor Statistics (2009) *Nonfatal Occupational Injuries and Illnesses Requiring Days Away from Work, 2009*, Washington, DC: U.S. BLS.

Williams, J. and Boushey, H. (2010) *The Three Faces of Work–Family Conflict*, Washington, DC: Center for American Progress and Center for Worklife Law.

World Health Organization (2006) *World Health Report 2006: Working Together for Health*, Geneva: WHO.

Young, I. (2000) *Inclusion and Democracy*, New York: Oxford University Press.

Young, I. (2006) "Responsibility and Global Justice: A Social Connection Model," *Social Philosophy and Policy* 23: 102–30.

35
BRAIN DEATH

Winston Chiong

"The boundaries which divide Life from Death are at best shadowy and vague. Who shall say where the one ends, and where the other begins?"

(Edgar Allan Poe, "The Premature Burial")

Introduction

In the history of medicine, debates and demands for greater precision regarding the determination of death have reflected technological advances in medical care as well as broader social concerns. Prior to the mid-1700s, physicians did not play a central role in pronouncing death; as Hippocratic tradition advised physicians to withdraw when death could not be delayed, this role was left largely to family, undertakers, and lay practitioners. The development of resuscitative techniques such as ventilation (advocated by the Amsterdam Society for the Recovery of Drowned Persons in 1767) and electrical resuscitation (first documented in 1774) raised public awareness that some people who had been presumed dead could be revived. Sensational press reports of people buried alive stoked widespread fears of premature burial, vividly represented by Poe and other Gothic writers, and uncertainty over the timing of death prompted laws requiring longer and longer observation periods prior to burial. Physicians of the period responded to demands for greater certainty in the determination of death by critically evaluating a variety of physical signs of death (often used in combination), such as rigor mortis, mottling of skin, pulseless arteries, absence of blood flow from transected blood vessels, hypothermia, pupillary dilation, and putrefaction (Powner et al. 1996). Laennec's invention of the stethoscope in 1819 eventually led to greater confidence in physicians' ability to discern even minimal heart and lung function, and thereby to consensus on the application of circulatory and respiratory tests for death.

In the twentieth century, two further advances disrupted this consensus: Intensive care (including mechanical ventilation) and organ transplantation. While spontaneous breathing depends on the brainstem, mechanical ventilation could maintain oxygen exchange and thereby continue heart function and blood flow for extended periods following the destruction of the brain, a condition originally characterized as *coma dépassé*, or "beyond coma" (Mollaret and Goulon 1959). Such artificially supported circulation despite permanent brain injuries incompatible with natural life raised the question of whether these patients were still truly alive.

The development of organ transplantation added further pressure to resolve this question, since procurement of vital organs for transplantation presented a practical dilemma. On one hand, removing vital organs from a potential donor prior to death would effectively sacrifice a living donor in order to save recipients' lives; on the other hand, delaying organ procurement until after the cessation of circulation would risk permanent injury to organs from prolonged lack of blood flow, limiting their usefulness in transplantation. An Ad Hoc Committee of the Harvard Medical School (1968) proposed new criteria for pronouncing death based on irreversible coma due to loss of all brain function; this would allow mechanical ventilation to be discontinued from brain-dead bodies without the threat of legal sanctions against physicians, and would also allow vital organs to be removed for transplantation from brain-dead bodies while circulation continued. In 1970, Kansas adopted a statute allowing for the declaration of death following either the loss of circulatory and respiratory function, or the loss of brain function. Following the recommendation of the President's Commission (1981), a uniform statute with a similarly bifurcated standard for determining death was adopted by most U.S. states, and similar laws have been adopted throughout the world (Wijdicks 2002).

While neurological criteria for the determination of death were rapidly adopted, there is continuing controversy and unease regarding the conceptual foundations and justification for this change. First, brain-dead bodies maintained with modern intensive care can *look* very much alive: They have a continued pulse and heartbeat, they are warm to the touch, and their chests rise and fall as air is mechanically forced into their lungs at set intervals. Furthermore, Alan Shewmon (1998b) documented remarkable cases in which the bodies of people reliably diagnosed as brain dead have exhibited other characteristic signs of biological life, including cardiovascular stress responses to incision for organ retrieval, successful gestation of fetuses in women who were pregnant at the time of brain death, and proportional growth and sexual maturation (in brain-dead children). Some critics of brain death have argued that the preservation of these functions demonstrates that these people are not truly dead, suggesting that brain death may be merely a useful fiction allowing for withdrawal of mechanical ventilation and procurement of organs from people who are permanently unconscious, but not dead. Finally, further advances in organ transplantation, including protocols for procuring organs from donors after the cessation of circulation, have raised questions about legal standards that accommodate both circulatory–respiratory and brain-based criteria for death.

In this chapter, I will consider the standard arguments offered for neurological criteria for death, and for the prevailing alternative views. I will also present a more recent challenge to a widely accepted argumentative framework accepted by proponents of these different criteria, and will conclude by considering a controversy over whether death should matter for organ procurement.

Criteria and Definitions

According to proponents of the whole-brain criterion of death, we die when our whole brains irreversibly cease to function. Coma, absence of respiratory effort, and absence of brainstem reflexes are the standard clinical tests for the loss of whole-brain function. The two main alternatives to the whole-brain criterion are the traditional circulatory–respiratory criterion and the higher-brain criterion of death. Proponents of the circulatory–respiratory criterion for death claim that death occurs when circulatory and respiratory function together are irreversibly lost; as this criterion is usually interpreted, it does not matter whether these functions are carried out spontaneously or via external measures (such as mechanical ventilation or chest compressions). Meanwhile, proponents of the higher-brain criterion claim that death does not require the irreversible loss of the entire brain's function, but only of the cerebrum—the "higher" part of the brain responsible for consciousness, memory, personality, and perception. This criterion would only require permanent unconsciousness to determine that death has occurred, dismissing the functions of the "lower" brainstem, such as respiratory drive and brainstem reflexes, as irrelevant. Finally, a view that is closely related to the whole-brain criterion of death is the brainstem criterion of death, which has been adopted in the United Kingdom—this criterion only requires the permanent loss of brainstem function, supported by the rationale that while cerebral function is necessary for consciousness, consciousness also requires brainstem activation of cerebral structures. For this reason, the clinical tests for the whole-brain criterion and the brainstem criterion of death are the same, and both will be grouped together in this chapter as accounts of "brain death."

These criteria can be illustrated by considering cases that they would classify differently. Prior to the advent of mechanical ventilation, destruction of the entire brain (including the brainstem) would lead to loss of respiratory function, and the resulting loss of oxygenation and buildup of carbon dioxide would quickly lead to cardiac arrest and the loss of circulatory function; however, in modern intensive care settings, respiration and circulation can be artificially maintained in the absence of brain function. Patients maintained in this way would be classified as still living according to the circulatory–respiratory criterion, but as dead according to the whole-brain and higher brain criteria. Meanwhile, other people have suffered the destruction of the cerebrum, while the brainstem remains intact; this condition leads to a persistent vegetative state, in which the patient is permanently unconscious but may retain brainstem-mediated functions such as spontaneous breathing, sleep/wake cycles (when "awake" they are not conscious, but generally more active), swallowing food placed in their mouths, and blinking when their corneas are touched. (For simplicity in this example I exclude cases in which patients diagnosed as persistently vegetative on clinical grounds might have undetected cerebral function—this example is limited to patients known to have suffered the destruction of the cerebrum.) These patients would be classified as still living according to both the circulatory–respiratory and whole-brain criteria, but as dead according to the higher-brain criterion.

How should we decide among these different accounts of death? In a series of influential articles, proponents of the whole-brain criterion have advanced a theoretical framework for these debates that has become widely accepted, even by proponents of the other criteria. This *definitions–criteria–tests* framework has three stages:

> This analysis of brain death should be conducted in three sequential phases: (1) the philosophical task of making explicit the *definition* of death that is implicit in our traditional conception of death; (2) the combined philosophical and medical task of identifying the *criterion* of death—that generally determinable standard that shows that the definition is satisfied by being both necessary and sufficient conditions for death; and (3) the medical task of devising a set of bedside *tests* to show that the criterion of death has been fulfilled. Thus, the optimal sequence of argument must proceed from the intangible and conceptual to the tangible and measurable.
>
> (Bernat 1992: 21–2)

This framework begins with the linguistic and conceptual project of explicating the shared meaning of words like "death," and then looks out into the world to see what actual phenomena satisfy the conditions implicit in that shared meaning. As such, this framework reflects the influence of the philosophical tradition of *conceptual analysis*, developed by Gottlob Frege, Bertrand Russell, and G. E. Moore in the early twentieth century. Within this structure, we may observe that arguments in favor of one criterion over others may occur at either phase 1 or phase 2. At phase 1, proponents of different criteria might disagree about what definition or analysis of "death" best captures the shared meaning of death; alternatively, proponents of different criteria might agree about the proper definition or analysis of "death," but might still disagree about which criterion is both necessary and sufficient for satisfying this definition. In fact, the disagreement between proponents of the whole-brain and higher-brain criteria typically is at phase 1, while the disagreement between proponents of the whole-brain and circulatory–respiratory criteria typically is at phase 2.

Higher-Brain and Whole-Brain Criteria: Disputes over Definitions

On this widely accepted *definitions–criteria–tests* framework, we must begin by analyzing our shared concept of death, so as to understand what findings indicate death. As a first step, we may note that our ordinary thinking about death incorporates both physical and psychological aspects. On the physical side of death, we associate death with bodily changes such as pulselessness, cessation of breathing, loss of warmth, and eventually decay and putrefaction. On the psychological side of death, we associate death with the end of conscious experience; thus, traditional philosophical discussions of the badness of death (as in Nagel 1970) focus on the deprivation of experience rather than the loss of biological function. Indeed, in some dualistic religious traditions the promise of "life after death" is understood as the persistence of our conscious experiences, memory, personality, and other psychological features in immaterial souls that survive the death and decay of our physical bodies.

Philosophers often mark this dichotomy by distinguishing the life and death of *organisms* from the life and death of *persons*—where "person" is used in a technical sense to refer to an entity possessing psychological continuity, or reflexive self-awareness, or some other mental property. These categories are not coextensive: Many organisms lack the psychological capacities constitutive of personhood (such as members of many if not all non-human species, and also some human organisms following severe brain injury or abnormal brain development), while there could be persons that are not organisms (such as disembodied souls or sophisticated robots).

In ordinary usage, we often do not distinguish between these two different senses of death—that is, between the death of the human organism and the death of the person. However, when trying to characterize death precisely for the purposes of death determination, this distinction is of great importance. Typically, proponents of the whole-brain and circulatory–respiratory criteria maintain that the sense of death relevant in this context is the death of the organism; thus, they propose definitions of death such as *the irreversible cessation of the functioning of the organism as a whole* (Bernat et al. 1981). Meanwhile, proponents of the higher-brain criterion argue that the relevant sense of death is the death of the person, and have proposed definitions of death such as *the irreversible loss of consciousness and cognition* (Youngner and Bartlett 1983). This difference explains why proponents of the whole-brain and circulatory–respiratory criteria classify patients in persistent vegetative states as still living, while proponents of the higher-brain criterion would classify them as dead.

While proponents of the higher-brain criterion might still acknowledge that heartbeat or continued spontaneous breathing and brainstem reflexes indicate the persistence of an organism, the loss of cerebral function in these patients means that their personhood has been irrevocably lost.

Some proponents of the higher-brain criterion, in supporting their preferred account of the definition of death, have appealed to philosophical work on the metaphysics of personal identity. One way of motivating this appeal is to note that, when we distinguish between organisms and persons as two different types of entity, it becomes natural to ask whether *we* are essentially organisms, or are essentially persons. As an example, consider persistent vegetative states in which patients are left permanently unconscious after the destruction of the cerebrum. We might describe this situation as one in which the person has ceased to exist, but the organism survives. If you were to suffer this sort of injury, would *you* then be alive or dead? Some people believe that after losing the capacity for conscious experience, *you* would be dead regardless of whether there was a remaining living organism; this view suggests that even now in the healthy state, *you* are essentially a person and not an organism. Other people believe that the surviving unconscious organism would still be *you*, though in a permanently unconscious state. This view suggests that even now in the healthy state, *you* are essentially an organism rather than a person.

Several philosophers have argued that we are essentially persons (Shoemaker 1984; Parfit 1984). This account of our identity has been taken to support the higher-brain criterion as an account of death that addresses what we essentially are, and some proponents of the higher-brain criterion have proposed other, related accounts of personal identity. Green and Wikler (1980) have proposed that our identity over time depends not on psychological continuity itself, but instead on the persistence of the causal processes (in the case of persons like us, neural mechanisms) that underlie our psychological continuity. (This account is closely related to what Parfit calls the Narrow psychological criterion of identity.) Similarly, Jeff McMahan (1995) has argued that we are neither persons nor organisms, but instead are essentially embodied minds; that is, brains with the capacity to support consciousness (regardless of psychological continuity, reflexive awareness or other persisting psychological traits). According to both accounts, conditions like persistent vegetative states, in which the brain structures responsible for consciousness and cognition are destroyed, are conditions in which *we* have died.

Some proponents of the whole-brain criterion have responded by arguing that death is a purely biological phenomenon that should be kept separate from questions of personal identity. For instance, Bernat has claimed that only organisms can die in the strict sense, while persons cannot die except in a metaphorical sense. However, it seems unclear how this very strong claim can be justified merely by appealing to an analysis of our shared understanding of death; after all, as previously mentioned, much of the long philosophical literature about death has been principally concerned with the cessation of conscious experience rather than with the cessation of any biological process.

There are other reasons, however, why the higher-brain criterion of death has not been widely adopted. First, philosophical debates over the nature of personal identity, or what we essentially are, have proven controversial and complex. While many philosophers accept psychological or embodied mind accounts of our identity over time, philosophers like Eric Olson (1997) have presented strong arguments for the claim that we are essentially organisms. (See DeGrazia (2005) for the implications of these and similar arguments for debates over brain death.) Second (perhaps especially given these unresolved philosophical questions), it is not obvious why medical practice and the law concerning the determination of death must reflect metaphysical claims about what we essentially are. Given that medical practice is principally concerned with the biology and health of the human body, proponents of the whole-brain and circulatory–respiratory criteria could grant that *we* are essentially persons while insisting that the appropriate sense of death in this context is the biological death of the human organism. Third, as we lack direct access to the conscious experiences of other people (the *other minds problem*), physicians and neuroscientists have faced serious difficulties in developing reliable *tests* to distinguish unconsciousness in persistent vegetative states from, e.g., conscious unresponsiveness in a paralyzed brain-damaged patient (Owen et al. 2006; see Chapter 36 in this volume).

Finally, some of the intuitive support for the higher-brain criterion reflects normative intuitions, such as the idea that being permanently unconscious would be just as bad as dying, or that we should not expend scarce medical resources to prolong the life of the permanently unconscious, or that we should use the organs of the irreversibly unconscious for transplants to save the lives of conscious people. While some early proponents of the higher-brain criterion explicitly introduced such normative considerations as part of their definition of death (Veatch 1993), other scholars who had previously advocated the higher-brain criterion now argue that the medical question of whether someone has died should be distinguished from the ethical questions of whether permanently unconscious people should be kept alive artificially, or whether their organs should be used for transplantation (e.g., Youngner and Arnold 2001). If so, then it may not have been necessary to adopt neurological criteria for death in order to remove permanently comatose patients from mechanical ventilation, or to use their organs for transplantation. Thus, many of these former proponents of the higher-brain criteria have returned to the circulatory–respiratory criterion as an account of how to determine death, but maintain that these practices can still be justified (as will be discussed in the final section).

Whole-Brain and Circulatory–Respiratory Criteria: Disputes on Criteria Meeting a Shared Definition

As we have seen, traditional proponents of the whole-brain criterion of death have adopted definitions of death that appeal to the loss of integrated functioning of the organism as a whole. The next step in the argument, applying the *definitions–criteria–tests* framework, is to argue that the destruction of the whole brain is necessary and sufficient for satisfying this definition in human beings. Meanwhile, this same definition could plausibly be adopted by defenders of the circulatory–respiratory criterion of death, who would then bear the same argumentative burden. Which criterion best fits with this definition?

Consider a paradigmatic case of disagreement between these criteria: A patient on mechanical ventilation, whose entire brain has been irreversibly injured and can no longer function. This patient, like those in persistent vegetative states, is permanently unconscious. In addition, due to the loss of respiratory control centers in the brainstem, the brain-dead body does not breathe on its own, depending on a mechanical ventilator that forces air into its lungs at set intervals for gas exchange. Protective reflexes such as the corneal blink reflex, the gag reflex, and the cough reflex are also lost; as are the regulation of body temperature and numerous hormonal systems by the hypothalamus, and autonomic regulation of the heart, blood pressure, gastrointestinal system, urination, and skin by the brainstem. Proponents of the whole-brain criterion have adduced these myriad regulatory functions of the brain to argue that the brain is the "master organ" or "critical system" that integrates the disparate activities of the other organs into a cohesive whole. In the brain-dead patient, it is argued, while individual organs may continue to carry out their respective functions for a while (so the heart continues to beat, the kidneys continue to filter blood, the pancreas continues to secrete insulin and digestive enzymes) they are no longer able to work together as a unified organism.

Until recently, most physicians believed that the organs in a brain-dead body could continue to function in this way for only one or two weeks. But as mentioned in the introduction, the neurologist Alan Shewmon has since documented 175 cases in which the bodies of patients reliably diagnosed as fulfilling the whole-brain criterion were maintained for at least one week (and in rare cases years), often with few aggressive interventions beyond mechanical ventilation. These cases exhibit a "litany of non-brain-mediated somatically integrative functions," including:

- homeostasis of a limitless variety of physiological parameters and chemical substances;
- assimilation of nutrients;
- elimination, detoxification, and recycling of cellular wastes;
- energy balance;
- maintenance of body temperature (albeit subnormal);
- wound healing;
- fighting of infections and foreign bodies;
- development of a febrile response to infection (albeit rarely);
- cardiovascular and hormonal stress responses to incision for organ retrieval;
- successful gestation of a fetus (as in thirteen pregnant women of the prolonged survivors);
- sexual maturation (in two prolonged-surviving children);
- proportional growth (in three children).

(Shewmon 1998a)

An important observation from this series is that patients do pass through a period of severe physiological instability after brain death requiring highly aggressive care to support blood pressure and maintain other basic physiological functions; physicians' experiences in managing this unstable period may have led them to believe that brain-dead patients have irreversibly lost the ability to regulate these physiological functions. However, in patients who have been successfully maintained through this period, this instability eventually subsides, allowing for persistent maintenance of circulation and other functions with less invasive care (other than mechanical ventilation). Shewmon argues that these cases suggest a more modest role for the brain in enhancing and fine-tuning an integrative unity that is distributed throughout the body rather than centralized in any critical organ, and which in these cases persists even in the absence of the brain.

These cases, then, seriously undermine the standard rationale offered for the whole-brain criterion, and have been taken by many scholars to support a return to the circulatory–respiratory criterion of death. In response, the U.S. President's Council on Bioethics (2008) offered an entirely new conceptual justification for the whole-brain criterion. This new justification rejected an analysis of death in terms of the loss of integrated functioning, instead analyzing death as the loss of an organism's ability to perform its "fundamental vital work." According to the President's Council, the work of the organism is self-preservation, and the mark of organisms is that they are driven by their needs to interact with the outside world. In human organisms, one form that this interaction takes is conscious awareness and action selection; while another form is spontaneous breathing to satisfy the need for oxygen.

This account has struck many commentators as an *ad hoc* attempt to preserve the whole-brain criterion in the face of counterexamples, rather than as a compelling account of death in its own right. The central notion of an organism's *work* is underspecified, and the President's Council makes no attempt to show that our shared, implicit understanding of life and death encompasses this idea (as would be required in the *definitions–criteria–tests* framework). It would also allay suspicions if this notion had an explanatory or conceptual role outside of this defense of the whole-brain criterion; however, it seems to play no explanatory role in physiology or evolutionary theory, and also seems to have no counterpart in the philosophy of biology (although it appears to be informed by an Aristotelian account of vital function). Finally, some defenders of the circulatory–respiratory criterion have been puzzled by the fact that this account of an organism's survival is disjunctive. According to this view, conscious human organisms that have lost the ability to breathe (for instance, due to paralysis) remain alive in virtue of their continued consciousness, while permanently unconscious human organisms that retain the ability to breathe (as in the vegetative state) are also alive in virtue of spontaneous breathing. How can it be that both of these count as cases in which the organism continues to perform its vital work, when the vital work performed by one organism is completely different from the work performed by the other (Shewmon 2009; Miller and Truog 2009)?

Criticisms of the *Definitions–Criteria–Tests* Framework

One irony of this controversy is that the *definitions–criteria–tests* framework initially proposed by proponents of the whole-brain criterion, along with their preferred definition of death in terms of the loss of integrated functioning, appears instead to support the circulatory–respiratory criterion that brain death was initially formulated to replace. Meanwhile, some authors have criticized this framework itself; for instance, by challenging the claim that there is any determinate standard that gives necessary and sufficient conditions for the death of the organism. In a famous exchange with Leon Kass, Robert Morrison (1971) argued for a view of death as a process rather than an event, alluding to the fact that some characteristically vital functions such as circulation and respiration can continue for long periods after the loss of others (such as the capacity for consciousness). Halevy and Brody (1993) have similarly proposed that there is no sharp line demarcating the boundary of life and death for all practical purposes; instead, given that some key functions can be present or absent in different combinations, some patients may exist upon a continuum across which different behaviors and ethical protocols may be appropriate at different stages. And Linda Emanuel (1995) has argued for a "bounded zone" account of death between clear cases of life and death, in which it may be appropriate to treat a patient either as still living or as dead depending upon his or her values and previously expressed preferences.

These challenges to the determinacy of the boundary between life and death are grounded in the physiological diversity observed in patients in different stages of dying. These observations may make us skeptical of the claim that we should identify any unified criterion that can clearly distinguish the dead from the living. In previous work (Chiong 2005, 2014) I have challenged the methodological assumptions underlying the *definitions–criteria–tests* framework. Within the framework advanced by Bernat and his colleagues, disputes about death should be resolved by explicating an implicit definition of the term "death" that yields necessary and sufficient conditions for its application. Some terms in the English language may admit of such definitions—for instance, we can define the term "bachelor" as "an unmarried adult male person," which would provide us with necessary and sufficient conditions for the term's application. However, there are many other important terms and concepts that do not fit this framework as neatly.

As an important and influential example, we may consider the case of biological species. First, it is unclear whether species terms such as "bottlenose dolphin" admit this sort of informative definition (Kripke 1972; Putnam 1973). Here a particular worry is that people who correctly use such a term could still be mistaken about the appropriate conditions for the term's application; for instance, the shared implicit conception of bottlenose dolphins in pre-Linnean times might have included that they are a type of fish. More problematically, there are evolutionary grounds for denying the claim that there are any necessary and sufficient features of bottlenose-dolphinhood shared by all bottlenose dolphins that all non-members of the species lack (Hull 1978). Species comprise myriad individuals with tremendous genetic and phenotypic diversity, including individuals with novel mutations and damaged individuals unable to carry out many of the characteristic functions of the species that nonetheless belong to the relevant species. Consider also speciation—bottlenose dolphins evolved from some ancestral species of dolphin via a gradual process over hundreds of generations, and it would be implausible to claim that there is any set of necessary and sufficient conditions that clearly demarcate bottlenose dolphins from members of the ancestral species.

Similarly, I have argued against the requirement for a definition that explicates the shared meanings that we associate with death, and have argued that we should not expect to find any unique set of features that is both necessary and sufficient for death. Following Richard Boyd's (1999) work on scientific categories, I have proposed a *cluster account* of life and death that does not attempt to identify some physiological functions (such as circulation or consciousness or spontaneous breathing) as essential to death while dismissing others as irrelevant. Instead, life and death involve a variety of functions including (in some species) the capacity for consciousness and behavior, circulation, spontaneous breathing, integration, reproduction, and nutrition. In typical cases these features reinforce and sustain one another, and thus tend to be present together (in living organisms) or absent together (in dead organisms). In some cases, one or two features might be missing (as with postmenopausal women and reproduction), but the presence of other features makes it obvious that something still is a living organism. (Just as some individual bottlenose dolphins may lack some features that are typically characteristic of bottlenose dolphins, without ceasing to belong to the species.)

However, there will also be cases of true indeterminacy, in which some but not all of the relevant features are present. On my view, persistent vegetative states are not cases of true indeterminacy; instead, as implied by the term, the mode of life of these unfortunate patients is comparable to many other indisputably living organisms such as plants. Meanwhile, on my view, a brain-dead pregnant woman that gestates a fetus while on mechanical ventilation is a borderline case between life and death. In such borderline cases, I believe that a number of policy approaches may be reasonable. One approach would be to adopt a standard, such as the whole-brain criterion, as an artificial cutoff, analogous to adopting an artificially determinate threshold for adulthood at age 18 or 21 years. Another approach might be to adopt a more pluralistic view such as Emanuel's, allowing for variation in patients' and families' preferences; although as a practical matter heterogeneity in our practices of determining death may also introduce new difficulties.

Is Death Important?

Finally, some authors (particularly those who accept the circulatory–respiratory criterion of death) have questioned an assumption at the root of the Ad Hoc Committee's original proposal of the whole-brain criterion as an account of death: Namely, that the determination whether or not someone has died is relevant to the ethical permissibility of discontinuing mechanical ventilation or removing their organs for transplantation. In the first case, while many at the time believed that physicians are obligated to do everything in their power to prolong the life of the patient, there is now widespread consensus that life-sustaining treatment can and in some cases should be withdrawn from still-living but moribund patients. Therefore, even if we were to adopt the circulatory–respiratory criterion, classifying brain-dead individuals as still biologically alive, we would remain well within prevailing ethical standards to withdraw mechanical ventilation from such patients (particularly in cases where the patient himself or herself, when still conscious, would not have valued continued existence in a permanently unconscious state).

Several authors have gone a step further, and proposed that we should in some cases procure vital organs for transplantation from permanently unconscious but still-living individuals (for instance, cases in which the individual, while still conscious, expressed the desire to become an organ donor and not to have his or her life prolonged in a vegetative state). In other words, these authors propose that we reject the "dead donor rule" that vital organ donors must die before their organs can be removed for transplantation. Such a transition would be a radical one, with legal and public policy ramifications. First, rejecting the dead donor rule would require changes in existing law, as a surgeon who removes a vital organ from a still-living patient would (given the present legal understanding) commit a homicide, even if done with the full prospective consent of the organ donor when he or she was conscious. Second, strong protections would be necessary to protect persistently vegetative patients (or more precisely, their families) from undue pressure to undergo a fatal organ procurement. This is made more critical by the recent finding that some patients who are reliably diagnosed as persistently vegetative may continue to have conscious experiences while being unable (due to paralysis or other limitations) to signal their consciousness to their physicians (Owen et al. 2006; see Chapter 36 in this volume). Finally, there is a concern that rejecting the dead donor rule might undermine public trust in organ transplantation, as it would allow procedures in which a living but permanently unconscious individual is killed in order to provide organs for others. If fear or misunderstanding about this prospect reduces healthy people's willingness to become organ donors, this might restrict rather than increase the supply of organs available for transplantation. Considering these difficulties, some authors who reject the dead donor rule have expressed pessimism that these legal and policy changes can be effected in the current political environment (Miller et al. 2010).

Of course, the urgency of rejecting the dead donor rule depends in part on one's view of the justifiability of current practices. If the circulatory–respiratory criterion instead of the whole-brain criterion is the only *true* standard for determining death in human organisms, then we are *already* violating the dead donor rule (because brain-dead organ donors are still living), but only doing so dishonestly. However, the strongest arguments against the whole-brain criterion presuppose a *definitions–criteria–tests* framework that itself lacks philosophical justification. A more modest defense of the whole-brain criterion, as an admissible though artificial cutoff for determining death in borderline cases, could be combined with a more modest version of the dead donor rule. Such a rule would still prohibit vital organ procurement from people who are determinately alive, but would allow vital organ procurement in borderline cases as long as these cases met the generally agreed-upon standard for determining death.

Appropriate criteria for the determination of death have been a rich topic for debate in bioethics, as they may depend on otherwise abstract issues of ontology and philosophical method, but have direct implications for life-and-death practices such as the discontinuation of intensive care or vital organ donation. One focus for future work on this topic may be its connections with other central philosophical questions, such as the question of whether we are essentially persons or organisms, or the question of what constitutes biological life.

Related Topics

Chapter 36, "From the Persistent Vegetative State to the Minimally Conscious State: Ethical Implications of Disorders of Consciousness," Joseph J. Fins

Chapter 43, "Organ Transplantation Ethics from the Perspective of Embodied Personhood," Fredrik Svenaeus

References

Ad Hoc Committee of the Harvard Medical School to Examine the Definition of Brain Death (1968) "A Definition of Irreversible Coma," *Journal of the American Medical Association* 205: 337–40.

Bernat, J.L. (1992) "How Much of the Brain Must Die in Brain Death?" *Journal of Clinical Ethics* 3: 21–8.

Bernat, J.L., Culver, C.M. and Gert, B. (1981) "On the Definition and Criterion of Death," *Annals of Internal Medicine* 94: 389–94

Boyd, R. (1999) "Homeostasis, Species, and Higher Taxa," in R.A. Wilson (ed.) *Species: New Interdisciplinary Essays*, Cambridge, MA: MIT Press.

Chiong, W. (2005) "Brain Death without Definitions," *Hastings Center Report* 35: 20–30.

Chiong, W. (2014) "Against Definitions, Necessary and Sufficient Conditions, and Determinate Boundaries in Debates about Death," in A.L. Caplan and R. Arp (eds.) *Contemporary Debates in Bioethics*, Malden, MA: Wiley-Blackwell.

DeGrazia, D. (2005) *Human Identity and Bioethics*, Cambridge: Cambridge University Press.

Emanuel, L.L. (1995) "Reexamining Death: The Asymptotic Model and a Bounded Zone Definition," *Hastings Center Report* 25: 27–35.

Green, M.B. and Wikler, D. (1980) "Brain Death and Personal Identity," *Philosophy and Public Affairs* 9: 105–33.

Halevy, A. and Brody, B. (1993) "Brain Death: Reconciling Definitions, Criteria, and Tests," *Annals of Internal Medicine* 119: 519–25.

Hull, D.L. (1978) "A Matter of Individuality," *Philosophy of Science* 45: 335–60.

Kripke, S. (1972) *Naming and Necessity*, Cambridge, MA: Harvard University Press.

McMahan, J. (1995) "The Metaphysics of Brain Death," *Bioethics* 9 (2): 9–126.

Miller, F.G. and Truog, R.D. (2009) "The Incoherence of Determining Death by Neurological Criteria," *Kennedy Institute of Ethics Journal* 19: 185–93.

Miller, F.G., Truog, R.D. and Brock, D.W. (2010) "The Dead Donor Rule: Can it Withstand Critical Scrutiny?" *Journal of Medicine and Philosophy* 35: 299–312.

Mollaret, P. and Goulon, M. (1959) "Le coma dépassé," *Revue Neurologique* 101: 3–15.

Morrison, R.S. (1971) "Death: Process or Event?" *Science* 173: 694–8.
Nagel, T. (1970) "Death," *Noûs* 4: 73–80.
Olson, E. (1997) *The Human Animal*, Oxford: Oxford University Press.
Owen, A.M., Coleman, M.R., Boly, M., Davis, M.H., Laureys, S. and Pickard, J.D. (2006) Detecting Awareness in the Vegetative State," *Science* 313: 1402.
Parfit, D. (1984) *Reasons and Persons*, Oxford: Oxford University Press.
Powner, D.J., Ackerman, B.M. and Grenvik, A. (1996) "Medical Diagnosis of Death in Adults: Historical Contributions to Current Controversies," *Lancet* 348: 1219–23.
President's Commission for the Study of Ethical Problems in Medicine and Biomedical and Behavioral Research (1981) *Defining Death: Medical, Legal and Ethical Issues in the Determination of Death*, Washington, DC: U.S. Government Printing Office.
President's Council on Bioethics (2008) *Controversies in the Determination of Death*, Washington, DC: President's Council on Bioethics.
Putnam, H. (1973) "Meaning and Reference," *Journal of Philosophy* 70: 699–711.
Shewmon, D.A. (1998a) "'Brainstem Death,' 'Brain Death' and Death: A Critical Re-Evaluation of the Purported Equivalence," *Issues in Law and Medicine* 14: 125–45.
Shewmon, D. A. (1998b) "Chronic 'Brain Death': Meta-analysis and Conceptual Consequences," *Neurology* 51: 1538–45.
Shewmon, D.A. (2009) "Brain Death: Can it be Resuscitated?" *Hastings Center Report* 39 (2): 18–24.
Shoemaker, S. (1984) "Personal Identity: A Materialist's Account," in S. Shoemaker and R. Swinburne (eds.) *Personal Identity*, Oxford: Blackwell Publishers.
Veatch, R.M. (1993) "The Impending Collapse of the Whole-Brain Definition of Death," *Hastings Center Report* 23 (4): 18–24.
Wijdicks, E.F.M. (2002) "Brain Death Worldwide: Accepted Fact But No Global Consensus in Diagnostic Criteria," *Neurology* 58: 20–5.
Youngner, S.J. and Arnold, R.M. (2001) "Philosophical Debates about the Definition of Death: Who Cares?" *Journal of Medicine and Philosophy* 26 (5): 527–37.
Youngner, S.J. and Bartlett, E.T. (1983) "Human Death and High Technology: The Failure of the Whole-Brain Formulations," *Annals of Internal Medicine* 99: 252–8.

36

FROM THE PERSISTENT VEGETATIVE STATE TO THE MINIMALLY CONSCIOUS STATE

Ethical Implications of Disorders of Consciousness

Joseph J. Fins

Introduction

The editors of this volume invited me to write a chapter about the "persistent vegetative state." It was an understandable request, but only when we consider the diagnosis as part of a larger story involving the relationship between brain injury and the evolution of American bioethics. Seldom has a clinical category done more to transform medical practice than the vegetative state and its related conditions. The debate over these brain states helped to transform the discussion of death and dying in America and to launch the place of bioethics in our society. Indeed, it would not be hyperbole to assert that this discourse played a key role in the birth of bioethics (Jonsen 1998).

In this chapter I will trace the origins of the vegetative state, its importance to prominent right-to-die cases, and differentiate its characteristics from brain death and related disorders of consciousness, such as coma and the more recently named minimally conscious state (MCS) (Giacino 2005). I will then discuss the diagnostic challenges and therapeutic opportunities presented by these conditions and how technologies like neuroimaging and neuromodulation are refining our understanding of this population and our ethical obligations to them (Fins Under Contract).

Jennett, Plum, and the Vegetative State

The persistent vegetative state was first described by the Scottish neurosurgeon Bryan Jennett and American neurologist Fred Plum in a landmark 1972 *Lancet* article (Jennett and Plum 1972). In a most elegant phrase, Jennett and Plum described the vegetative state as a state of "wakeful unresponsiveness." By that they meant a condition in which the patient appeared awake but was unresponsive and unconscious.

The vegetative state contrasts with a coma, which is an eyes-closed state of unresponsiveness and represents the recovery of the lowest part of the brain, just above the spine, called the brain stem. The brain stem is responsible for autonomic functions that do not require consciousness, for example causing one to breathe or maintaining the rhythmic neural input to the heart. These "lower" functions are in the brain stem which, when recovered, causes the eyes to open and sleep–wake cycles to resume out of the unbreachable "sleep" of coma. The vegetative state thus represents the recovery of the non-sentient, non-cognitive parts of the brain. And because the brain stem functions without the involvement of "higher" cortical areas, the brain is wakeful but unresponsive (Posner et al. 2007).

This wakeful unresponsiveness makes for a paradoxical and confusing state. We are accustomed, even acculturated, to equate an eyes-open state with awareness and a capability for engagement and awareness. Yes, the eyes are the windows to the soul, but not in the case of the vegetative state, wherein the patient stares blankly, though her eyes can move about randomly and autonomically without purposeful intent. Families can be devastated when their loved one's eyes open and they expect recovery only to be told that the patient is not aware but vegetative, nomenclature that Plum has been said to have obtained from Aristotle's *De Anima* (Aristotle 1986).

By the time they described the vegetative state, Jennett and Plum were prominent physicians. Jennett would be known for the Glasgow Coma (Teasdale and Jennett 1974) and Glasgow Outcome Scales (Jennett and Bond 1975) assessment measures to describe the severity of brain injury and predict the likelihood of recovery. Plum in 1966 had already described the Locked-In Syndrome (LIS) (Plum and Posner 1972), a condition of normal consciousness in which the spine or brain stem is injured so that there is no motor output below the lesion. These patients typically can only move their eyes whose muscles are ennervated higher up in the brain stem than is generally affected in the LIS.

Although patients with LIS have a paucity of motor output and can easily be confused with vegetative patients, unlike vegetative patients those who are locked in have normal cognition, as anyone who has read Jean-Dominique Bauby's *The Diving Bell and the Butterfly* can attest (1997). Bauby, the former editor of French *Elle*, wrote a brief but eloquent memoir by blinking the alphabet with his one functioning eye. Seldom has so much been said with so tenuous a communication vector. The point of the differential diagnosis is critical here lest LIS and the vegetative state be confused by errors in assessment.

Jennett's work as a neurosurgeon and Plum's practice as a neurologist positioned them to recognize the vegetative state as what they described as "a syndrome without a name" (Jennett and Plum 1972). They had seen cases like it before and they needed to name it. But they did not describe it as a diagnosis without a name. They considered it a syndrome and not a proper diagnosis. The former is less precise than the latter, whose cause, nature, and duration are fully described. Consider the diagnosis of pneumococcal pneumonia, an infection of the lung by the bacterium *Streptococcus pneumoniae*. The condition is stereotypic and can be induced by a known causative agent, which itself can be precisely distinguished from other pathogens, satisfying *Koch's Postulate*, an important criterion for ascribing an infection to a particular etiology (Fins Under Contract).

No such precision exists for the syndromic vegetative state. Its etiology is diverse: It can be caused by anoxia (prolonged oxygen deprivation), trauma, stroke, or metabolic derangements (hypoglycemia). While patients in the vegetative state share a behavioral profile of "wakeful unresponsiveness," once we look under the hood, as it were, via neuroimaging studies of vegetative states, we see that not all vegetative scans look the same. Finally, we also see that the vegetative state, unlike a diagnosis, can be transient or permanent (Posner et al. 2007). This is not the stuff of which confident diagnoses are constructed.

Quinlan and the Right to Die

Clinical interest in the vegetative state intensified because of a brain injury case in New Jersey involving Karen Ann Quinlan (Matter of Karen Quinlan 1976; Fins 2010a). Ms Quinlan had lapsed into a coma and then moved to the vegetative state after a presumptive drug overdose at a party. The exact cause of her condition was never determined (Quinlan 2005).

Quinlan required life-sustaining measures, including a ventilator. After a protracted period, her parents asked that her ventilator be removed and that she be allowed to die. They were devout Catholics, had consulted with their church, and felt that ongoing ventilation was an "extraordinary measure" not required by Catholic teaching. So they asked that the ventilator be withdrawn. When Karen's doctors and the nursing home where she resided objected, the case went to court.

Ultimately, the New Jersey Supreme Court determined that Karen's parents could remove her ventilator. Informed by testimony from the court-appointed expert witness, Dr Fred Plum, who had examined Ms Quinlan, Chief Judge Hughes wrote:

> . . . It was indicated by Dr. Plum that the brain works in essentially two ways, the vegetative and the sapient . . . We have no hesitancy in deciding . . . that no external compelling interest of the State should compel Karen to endure the unendurable, only to vegetate a few more measurable months with no realistic possibility of returning to any semblance of *cognitive or sapient life*.
>
> (Matter of Karen Quinlan 1976)

It is an interesting decision that forever linked the right to die to the utter futility of the vegetative state, in which Karen's existence would be destined to have "no realistic possibility of returning to any semblance of cognitive or sapient life" (Matter of Karen Quinlan 1976). But it was also an internally contradictory decision. If Karen was forever without cognition, sapience, or consciousness, how was it that she was *enduring anything*, much less the unendurable? That error in logic was overlooked at the time but it demonstrates how easy it is to project one's own feeling onto a state in which thoughts and feelings are absent (Fins 2010a). As we shall see later in this chapter as we consider the cases of Nancy Cruzan and Terri Schiavo, the vegetative state throughout the history of bioethics—and American political life—has stirred the passions but often confused our thinking. This is just one early example from the pen of a distinguished jurist.

The Quinlan decision was also important to bioethics for another *institutional* reason. Judge Hughes, in his opinion, also suggested that the courts were not the best place to adjudicate such cases. Instead, he thought the deliberative process should be closer to the patient's bedside, recommending a role for then nascent hospital ethics committees (Matter of Karen Quinlan 1976).

When the ventilator was removed, however, Karen did not die. Although this was a surprise given all the talk about the right to die, it was not unexpected by the court-appointed expert, Dr Plum, who had examined Karen to provide information to the presiding judge (Fins Under Contract). He knew that she had an intact brain stem and maintained respiratory drive. Thus she was able to breathe on her own. Indeed if she had lost her respiratory drive, she would have been brain dead, as defined by whole brain death—i.e., death of the entire brain, both the brain stem and higher cortical functions. This contrasts with the vegetative state in which the brain stem remains intact (Posner et al. 2007). These observations about the vegetative state, and the criteria defining this condition, would be codified by a group of experts in the mid-1990s.

The Multi-Society Task Force Report on the Vegetative State

The paradoxical nature of the vegetative state led experts from diverse specialties to gather as a Multi-Society Task Force (MSTF) to reach a consensus on the condition. In 1994, the MSTF had two key articles published in the *New England Journal of Medicine* further clarifying the parameters of the vegetative state (Multi-Society Task Force on PVS 1994). These authors came to a consensus agreement that remains useful today. They maintained that if the vegetative state lasts a month it is defined as being persistent. If it persists longer than that, it is designated as being permanent. Unlike the persistent vegetative state that may be transient and lead to recovery, the permanent vegetative state is irreversible and cannot be ameliorated.

Experts, drawing upon epidemiologic data, also distinguished the etiology or cause of the vegetative state as it relates to the question of when the state becomes permanent or irreversible. It was determined that permanence is reached three months after anoxic injury, or profound oxygen deprivation that occurs following a cardiac arrest, and one year after traumatic brain injury. The difference in time courses reflects the different mechanisms of injury and possible recovery that attend these etiologies.

The authors realized that from a clinical perspective, when one advises families about the nature and duration of the condition and about the potential for recovery, the most important historical fact the physician can ascertain is how the injury occurred and how long ago it happened. Because not all vegetative states were created equally, the answer would depend upon the cause of the insult and how long that condition had continued. According to the MSTF, a patient four months post-anoxic injury would be considered permanently vegetative while one who had reached that point after traumatic injury would still have months to experience a recovery before the specter of permanence set in. This remains true today, although patients who receive therapeutic hypothermia (or cooling) following the anoxic brain injury of cardiac arrest have a more favorable prognosis than that outlined in 1994, however its details are still not fully defined.

The Right to Die: From Cruzan to Schiavo

The vegetative state figured prominently in two additional national debates over the right to die. The first was the Nancy Beth Cruzan case in Missouri, in which the parents of a woman in the vegetative state petitioned to have her *feeding tube* removed (Annas 1990). The request was refused by officials at the nursing home where Ms Cruzan was receiving care. The case differed from Quinlan because it involved a feeding tube instead of a ventilator. Was the delivery of artificial nutrition life support or ordinary care? Should it be treated just like a ventilator or should feeding always be morally obligatory? The case was also distinct from Quinlan because it made national law, adjudicated in federal court.

After battles in lower courts, the case went up to the U.S. Supreme Court, which ruled in 1990 that adult competent patients have a constitutional right to refuse life-sustaining therapy based on a liberty interest ensconced in the 14th amendment (Cruzan v. Director 1990). But Ms Cruzan was not a competent individual and unable to express preferences. So the second point of the decision was that *each* state could set an evidentiary standard to determine what degree of evidence was necessary to empower surrogate (or alternate) decision-makers to make a decision to withdraw life-sustaining therapy. Finally, the Court ruled that food and water was a medical treatment and was no different than other life-sustaining therapies. Ultimately, the case was returned to Missouri where evidence was presented to a new court that found that its evidentiary standard was met, thus enabling the removal of Ms Cruzan's feeding tube.

One of the challenges of the case was ascertaining the presence and accuracy of any prior wishes about life-sustaining therapies. The court did not require a specific level of information, but instead ceded that judgment to each state to determine for itself according to its own laws, traditions, and values. To avoid the challenge of unclear, uncertain or absent prior wishes, Justice Sandra Day O'Connor raised the question of whether it might be a good idea for adult competent individuals to articulate their preferences in an advance directive before the onset of decisional incapacity (McCloskey 1991).

These recommendations eventually found their way into federal legislation, the *Patient Self-Determination Act* (PSDA) authored by Senators John Danforth of Missouri, an ordained minister, and Daniel Patrick Moynihan, a sociologist (McCloskey 1991). Physician-ethicist, Mark Siegler termed this law the high water mark of patient autonomy, eclipsing the age-old traditions of paternalism and beneficence which had determined the doctor–patient relationship (Siegler 1993).

The PSDA legislation required that each state set out a mechanism in law to engage in advance care planning either through the use of a living will or designation of a health care agent (DPAHC) or durable power of attorney for health care who speaks with the authority of the patient (*Omnibus Budget Reconciliation Act* 1990). The hope was that through this process a patient's wishes would outlive his or her ability to articulate a preference, thus directing care either through a document outlining wishes (a living will) or through the delegated agency of a surrogate (DPAHC).

That was the state of the law and the national consensus on end-of-life care until the right to die was expanded to a right to physician-assisted suicide. Some viewed this as the natural extension of the negative right to refuse life-sustaining therapy, while others saw it as a distinct positive right, upon which there was not wide agreement. Indeed, the broad consensus within the bioethics community in *Cruzan*, in which there was one bioethics *amicus curiae*—or friend of the court brief—was fractured in the cases brought to the Supreme Court to assess the constitutionality of physician-assisted suicide in 1997. In that fractious debate, there were two bioethics briefs, both pro and con (Transcript of Oral Arguments 1997; Vacco v. Quill 1997; State of Washington v. Glucksberg 1997).

The details of that debate are off-point to our discussion, but the split in views anticipated the political divide that occurred in the Terri Schiavo case (Annas 2005). This case involved another woman in the vegetative state. And like the Cruzan case, it centered on the removal of her feeding tube. Cast against the conservatism of the times, the case challenged ethical and legal norms that had seemingly been codified in Cruzan and subsequent medical practice.

But the Schiavo case was different because there were growing doubts about the vegetative state, with some arguing that Ms Schiavo, and patients like her, were actually aware. As such they were entitled to a different sort of consideration given the provision of food and water, which is considered "ordinary care" in some religious traditions and thus obligatory. Although the question of awareness in the vegetative state had been settled by Dr Plum's testimony as a clinical question in Quinlan, and the distinctiveness of artificial nutrition and hydration had been litigated as a judicial question in *Cruzan*, these matters were brought to the fore once again in the contentious debate surrounding Terri Schiavo (Fins 2006).

From an historical perspective, the image that captures both issues is the video of Ms Schiavo and her mother in which Terri seems to be looking at her mother. That six second video clip, excerpted from hours of tape, was shown as a loop on television. It was powerful stuff raising the question whether her glance was intentional, and thus an indication of preserved awareness and consciousness. Just as in Quinlan, the paradox of the wakeful unresponsive nature of the vegetative state had an emotional impact on society and the ensuing right to die debate. In the context of the polemics of the day, the video depicting Ms Schiavo's condition took on greater meaning. Forces that sought to prevent the withdrawal of her feeding tube sought to assert that her diagnosis was not vegetative but MCS, a category that entered the medical literature in 2002 (Giacino 2005).

The Minimally Conscious State

MCS is a newly described disorder of consciousness in which patients exhibit definitive evidence of consciousness, intention, attention, memory, and awareness of self, others, or the environment. The diagnostic challenge is that patients manifest these actions or behaviors in an intermittent and episodic manner. They are not reliably reproducible. When families see these behaviors and report them to physicians caring for their loved ones, these actions are often not repeated. The common result: Clinicians may chalk it up to wishful thinking or the denial of the families, not appreciating that the episodic and intermittent nature of these actions is part and parcel of MCS. To further complicate evaluation, when these patients are *not* following commands, they are indistinguishable from the vegetative patient on bedside examination, especially on a single examination. Finally, there are medical power dynamics. If a patient arrives from the hospital at a nursing home in the vegetative state, as assessed by physicians at an academic medical center, and then morphs into MCS, will the doctors working in chronic care make a diagnosis against hospital-based experts? Will they know of the recent category of MCS? And if so, will they go against the diagnostic assessment of referring doctors who are more specialized than they are? Probably not.

In the aggregate all these factors translate into a staggering misdiagnosis rate of 20–40 percent for these patients (Childs et al. 1993; Wilson et al. 2007). The most recent diagnostic error rate for nursing home patients with traumatic brain injury diagnosed as vegetative, but who actually are in MCS, is 41 percent (Schnakers et al. 2009).

Biology of the Vegetative *versus* Minimally Conscious State: Ethical and Clinical Salience[1]

The clinical and ethical imperative to distinguish the vegetative from the minimally conscious has it roots in the biologies of these two conditions (Fins 2008). In contrast to vegetative patients, those who are minimally conscious have retained or regained the ability for *integrative* function. MCS brains can activate internal networks that form the basis, in a sufficient aggregation, for consciousness. This is not the case for patients who are permanently vegetative.

This distinction was clearly underscored in a paper on positron emission tomography by Laureys and colleagues, examining the pain response in patients in the vegetative state (Laureys et al. 2002). Unlike normal patients, who activate a broad pain network mapped widely on the brain, patients in the vegetative state only activate the first way station or the primary sensory area. Activation of subsequent areas are "*functionally disconnected*" from secondary somatosensory areas and higher-level associative areas (Fins and Schiff 2007).

This is in contrast to the network-level activations seen in the processing of language in patients in MCS. Using a passive language paradigm, Nicholas Schiff and his colleagues published a paper in 2005 that showed that when spoken narratives were read to patients in MCS, large-scale network activation or integration resulted, as they did in control subjects (Schiff et al. 2005). This response seemed to relate specifically to language; it did not occur when the same narratives were played backwards, with the same frequency spectrum.

The epistemic and ethical salience of these findings—i.e., the differential responses of subjects in MCS and vegetative state—cannot be overstated. Although they appear overtly similar, at the level of neuroimaging patients in MCS respond to the outside world and seem to do so in response to language. This suggests that these patients may retain or have regained the ability to process language, grammar, and speech. When patients with these capabilities are conflated and confused with patients in the vegetative state, it comes at the cost of discounting conscious individuals who at some level may have the ability to appreciate their isolation and segregation from the rest of us. Such diagnostic errors also preclude efforts to develop a rationale for a neuro-palliative ethic of care for this long neglected population (Fins 2005). Making the diagnosis of MCS is very important from a clinical perspective. First, if a patient reaches that level of consciousness before the permanence of the vegetative state precludes additional recovery, then the prospect remains for the return of functional communication. Patients who regain reliable functional communication are said to have *emerged* from MCS. That evolution is not well understood, and to date we are unable to predict who will make this transition. But the key point is that if a patient reaches MCS, they have the prospect of recovery, even years and decades after their injury (Lammi et al. 2005).

This was the case with Terry Wallis, who emerged from MCS some 19 years after traumatic brain injury (Fins and Schiff 2007). Such variability in time course, and even the likelihood of additional recovery, points to the heterogeneity of these brain states and the difficulty of prognostication.

The diagnosis of MCS is also important from an ethical point of view, regardless of whether or not patients have the capability for additional recovery and emergence. It is important to identify patients in MCS so as to distinguish them from those in the vegetative state (Fins and Plum 2004). The difference may seem marginal at the bedside but patients in MCS are conscious. Those who are truly in the vegetative state are not. And if patients in MCS are conscious, then it raises a rather fundamental question of what is owed to them.

It would seem self-evident that our moral obligations to a sentient being, able to interact with and be aware of herself and others (a patient in MCS), should be different than what is owed to patients who are unconscious and vegetative. The potential of the former to perceive pain, feel lonely, sense isolation and abandonment—while unexpressed —is plausible given the biology underlying the MCS. At the very least, we have an ethical obligation to clearly and properly distinguish those who are in the vegetative state from those who are minimally conscious (Banja and Fins 2007). By doing so, patients in MCS with a more favorable prognosis, i.e., a retained capacity for communication, might be further engaged through diagnostic and therapeutic interventions geared towards their reintegration into their families (Fins 2009).

Neuroimaging and Neuroethics of Disorders of Consciousness

If the aforementioned work were to mark the extent of progress in neuroimaging relating to disorders of consciousness, there would already be much to debate and discuss. But these mid-decade papers were only the start of a revolution in neuroimaging that is demonstrating the potential for diagnostic discordance between what one sees at the bedside and what one observes on neuroimaging scans. It raises the question of which criteria should be used—behavioral or neuroimaging—to make a diagnosis. And if there is a difference in assessment, with one method calling for a vegetative diagnosis and the other the MCS, which diagnosis should the patient carry? This is not a trivial question. Conscious individuals should not be treated as though they were unconscious and forever uncommunicative.

These questions quickly came into stark relief in 2006 when Adrian Owen and colleagues at the Universities of Cambridge and Liege published a paper that showed that a "*vegetative*" patient could respond to *active* language paradigms (Owen et al. 2006). Investigators asked a 25-year-old woman in the vegetative state, six months out from traumatic brain injury, a series of questions while she was undergoing functional magnetic resonance imaging (fMRI). She was asked to imagine playing tennis in her head, walking through her home, and disambiguating two linguistically similar words. The results were quite amazing and brought international press coverage and widespread commentary. Even though she was vegetative by behavioral criteria, she had neuroimaging activations in motor, spatial, and language networks that were identical with controls.

Her "responses" raised serious questions regarding her diagnosis. As we saw with Plum and Jennett, the word "diagnosis" needs to be used with caution; so more precisely, we must ask what was the nature of her brain state? If the vegetative state is one of wakeful unresponsiveness and she responded, how could she be viewed as vegetative? On the other hand, her response was not a response by conventional standards but through the prism of neuroimaging, which might be less reliable than an overt behavioral response. So how should her brain state be described?

My colleague, Nicholas D. Schiff, and I have suggested that patients who are *behaviorally* vegetative but who demonstrate active responses on neuroimaging should be placed in a new category of *non-behavioral* MCS (Fins and Schiff 2006). We believed that the subject's highest level of function should dictate the description, given the prognostic importance of the potentiality of being MCS and not vegetative. Interestingly, five months later the patient described by Owen et al. met behavioral criteria for MCS (Owen et al. 2006), although that need not have occurred for her to occupy the non-behavioral MCS category. It is possible that other patients will be stuck there and not progress to MCS.

More recent papers by Monti et al. and Bardin et al. further complicate—or enrich—the terrain. Building upon the active language paradigm of Owen, in 2010 Monti et al. asked subjects to toggle yes or no responses to playing tennis (yes) and walking in their home (no) (Monti et al. 2010). One patient with traumatic brain injury who was diagnosed as vegetative by behavioral criteria was able to reliably answer yes/no questions using this method of willful modulation, providing a narrow band communication channel for someone otherwise thought to be vegetative and unreachable.

Before we get overly enamored with the technology of neuroimaging, it is important to note that this patient was subsequently identified to be MCS by behavioral criteria with redoubled efforts of assessment after investigators knew of the response on fMRI. And it should be noted that behavioral assessment remains the most reliable mode of assessment when the proper Coma Recovery Scale-Revised assessment tool is used to evaluate patients (Giacino et al. 2009).

A 2011 paper by Bardin et al. used a similar method as Owen and found inconsistent responses in subjects who were behaviorally able to respond at the bedside but did not always produce the expected images on fMRI (Bardin et al. 2011). This was just the opposite of the Monti patient. Behavioral output was not consistently followed by evidence on scanning based on prior spatial and temporal expectations (Bardin et al. 2012; Fins 2012).

A Prudential Ethic

By this juncture it should be clear to the reader that neuroimaging is an evolving and still unperfected technology, and that we need to be cautious in applying it outside of the research context. We still must determine as a scientific and ethical community how to reconcile behavioral findings with data obtained on neuroimaging. Until we break that code, it will be as if we are trying to understand the relationship of genotype and phenotype without an appreciation that there is an inheritable and mutable biological material that can effect multigenerational changes in the phenotype (Fins 2007).

Neuroimaging will be an important tool in diagnosing and assessing these brain states, but for now it is best if they remain investigational tools, lest false information or false hope be disseminated to families desperate for information about their loved ones (Fins et al. 2008). We need to do large-scale studies correlating what is currently known with a relatively small sample of patients and developing the test characteristics of sensitivity and specificity for discrete populations of patients, before these methods are brought to routine clinical practice (Fins and Shapiro 2007).

Until then, we need to balance the vast potential of these methods against their limitations, appreciating the importance of attending both to the history of how patients came to be injured and the remainder of the clinical exam, to place neuroimaging—and all the clinical data—into a proper context. Only then can these methods realize their full potential to provide useful information.

Most importantly, we need to be careful to avoid premature adoption of these "communication" technologies, which have the potential for profound misconstrual in patients who are at the edge of consciousness and can neither reliably speak nor interact.

To turn to scanners to ask patients whether they want to live or die, as has been done, is to open up the possibility of generating wrong or inauthentic answers that have the potential to do great harm (Fins and Schiff 2010). Given the state of our technology, responses from patients will be totally dependent upon the questions that are asked and who asks them. These patients cannot initiate queries. Moreover, given the state of technology, we must be cautious about how a non-response is interpreted. Although a pause or hesitancy may be *interpreted* by a listener, it is important to appreciate that there are many reasons why a non-response might occur: Latency of response, distraction, fear, consideration of choices, fatigue, or a failure of the methodology itself. All of these variables need to be better understood and characterized lest we be overconfident in thinking that we are giving voice to patients through these prosthetic devices. The more worrisome paradox is that we might be hearing only part of what they want to say and silencing their true expressions, if indeed they have a requisite level of cognitive, sapient thought.

Conclusion

As we have seen, the study of disorders of consciousness helps illuminate the evolution of the right to die in America. It is also an important focus of study for students in the emerging field of "neuroethics"—a domain of knowledge made possible by technology and utterly dependent upon it (Fins 2011).

Acknowledgement

The author notes with appreciation the editorial assistance of Barbara Pohl, MA.

Related Topics

Chapter 35, "Brain Death," Winston Chiong
Chapter 37, "Disability and Assisted Death," Leslie P. Francis and Anita Silvers

Note

1 This section is drawn from Fins (2010b).

References

Annas, G. (1990) "Nancy Cruzan and the Right to Die," *New England Journal of Medicine* 323: 670–3.

Annas, G. (2005) "'Culture of Life' Politics at the Bedside: The Case of Terri Schiavo," *New England Journal of Medicine* 352: 1710–15.

Aristotle (1986) *De Anima (On the Soul)*, New York: Penguin Classics.

Banja, J.D. and Fins, J.J. (2007) "Ethics in Brain Injury Medicine," in N. Zasler, D.I. Katz and R.D. Zafonte (eds.) *Brain Injury Medicine*, 2nd edition, New York: Demos Medical Publishing.

Bardin, J., Fins, J.J., Katz, D., Hersh, J., Heier, L.A., Tabelow, K. et al. (2011) "Dissociations Between Behavioral and Functional Magnetic Resonance Imaging-Based Evaluations of Cognitive Function After Brain Injury," *Brain* 134: 769–82.

Bardin, J.C., Schiff, N.D. and Voss, H.U. (2012) "Pattern Classification of Volitional Functional Magnetic Resonance Imaging Responses in Patients with Severe Brain Injury," *Archives of Neurology* 69: 176–81.

Bauby, J. (1997) *The Diving Bell and the Butterfly*, New York: Knopf.

Childs, N.L., Mercer, W.N. and Childs, H.W. (1993) "Accuracy of Diagnosis of Persistent Vegetative State," *Neurology* 43: 1465–7.

Cruzan v. Director (1990) 110 S. Ct. 2841.

Fins, J.J. (2005) "Clinical Pragmatism and the Care of Brain Damaged Patients: Toward a Palliative Neuroethics for Disorders of Consciousness," *Progress in Brain Research* 150: 565–82.

Fins, J.J. (2006) "Affirming the Right to Care, Preserving the Right to Die: Disorders of Consciousness and Neuroethics After Schiavo," *Palliative and Supportive Care* 4: 169–78.

Fins, J.J. (2007) "Border Zones of Consciousness: Another Immigration Debate?" *American Journal of Bioethics-Neuroethics* 7 (1): 51–4.

Fins, J.J. (2008) "Neuroethics & Neuroimaging: Moving Towards Transparency," *American Journal of Bioethics* 8: 46–52.

Fins, J.J. (2009) "Neuroethics and Disorders of Consciousness: A Pragmatic Approach to Neuropalliative Care," in S. Laureys and G. Tononi (eds.) *The Neurology of Consciousness, Cognitive Neuroscience and Neuropathology*, Burlington: Elsevier, pp. 234–44.

Fins, J.J. (2010a) "Minds Apart: Severe Brain Injury, Citizenship, and Civil Rights," in M. Freeman (ed.) *Law and Neuroscience: Current Legal Issues 2010*, New York: Oxford University Press.

Fins, J.J. (2010b) "Neuroethics, Neuroimaging & Disorders of Consciousness: Promise or Peril?" *Transactions of the American Clinical and Climatological Association* 122: 336–46.

Fins, J.J. (2011) "Neuroethics and the Lure of Technology" in J. Illes and B. Sahakian (eds.) *The Oxford Handbook of Neuroethics*, New York: Oxford University Press.

Fins, J.J. (2012) "Wait, Wait . . . Don't Tell Me: Tuning into the Injured Brain," *Archives of Neurology* 69: 158–60.

Fins, J.J. (Under Contract) *Rights Come to Mind: Ethics and the Struggle for Consciousness*, New York: Cambridge University Press.

Fins, J.J. and Plum, F. (2004) "Neurological Diagnosis Is More Than a State of Mind: Diagnostic Clarity and Impaired Consciousness," *Archives of Neurology* 61 (9): 1354–5.

Fins, J.J. and Schiff, N.D. (2006) "Shades of Gray," *New Insights into the Vegetative State* 36 (6): 8.

Fins, J.J. and Schiff, N.D. (2007) "Hope for 'Comatose' Patients," in C. Read (ed.) *The Dana Foundation's Cerebrum 2007*, New York: Dana Press, pp. 185–203.

Fins, J.J. and Schiff, N. (2010) "In the Blink of the Mind's Eye," *The Hastings Center Report* 40: 21–3.

Fins, J.J. and Shapiro, Z. (2007) "Neuroimaging and Neuroethics: Clinical and Policy Considerations," *Current Opinion in Neurology* 20 (6): 650–4.

Fins, J.J., Illes, J., Bernat, J., Hirsch, J., Laureys, S., Murphy, E. and Participants of the Working Meeting on Ethics (2008) "Neuroimaging and Disorders of Consciousness: Envisioning an Ethical Research Agenda," *American Journal of Bioethics* 8 (9): 3–12.

Giacino, J. T. (2005) "The Minimally Conscious State: Defining Borders of Consciousness," *Progress in Brain Research* 150: 381–95.

Giacino, J.T., Schnakers, C., Rodriguez-Moreno, D., Kalmar, K., Schiff, N. and Hirsch, J. (2009) "Behavioral Assessment in Patients with Disorders of Consciousness: Gold Standard or Fool's Gold?" *Progress in Brain Research* 177: 33–48.

Quinlan, J.D. (2005) *My Joy, My Sorrow: Karen Ann's Mother Remembers*, Cincinnati: St Anthony Messenger Press.

Jennett, B. and Bond, M. (1975) "Assessment of Outcome After Severe Brain Damage: A Practical Scale," *Lancet* 305 (7905): 480–4.

Jennett, B. and Plum, F. (1972) "Persistent Vegetative State after Brain Damage: A Syndrome in Search of a Name," *Lancet* 299 (7753): 734–7.

Jonsen, A. (1998) *The Birth of Bioethics*, New York: Oxford University Press.

Lammi, M.H., Smith, V.H. and Tate, R.I. (2005) "The Minimally Conscious State and Recovery Potential: A Follow-Up Study 2 to 5 Years After Traumatic Brain Injury," *Archives of Physical and Medical Rehabilitation* 86: 746–54.

Laureys, S., Faymonville, M.E., Peigneux, P., Damas, P., Lambermont, B., Del Fiore, G. et al. (2002) "Cortical Processing of Noxious Somatosensory Stimuli in the Persistent Vegetative State," *NeuroImage* 17: 732–41.

Matter of Karen Quinlan (1976) 70 N.J. 10, 355 A.2d 677.

McCloskey, E. (1991) "The Patient Self-Determination Act," *Kennedy Institute of Ethics Journal* 1(2): 163–9.

Monti, M., Vanhaudenhuyse, A., Coleman, M., Boly, M., Pickard, J., Tshibanda, F. et al. (2010) "Willful Modulation of Brain Activity in Disorders of Consciousness," *New England Journal of Medicine* 362: 579–89.

Multi-Society Task Force on PVS (1994) Medical Aspects of the Persistent Vegetative State," *New England Journal of Medicine* 330: 1499–508; 1572–9.

Omnibus Budget Reconciliation Act (1990) Public law no. 101-508 §§ 4206, 4751 (codified in scattered sections of 42 U.S.C., especially §§ 1395cc, 1396a (West Supp. 1991)).

Owen, A.M., Coleman, M.R., Boly, M., Davis, M.H., Laureys, S. and Pickard, J.D. (2006) "Detecting Awareness in the Vegetative State," *Science* 313: 1402.

Plum, F. and Posner, J.B. (1972) *The Diagnosis of Stupor and Coma*, 2nd edition, Philadelphia, PA: F.A. Davis Co.

Posner, J.D., Saper, C.B., Schiff, N.D. and Plum, F. (eds.) (2007) *Plum and Posner's Diagnosis of Stupor and Coma*, New York: Oxford University Press.

Schiff, N.D., Rodriguez-Moreno, D., Kamal, A., Kim, K.H., Giacino, J.T., Plum, F. et al. (2005) "fMRI Reveals Large-Scale Network Activation in the Minimally Conscious State," *Neurology* 64: 514–23.

Schnakers, C., Vanhaudenhuyse, A., Giacino, J., Ventura, M., Boly, M., Majerus, S. et al. (2009) "Diagnostic Accuracy of the Vegetative and Minimally Conscious State: Clinical Consensus Versus Standardized Neurobehavioral Assessment," *BMC Neurology* 9: 35.

Siegler, M. (1993) "Falling Off the Pedestal: What Is Happening to the Traditional Doctor–Patient Relationship?" *Mayo Clinic Proceedings* 65 (5): 401–67.

State of Washington v. Glucksberg (1997) No. 96-100, U.S. Lexis 4039.

Teasdale, G. and Jennett, B. (1974) "Assessment of Coma and Impaired Consciousness: A Practical Scale," *Lancet* 2: 81–4.

Transcript of Oral Arguments before the US Supreme Court. Justices Hear Arguments on Laws Barring Physician-Assisted Suicide (1997) *Chicago Daily Law Bulletin* 143 (7).

Vacco v. Quill (1997) No. 95-1858, U.S. Lexis 40388.

Wilson, F.C., Harpur, J., Watson, T. and Morrow, J.I. (2007) "Vegetative State and Minimally Responsive Patients: Regional Survey, Long-Term Case Outcomes and Service Recommendations," *NeuroRehabilitation* 17: 231–6.

37

DISABILITY AND ASSISTED DEATH

Leslie P. Francis and Anita Silvers

Introduction

The Disability Critique

For the past quarter century, disability rights organizations have joined sanctity-of-life proponents so regularly in opposing the practice of helping people to die that such advocacy has become a hallmark of the organized disability movement. These disability activists have advanced political rather than theological considerations to the forefront of the debate. They have argued that practices permitting medical professionals to assist in enabling patients' deaths unavoidably discriminate against people with disabilities, an especially vulnerable group (Coleman 2010). By advancing this argument, they give opposition to the practice of assisting dying additional weight by characterizing it as a violation of justice, and therefore as a collective political concern rather than as a violation of individual moral conscience.

A tri-partite generalization about social realities that make the practice of assisting death threatening to disabled people lies at the heart of this disability critique. First is the fear that individuals whose disabilities render them unable to articulate decisions about living and dying for themselves will be sacrificed, supposedly in the name of compassionately relieving them of the burdens of their lives. Second, permitting medical professionals to aid in dying invites the health care system to become more aggressive about reducing society's burden of care for people with disabilities by viewing at least some medical interventions as futile for them, as unlikely to succeed in addressing underlying conditions or bringing them a normal quality of life, or as unjustifiably risky and therefore not medically indicated. Third, even individuals with disabilities who can formulate and express their own decisions about living or dying may not be truly free to make such choices. Because their everyday existence unremittingly exposes them to negative assessments of their worthiness, persons marked by disability cannot help but be coerced or manipulated into devaluing their lives. Moreover, the contingencies of social and economic circumstances may deprive them of control, deepening dependency and restricting meaningful access to important human goods such as companionship or work. These generalizations—about misplaced compassion, problematic medical assessments, and thwarted autonomy—have been deployed to raise different but related disability concerns (Menzel and Steinbock 2013) about aid in dying.

A Pressing Paradox

To the extent that disability activists defend disability rights, but condemn offering people with disabilities the right to obtain aid in dying, they might be expected to acknowledge a pressing paradox. On the one hand, choosing one's manner of dying seems an important exercise of autonomy. On the other hand, if for people with disabilities making this choice ineluctably and irreversibly results from their devaluing themselves, just having the choice unavoidably exposes them to manipulation and coercion that compromise their autonomy.

This paradox has not deterred disability critiques of assisting dying. A common resolution from a disability perspective is to dissolve the paradox by denying that autonomy rights hold value for people with disabilities. Denials of this sort typically take being autonomous as being incompatible with being dependent and therefore as irrelevant to the kind of individual most people with disabilities are. From this assumption it seems to follow that establishing practices of assisting dying to allow self-determination for persons at the end of life endanger rather than emancipate people with disabilities because autonomy is not a possibility for them. This rejoinder, however, divorces disability from autonomy in a manner that is potentially deeply problematic and undoubtedly paternalistic.

The paradox has not gone unnoticed by political theorists. For example, Katharina Heyer (2011; see also Bagenstos 2006) examines potential legal and political consequences of the disability opposition's rejection of a right framed by its proponents as a fundamental liberty interest or a right to privacy. Heyer posits an inherent conflict between such anti-rights rhetoric and a global disability civil rights movement energized by an emphasis on the autonomy of people with disabilities (Degener 2013) and by aspirations for self-determination in regard to where and how people with disabilities live their lives (Harnacke and Graumann 2012).

This chapter explores tensions between end-of-life liberty and life course safety in regard to people with disabilities. We address the dilemma by demonstrating that its drivers are contextually nuanced and therefore conditional on contingencies about economic dependency and the lack of meaningful options for health care and social services, as well as on biased assessments about quality of life, suffering, and the likely efficacy of medical interventions. In this regard, we consider the potential for improving such circumstances, as well as whether doing so would help secure people with disabilities against any special dangers that practices of assisting dying may pose for them. We hope that dissolving the paradox in the ways we propose will provide an enlightening guide to a fair and safe approach for end-of-life practices.

People with Disabilities and Life-Ending Medical Practice: Compassion Misplaced?

Life-Ending Decision-Making

More than people in most other walks of life, medical professionals are positioned to influence or decide when others shall die. They can exercise this capacity in several ways: By not presenting options to patients or their decision makers because they are judged not medically indicated, by not initiating essential treatment or other life-sustaining support, by withdrawing previously provided treatment or life support, by arranging for patients' self-administration of lethal substances, or by actively undertaking fatal pharmaceutical or surgical interventions (Robinson et al. 2006). It is commonly supposed that there are circumstances in which death at a doctor's hands, through at least one of these means, is allowable and perhaps even advisable. But assisting dying in any of these ways is not free of moral or legal concerns.

The standard position about the legitimacy of end-of-life decisions is that they must be based on the patient's choices and values, so far as these are known, or the patient's best interests, when information is incomplete or completely missing about what the patient would have chosen. Concerning patients' interests, a core question is whether inhumane suffering will be the prevailing result of the intervention that extends the patient's life, so that the person himself would escape from further life if he could. Other questions may lurk in the background, less acknowledged but playing important roles in the decisions made. Is a decision not to intervene in such a circumstance motivated solely by what the patient would decide if she herself could act or refrain from acting, or by the patient's interests as perceived by the patient to the extent this is possible, rather than by someone else's judgment of what would be good for the patient? And, are decisions about what would be good for the patient influenced by physicians' interests, by reference to benefitting other individuals, or by considerations of the collective good?

When these further questions elicit a positive response, or even a hesitant moment of recognition, confidence that the patient's choices or best interests are the paramount incentives for ending life is clouded. Disability critiques of life-ending medical practice are especially trenchant because they contend that, at least in medical contexts, people with disabilities are systematically subjected to judgments that deny their own points of view. Life-ending action intended for the sake of someone else provokes suspicions that third-party judgments are being substituted for the patient's own choices and thus is especially challenging—perhaps impossible—to legitimize. If accurate, this complaint illustrates the challenges of securing autonomous life-ending decision-making for people with disabilities, and perhaps for others as well.

Euthanasia in the broadest sense includes intervening in dying and withdrawing or withholding care in order to intentionally and mercifully hasten death. Although distinctions between actions and omissions, or intention and foresight, are often drawn in this context,[1] the issues discussed below are similarly implicated across the spectrum of euthanasia broadly construed. Euthanasia is defined as benefitting individuals by offering them death. Euthanasia also may be thought to benefit whoever is burdened by, or otherwise disadvantageously implicated in, the lives of the aforementioned sufferers. Thus, euthanasia divides populations into two classes of people: Those who are supposed to benefit from their own quick deaths and those who are supposed to benefit from others' quick deaths. These benefits may be portrayed as aligned, with the relief of suffering of the patient also relieving burdens on others. History cautions, however, that such supposed alignment of interests may be self-serving on the part of the latter group and therefore spurious.

Euthanasia and Disability: Warnings from History

The history of euthanasia programs targeting people with disabilities stands as a warning about the threats life-ending practices pose to these individuals. While some such practices have been open, others have been carried on at the periphery of public scrutiny. For example, allowing neonates with Down syndrome or other congenital anomalies to die from lack of hydration/nutrition or basic therapeutic intervention was assumed to be good medical practice by some U.S. and U.K. physicians up until the last decade of the twentieth century (Wilkinson 2011; Wilkinson et al. 2006; Duff and Campbell 1973).

The Nazis conducted the most often cited and clearest example of euthanizing people because they were physically or mentally anomalous and deemed thereby to be disabled and unfit (Florida Center for Instructional Technology 2012). The formal program was presented as prompted by the best medical judgment, and the process included review of cases by committees of physicians (Gallagher 2001). Authorized by this program, physicians ordered people who were diagnosed with incurable illnesses, including those with impairments who were far from dying of natural causes, to be put to involuntary, but supposedly merciful, deaths. On October 6, 1939, Hitler issued an order to "relieve through death" those mentally ill individuals who could not "take any conscious part in life" (Schmidt 2007: ch. 5)

The Nazi program put people with disabilities to death against their interests and without their consent, under the guise of relieving their suffering but actually to relieve and thereby benefit non-disabled people who otherwise would have had to care for them. Other benefits were realized as well; for example, institutionalized individuals with psychiatric illnesses were euthanized to enable transition of mental hospitals into acute trauma facilities for wounded troops. At the Nuremberg trials, however, the physician who administered the Nazi program for euthanizing people with disabilities claimed explicitly that the standard of practice among medical professionals in all nations understood people with disabilities to be burdensome to themselves, their families, and society in general (Morris 1992).

Knowledge of this historical practice of euthanizing people with disabilities, by no means unique to the Nazis, fuels the disability critique of life-ending medical practice by evoking fear of medical professionals' self-serving or paternalistic assessments of the value of the lives of people with disabilities and the supposed benefits for them of relieving their suffering. Among the theoretically benevolent, but practically malignant, ideas that have been applied to people with disabilities, euthanasia probably is the most prominent. However, problematic judgments about the supposed unhappiness and poor quality of life of people with disabilities, as well as about the limited benefits of treatment for them, have generated support for decisions to withhold or to withdraw treatment that go far beyond practices of involuntary active euthanasia.

Judgments of Suffering and Quality of Life

Suffering

The Nazi contentions that people with disabilities would welcome relief from suffering were chillingly disingenuous. But from the point of view of the disability critique of end-of-life practices, they echo eerily in contemporary practices. Euthanasia in the Netherlands is premised on the justifiability of compassionate relief of intolerable suffering, when that is the patient's choice. The Swiss organization Dignitas announces on its web site that:

> Anyone suffering from an illness which will lead inevitably to death, or anyone with an unendurable disability, who wants voluntarily to put an end to their life and suffering can, as a member of DIGNITAS, request the association to help them with accompanied suicide.
>
> (Dignitas 2013)

Physicians in Belgium construed their euthanasia law as permitting the practice in the case of 45-year-old identical twins with deafness who judged the loss of their sight "unbearable" (Reuters 2013). An Irish High Court decision rejecting aid in dying as an autonomy right nonetheless invited prosecutors to avail themselves of the "fullest opportunity to consider . . . the special and extenuating factors arising from the harrowing experiences being endured by the plaintiff," a woman rendered largely immobile by multiple sclerosis and seeking assistance in dying.[2] But the assumptions that underlie these claims—that these judgments of intolerable suffering are accurate reflections of the patient's own experiences—are precisely what concern the disability advocates who oppose aid in dying.

In many court cases in the U.S., Canada, the U.K., and elsewhere, people with chronic or life-limiting illnesses have sought assistance in death as their autonomous choice, claiming that they would rather have their lives end than continue to endure their current suffering. In the U.S. in the 1980s, Elizabeth Bouvia, whose cerebral palsy and arthritis led her to want to cease eating, obtained a court order to prevent nutrition being forced on her.[3] Larry McAfee, a respirator-dependent quadriplegic, designed a device that enabled him to turn off his respirator independently; he obtained a ruling from the Georgia Supreme Court that he had the right to refuse continued ventilator support and to receive pain medication from physicians during the process of withdrawal (*New York Times* 1995).[4] In Quebec in 1992, a patient with paralysis from Guillain–Barré syndrome sought discontinuation of ventilator support, and the court agreed that she was a competent patient who had the right to refuse treatment.[5] In British Columbia in 1993, Sue Rodriguez unsuccessfully petitioned to enable a physician to provide a device permitting her to self-administer a lethal dose when she believed her motor neuron disease (MND) had reached an intolerable stage.[6] Also in British Columbia, in 2012 Gloria Taylor won an exemption from the principle of opposition to assisted suicide established in *Rodriguez*.[7] The British Columbia Supreme Court declared the equality rights of patients were infringed by treating differently patients who can refuse treatment and patients who require an active intervention to end their lives, an issue not reached in *Rodriguez*. The Court suspended its judgment for a year, granting the exception to Taylor, to allow for appeal as *Rodriguez* is binding Canadian Supreme Court precedent. Despite Taylor's death from an acute infection, the Canadian government is continuing the appeal (Global Montreal 2012).

The U.K. has also decided significant cases involving the decision to die by competent people with disabilities. In 2000, 19-year-old "AK," a patient with degenerative MND, won the right to have his ventilator removed when he became "locked in" and no longer able to communicate even by blinking (BBC News 2000). Another patient with MND, Diane Pretty, sought a legal shield against her husband's prosecution, should he help her to kill herself, but was not granted the shield in the U.K. courts or the European Court of Human Rights.[8] More recently, the British courts denied stroke patients Tony Nicklinson and "AM" assistance in dying (BBC News 2012).

The arguments pressed in court by many of those seeking aid in dying rest heavily on the intolerability of their circumstances. For example, the recent *Taylor* decision in British Columbia quotes expert witnesses on the moral importance of choosing relief from suffering:

> "[N]eedless suffering" should be avoided (Wayne Sumner).
>
> "[N]o one should be deprived of liberty or forced to suffer, without adequate cause" (Margaret Battin).

> "Nor do I think it is right to allow grievously and irremediably ill patients to suffer against their wishes if they are far from death but their suffering is protracted over time and life is no longer bearable to them as may be the case for bedridden individuals or those facing major loss of autonomy" (Dr Cohen).[9]

What, from the standpoint of observers, does suffering that makes life itself unbearable consist of? And from the standpoint of the suffering parties themselves, does such suffering make death appear the best choice? As we shall argue, inappropriate epistemic privileging of an observer standpoint over a sufferer standpoint, along with normative biases and contingencies of social injustice, shape these judgments of the nature and profundity of suffering (Silvers 1997). Attention is required to guard against special dangers assisted dying may pose for people with disabilities.

Quality of Life

A number of studies indicate the frequency with which the able-bodied project judgments concerning the poor quality of life of persons with disabilities (NCD 2009: 47; Adelman 2004; Boslaugh et al. 2009; Bryant and Fernandes 2010; McPhail and Haines 2011; Sandel 2011; White-Koning et al. 2008). Correlations between chronic conditions causing disability and perceived low quality of life are imperfect at best and may reflect remediable circumstances or depression (Patrick et al. 2000). Studies also document the increasingly positive or accepting views that many persons acquiring disabilities during their lives have to their circumstances (Patrick et al. 1997). But, particularly when held by physicians, disparaging views about the quality of life of people with disabilities may significantly influence life-ending decisions about continuing to receive treatment or withdrawing it.

In a recent essay in the *Hastings Center Review*, anthropologist William Peace, who has been paraplegic since 1978, reports how a physician approached him about consent to receive aggressive antibiotic treatment:

> What transpired after the nurse exited the room has haunted me. Paralyzed me with fear. The hospitalist . . . grimly told me I would be bedbound . . . most likely a year or more. . . . there was a good chance the wound would never heal . . . I would never sit in my wheelchair . . . I would never be able to work again . . . I was looking at a life of complete and utter dependence. My medical expenses would be staggering. Bankruptcy was . . . likely. Insurance would stop covering wound care well before I was healed. Most people with the type of wound I had ended up in a nursing home.
>
> This litany of disaster is all too familiar to me and others with a disability. The scenario laid out happens with shocking regularity to paralyzed people. The hospitalist went on to tell me I was on powerful antibiotics that could cause significant organ damage . . . Many paralyzed people die from such a wound.
>
> (Peace 2012: 14)

It's no accident that Peace chooses the word "litany"—a prolonged or tedious account—to characterize the "consenting" to which he was subjected. What he had to listen to while being "consented" are words prompted by a health care professional's compulsion to relieve his own discomfort about the dubiousness of success. The two have profoundly different perspectives on the risks involved. The physician measures the risk of a bad outcome, and the degree of badness this potential outcome bears, against his experience of patients generally. But Peace's attitude and assessment differ from the usual patient's. His life's history is one of overcoming intimidating odds, often painfully. He is expert at picking up and functioning even if treatment outcomes fall far short of optimal. To succeed, he knows, calls not only for determination, but also for the kind of hope the physician's litany seems aimed to destroy.

The ethical question is which view of Peace's future should prevail. It's hard to see why the prognosis should not be Peace's hopeful one, as it is epistemologically superior; his intentions not only best serve his interest but are better informed about achievable gain as the actual outcome—his recovery—shows. Peace and other people with disabilities like him (not all people with disabilities are like him, of course) are knowledgeable about themselves, are responsive to their specific physiological situation rather than to that of the typical patient, and are well informed about health dangers that might befall them as well as medical services they might need.

Individuals with chronic illness or disability often are experienced at functioning under adverse health conditions and thus have developed not only knowledge, but also adaptive skills, capacity to maintain morale, and endurance that surpass those of the "normal" patient. These are strengths that equally often health care professionals do not fully understand or appreciate. Consequently, these biased approaches to risk, and to restrictions on activity as well, can gnaw at patients' confidence in pursuing treatment and become further barriers to overcome.

Misplaced Judgments of Futility

Problematic judgments about quality of life are entangled with problematic judgments about medical futility. It is a principle of medical ethics that medically futile interventions need not be provided, absent strong countervailing reasons. Understanding this principle demands recognition that "futility" is a slippery concept. "Medical futility" in the strictest (and, we believe, most appropriate) sense should be reserved for interventions that simply will not work: An antimicrobial against an organism that is resistant to it, a blood transfusion for a person with an unrepaired aortic aneurism, or ventilator support for a patient whose lungs can no longer exchange oxygen at all. For purely physiological reasons, these interventions will not achieve their intended purpose. But medical futility in this sense is often blurred with concepts such as low probability, inability to alter underlying conditions that are judged to affect quality of life, or high cost (Schneiderman et al. 1990; Jecker 1995). Each of these latter conceptions involves a value judgment: How high a probability of success is needed to offset the risks of an intervention? Must goals of treatment address the patient's underlying condition in addition to the problem to which the intervention at hand is directed? Should costs be considered in treatment decisions, by whom, and in what ways? The American Medical Association's (2012) ethics opinion on futility in end-of-life care judges that "there are necessary value judgments involved in coming to the assessment of futility" and recommends a "due process" approach to futility judgments.

Conceptualized as physiological claims, judgments of medical futility must rely on the best scientific evidence. Unfortunately, disability rights advocacy may at times become entangled with problematic attitudes toward scientific evidence. For example, some advocates in the case of Teresa Marie Schiavo advanced questionable beliefs about the potential efficacy of hyperbaric therapy as well as refusals to believe the findings in autopsy reports about Schiavo's capacity for cognitive functioning (Francis and Silvers 2007).

This said, people with disabilities all too often find themselves subjected to harm from bias masquerading as scientific fact or from supposedly objective claims that are infected by conflicts of interest (NCD 2009: 10). Moreover, judgments of medical futility prompted by medical professionals' personal values and attitudes are especially problematic when decisions involve patients with disabilities. Patients or their personal representatives may be told by health care providers that interventions would be "futile," without disaggregation of whether this is a judgment of medical futility in the strict sense or some kind of additional value judgment that the intervention has a small probability of success, that it will not reach to an underlying disabling condition, or that it may be very costly in comparison to the likely benefits in overall quality of life to be achieved. But if patients or their representatives are to weigh what is at stake in recommendations about futility, these distinctions are exactly what they need to understand.

Autonomy and Loss of Self-Determination

In Oregon where physician-assisted suicide is permitted, most of those who seek it are not economically disadvantaged. For the most part, the same is true of euthanasia in the Netherlands. One recent study interviewed patients seeking aid in dying about their reasons for the request. Loss of independence and the desire for control over circumstances of dying (especially the ability to die at home) were paramount reasons (Pearlman et al. 2005). Also important were perception of self as a burden, the prospect of worsening pain or quality of life, and the inability to care for self. Physical symptoms such as pain or loss of bladder or bowel control were rated as much less important (Ganzini et al. 2009a, 2009b).

From the demography of choice in Oregon and the Netherlands, some scholars have concluded that, as practiced at present, assisted death presents little risk to the vulnerable in these jurisdictions (Battin 2008; Battin et al. 2007). The data about patients who seek active intervention in dying indeed do not indicate over-representation of patients who fall into selected "vulnerable" groups: The elderly, women, the uninsured (inapplicable in the Netherlands, where all are insured), people with low educational status, the poor, the physically disabled or chronically ill, minors, people with psychiatric illnesses including depression, or racial or ethnic minorities, compared with background populations. People with HIV/AIDS are over-represented, the only potentially vulnerable group identified. This research strategy, of searching for over-representation of members of vulnerable groups among those seeking active intervention, has limits, however. It does not identify ways in which problematic judgments such as those that underestimate quality of life, or those that exaggerate profundity of suffering, might be affecting non-treatment decisions more generally, including those of persons both within and outside of the groups identified as vulnerable.

It also looks only at the patterns with which intervention is obtained—the conclusions—and not at counter pressures that might, for a time, be functioning protectively for certain of these groups. Notably, the authors' discussion distinguishes between pre-existing disability (e.g., paralysis or chronic illness) and terminal illness (which surely also is a source of disability or vulnerability), arguing that there is no over-representation in the first group among those choosing aid in dying.

The core to the disability critique is that end-of-life practices only apparently reflect autonomous patient choice. If people with disabilities are subject to frequent negative judgments by others about their supposed quality of life, they may be coerced or deluded into embracing the view that their lives should not be prolonged. Compounding the assault of quality-of-life judgments on autonomy are the problematic social and economic circumstances in which many people with disabilities must lead their lives.

It is far from clear, however, whether such oppressive societal disregard prevents people from autonomously forming ideas of their good and thereupon exercising, attempting to exercise, or wishing they could exercise self-determination.

Recall the case of Larry McAfee, described in detail by Alicia Ouellette (2010). McAfee was a person with quadriplegia who required ventilator support. For almost a year after his accident, McAfee was able to live in an apartment near friends and family; round-the-clock nursing care was paid for by his Blue Cross insurance policy, his Social Security disability check, and his parents. When the private insurance ran out, McAfee became eligible for Medicare, which with Social Security disability payments and contributions from the hospital that cared for him in Georgia, paid for $650-a-day nursing home care. However, as there were no nursing homes in Georgia that would accept patients on ventilators (Applebome 1990), all McAfee could find for his care was an institution in Ohio. Eventually the Ohio nursing home decided that he should be discharged and he was sent to Grady Memorial Hospital in Atlanta, where he was placed in the ICU. Then the *Medicare Catastrophic Coverage Act*, which had been paying for McAfee's nursing home care, was repealed, and McAfee was faced with a shift to Medicaid, the health insurance plan for the poor, with payments substantially less than Medicare. Moreover, neither government program would pay for care in the community, outside an institution, even though the cost was substantially less than hospital care.

At this point, McAfee decided that he had had enough and sought the installation of a device that would enable him to turn off his own ventilator. "I've been moved from place to place with no say-so on why or where or how," he said. "I'm just tired of it. I'm fed up. I have no control over what's done to me, how it's done or by whom." A Georgia Superior Court judge decided in his favor and the Georgia Supreme Court affirmed.[10]

McAfee did not avail himself of the right to die he had won, however. As a result of the attention he gained by going to court, he was able to move to a nursing home in Birmingham, Alabama, where the director of the Injury Prevention Research Center at the University of Alabama assisted him in learning to operate adapted computer equipment. Subsequently, he moved again, this time to a personal care home in Augusta, where he lived until hospitalized with pneumonia, from which he died in 1995.

McAfee's story was made into a television drama in 1993. The theme was his conversion from choosing death to choosing life; the insight was the crucial role gaining some control over his living conditions played. By no means was McAfee's autonomy compromised by his socially devalued situation. His own idea of his good drove his campaign to regain self-determination over the details of his daily life. Absence of control is well known to be correlated with and to create anxiety, frustration, and despair (WomenWorld 2012). But whether an individual who is disabled experiences such hopelessness depends in part upon the person's social circumstances, and especially on whether the individual can command respectful living conditions or whether instead demeaning conditions are imposed either deliberately or through the impact of social policies and circumstances. McAfee's gaining more secure governance of his living conditions clearly shifted his choice from dying to living. The key to his choice to live was a change of circumstance that expanded his opportunity to self-determine his daily life (California Advocates for Nursing Home Reform 2010). But how to facilitate the requisite social responsiveness for disabled people generally remains a stubborn dilemma, as we explain more fully below.

Commanding funding for support services will alleviate despair in some circumstances, but not in all. For example, a reason frequently given by members of eligible populations for seeking physician-assisted suicide is the loss of dignity occasioned by not being able to perform intimate functions of ingestion and excretion in privacy by one's self. In this case, it is the presence of assistants rather than their absence due to lack of funding that is experienced by the person with a disability as powerlessness. So there are different ways of altering context to reduce the anxiety of dependence. In some cases, changing an individual's economic situation may do the trick but in others changing psychological or cultural attitudes will be more important.

These are all contingencies, even though of different kinds. As such, they can in principle be addressed and ameliorated. Dependence in its various forms is not necessarily a trigger for wanting to die, although for some individuals it may reasonably be. Individuals with disabilities who seek assistance to die may or may not be motivated by the constraints of their biological conditions, but by features of the social context. The patients with MND who went to court stated that they found declining physical functioning intolerable, especially without any control over means of potential escape. However, Larry McAfee sought to die because, while his post-injury physical state was stable, his economic support and his living situation, and therefore the texture of his experienced life, appeared to be plummeting in an unstoppable downward spiral.

People prefer to live at home and in communities they value; data are overwhelming that people with disabilities are no different in this respect (NCD 1997; Shapiro 1994). Yet U.S. health care and social services are structured counter-productively with respect to these goals. Many states have long waiting lists for community-based services. The result in these states is that the only way people can receive personal care services is to be institutionalized (Watson 2009). Long state waiting lists have survived challenges brought in court under the *Americans with Disabilities Act*, so long as states structure their programs reasonably in light of resources available and the needs of all with disabilities (Olmstead v. L.C., 527 U.S. 581 1999). Paul Longmore (1995) and other critics draw linkages between former Colorado Governor Richard Lamm's opposition to paratransit, needed by people with the most severe disabilities to travel outside their homes, and his opposition to providing for the educational needs of children with profound disabilities, to his views that constrained resources may portend recognition of a duty to die. Not surprisingly, some may find these circumstances intolerable. If state budget crises continue, the situation will be unlikely to improve and indeed may worsen as pressures on state funds continue to grow (Bird (2012) about Worcester, Massachusetts).

The U.S. is not alone in presenting challenges to those in need of home- and community-based services. The United Nations Convention on the Rights of Persons with a Disability, Article 19 (2008) provides for:

> the equal right of all persons with disabilities to live in the community, with choices equal to others, and . . . effective and appropriate measures to facilitate

> full enjoyment by persons with disabilities of this right and their full inclusion and participation in the community . . .

However, many nations appear not to meet this rights-based provision. To take one example, Parker and Fisher (2010) document the inadequacies of disability housing support in Australia. In the U.K., cost concerns have generated controversial proposals to cap expenditures for care at home (Murray 2012). Despite an overall government commitment to independent living, home care is funded by local authorities and access to services varies significantly (Department of Health (U.K.) 2012).

Conclusion

In this chapter, we have argued that the disability critique of current end-of-life practice is often exaggerated and paternalistic, but nevertheless raises issues that have not been well addressed in social policy. Epistemic problems are raised by the imposition of judgments (often in the guise of medical judgments), especially by medical professionals who are unqualified to judge the value of life with disability, or who are weighing in their own or third-party interests. In practice, the medical standpoint is given more weight than epistemic standards should permit. In addition, judgments of quality of life made about persons with disabilities may be invoked in ways that devalue the lives of such persons. Finally, the reality of lives faced by many people with disabilities—the absence of supports needed for them to have meaningful access to goods such as life in the community, the companionship of family and friends, or useful work—may lead people with disabilities to opt—apparently autonomously—for choices to forego care that are contingent on their remediable social circumstances. Dissolving the paradox embedded in the disability critique of assistance in dying thus requires changes in current epistemic, normative, and socio-economic practice, so that people with disabilities can be free of coercion and securely exercise the autonomy the medical system owes every individual alike.

Related Topics

Chapter 21, "Autonomy," Catriona Mackenzie
Chapter 22, "Capacity and Competence," Jessica Berg and Katherine Shaw Makielski
Chapter 32, "Reproductive Testing for Disability," Adrienne Asch and David Wasserman
Chapter 38, "End-of-Life Decisions for Newborns," Marian Verkerk and Hilde Lindemann

Notes

1 Vacco v. Quill, 521 U.S. 793 (1997).
2 Fleming v. Ireland, [2013] IEHC 2.
3 Bouvia v. Superior Court, 179 Cal.App.3d 1127, 225 Cal.Rptr. 297 (1986).
4 Georgia v. McAfee, 385 S.E. 2d 651 (Ga. 1989).
5 Nancy B. v. Hotel Dieu de Quebec (1992), 86 D.L.R. (4th) 385 (Que. S.C.).
6 Rodriguez v. British Columbia, [1993] 3 S.C.R. 519.
7 Carter v. Canada (Attorney General), [2012] B.C.J. No. 1196.
8 Pretty v. United Kingdom, [2002] European Court of Human Rights (4th Division).
9 Carter v. Canada (Attorney General), [2012] B.C.J. No. 1196, 165–172.
10 Georgia v. McAfee, 385 S.E.2d 651 (Ga. 1989).

References

Adelman, E.E.E. (2004) "Disparities in Perceptions of Distress and Burden in ALS Patients and Family Caregivers," *Neurology* 62 (10): 1766–70.

American Medical Association (2012) Opinion 2.037—Medical Futility in End-of-Life Care. Available at: http://www.ama-assn.org/ama/pub/physician-resources/medical-ethics/code-medical-ethics/opinion2037.page (accessed August 2, 2014).

Applebome, P. (1990) "An Angry Man Fights to Die, Then Tests Life," *New York Times* February 7. Available at: http://www.nytimes.com/1990/02/07/us/an-angry-man-fights-to-die-then-tests-life.html?pagewanted=all&src=pm (accessed August 2, 2014).

Bagenstos, S.R. (2006) "Disability, Life, Death, and Choice," *Harvard Journal of Law & Gender* 29: 425–63.

Battin, M.P. (2008) "Physician Assisted Dying and the Slippery Slope: The Challenge of Empirical Evidence," *Willamette Law Review* 45 (1): 91–136.

Battin, M.P., van der Heide, A., Ganzini, L., van der Wal, G. and Onwuteaka-Phillipsen, B.D. (2007) "Legal Physician-Assisted Dying in Oregon and the Netherlands: Evidence Concerning the Impact on Patients in 'Vulnerable' Groups," *Journal of Medical Ethics* 33 (10): 591–7.

BBC News (2000) "Motor Neuron Sufferer Wins Right to Die," August 11. Available at: http://news.bbc.co.uk/2/hi/health/875584.stm (accessed August 2, 2014).

BBC News (2012) "Tony Nicklinson right-to-die refused Court of Appeal hearing," October 2. Available at: http://www.bbc.co.uk/news/uk-england-wiltshire-19797634 (accessed August 2, 2014).

Bird, W., Jr (2012) "State Budget Cuts Devastate the Elderly," *GoLocalWorcester Reporter* [online], May 3. Available at: http://www.golocalworcester.com/news/budget-crisis-leaves-area-seniors-play-waiting-game/ (accessed August 2, 2014).

Boslaugh, S.E., Andresen, E.M., Reckfenwald, A. and Gillespie, K. (2009) "Evidence for Potential Bias in the Health and Activity Limitation Index as a Health Preference Measure for Persons with Disabilities," *Disability & Health Journal* 2 (1): 20–6.

Bryant, D. and Fernandes, N. (2010) "Measuring Patient Outcomes: A Primer," *Health and Quality of Life Outcomes* 10 (8): 65.

California Advocates for Nursing Home Reform (2010) "Physician Orders for Life Sustaining Treatment ('POLST'): Problems and Recommendations." Available at: http://www.canhr.org/reports/2010/POLST_WhitePaper.pdf (accessed August 2, 2014).

Coleman, D. (2010) "Assisted Suicide Laws Create Discriminatory Double Standard for Who Gets Suicide Prevention and Who Gets Suicide Assistance: Not Dead Yet Responds to Autonomy, Inc," *Disability and Health Journal* 3 (1): 39–50.

Degener, T. (2013) "Challenges and Compliance of the UN CRPD," forthcoming working paper of the European University Florence.

Department of Health (U.K.) (2012) *Caring for Our Future: Reforming Care and Support*. Available at: https://www.gov.uk/government/publications/caring-for-our-future-reforming-care-and-support (accessed August 22, 2014).

Dignitas (2013) http://www.dignitas.ch/index.php?option=com_content&view=article&id=6&Itemid=47&lang=en (accessed August 2, 2014).

Duff, R.S. and Campbell, A.G.M. (1973) "Moral and Ethical Dilemmas in the Special-Care Nursery," *New England Journal of Medicine* 289: 890–4.

Florida Center for Instructional Technology (2012) "A Teacher's Guide to the Holocaust: Extermination of People with Mental Disabilities," Letter from Dr Wurm, of the Wuerttemberg Evangelical Provincial Church, to Reich Minister of interior Dr Frick September 5 1940. Nazi Conspiracy and Aggression—Washington, U.S. Govt. Print. Off., 1946, Suppl. A, p. 1223. Available at: http://fcit.coedu.usf.edu/holocaust/resource/document/DocEuth.htm (accessed August 2, 2014).

Francis, L.P. and Silvers, A. (2007) "(Mis)framing Schiavo as Discrimination against People with Disabilities," *University of Miami Law Review* 61: 789–820.

Gallagher, H. (2001) "What the Nazi 'Euthanasia Program' Can Tell Us About Disability Oppression," *Journal of Disability Policy Studies* 12 (2): 96–9.

Ganzini, L., Gov, E.R., Dobscha, S.K. and Prigerson, H. (2009a) "Mental Health Outcomes of Family Members of Oregonians Who Request Physician Aid in Dying," *Journal of Pain & Symptom Management* 38 (6): 807–15.

Ganzini, L., Goy E.R. and Dobscha, S.K. (2009b) "Oregonians' Reasons for Requesting Physician Aid in Dying," *Archives of Internal Medicine* 169 (5): 489–92.

Global Montreal (2012) "Murder or Mercy? Euthanasia and Assisted Suicide in Canada," October 25. Available at: http://www.globalmontreal.com/timeline/6442457485/story.html (accessed August 2, 2014).

Harnacke, C. and Graumann, S. (2012) "Core Principles of the UN Convention on the Rights of Persons with Disabilities: An Overview," in J. Anderson and J. Phillips (eds.) *Disability and Universal Human Rights: Legal, Ethical, and Conceptual Implications of the Convention on the Rights of Persons with Disabilities*, Utrecht: Netherlands Institute of Human Rights.

Heyer, K. (2011) "Rejecting Rights: The Disability Critique of Physician Assisted Suicide," in A. Sarat (ed.) *Special Issue Social Movements/Legal Possibilities (Studies in Law, Politics, and Society, Volume 54)*, Bingley, UK: Emerald Group Publishing Limited, pp. 77–112.

Jecker, N.S. (1995) "Medical Futility and Care of Dying Patients," *Western Journal of Medicine* 163 (3): 287–91.

Longmore, P.K. (1995) "Medical Decision Making and People with Disabilities: A Clash of Cultures," *Journal of Law, Medicine & Ethics* 23: 82–7.

McPhail, S. and Haines, T. (2011) "Response Shift, Recall Bias and Their Effect on Measuring Change in Health-Related Quality of Life Amongst Older Hospital Patients," *Injury* 42 (3): 232–5.

Menzel, P.T. and Steinbock, B. (2013) "Advance Directives, Dementia, and Physician-Assisted Death," *Journal of Law, Medicine & Ethics* 41: 484–500.

Morris, J. (1992) "Tyrannies of Perfection," *The New Internationalist* (July 1): 16–17.

Murray, K. (2012) "Cap on Care at Home Could Force Under-65s into Institutions," *Guardian* [online], July 17. Available at: http://www.guardian.co.uk/society/2012/jul/17/social-care-disability (accessed August 2, 2014).

National Council on Disability (NCD) (1997) *Assisted Suicide: A Disability Perspective Position Paper*. Available at: http://www.ncd.gov/publications/1997/03241997 (accessed August 2, 2014).

National Council on Disability (NCD) (2009) *The Current State of Health Care for People with Disabilities*. Available at: http://www.ncd.gov (accessed August 2, 2014).

New York Times (1995) Larry McAfee, 39; Sought Right to Die (online), October 5. Available at: http://www.nytimes.com/1995/10/05/obituaries/larry-mcafee-39-sought-right-to-die.html (accessed August 2, 2014).

Ouellette, A. (2011) *Bioethics and Disability*, New York: Cambridge University Press.

Parker, S. and Fisher, K.R. (2010) "Facilitators and Barriers in Australian Disability Housing Support Policies: Using a Human Rights Framework," *Disability Studies Quarterly* 30 (3/4): 1283–310.

Patrick, D.L., Kinne, S., Engelberg, R.A. and Pearlman, R.A. (2000) "Functional Status and Perceived Quality of Life in Adults with and without Chronic Conditions," *Journal of Clinical Epidemiology* 53 (8): 779–85.

Patrick, D.L., Pearlman, R.A., Starks, H.E., Cain, K.C., Cole, W.G. and Uhlmann, R.F. (1997) "Validation of Preferences for Life-Sustaining Treatment: Implications for Advance Care Planning," *Annals of Internal Medicine* 127 (7): 509–17.

Peace, W.J. (2012) "Comfort Care as Denial of Personhood," *Hastings Center Report* 42 (4): 14–17.

Pearlman, R.A., Hsu, C. and Battin, M.P. (2005) "Motivations for Physician-Assisted Suicide," *Journal of General Internal Medicine* 20 (3): 234–9.

Reuters (2013) "Deaf Belgian Twins, 45, Helped to Die after Losing Sight." Available at: http://www.reuters.com/article/2013/01/14/us-belgium-euthanasia-idUSBRE90D0W620130114 (accessed August 2, 2014).

Robinson, E.M., Phipps, M., Purtilo, R.B., Tsoumas, A. and Hamel-Nardozzi, M. (2006) "Complexities in Decisionmaking for Persons with Disabilities Nearing End of Life," *Topics in Stroke Rehabilitation* 13 (4): 54–67.

Sandel, E.M. (2011) "Stroke, Disability, and Unconscious Bias: Interrelationships and Overdetermination in Medical Decisions," *Topics in Stroke Rehabilitation* 18 (1): 70–3.

Schmidt, U. (2007) *Karl Brandt: The Nazi Doctor—Medicine and Power in the Third Reich*, London: Hambleton Continuum.

Schneiderman, L.J., Jecker, N.S. and Jonsen, A.R. (1990) "Medical Futility: Its Meaning and Ethical Implications," *Annals of Internal Medicine* 112: 949–54.

Shapiro, J.P. (1994) *No Pity: People with Disabilities Forging a New Civil Rights Movement*, New York: Three Rivers Press.

Silvers, A. (1997) "Protecting the Innocents: People with Disabilities and Physician Assisted Dying," *Western Journal of Medicine* 166 (6): 407–9.

United Nations (2008) *Convention on the Rights of Persons with a Disability*. Available at: http://www.un.org/disabilities/default.asp?id=259 (accessed August 2, 2014).

Watson, S.D. (2009) "From Almshouses to Nursing Homes and Community Care: Lessons from Medicaid's History," *Georgia State University Law Review* 26 (3): 936–69.

White-Koning, M., Grandiean, H., Colver, A. and Arnaud, C. (2008) "Parent and Professional Reports of the Quality of Life of Children with Cerebral Palsy and Associated Intellectual Impairment," *Developmental Medicine & Child Neurology* 50 (8): 618–24.

Wilkinson, D.J. (2011) "A Life Worth Giving? The Threshold for Permissible Withdrawal of Life Support from Disabled Newborn Infants," *American Journal of Bioethics* 11 (2): 20–32.

Wilkinson, D.J., Fitzsimons, J.J., Dargaville, P.A., Campbell, N.T., Loughnan, P.M., McDougall, P.N. et al. (2006) "Death in the Neonatal Intensive Care Unit: Changing Patterns of End of Life Care Over Two Decades," *Archives of Disease in Childhood: Fetal & Neonatal* 91: F268–71.

WomenWorld (2012) "Health: Stress Mastery on the Job—Factors Leading to Increased Workplace Stress." Available at: http://womenworld.org/health/stress-mastery-on-the-job---factors-leading-to-increased-workplace-stress.aspx (accessed August 2, 2014).

38

END-OF-LIFE DECISIONS FOR NEWBORNS

Marian A. Verkerk and Hilde Lindemann

In *Neonatal Bioethics: The Moral Challenges of Medical Innovation*, John Lantos argues that neonatology should be viewed not as "one of the pinnacles of modern medical success, but instead as one of the best examples of modern medicine's moral ambiguity or hubris" (Lantos and Meadow 2008: 4). On the one hand, its successes cannot be denied: Every year in neonatal intensive care units (NICUs) around the world, thousands of newborns are saved who, had they been born 50 years ago, would have died. On the other hand, the cost to these infants in what might be years of suffering, disability, or fragile health can sometimes be so high that it might have been better had they not been saved. Then too, there are moral puzzles that arise in the NICU that have nothing to do with end-of-life decisions. Given the moral ambivalence that characterizes all the decisions that must be made, ethics is an inseparable part of neonatology. In this chapter we focus on end-of-life decisions, examining many of the considerations that matter morally when they must be made, paying special attention to recent developments in The Netherlands. We'll argue that the best ethical response to mortally ill newborns is to set treatment decisions into the context of palliative care.

A New Neonatal Ethics?

NICUs are a fairly recent medical innovation and an instance of scientific progress. Respirators, the routine use of surfactants to keep the baby's lungs working properly, and other relatively new biomedical technologies mark a kind of medical progress: They make it possible to save the lives of babies born as prematurely as 24 weeks' gestation, although with a considerable risk of damage to the lungs and brain. Such innovations do not necessarily give rise to new ethical complications, nor do they routinely give rise to dramatic, life-or-death moral dilemmas, but they do require an approach to ethics that can capture all the considerations that are salient in a given set of morally puzzling circumstances.

On our view, approaches that apply moral principles deduced from idealized moral theories to hard cases are not up to the task, as they leave us with guidance that is either too vague to be useful or so precisely specific that we would constantly have to wonder about legitimate exceptions. So we favor a neonatal ethics that draws on the best moral knowledge we can find in the actual world—where "best" means critically reflective, politically skeptical, and aimed at ways of life that are good for everyone concerned

(Walker 1998; Verkerk and Lindemann 2008). Because we conceive of morality as something the members of a moral community do together, we endorse an ethics that proceeds by means of conversations in which all those with a stake in the outcome try to reach a consensus about what should be done, from whose point of view it should be done, and who is responsible for doing it. The process of decision-making takes time and must be negotiated by all those involved. We will show how end-of-life decisions for newborns should be the result of exactly this collaborative morality: The medical team and the parents all deliberate to make the morally best response to an often very difficult situation focusing on the suffering of a newborn.

The Central Moral Question

The focus of this article is on the morality of end-of-life decisions for neonates. These include decisions about letting a newborn die or sometimes even deliberately killing them; they encompass deciding whether to withdraw or withhold treatment where the foreseen or intended outcome is the infant's death. Palliative sedation and other interventions to relieve suffering are also part of the palliative care process. Any decision about stopping or sustaining a neonate's life should be considered an end-of-life decision.

Health care professionals evaluate various kinds of decisions differently. Between one-third and two-thirds consider withdrawing treatment to be morally more serious than withholding treatment (Wilkinson 2013). Others act on what Wilkinson and Savulescu have dubbed the Equivalence Principle, which states that "other things being equal, it is permissible to withdraw a medical treatment that a patient is receiving, if it would have been permissible to withhold that same medical treatment and vice versa" (Wilkinson and Savulescu 2014: 128; see also Sulmasy and Sugarman 1994). While many bioethicists dismiss the moral distinction between withholding and withdrawing treatment as not ethically justified, one way the professionals' feelings can be explained is as a cognitive bias based in the perception that acts carry greater moral weight than omissions (Kordes de Vaal 1996; Baron and Ritov 2004). In any case, as long as there is a gap between ethical analysis and professional practice, there is something here that is worthy of investigation (Wilkinson and Savulescu 2014). It is worth asking whether professionals' feelings about this should be taken more seriously, as an indication that something morally more complex might be going on than bioethicists typically recognize.

The question, "Are we justified in ending this baby's life?" touches on several delicate and difficult issues. First of all, there is the question whether it is ever morally permissible to end any human life. The *sanctity of life* doctrine, usually defended with religious arguments, proclaims that all human life is sacred, no matter what its quality. So from a sanctity-of-life perspective, there can be no serious moral discussion about direct killing of infants. Some defenders of the doctrine find it morally permissible to withhold or withdraw "extraordinary means" of sustaining life—means that cause disproportionate amounts of suffering—but all partisans of this doctrine agree that it is wrong to act with the deliberate intention of ending the patient's life.

The sanctity-of-life view can be contrasted with a *quality of life* view, which does not recognize an absolute right to life or an absolute duty to preserve it, but rather judges whether a life is worth preserving (or having in the first place) in terms of its quality (see, among many others, Arras 1987). From this viewpoint, the end-of-life decision is shaped by at least three different considerations. (1) The medical intervention does not improve the situation; it isn't effective (this is a question about medical futility); (2) it might be effective, but it would cost the child and perhaps others too much to get to the improvement (this is a question about disproportionality); (3) the ultimate quality of life achieved would be very poor. So what we'll do now is focus on the quality of life, but also on the disproportionality of the intervention.

Consideration 1, about medical futility, can only be answered by physicians. Considerations 2 and 3 contain value judgments and raise three sets of moral issues: *How* we can decide someone's quality of life, *who* is to do the deciding, and *from whose point of view* the decision should be made. Newborns are not in a position to assess their own quality of life, so others will have to do this for them. The judgment could be a comparative one, from the point of view of the parents or the health professionals or both: "This level of quality is not good enough for anyone." More typically, however, the judgment is a non-comparative judgment based on the child's own subjective experience; it is made by taking the child's own point of view. So, for example, the parents might ask, "Is it in our baby's best interest to continue all these treatments if the outcome for her is an intolerable life?" Or the physicians might ask, "Is there any point to subjecting this neonate to painful treatments if his death is inevitable?" In addition, however, acting in the baby's interest may be legitimately constrained by other people's interests, or by considerations of justice. In such cases, the salient question from the parents might be, "Would it be permissible to keep our dying baby on a ventilator and morphine drip until tomorrow, when his grandparents from out of town arrive?" Or even, "We have five other young children at home and live too far away to manage the repeated surgeries you say our baby will need, if she survives at all. Is it fair to the others to devote all our resources to this baby?" In perhaps the saddest cases, the infant is so badly damaged that it may be said to have no interests at all, save the interest all humans have in being treated with respect (see McDougall and Notini 2013).

The Moral Status of the Newborn

How the treatment decision is made depends in part on the infant's moral status. The quality-of-life position presupposes that the infant has a moral status, but that fact alone does not tell us much. Moral status is sometimes discussed as if it were an all-or-none phenomenon: "Does Baby Doe have moral status?" But for those of us who share the intuition that older children and adults have a different moral status from, say, an infant born at 24 weeks' gestation, it arguably makes more sense to conceive of moral consideration as admitting of degrees, and for the appropriate question to be, "What moral status does Baby Doe have?" (Wilkinson 2011: 26; see also DeGrazia 2008). An important reason for considering the moral status of newborns differently is that their interest in their future wellbeing may be diminished by their reduced awareness of themselves, and of that future (McMahan 2002: 170). On this view, it is not future levels of wellbeing that determine the infant's moral status, but, rather, the other way around: The infant's moral status determines how we should take its future wellbeing into account (Wilkinson 2011: 26).

Quality of Life and Suffering

According to Great Britain's Nuffield Council on Bioethics, "It would not be in the baby's best interests to insist on the imposition or continuance of treatment to prolong the life of the baby when doing so imposes an *intolerable* burden on him or her" (Nuffield Council on Bioethics 2006: 12). There are at least three ethical difficulties here.

The first is that babies cannot judge for themselves when their suffering is so great as to be intolerable. Although they can have a somatic experience of pain (Fabrizi et al. 2011), they do not conceptualize it as pain, much less as their own pain. Slowly, as babies acquire a self, they also acquire a dimension that may be called "subjectivity"—the special understanding we have of ourselves as subjects of our lives, a sense of agency that arises out of the operation of our identities within the social world (Scully 2008). As they gain subjectivity, they develop a sense of a past and future. Then comes self-awareness: The pain the growing child feels becomes "my pain" (Kluge 2009). Only when the child becomes self-aware can she judge that her pain is intolerable.

This last point is connected with a second ethical worry. Even if pain seems to be measurable, and it seems fairly clear that neonates can experience pain, the idea of babies' suffering is complicated. According to Eric Cassel, suffering is "the state of severe distress associated with events that threaten the intactness of the person" (Cassell 1982). It is awareness of the disintegration, or the danger of disintegration, of one's sense of self. According to this definition, infants cannot suffer, as they do not yet have a sense of self.

However, there is a perfectly ordinary sense of the word in which one can suffer pain—just as one can suffer humiliation, cold, fools gladly, or the consequences. Babies, being babies, are severely limited in the range of things they can suffer, but they can certainly suffer from pain, air hunger, restricted mobility, and perhaps also isolation and fear. In this article, we use *suffering* in its more extended sense rather than in Cassell's restricted sense of the term.

Third, the experiential framework of the developing infant is not static—it extends into the future. The question, therefore, is whether we are to take into account only the neonate's current suffering, or whether we also have a reason to withhold or withdraw treatment if the infant is not suffering now but later will surely suffer unbearably, as can happen, for example, to babies born with necrotic bowel syndrome. Is it humane to keep such a baby alive until it begins to experience treatment as an intolerable burden? Because newborns lack subjectivity and self-awareness, they can have no conception of their future wellbeing, although their current state might be something they care about. So the decision whether to subject them to future unbearable suffering must be made by those who care for them.

On the line of argument we favor, any human being capable of expressing hunger, alertness, or some other mental state can and should be held in personhood—the special moral status we reserve for entities of our kind—by being treated the way we treat persons as opposed to the way we treat pets, plants, or inanimate objects (Lindemann 2002). But we also think that personhood admits of degrees. We contend that while extremely premature neonates are persons, and therefore cannot, for example, be killed merely for others' convenience, their hold on life is of such a short duration and so tenuous that they cannot properly be said to be persons in the fullest sense. Indeed, it takes interaction with many other persons over the first two years of life for even healthy children to participate completely in the human practice of personhood; before that, they depend on others to hold them in that status. This is not to imply that some persons are better than others or morally more valuable. Rather, it means that some persons have less at stake in their lives than others do, because they have only just started to live them.

Whose Interests?

Another question to be considered in end-of-life decision-making is, *whose* interests count? Parents are ordinarily the initiators and major contributors to the long process by which their children attain selfhood, enveloping their children with their own sense of what matters and what does not, what one must do, what is forbidden, what is admirable, and in general, how life is to be lived. The parental selves are the closest thing the newborn has to a self of its own. When parents make decisions about the treatment of babies who are very badly damaged, then, they do not and should not decide on the basis of some impersonal and impartial best-interests standard. They do it out of the relationship that holds this particular baby inside the value structure of these particular parents. This could be the basis for an argument that the parents—at least, if they are decent, engaged, and loving parents—have the greatest authority to decide about the infant's quality of life. But parents are not the only players here. The physicians and other health care professionals involved in the care of the infant are also moral agents, and their knowledge and experience of end-of-life care generally surpasses that of the parents. If the parents have unrealistic expectations or make morally dubious demands on the staff, their authority to decide what should be done is diminished, and the health care professionals should base their decisions on the interests of the child.

The Groningen Protocol

Especially relevant to quality-of-life discussions regarding newborns is the Groningen Protocol, which lays out the conditions for legally tolerated infanticide in The Netherlands. The protocol allows doctors, at parental request, to kill neonates if they are experiencing unbearable suffering. This form of infanticide can be distinguished from the active withdrawal of life-sustaining medical care (an intentional act, often referred to as an omission, that kills), which is a standard part of the care of newborns with severe disability and suffering in the U.K., the U.S., the rest of Europe, and nearly all of the world, and which is sometimes called passive euthanasia.

To explain the practice the protocol governs, it is important to draw distinctions among categories of newborns for whom euthanasia might be ethically justified. Eduard Verhagen and Pieter Sauer, the two pediatricians at the University Medical Center in Groningen most intimately involved in developing and publicizing the protocol, distinguish three groups.

Group 1 consists of newborns with no chance of survival. Typically, they have a fatal disease such as severe lung or kidney hypoplasia (the organ is badly underdeveloped), and can only live for one or two days. They are put on life support immediately after birth while their physicians determine the extent of the damage. Once it is clear that treatment is useless, life support is removed. However, if the baby does not die immediately, the doctors may feel they should intervene directly to end the infant's life. Because infants belonging to group 1 cannot live very long no matter what, the decision concerns only the time of dying, not whether it is better for the newborn to die. They will die soon in any case. For that reason, no quality-of-life judgments are needed for this group.

Group 2 comprises neonates who "may survive after a period of intensive treatment, but expectations regarding their future condition are very grim" (Verhagen and Sauer 2005b: 959). This category includes infants with severe brain abnormalities or extensive organ damage caused by lack of oxygen. The dilemma for professionals is whether such an infant is so badly off that death is preferable. If neither withholding nor withdrawing intensive treatment will end the infant's life quickly, many Dutch physicians would feel compelled to intervene directly and kill the infant. In the U.S. this would count as a serious breach of medical ethics, as it also would in the U.K. The Nuffield Council makes it very clear that "the active ending of neonatal life even when that life is 'intolerable' is rejected" (Nuffield Council on Bioethics 2006: 20). But in The Netherlands, there seems to be moral room for this option, perhaps because physicians there feel that, having subjected the neonate to intensive medical treatment, they are responsible for extricating it from its present predicament. The end-of-life decision for a group 2 baby is not merely about *when* death should occur, as it is for babies in group 1, but also about the infant's quality of life: Would this baby be better off dead than forced to endure the only kind of life it can ever have?

While actively ending the life of group 2 babies is not morally countenanced in most countries, from the Dutch point of view the controversy centers on group 3. This group is made up of babies with an extremely poor prognosis "who do not depend on technology for physiologic stability and whose suffering is severe, sustained, and cannot be alleviated" (Verhagen and Sauer 2005a: 736). These infants are not and never were dependent on intensive medical treatment. In fact, with proper care, some of them can survive for many years, even into adulthood. A prime example would be a baby with epidermolysis bullosa, which, at its most severe, covers the entire body with fluid-filled blisters, creating continual scarring that fuses the fingers and toes as well as making it terribly difficult to swallow. Progressive paralysis, permanent inability to communicate in any way, and complete lifelong dependency might be other examples of conditions severe enough to put a baby in this group.

Although the decision for group 3 has given rise to the most controversy, the Groningen Protocol, developed in 2002, is applicable to all three groups. It consists of two sections, one setting out the conditions necessary for euthanasia to be performed in a responsible manner, and the other detailing the kinds of records that should be kept "to clarify the decision and facilitate assessment" (Verhagen and Sauer 2005a: 738). The committee that created this standard borrowed heavily from the "due care" criteria that in The Netherlands serve as moral and legal safeguards for physicians who perform active voluntary euthanasia on adults, but they also relied on previous court decisions in which doctors were acquitted in two cases: One dealt with a newborn who had an extreme form of spina bifida (a neural tube defect in which the fetal spinal column fails to close in the first month of pregnancy, causing nerve damage and permanent disability) and the other a severe trisomy 13 (a disorder in which a baby's extra genetic material interferes with normal development, causing over 80 percent of those who have it to die within the first year). Despite the palliative care these infants received, they endured intense suffering that ended only when doctors gave them lethal drugs. "The courts accepted," wrote Verhagen and Sauer, "that the physicians had to choose between the duty to retain life (and accept the severe suffering) and the duty to limit the suffering (and end the life of the child). They considered the choice to end the life of the infants justified because there was no alternative" (Verhagen and Sauer 2005a: 738). Strictly speaking, of course, there was an alternative—to let the child suffer—but the physicians clearly thought it was morally unacceptable. In both court cases, the decision to end life was made only after the decision to withdraw all other medical treatments had been made.

According to the Groningen Protocol, direct physician killing of a neonate is legally justifiable only under these conditions: (1) The diagnosis and prognosis must be certain; (2) hopeless and unbearable suffering must be present; (3) the diagnosis, prognosis, and unbearable suffering must be confirmed by at least one independent doctor; (4) the parents must give informed consent; (5) the procedure must be performed in accordance with the accepted medical standard. The diagnosis, decision to end the baby's life, consultation, and implementation must be fully documented; after the death, similar documentation must include the coroner's findings, how the death was reported to the prosecutor's office, how the parents are being counseled and supported, the case review, postmortem examination, and genetic counseling.

Problems with the Groningen Protocol

The publication of the protocol in the English-language press in 2005 created a small uproar. The criticisms—which were not so much of the protocol itself as of its complicity in countenancing non-voluntary euthanasia in a highly vulnerable patient population—can be divided roughly into two sets of claims: That infanticide is wrong, and that end-of-life decisions should never be based on judgments of another person's quality of life. It was claimed, for example, that the protocol allows parents to commit infanticide as a way of escaping the responsibility to give their child burdensome care (Chervenak et al. 2006). Quality-of-life concerns included the accusation that the protocol permits doctors to make judgments of what kind of life is acceptable, and that it targets mainly neonates with spina bifida, even though such children often have quite a decent quality of life (Chervenak et al. 2006; Curlin 2005). In addition, the criteria for determining quality of life were criticized as incoherent because they included "unbearable suffering," even though newborns cannot suffer (Chervenak et al. 2006; Jotkowitz and Glick 2006). Other charges were that the protocol fails to distinguish with clinical precision between neonates who will surely die and those who could continue to live (Chervenak et al. 2006), and that it leaves "doctors alone determining the morality of their actions" (Jotkowitz and Glick 2006: 157).

Here we focus on the quality-of-life criticisms. The protocol requires that "hopeless and unbearable suffering" be present, but hopelessness worries some critics of the protocol because it seems far too subjective for ending the life of another human being. Jack's reason for losing hope might be Jill's reason to press on; what seems hopeless to him may encourage her not to give up. We believe that the brunt of this criticism can be deflected by considering the Dutch word from which the English one was translated. That word is *uitzichtloos*, which literally means "outlook-less," or, in better English, "without prospect." While not all are hopeful who have reason to hope, and some continue to hope against all reason, agreement can be reached concerning a baby's prospects for improvement. It is true that the determination that there is no prospect is a judgment, not a self-evident fact, but it is a judgment that will have been based on clinical data and medical expertise, and it will have been confirmed by a second, independent opinion.

The harder quality-of-life judgment to establish is that of *unbearable suffering*. How can Jack know what Jill cannot bear unless she tells him, and if she is a newborn baby, how can she tell him? And then, what is it she cannot bear? Pain? Total lifelong dependency? Lack of any capacity for communication? Progressive paralysis resulting in total immobility? She might find in retrospect that she can, after all, bear what in prospect seemed so unbearable. And while some have collapsed under the slightest burden, others have borne a very great deal indeed. In the face of all these considerations, surely some argue that none of us has the right to judge another's quality of life.

But quality-of-life judgments for others cannot be evaded—we make them all the time. The routine use of life-sustaining technologies requires that comparative judgments be made as to whether the quality of life the technologies sustain is good enough to be continued. It is one of the harsh realities of twenty-first-century medicine that these judgments must be made. There is something disingenuous about pretending that we do not already make them, not only for competent adults but also for newborn babies.

After the Upheaval

While the Dutch euthanasia law was passed in 2001, exempting from prosecution doctors who followed the "due care" criteria for administering euthanasia to competent adults, the government was reluctant to extend the same exemption in cases of non-voluntary euthanasia. However, because of the international attention the Groningen Protocol attracted in 2005, the government decided to keep the direct killing of newborns illegal but to set up a review committee similar to the ones that already reviewed cases of voluntary adult euthanasia. It was expected that several cases would be reported annually. To date, however, it appears that only one case has been brought to the review committee's attention (Buiting et al. 2010).

While there may be a number of explanations for this, the most plausible is that the introduction in 2006 of ultrasound at 20 weeks' gestation has probably resulted in higher detection rates of congenital abnormalities, which seems to have led to more such fetuses being aborted. The fact that the number of abortions per 1000 live births is still rising in The Netherlands supports this assumption (Buiting et al. 2010). We note in passing that the decision to abort for these reasons is no more exempt from quality-of-life judgments than are end-of-life decisions for neonates.

The Role of Culture

It could be argued that active physician intervention to end the lives of profoundly damaged neonates is ethically permissible, if at all, only in a culture whose institutions and practices are morally sound. It matters, for example, that Dutch people enjoy a fairly robust social safety net, including universal access to health care. Possibly as a result of this, they are much more inclined to trust their health care system, and their own doctors, than are people in, say, the U.S. Moreover, since there is good reason to suspect that physicians everywhere occasionally feel compelled to end an infant's dreadful suffering even if they must do so surreptitiously, the Dutch attempt at transparency and accountability here might strike skeptics as admirable. In these and other ways, the ethical permissibility of direct physician killing of severely damaged neonates can be relativized to specific cultures (Lindemann and Verkerk 2008; for another view, see Swinton and Lantos 2010). Not every society, then, should permit physicians directly to hasten the death of its most severely afflicted infants. Even within a particular society, there may be a number of different hospital cultures, not all of them, perhaps, morally suited to this extreme measure for ending the worst neonatal suffering.

Palliative Care for Neonates

As a result of the Groningen Protocol there has been an increased awareness in The Netherlands of the importance of palliative care for neonates. According to the World Health Organization:

> Palliative care is an approach that improves the quality of life of patients and their families facing the problem associated with life-threatening illness, through the prevention and relief of suffering by means of early identification and impeccable assessment and treatment of pain and other problems, physical, psychosocial and spiritual.
>
> (World Health Organization 2001)

Yet while palliative and hospice care are well recognized options for adult patients (even if, in practice, patients do not always receive this care when it would do the most good), health care professionals have been slow to adopt palliative measures for the pediatric population (Romesberg 2007). As with adults, its use for children and neonates encompasses the care of families.

In June 2013, the Royal Dutch Medical Association (RDMA) issued a position paper on end-of-life decisions for newborns. In this paper they stress the idea that end-of-life decisions for neonates should be made within the context of palliative care, a form of caregiving that is a process that unfolds over time. The decision to end the baby's life should therefore not be considered in isolation, but as one that takes its shape and meaning from the ongoing process of giving care when an infant is desperately ill.

Most end-of-life decisions start with decisions about withholding or withdrawing treatment, but it is important that parents realize what will happen after that. Sometimes the dying process will take time—often more time than the family imagined. Sometimes the baby experiences discomfort or pain. When that happens, palliative sedation or muscle relaxants can be an option. Interestingly, the RDMA suggests that when the dying process is a lengthy one, muscle relaxants may be given to hasten death, not so much to end the baby's discomfort as to ease the distress of the parents who are witnessing it. Here the ethos of palliative care is particularly visible, as the ambit of care extends beyond the neonatal patient to the suffering family.

Palliative care requires great skill, sensitivity, and compassion, imposing obligations regarding both decision-making and caregiving on the professional staff. Obligations in decision-making include communicating clearly with parents and other health team members and engaging in fully shared decision-making with parents. Obligations in caregiving include providing options, preparing parents, being with, advocating, creating peace and normalcy, and providing comfort (Epstein 2010: 582–5).

Unfortunately, most doctors and nurses working in NICUs are not required to learn how to give palliative care and have severely limited access to caregivers who are specially trained in such care (Nuffield Council on Bioethics 2006). This needs to change. Good empirical research on the effect of palliative sedation, muscle relaxants, and other palliative measures on neonates is also badly needed, as is a neonatal ethics that specifically includes an important role for families. If NICUs are to divest themselves of the moral ambiguity that currently characterizes them, they must do a better job of not merely saving babies' lives, but also abiding with, comforting, and caring for the suffering ones who cannot or should not be saved.

Related Topics

Chapter 36, "From the Persistent Vegetative State to the Minimally Conscious State: Ethical Implications of Disorders of Consciousness," Joseph J. Fins
Chapter 37, "Disability and Assisted Death," Leslie P. Francis and Anita Silvers

Bibliography

Arras, J.D. (1987) "Quality of Life in Neonatal Ethics: Beyond Denial and Evasion," in W. Weil and M. Benjamin (eds.) *Ethical Issues at the Outset of Life*, Boston, MA: Blackwell Scientific Publications, pp. 151–86.
Baron, J. and Ritov, I. (2004) "Omission Bias, Individual Differences and Normality," *Organic Behavior in Humans Dec Proc* 94: 74–85.
Bellieni, C. (2005) "Pain Definitions Revised: Newborns Not Only Feel Pain, They Also Suffer," *Ethics and Medicine: An International Journal of Bioethics* 21 (1): 5–9.
Bellieni, C., Bagnoli, F. and Buonocore, G. (2003) "Alone No More: Pain in Premature Children," *Ethics and Medicine: An International Journal of Bioethics* 19 (1): 5–10.
Buiting, H.M., Karelse, M.A.C., Brouwers, H.A.A., Onwuteaka-Philipsen, B.D., van der Heide, A. and van Delden, J.J.M. (2010) "Dutch Experience of Monitoring Active Ending of Life for Newborns," *Journal of Medical Ethics* 36 (4): 234–7.
Cassell, E. (1982) "The Nature of Suffering and the Goals of Medicine," *New England Journal of Medicine* 306: 639–45.
Chervenak, F.A., McCullough, L.B. and Arabin, B. (2006) "Why the Groningen Protocol Should Be Rejected," *Hastings Center Report* 36 (5): 30–3.
Curlin, F.A. (2005) "Letter to the Editor," *New England Journal of Medicine* 352: 2354.
DeGrazia, D. (2008) "Moral Status as a Matter of Degree?" *Southern Journal of Philosophy* 46 (2): 181–98.
Epstein, E.G. (2010) "Moral Obligations of Nurses and Physicians in Neonatal End-of-Life Care," *Nursing Ethics: An International Journal for Health Care Professionals* 17 (5): 577–89.
Fabrizi, L., Slater, R., Worley, A., Meek, J., Boyd, S., Olhede, S. et al. (2011) "Shift in Sensory Processing that Enables the Developing Human Brain to Discriminate Touch from Pain," *Current Biology* 21: 1552–8.
Janvier, A., Bauer, K.L. and Lantos, J.D. (2007) "Are Newborns Morally Different from Older Children?" *Theoretical Medicine and Bioethics: Philosophy of Medical Research and Practice* 28 (5): 413–25.
Jotkowitz, A.B. and Glick, S. (2006) "The Groningen Protocol: Another Perspective," *Journal of Medical Ethics* 32: 157–8.
King, N.M.P. (1992) "Transparency in Neonatal Intensive Care," *Hastings Center Report* 22 (2): 18–25.
Kipnis, K. (2007) "Harm and Uncertainty in Newborn Intensive Care," *Theoretical Medicine and Bioethics: Philosophy of Medical Research and Practice* 28 (5): 393–412.
Kluge, E.W. (2009) "Quality-of-Life Considerations in Substitute Decision-Making for Severely Disabled Neonates: The Problem of Developing Awareness," *Theoretical Medicine and Bioethics: Philosophy of Medical Research and Practice* 30 (5): 351–66.
Kordes-de Vaal, J.H. (1996) "Intention and the Omission Bias: Omissions Perceived as Nondecisions," *Acta Psychologia* (Amst) 93: 161–72.
Lagercrantz, H. (2007) "The Emergence of the Mind: A Borderline of Human Viability?" *Acta Paediatrica* 96: 327–8.
Lantos, J. and Meadow, W. (2008) *Neonatal Bioethics: The Moral Challenges of Medical Innovation*, Baltimore, MD: Johns Hopkins University Press.
Lindemann, H. (2002) "What Child Is This?" *Hastings Center Report* 32 (6): 29–38.
Lindemann, H. and Verkerk, M.A. (2008) "Ending the Life of a Newborn: The Groningen Protocol," Hastings Center Report 38 (1): 42–51.
McDougall, R.J. and Notini, L. (2014) "Overriding Parents' Medical Decisions for Their Children: A Systematic Review of Normative Literature," *Journal of Medical Ethics* 40: 448–52.
McMahan, J. (2002) *The Ethics of Killing: Problems at the Margins of Life*, New York: Oxford University Press.
Nuffield Council on Bioethics (2006) "Critical Care Decisions in Fetal and Neonatal Medicine," November. Available at: http://nuffieldbioethics.org/project/neonatal-medicine/ (accessed August 22, 2014).
RDMA (2013) "KNMG-standpunt Medische beslissingen rond het levenseinde bij pasgeborenen met zeer ernstige afwijkingen, Koninklijke Nederlandsche Maatschappij tot bevordering der Geneeskunst."
Romesberg, T.L. (2007) "Building a Case for Neonatal Palliative Care," *Neonatal Network: The Journal of Neonatal Nursing* 26 (2): 111–15.

Ross, L.F. (2007) "The Moral Status of the Newborn and Its Implications for Medical Decision Making," *Theoretical Medicine and Bioethics: Philosophy of Medical Research and Practice* 28 (5): 349–55.
Scully, J.L. (2008) *Disability Bioethics: Moral Bodies, Moral Difference*, Lanham, MD: Rowman and Littlefield.
Sulmasy, D.P. and Sugarman, J. (1994) "Are Withholding and Withdrawing Therapy Always Morally Equivalent?" *Journal of Medical Ethics* 20: 218–22; discussion 23–4.
Swinton, C.H. and Lantos, J.D. (2010) "Current Empirical Research in Neonatal Bioethics," *Acta Paediatrica* 99 (12): 1773–81.
Verhagen, A.A., Dorscheidt, J.H., Engels, B., Hubben, J.H. and Sauer, P.J. (2009) "End-of-Life Decisions in Dutch Neonatal Intensive Care Units," *Archives of Pediatric and Adolescent Medicine* 163: 895–901.
Verhagen, E. and Sauer, P.J. (2005a) "End-of-Life Decisions in Newborns: An Approach from the Netherlands," *Pediatrics* 116: 736–9.
Verhagen, E. and Sauer, P.J. (2005b) "The Groningen Protocol: Euthanasia in Severely Ill Newborns," *New England Journal of Medicine* 352: 959–62.
Verkerk, M.A. and Lindemann, H. (2008) "Epilogue: Naturalized Bioethics in Practice," in H. Lindemann, M.A. Verkerk and M. Walker (eds.) *Naturalized Bioethics: Toward Responsible Knowing and Practice*, New York: Cambridge University Press.
Walker, M. (1998) *Moral Understandings: A Feminist Study in Ethics*, New York: Routledge.
Wilkinson, D.J. (2011) "A Life Worth Giving? The Threshold for Permissible Withdrawal of Life Support from Disabled Newborn Infants," *American Journal of Bioethics* 11 (2): 20–32.
Wilkinson, D.J. (2013) "Which Newborn Infants Are Too Expensive to Treat? Camosy and Rationing in Intensive Care," *Journal of Medical Ethics* 39: 502–6.
Wilkinson, D.J. and Savulescu, J. (2014) "A Costly Separation Between Withdrawing and Withholding Treatment in Intensive Care," *Bioethics* 28: 127–37.
World Health Organization (2001) "WHO Definition of Palliative Care." Available at: http://www.who.int/cancer/palliative/definition/en/ (accessed August 2, 2014).

Part VIII

EMBODIMENT

The human body is at the center of some of the most challenging debates in bioethics, yet is rarely singled out as a topic of discussion in itself. This section attempts to bring together a number of issues regarding the ways in which human bodies are perceived, understood, treated, and imagined in health and health care settings. Two themes emerge from the chapters in this section. The first is the difficulty of defining the topics being explored here. Rebecca Kukla's chapter, for example, reminds us that although everyone has an intuitive idea of what "health" is, there exists no rigorous definition of it. The term "enhancement" can be applied to everything from cosmetic procedures and neuroscientific interventions to efforts to improve one's moral capacity or status. The concept of "transgender" is just as fluid, and the question of how and whether someone can label a being along gender lines informs the ethical analysis of transgender issues.

This trouble with labeling, diagnosing, and even studying how beings see themselves as selves—how they are embodied—leads to the second theme: The importance of social justice. The limitations the authors in this section see in narrow or outmoded approaches to their topics tend to result from a lack of attention to justice considerations. In her chapter on race and bioethics, for example, Alexis Shotwell finds traditional understandings of "race" and "racism" simplistic because they fail to account for the social contexts in which those terms arose and continue to manifest themselves. And Nikki Sullivan's chapter criticizes traditional bioethical thinking for being too narrow to humanely and justly reckon with newer issues of embodiment, such as those surrounding body integrity and gender identity disorders.

The chapters in this section demonstrate that there are as many ways of thinking about embodiment as there are thinkers about it. And because one cannot think about the body without also thinking about the condition—the health—of that body, it is fitting that the opening chapter establishes a solid account of how "health" should be understood. The institutional definition of health Kukla develops accommodates current concepts of ill- and wellbeing while shedding the theoretical or practical motivations behind many accounts of those concepts. More than a purely biological/functional or purely social constructionist way of defining the term, Kukla's institutional account places health firmly within the context of collective wellbeing and presumes that bodies function *only* within a material environment; the result is a definition that automatically incorporates the social considerations that are essential to a just state. As she tests the institutional account on the problematic diagnostic label of gender dysphoria, Kukla provides a guide to understanding health and disease theory that is especially illuminating for the five chapters that follow hers.

Human enhancement is an increasingly controversial topic in bioethics, as technology continues to make real what was once only imaginable. Nicholas Agar and Felice Marshall propose a way of understanding enhancement that is broad enough to encompass the ethical intricacies of the different means, degrees, and targets of enhancement. The first part of their pluralist conception, enhancement through the alteration or selection of genetic material, has been the traditional focus of bioethicists. Yet that focus has meant that other ways of considering enhancement have been overlooked; thus, the second part of their definition of enhancement: Modification or alteration through environmental means (prostheses, neuroenhancement, even education). The authors then offer a "human enhancement consistency test" to help sort through the ethical issues surrounding the enhancement debate, from how to define the term to whether it is ever ethically permissible to enhance beyond human norms. According to the consistency test, a practice or procedure is ethical if it is comparable to—consistent with—a practice or procedure that has already been deemed ethical. Agar and Marshall apply the test to several scenarios, acquainting readers with historical and contemporary enhancement arguments, both pro and con, along the way. Proponents of genetic modification, for instance, would do well to remember last century's eugenics movement, while defenders of morally enhanced "post-persons" must keep in mind concepts of human moral status and where they situate humans among all living beings. This latter concern also arises in Fredrik Svenaeus's discussion of the ethics of organ transplantation, in which he wonders whether those who undergo radical moral enhancement ("those who have left the current limits of human embodiment behind") will possess traditional human ethics at all.

Many of the underpinnings of bioethics are interwoven with cultural and legal ideas of race. Alexis Shotwell and Ami Harbin employ the concept of "racialization," the process through which groups come to be identified as racial groups, to describe *how* bioethics and race are entwined. Using the syphilis study in Tuskegee as a backdrop, the authors show that although bioethicists have long known that race matters in every scholarly and professional endeavor, they have failed adequately to explore the ways in which it matters. Bioethicists must both move beyond simple biological constructs of race and racism (evil white doctors exploiting vulnerable black sharecroppers) and see that racial sensitivity is much more than cultural competency. They must acknowledge and evaluate the morality of an era's prevailing systems of inequality; failure to do so can let an entire unjust system off the hook. This mode of thinking is important if the field of bioethics is to successfully confront implicit bias and stereotyping that occurs in certain sectors of health care, and it is essential if bioethicists are to understand how modern technologies (such as biobanking) intersect with racialization.

Jamie Lindemann Nelson also urges bioethicists to expand their traditional ways of thinking. Like the simplistic constructs of race that Shotwell and Harbin take to task, traditional ethical queries about transgender issues have tended to focus on the medical arena—pondering the morality of doctors "doing harm" on healthy tissue, performing "gender normalization" procedures. This has left unexplored how transgender people identify themselves, how the medical and mental health fields consider them (and whether they should be subjects of their consideration in the first place), and what can even be regarded as an "authentic" embodiment of one's gender. Bioethical thinking would have been especially welcome, Nelson argues, in discussions of stigma resulting from transgender-oriented research, whether gender dysphoria ought to be classified as a mental disorder, and the contemporary and rapidly evolving moral issues, such as those surrounding transgender parenthood. He also questions, however, whether the time for bioethics' influence has passed, as some transgender people today have achieved political power similar to that of the disability movement and may not need bioethicists to advocate for them against, say, the medical establishment. Still, Nelson sees a place for the bioethicist—not as an analyst of transgender issues but as a contributor to ongoing conversations about them.

Fredrik Svenaeus's development of a guide to ethical thinking about organ transplantation incorporates the themes raised throughout this section. First, transplantation touches on virtually every bioethical principle (notions of consent; the ethics of buying and selling organs and "living" donations, including the medical profession's role in removing healthy tissue; definitions of death and the interests of potential donors; and what, if anything, we may owe fellow humans in need of organs). Second, the ethics of organ transplantation cannot be investigated independent of considerations of embodiment. Once again the problem of definition arises: Are our organs commodities that we own, or do they comprise who we are? Svenaeus favors the latter view, which he calls a phenomenological idea of selfhood. It allows an understanding of self as something connected to others; organs, then, are identity-bearing parts of the processes of selfhood, and donation can be regarded as a humane act of sharing a gift rather than a commercial enterprise.

The section concludes with a discussion of body integrity identity disorder (BIID), defined by Nikki Sullivan as the feeling of non-contiguity between the body and the self. By exploring desires for elective amputation, Sullivan surveys the ethics of "non-normative"-embodiment desires—for amputation, varying degrees of paralysis, deafness, blindness, and the like—and strives to lay bare troublesome assumptions of "conventional bioethics," including classic bioethics principles and definitions of "disability" and "normal." Sullivan asks ethicists to step back and take a meta-analytical view of BIID, questioning, for example, why it is that a disability is automatically considered undesirable. This inquisitive orientation, as opposed to more results-driven approaches, can foster a more expansive and humane way of understanding BIID. Sullivan's review of efforts over the last decade to define, label, diagnose, and ethically evaluate those with BIID, especially her insights into analogies with gender identity disorder and the mental competency of those seeking elective amputation, have important resonances with earlier chapters in this section on transgender and human enhancement.

39

MEDICALIZATION, "NORMAL FUNCTION," AND THE DEFINITION OF HEALTH

Rebecca Kukla

Introduction

"Health" is an intuitive notion and not a technical term. The institutions of medicine are designed, first and foremost, to promote, restore, and protect health. The protection of health and distribution of health services is, almost all societies would agree, an important component of justice. Yet it has proven surprisingly difficult to come up with a rigorous definition of health that accommodates all of our core intuitions about what work the notion should do for us. Some theorists have tried to carve out a biological notion of health and disease based in one way or another on the "normal functioning" of the body and its systems and parts. Others have tried to understand health and disease as socially constructed notions, and have focused upon social and institutional processes of "medicalization," wherein clusters of symptoms are identified as unified diseases and brought under medical surveillance and management. Both the biological and the social approaches to defining health face serious roadblocks and objections, as do various hybrid accounts. In this chapter, I will look at some influential attempts to define health, explore exactly why it is so difficult to come up with a satisfactory definition, and finally, propose a tentative alternative definition of health.

One reason why the various attempts to define health and disease have been so unsatisfactory is that those using the notion are driven by deeply diverse theoretical and practical goals. It seems to me that there is no reason why we should expect to be able to find a single, unified account of health or disease that meets all these disparate goals and captures the "true" meaning or essence of the terms; we may need to understand health and disease differently in the context of different kinds of projects and goals.

Consider two different kinds of theoretical projects that centrally employ a conception of health:

1. *Scientistic* projects: The primary goal of such projects is to understand health and disease as respectable concepts from the point of view of the natural sciences. This is possible only if we can characterize what counts as a disease or a state of health independent of our specific, contingent social categories and practices. Such accounts avoid appeals to social or personal values, as these play no role in the

categories and explanatory strategies of the natural sciences. Instead, they appeal to notions such as statistical normalcy, adaptive fitness, and biological function.

2. *Social justice* projects. In this context, an understanding of health and disease is a part of a specific type of *normative* project—namely, that of determining the role that health *should* play in a larger theory of social justice. Political philosophers, policy makers, and others ask questions such as: To what extent and in what sense is there a universal right to health, or health care? What counts as a fair social distribution of health resources? When does a health inequity count as a justice issue in need of moral redress? How shall we balance health needs with other social needs in a just state? To answer such questions, we need an understanding of what health *is*. But not any old understanding will do: This has to be the kind of understanding that will guide and clarify health policy and normative questions about the role of health care in a just society.

Now it seems to me that there is no *prima facie* reason to think that our best attempts to specify a scientifically rigorous definition of health and our best attempts to specify a politically and normatively useful notion of health will correspond with one another. We neither can assume that a unified, universally satisfactory definition of health exists, nor, likewise, that there is a single essence of the notion that we just need to be clever enough to ascertain. For example, from a scientific perspective, it may well be that we are best off defining *disease* as some kind of biological pathology, and then understanding health as the absence of disease. But from the point of view of social justice, the notion of disease may be less central. We want to be able to understand why, for example, poor nutrition among low-income children is a socially pressing health problem, even if it does not plausibly constitute a shared disease (but rather a state that bears complex causal relations to a wide variety of diseases). Hence in considering the best definition of health, we need to keep clearly in view the theoretical and practical purposes to which we want to put the concept, while keeping an open mind as to how unified a definition is possible.

Two Different Ways of Thinking about Health: Normal Function and Medicalization

By far the most influential attempt at a scientistic definition of health and disease is Christopher Boorse's account, which focuses on the notion of statistically normal function. He defines the *normal function* of a part or process within biological members of a class as "a statistically typical contribution by it to their individual survival and reproduction" (Boorse 1977: 555). Within reference classes of members of a species of a particular sex and age, he defines health as "the readiness of each internal part [or process] to perform all its normal functions on typical occasions with at least typical efficiency" and disease as "a type of internal state which impairs health, i.e. reduces one or more functional abilities below typical efficiency" (Boorse 1977). In other words, roughly, health is statistically normal function and disease is a state leading to below-normal function.

There are various ways to challenge this definition or to demand further specification. The notion of a biological function is a vexed one (Godfrey-Smith 1993), and its place in biological science is non-obvious. Many have argued that a thoroughly naturalistic biology will eventually do away with teleological notions such as "function" and restrict itself to causal explanations (i.e., see Schaffner 1993, among others).

Others have questioned why we should accept that evolutionary adaptation for survival and reproduction are the right categories of analysis for understanding medical notions like health and disease. After all, our health goals can and often do involve both more and less than survival and reproduction (Cooper 2002). One might also wonder about how Boorse picked his reference classes. For instance, why we should accept that sex is a relevant way of constraining the reference class. Sex is a contested category to start with: Not everyone has one of the two sexes; it is not settled how to biologically define sex; sex may be changeable. For these reasons and others it is not obvious that our sex is a privileged feature of us when it comes to constraining what counts as normal function for us.

But for purposes of argument, let us assume that we can fix or fill out all the pieces of Boorse's definition and arrive at a solid definition of health as statistically typical function, as many have tried to do (for instance D'Amico 1995; Wakefield 1997). Such an account would be explicitly devoid of normative force or practical upshot. That is, as Boorse himself insists, if we accept his account we cannot assume that there are any ethical or practical implications that follow in any direct way from determining that something is a disease, or that someone (or some group of people) is (or is especially likely to be) in ill health. That something is a disease does not imply that it ought to be treated, that it is bad to have it, or anything of the sort. For instance, a part or process in me could function in a statistically below-normal way without affecting my life in any way that matters to me or to anyone else. Dysfunction, for Boorse, is a statistical notion indexed to certain evolutionary concepts that bear no direct connection to our practical or moral lives, and hence it comes along with no direct practical or ethical valence. His goal is to give a scientifically sound definition of health and disease, not an ethical or political tool. Given a pointedly non-normative, non-directive account of health, we cannot know what role the protection and promotion of health should play in a just state without adding in extra claims about how and when to value health, how health inequalities matter, what kind of a good health is, and so forth. None of this will be extractable from the definition of health itself.

At the other extreme from the scientistic approach to defining health is what I will call a social constructionist approach. This approach begins from the recognition that health and disease are phenomena that are embedded in social practices and fraught with social meanings. Diseases do not merely physically impair us or make us uncomfortable; they co-travel with a variety of social possibilities, barriers, and connotations, which shift and reconfigure over time. Health is not a socially neutral state; it varies demographically and takes on meanings that are shaped by class, race, and other social markers. Clusters of symptoms may start out having no unified medical meaning, and become "medicalized" over time (of which more below), and hardened into recognizable diseases. If we start from noticing these sorts of phenomena, we might be tempted to see health and disease as in the first instance *socially constructed* states, carved out by contingent institutional practices, rather than as given natural categories that can be understood at the level of biological organisms abstracted from their social contexts.

In its most extreme form, this takes the form of what we might call a *pure social constructionist* account of health and disease: *A condition or state counts as a disease if and only if it is medicalized, where medicalization is a social and institutional process, and health is the absence of disease.* There is no formal, agreed-upon definition of medicalization. But roughly, a condition or set of symptoms or bodily features is *medicalized* when health professionals and health institutions take substantial responsibility for understanding, identifying, managing, and/or mitigating it (Conrad 1992). The idea is that diseases are not natural kinds or biologically definable pathologies; rather, for something to be a disease is for it to be embedded within and taken up by the relevant social institutions as being one. Accordingly, on this view, something is a disease exactly when it is treated as being one by those with the social authority to settle the issue.

Which conditions are medicalized shifts over time: Clusters of behaviors and traits can come to have perceived unity and medical significance that they did not have before (as occurred with attention deficit hyperactivity disorder (ADHD) and fetal alcohol syndrome), and they can also lose this unity or this medical significance (as homosexuality did, for instance). Furthermore, typically, medicalization is not a normatively neutral process. On the one hand, it often effects a shift in moral valence: What was previously seen as a character flaw comes to be seen as a form of illness protected from the logic of personal responsibility, and requiring management by experts instead. (Consider what happened when we started thinking of alcoholism and other forms of addiction as diseases, or when we started conceiving of "hyper" children as having ADHD.) On the other hand, it can invest bodily parts and processes with direct normative statuses: The body is reconceived as a site of deformity, pathology, or dysfunction—it is to be fixed if possible. As Peter Conrad (1992) puts it, medicalization often involves a "move from badness to sickness," replacing moral stigma with functional stigma at the level of social meaning.

One of the purest defenders of the pure social constructionist account of health and disease is Tristram Engelhardt. Diseases, for him, are "clusters of phenomena *seen as* amenable to medical assessment, explanation, and up to a point, alleviation or cure . . . Their sense, significance, and reality are cast in terms of the social and intellectual institutions of medicine" (Engelhardt 1996: 189). For instance, Engelhardt infers from the fact that masturbation *was treated as* a disease in the nineteenth century directly to the conclusion that it *was* a disease: "As masturbation became subject to medical management in the 19th century . . . the moral offence of masturbation was transformed into a disease" (Engelhardt 1996: 234). For Engelhardt, "transformation" into a disease is an entirely social process—one marked by institutional power and moral meaning.

A pure social constructionist account has not been appealing to those who wish to use the concept of health to help ground a normative social justice account, and rightly so. The process of medicalization is clearly driven in part by political and cultural forces. It is no accident that drapetomania—the "disease" wherein a slave wants to escape his or her master—ceased to be a plausible or appealing diagnosis as we came to see slavery as archaic and abhorrent, or that the demedicalization of homosexuality correlated with the sexual civil rights movement. But if what counts as health or as disease is subject to the vagaries and contingencies of social history and attitudes, and is not directly constrained by discoverable natural facts, then it is hard to see how these notions could serve as stable grounds for normative claims about rights, just social arrangements, and so forth.

On the pure social constructionist account, our notions of health and disease are thoroughly infected by the very normative notions that we are interested in critiquing. We often decide, with the benefit of hindsight, that the medicalization of a condition reflected and reinforced *unjust* social conditions and arrangements; both drapetomania and homosexuality are excellent examples. Remember, on this account, being a disease *is* just being recognized as one by medical institutions; there is no room for saying that they are wrong about what counts (although later we might say that they were correct but unjust in counting something as a disease). Any principle that tries to specify when health inequalities are unjust, or whether treatment for disease is a human right, for instance, will have difficulties if the very existence of some diseases (but not others) is bound up with unjust social relations. Hence the pure social constructionist account seems an unpromising cornerstone for any normative project.

So far, both the scientistic and the social constructionist approach to understanding health and disease appear unsuited to the normative projects that concern many theorists. Yet theorists with these normative interests have been loath to give up on scientistic accounts. I suspect that this is because they wish to anchor their stories in a stable definition of health and disease that is constrained by natural facts about the world and not just the vagaries of value-laden, shifting social practices and attitudes. Several prominent bioethicists have tried to add normative principles to a naturalistic, scientistic account of health, in order to generate a normatively fecund account. I will argue that this approach is doomed. Luckily, we are not restricted to a stark choice scientism and social constructionism, as I will demonstrate later.

Some Important and Easily Forgotten Facts about the Body

Here are three important facts about bodies. These are often ignored or implicitly contradicted in contemporary discussions of the nature of health and disease, even though almost no one would deny them explicitly. Between them, they make it impossible to build a normative, social justice project on top of a scientistic conception of health and disease.

1. *No body ever functions in a vacuum—all bodily functioning happens in some material environment or other.* How a body and its parts and subsystems function is always and necessarily relative to short- and long-term material context. The functioning of the body will vary depending on nutrition, air quality, available technology (whether the body has access to eyeglasses, insulin shots, antibiotics) the built environment (transportation options, the availability of elevators, grocery stores), and more. What a body can do and how its parts work varies depending on such things in concrete ways. Thus there is literally no answer to the question of how the body functions independent of context—it must always be in *some specific context or other*, and there is no such thing as the "neutral" context. (Nor, notice, is there such a thing as the *ideal* context. One can always imagine a yet better environment that could enhance the functioning of the body.) The body is not a closed system.
2. Some health conditions cannot be causally traced to the malfunctioning of a single part or subsystem of the body. Whether or not we can generate a technical definition of disease as a kind of dysfunction, not everything we recognize, intuitively, as a health condition can be understood as a single dysfunction or even a unified and stable set of dysfunctions. For instance, depression, morbid obesity, and malnutrition all likely involve multiple subsystems and social determinants. Infertility can have its source in a variety of systems and social factors. The fact that we cannot tell a complete or unified story about the causal genesis of such conditions in malfunctioning parts and subsystems does not impede our recognition of them as health conditions.
3. Physicalism: Any capability or function of a *person* supervenes on her *body* in its material environment. That is to say, the body has no spiritual capacities that function independently of its material capacities. One's material body, in all its detail,

situated in its material environment, fully determines one's capacities. *Everything* I can do or be, I can do or be because of the body I have, in the context it is in. This includes my capacity for reasoning, my trained skills, my temperament, and so on. Physicalism is perhaps more contentious than my first two points, since there are those who believe in souls or other kinds of immaterial substance. However, it is not really contentious among most philosophers, and it is certainly not contentious among those seeking scientistic groundings for their theoretical accounts. I assume physicalism from hereon in without further discussion.

In the next two sections, I look in some detail at two recent, influential accounts of the role that health and health care should play in a just state, both of which rely upon a naturalistic definition of health. I will show why, in light of these three core facts about bodies, neither can ultimately achieve its goals. I suggest that their failures are exemplary of the general problems that will be faced by any such accounts.

Norman Daniels on Justice and Health

In his book, *Just Health: Meeting Health Needs Fairly* (2007) Norman Daniels seeks to answer three "focal questions": How is meeting health needs connected with other goals of justice? What is the special moral importance of health? When are health inequalities unjust? (Daniels 2007: 11). He develops a definition of health that is specifically designed to enable us to answer these three normative questions. This is a classic example of what I have called a social justice project. Furthermore, Daniels is explicit about his goal of building his conception of health by grounding it in a scientistic account and adding normative principles so as to make such an account practically useful. Hence he is a perfect test case for our purposes here.

Daniels' definition of health cleaves close to Boorse's statistical definition, modifying it only slightly for normative purposes. He defines health as the absence of *pathology*, where pathology is any *harmful* deviation of the normal functional organization of a typical member of the species, indexed to age and sex (Daniels 2007: 38–9). He is explicit about trying to stay close to the naturalistic, social-practice-independent understanding of health that Boorse offers us, while introducing just enough of an evaluative valence (through the idea of "harmfulness") to make the notion potentially useful within a normative account of justice with some practical import (Daniels 2007: 39).

Daniels' central normative move is to claim that health has distinctive moral import in a just society because pathology impacts people's access to a *normal range of opportunities*. Only those differences in opportunity that originate in *pathology* or its absence are the proper concern of a just health care system, he claims. He argues, for instance, that systematic health inequalities (as opposed to, say, systematic inequalities in ice-skating abilities or systematic hair luster inequalities) deserve social redress as a matter of justice specifically because they lead to systematic differences in opportunities. In moving from the notion of dysfunction to that of restricted opportunity range, Daniels makes the transition from the naturalistic to the normative that is supposed to enable him to place health and health care within an account of just social arrangements.

But can Daniels in fact sustain the distinctions he needs using his theoretical toolbox? Note that all sorts of features and functions of the body restrict opportunity. Having narrow hips and a thick waist restricts one's opportunity to win hula-hoop contests, for example. Daniels is not interested in *all* opportunity restrictions that issue from the body.

Rather, he needs to be able to specify which opportunity restrictions matter as a matter of justice, and he needs those to correspond in some non-accidental way with those that count as the proper concern of medicine and health institutions. Furthermore, it will not be enough for him to say that the opportunity restrictions that matter just are those that medicine can mitigate. For many seemingly non-health-related opportunity restrictions can be mitigated using medical techniques. Having small breasts restricts one's opportunities to be a stripper, *unless* one's body is altered using the tools of medicine. Yet we do not take it as the job of a just social system to mitigate these opportunity restrictions, with or without medical techniques.

So far, Daniels would agree with everything I just said. His goal is to use the notion of normal function in order to make the relevant cut between health issues that restrict our opportunities in ways that are the concern of a just state, and other sorts of opportunity restrictions. In order to make the cuts he needs, Daniels makes two important and unsupported assumptions.

First, he assumes that we can distinguish between those opportunity restrictions that are caused by pathology (given his definition of pathology) and those that are not. But remember our first and third facts about the body above. *Everything* we can do and be depends on how our body functions in a particular context—there is no such thing as how it functions independent of any context, or in a "neutral" context. Nor is there anything we do that isn't something our body does. I think that taking these uncontentious facts seriously makes it difficult or impossible to carve the health-related opportunity-restricting dysfunctions off from the others in any plausible or pragmatically fecund way.

For instance, consider illiteracy. Being illiterate clearly restricts opportunities in important ways. Furthermore, illiteracy is a matter of the body functioning atypically, and it involves specific brain and visual deficits. Yet we do not count it as a health condition. Why not? What is the relevant difference between illiteracy and, say, asthma, which is universally recognized as a health condition? We might argue that illiteracy is not a health condition because it is not an *inherent* feature of the body; typically, it is not explained just by genetics or other innate bodily features, but also by elaborate environmental influences and deficits. But the same goes for many health conditions, including asthma, which is triggered by a combination of genes and environment, not to mention contagious illnesses and much else. Thus, once we keep in mind the contextual complexity of bodily functioning and the fact that everything we do is embodied, it is not at all obvious that we can draw a clean distinction between pathology and other opportunity restrictors, given the contents of Daniels' toolbox.

Second, Daniels assumes that once we make the *scientific* distinction between opportunity restrictions grounded in pathology and other opportunity restrictions, it will in some important sense track a *moral* distinction: The opportunity restrictions based on pathology will be distinctively deserving of social attention in a just state. To be sure, having breasts too small for a stripper will not deserve social redress in the same way as having a muscle disorder that prohibits walking. But Daniels needs it to be *systematically* true that opportunity restrictions resulting from pathology have a special moral priority over those with other causes. This is key for him, as it is what allows his naturalistic definition of health to be sutured to the notion of a restricted opportunity range in a way that has normative or political consequences.

But consider one of Daniels' own central examples, which he uses in multiple publications: Shortness and human growth hormone (HGH) treatment. Being short is, he presumes, an opportunity disadvantage in our culture (Daniels 1992, 2007, and elsewhere).[1] Daniels claims that kids who suffer from hormonal disorders involving a HGH deficiency have a dysfunction of the right sort to count as a pathology, and hence that they have a justice claim on HGH treatment, whereas kids who are just genetically short but "healthy" have no such claim—giving them the HGH therapy would count as "enhancement" rather than treatment. This is supposed to exemplify how his scientistic definition of health can be used to make normative policy distinctions as to who is owed treatment. But the example seems to me to backfire severely. If one's abnormal height restricts opportunities, in a particular social and material context, how could the *cause* of that abnormal height have any moral significance? It is hard to imagine why or how either of two identical opportunity restrictions in two equally short kids, whose shortness has a different genesis, could possibly matter in terms of its moral or practical significance, on Daniels' own account.[2] Our opportunity range is always a product of what we can do *with our body, in our environment*, and the causal genesis of these abilities seems morally irrelevant.

In trying to show how he can use his naturalistic notion of pathology as the basis of a practically fecund account of health justice, by way of the impact of pathology on opportunity, Daniels has, I think, in fact accidentally done the opposite: He has demonstrated that if opportunity is what we care about, then—although surely pathology does cause opportunity restrictions—pathology or its absence become quite irrelevant to what justice owes people. And again, that's so even if we can stably distinguish between pathology and other opportunity-compromising bodily features, which is by no means clear.

I contend, then, that once we force ourselves to remember that everything we do is something we do with our body, and that bodily functioning is ineliminably context dependent, we can see that Daniels fails to ground a contentful theory of health justice in his scientistic definition of health and disease. Furthermore, this failure is located at exactly the junctures that matter for our purposes: At the point where we distinguish health conditions from other bodily conditions, and at the point where we assign moral significance with practical consequences to having a health condition as opposed to some other kind of condition.

Powers and Faden on Dimensions of Well-Being

In their book *Social Justice: The Moral Foundations of Health and Health Policy* (2006), Madison Powers and Ruth Faden develop a theory of justice, including health justice, built on the idea that there are at least six basic "dimensions of well-being." They argue that justice requires that society attempt to guarantee all its members a sufficiency of well-being in each dimension. These are dimensions that matter centrally to all people, regardless of their specific life plans; they are "weighty interests of special enough importance to be given protection as basic human rights" (Powers and Faden 2006: 85)· The six dimensions they identify are health, personal security, reasoning, respect, attachment, and self-determination. Each dimension is, in their view, "morally distinctive" as well as conceptually separable for the purpose of designing just policy and institutions; they are also causally intertwined and interdependent in a variety of ways. While the dimensions are distinct, Powers and Faden demonstrate in detail how they create densely woven systematic patterns of inequality and disadvantage. "Inequalities beget inequalities, and existing inequalities . . . can compound, sustain, and reproduce a multitude of deprivations in well-being" (Powers and Faden 2006: 8).

According to Powers and Faden, health is a distinct and irreducible dimension of well-being. They are concerned to carve it off from the other dimensions so that it can serve as a substantive tool for designing specific health policies and just health practices. In particular, they are concerned to set boundaries around the concept of health so that it doesn't become so vague that it swallows up every facet of well-being; they wish to push back against the notoriously broad definition of health in the constitution of the World Health Organization, namely "*a complete state of physical, mental, and spiritual well-being*." Powers and Faden point out that the WHO definition:

> conflates virtually all elements of human development under a single rubric and thereby makes almost any deficit of well-being into a health deficit. Were we to adopt the WHO definition, we would lose the human capacity to maintain any distinctive interest in dimensions of human well-being such as respect, affiliation, and reasoning that we believe have independent moral significance as matters of social justice, however intertwined with health they may be.
>
> (Powers and Faden 2006: 17)

If our notions of health and disease are to play substantive roles in normative accounts of just social institutions, then we have to be able to separate health from other forms of well-being, just as we have to be able to separate disease from other forms of dysfunction.

Given how much it matters to Powers and Faden that health be a distinct and identifiable dimension of well-being, they spend surprisingly little time defining it or defending and explaining their definition. Instead, they give a rough intuitive definition that invokes the scientistic language of biological function:

> We work with what is essentially an ordinary-language understanding of physical and mental health that is intended to capture *the dimension of human flourishing that is frequently expressed through the biological or organic functioning of the body*.
>
> (Powers and Faden 2006: 16–17, italics in the original)

If we try to sharpen their definition in a way that is consonant with their goals and the rest of their account, we get into trouble similar to that Daniels faced. Remember, *everything* we can do or be is something we can do or be *with our body*, and hence in a straightforward sense every possible kind of human flourishing is *expressed through the body*. So this part of their definition is not helpfully restrictive. Presumably this is why they introduce the qualifier that it is the "biological/organic functioning" of the body that matters for health. Of course, our biological body is the only one we actually have. Hence we need some other reading of the emphasis on the biological/organic functioning of the body. Presumably Powers and Faden are here trying to separate the functioning of the body *qua* biological entity from its functioning in social and technological context. But as we saw, *there is no such thing*. The states and functions of the body are environment dependent.

Thus far, Powers and Faden's definition of health does nothing to help us restrict the notion more narrowly than human flourishing in general; they do not seem to have gotten us farther than the WHO definition they denigrate. And without this, the concept of health does not give us a tool for making substantive claims about just health institutions and practices. In order to flesh out to this worry, it will be helpful for us to look at some of their other dimensions of well-being that are supposedly distinct from health, to see how the distinctions collapse in practice. Consider two of these dimensions: *Reasoning* and *attachment*.

Powers and Faden are surely right that impairments of reasoning and of attachment are serious compromises of human flourishing. Clearly, *some* such impairments are *also* health conditions. Consider clinical paranoia and attachment-impeding forms of autism, for instance. Just as clearly, *some* impairments of reasoning and attachment are not health conditions, in any intuitively recognizable sense. Closed-mindedness due to a narrow religious upbringing can impair reasoning (and probably attachment too). Moderate introversion can impair attachment. It should be the job of health policies to address the needs of citizens with clinical paranoia or autism; it's not specifically the business of *health* policies or institutions to address religious closed-mindedness or personality variations. Given the terms of their project, Powers and Faden must be able to distinguish the two types of case.

We cannot, of course, reason about anything or attach to anyone without our bodies; our bodies are what we reason and attach *with*. So the involvement of the body is not a criterion we can use for distinguishing health-related from non-health-related impairments of reasoning or attachment. Nor can we use the distinction between socially and biologically caused impairments to help us. One might suggest that religious closed-mindedness, for instance, is not a health condition because it is socially caused rather than properly biological, but this will not give us the cut we need. For instance, post-traumatic stress disorder and dissociative identity disorder are health conditions in which social factors play crucial causal roles (and they may impair reasoning and attachment as well).

Powers and Faden admit that any reasoning (and presumably any attachment) depends on a biological substratum—a "healthy brain." In order to try to sustain their claim that reasoning is not a subset of health, they write:

> Certain kinds of health states are necessary for reasoning, but they are not sufficient. What further distinguishes reasoning abilities from the healthy functioning of the brain is that the former also require an understanding of the world that must be *learned*.
>
> (Powers and Faden 2006: 21)

But this is unhelpful. For learning itself supervenes on brain function; changing brain function is the mechanism by which learning occurs. We cannot separate how the brain functions "in itself" from how it functions after learning, for learning is among its most central functions. Once again, there is no stable, contextually independent background state of "brain health" to which learning is added. (This becomes exceptionally clear if we note that a healthy infant brain would be very unhealthy indeed were it to reside in an adult, since enormous amounts of learning in between are essential.)

Thus Powers and Faden have not given us theoretical resources with which we can distinguish between compromises in reasoning and attachment *per se* and compromises in health. More generally, they have offered us no mechanism for telling when facts about the functioning of the body are relevant to our health as opposed to other dimensions of our well-being. For example, they cannot help us explain why poor reasoning due to poor education and parenting is not a health condition, whereas poor reasoning due to post-traumatic stress disorder is one. But this means that their (fairly minimal) scientistic definition of health does not enable them to carve out the dimensions of well-being as distinct and independent. But a central goal, for Powers and Faden, was to earn substantive practical conclusions about justice by keeping these dimensions distinct.

Kinds of Conceptual Categories and the Institutional Definition of Health

Here's where we are so far: We are apparently caught between a social constructionist understanding of health, wherein health and disease are whatever we take them to be, and a scientistic understanding of health, wherein health and disease are biological concepts. We have seen that neither yields a concept of health that is substantively useful within a normative project of deciding what just health institutions and policies would look like. As long as we think that health has to be either a natural, biological category or a mere social construction, the problem seems hopeless. Luckily, the dilemma is false.

Some conceptual categories are purely socially constructed. The independent material world does not constrain our usage of them, and our practices for using them are the only measure of their own correctness. Consider the concept of "cooties," or of "witch" in seventeenth century Salem. Nothing determines whether you count as having cooties or being a witch (in their sense) except social agreement. It's not like there could be new evidence that could confirm or falsify someone's cootie or witchy status.

Other categories mark out scientifically relevant distinctions in the natural world, completely apart from our practices or attitudes. We *discover* their properties rather than constituting them. Gold and atomic nuclei are good examples. Whether we are in the habit of counting something as gold (Au) is irrelevant to whether it is in fact that element.[3]

But plenty of our categories are constrained by both the world and our social practices (Weiskopf 2011). Artifactual categories such as "scalpel" or "prosthetic" are defined in terms of their intended function. Were there no human practices, nothing would be a scalpel; scalpels exist only because we design and make them. But at the same time, not any old thing we choose can count as a scalpel. An object must be organized in the right way to count as a scalpel, and only certain kinds of material (metal but not Styrofoam, for instance) will support such organizations. Saying something is a scalpel isn't like saying someone has cooties; there are natural constraints independent of us on what can count. But it also isn't like saying something is gold. An object has to be enmeshed in human intentions and practices in the right way to count as a scalpel.

Consider now *institutional* categories such as "voting," "paycheck," "convict," or "student." The existence of such things is thoroughly dependent upon elaborate social institutions, and to be such a thing is to be embedded in these institutions in the right way. You can't be a convict without a legislative, justice, and penal system. Nothing counts as a paycheck without elaborate labor and economic institutions. And yet, things don't become or cease to be convicts or paychecks just because we choose to classify or declassify them in that way. Being either one has definite empirical consequences and preconditions. We may slowly refine or shift these kinds in accordance with our social needs. But we cannot simply discover that we were totally wrong about what a convict or a paycheck is, since our practices carved these kinds out.

With all this in mind, let's return to the question of how we should most productively understand the concepts of disease and health. I suggest that we understand health as a special sort of *institutional* concept. I will propose a definition and then take some time to spell out its meaning and consequences:

> *The Institutional Definition of Health*: A condition or state counts as a *health condition* if and only if, given our resources and situation, it *would be best for our collective well-being* if it were medicalized—that is, if health professionals and institutions played a substantial role in understanding, identifying, managing and/or mitigating it. In turn, *health* is a relative absence of health conditions (and concomitantly a relative lack of dependence upon the institutions of medicine).

Both this definition and the pure social constructionist definition define health in terms of medicalization by health institutions. But my institutional definition differs from the pure social constructionist definition in that it talks about what we *should* medicalize, from the point of view of our collective flourishing, rather than what we *do* medicalize.

The essential idea here is that *real* health conditions are conditions for which the tools and methods and support of medicine and its institutional mechanisms are genuinely helpful, given both the natural and the social facts. This is something we can be *wrong about* and can *empirically discover*. That something is a health condition is a social fact, which is dependent on what medicine has to offer and the social context of the condition, but not a *purely* social fact. For example, it turned out that even though, as Engelhardt points out, people *thought* that the tools of medicine would be helpful when applied to masturbators, they were in fact wrong. And while many people used to think that people with schizophrenia were best served by exorcists, we now know that the tools of medicine are helpful in diagnosing and managing schizophrenia.

It is *not* a consequence of my account that all health conditions deserve medical treatment, or even that medical treatment is always the best option. Something might meet my definition of a health condition because it is best *diagnosed and classified* using the tools of medicine, but then best managed using non-medical strategies. Mild hypertension might be a candidate, for instance. Perhaps it is best, all things considered, for us to use medical tools to identify and label mild hypertension, but also best all-in to address it with lifestyle changes and self-monitoring (as opposed to pharmaceuticals, say).

It is also not a consequence of my account that an *individual* counts as having a health condition just because providing medical services to *that individual* would benefit *her or him*. I've defined health in terms of our *collective* well-being. So for example, just because an individual might personally benefit from cosmetic breast augmentation, this does not mean that having smallish breasts is properly categorized as a health condition. The question would be whether using the tools of medicine to manage small-breastedness would be better for our collective well-being, and this is much less plausible than that particular individuals might benefit.

Notice that I have left open how to understand "collective well-being." The question of what constitutes this is far beyond the scope of this chapter; it's roughly equivalent to the question of the nature of justice. My proposed definition of health is intended to be neutral between conceptions of collective well-being. Whether one is a consequentialist, a libertarian, a Rawlsian, or whatever else, one can be invested in what I have called the normative project of figuring out how a just state should manage health policy and health needs, and my definition of health can be slotted into any such project.

The institutional definition of health is a realist one, in the sense that one can *discover* that something is properly thought of as a health condition, by *learning* that the toolkit of medicine is helpful. But what we are discovering, in such a case, are not just natural facts that are independent of human interests and practices. Whether the toolkit of medicine turns out to be a good thing to bring to bear, all things considered, depends on all sorts of changeable and human-practice-dependent facts, including what medical techniques and interventions are available and the cultural context in which they will be used, among other factors. Whether something is rightly brought under the rubric of health institutions will change as the capacities, resources, technology, and knowledge base of medicine changes, and as the culture at large (including attitudes towards particular conditions and diseases, the self-understandings of those who have a particular condition, available resources and support networks, and so forth) changes as well.[4]

This means that even though there are all sorts of concrete facts that help determine whether something counts as a health condition, whether it counts is not a *fixed or natural fact* about it. Likewise what counts as being healthy will change as culture and medicine change; health is not an intrinsic property of a body, on this account, but only of a body in context. This is intuitively appealing: Surely what counted as being a healthy 60-year-old in medieval England is not the same as what counts as being a healthy 60-year-old in twenty-first century Norway.

Unlike Boorse, Daniels, and others, I have not defined health in contrast to "disease." I suspect that for normative purposes, carefully separating diseases from other health conditions will not turn out to be very important (in contrast to its importance within a scientistic account of health). Roughly, we can think of a disease as a repeatable, relatively stable bodily state or process that systematically causally contributes to one or more health condition. Notice that, on this definition, particular diseases may be natural kinds, definable and identifiable apart from human practices (in terms of their viral or genetic underpinning, say). But *that* a condition is a disease is an institutional fact, not a purely natural fact, as this depends on its relationship to health conditions, which are institutional concepts. And the concept of disease *itself* is likewise, here, an institutional concept.

In short, health and concomitant concepts like disease are not *natural kinds*, on my institutional account, even though they are largely *materially determined kinds*, whose extension is not simply up to us. Understanding health inherently requires more than the tools of the natural sciences; it needs the human sciences as well.

How does my account constitute an improvement over the pure social constructionist account? The key lies in my shift to a *counterfactual* definition; this shift, I claim, creates the room we need to allow the concept of health to have some substantive normative punch. For remember, on the social constructionist account, diseases are whatever is medicalized, even though we know that sometimes this medicalization does more harm than good from the point of view of justice and the promotion of collective well-being, as in the cases of homosexuality and drapetomania. On my account, unlike the pure social constructionist account, such things *never were* actually health conditions. Our classification and treatment of them as health conditions were *mistakes*; they got the world wrong. Likewise, sometimes we discover that as an empirical fact, a condition that used to be seen as non-medical is actually best medicalized—that more justice and human flourishing results from medicalizing it. Alcoholism—which used to be cast as simply a moral failing—is a plausible example. On the institutional account I have proposed, determining that something is a health condition has direct consequences for deciding how the tools of medicine ought to be used. Thus we can use health and its absence as stable normative notions for the purposes of building an account of just social arrangements.

A Brief Test Case: Gender Dysphoria

Let's look at how the institutional definition of health works in a contentious case: Gender dysphoria, also known as gender identity disorder. This is the official diagnostic category for transgender people; it marks out transgender as a unified *health condition*. The medicalization of transgender identity has rightly been contentious from the start. To simplify the debate dramatically: On the one hand, a large percentage of trans*[5] people claim that access to the tools and techniques of medicine (hormone therapy, plastic surgery, etc.) is crucial to their embodied flourishing and mental well-being. On the other hand, first, trans* folks have been understandably resistant to the idea that they have a *disorder* or a *disease*, as opposed to just a configuration of identity that needs social and technical support in order to be successfully maintained (as do all configurations of identity, although sometimes to a less heightened degree). And second, the medicalization of trans* identity is worrisome insofar as it gives doctors the power to serve as identity "gatekeepers," who can enforce rigid criteria and set up practical hurdles that "patients" must meet before they can "count as" officially having access to the identity they experience themselves as having.

On the account I have proposed, we can find a way out of this dilemma. Whether gender dysphoria is a "real" health condition, on my account, is not a question of whether it corresponds to some substantial biological dysfunction (as on a scientistic account), nor is it simply answered by noting that we treat it as one (as on a social constructionist account). Rather, the question of the "reality" of the diagnostic category is a question about whether we *should* use the tools and techniques of medicine for addressing the needs of trans* folks. And this, in turn, is a contingent empirical question that depends on the current treatments available, the specific standards of diagnosis and care, the culture and support networks available to trans* folks, and more. These are facts that are *changing* rapidly.

Not very long ago, medical interventions available for trans* folks seeking them were fairly coarse grained, and among other limitations did little to preserve sexual pleasure and function. Furthermore, access to such interventions depended on meeting a rigid set of standards for what counted, medically, as "truly" being transgender. Patients had to present as having lived out a formulaic narrative, in which they had felt "trapped in the wrong body" since early childhood and had consistently manifested highly stereotyped gendered behavior. They had to desire to "pass" as their preferred gender and be able to do so fairly successfully, and they had to crave the genitals of their preferred gender. If they did not meet all these requirements and more, they weren't "really" transgender and did not qualify for medical interventions. All this served to make the medical management of sex identity a mixed blessing at best.

There have been seismic changes recently, however (see Chapter 42 in this volume). Diagnostic criteria have broadened and become more patient centered. There is widespread medical recognition that not all trans* patients are simply interested in approximating the "normal" body of a sex other than the one they were assigned at birth; some patients may only need or desire hormone therapy, or chest surgery, or any combination of interventions, and trans* identities run the full spectrum of gender identities. A teleological march towards genital reconstruction is no longer the norm, nor is the desire to have this surgery treated by medicine as the "true" measure of sexual identity. Concomitantly, the trans* community now embraces a much wider range of body formations and self-presentations, with much less emphasis on policing a "proper" trans narrative.

On the institutional account, gender dysphoria is a legitimate medical diagnosis just insofar as bringing it under the purview of medical institutions enhances human flourishing and the ends of justice. I hypothesize (though I certainly cannot thoroughly prove here) that, *as a matter of contingent, historical fact,* it has turned out that the diagnostic category of gender dysphoria, and the medical tools and procedures that it gives access to, have increased the well-being of trans* folks (and indeed people in general), all things considered. We now have substantial experience with how trans* folks do when they have access to the medical interventions they feel they need, and it seems fairly clear that more people are able to flourish and be happy in virtue of this access. Meanwhile, public consciousness and acceptance of trans* folks and medically altered trans* bodies have skyrocketed forward. (Of course, none of that is to deny the very serious forms of discrimination and danger still faced by many trans* people.)

Thus on my account, gender dysphoria counts as a legitimate, bona fide *health condition*—a condition that is in the running for various rights of access to health services in a just state. But crucially, this is not because there is some unified, underlying *pathology* that explains or undergirds the "symptoms" of gender dysphoria. There is no reason for the claims of trans* folks on health resources, or the reality of their condition, to depend in any way on finding some sort of stable dysfunction that "legitimates" their condition. There is no underlying natural fact that would determine whether gender dysmorphia is *truly* a health condition, and hence no reason to hook claims to health services to any story of disease etiology. Nor, however, does gender dysphoria count as a disease just because it is pathologized by the practices of medicine, as it would on a pure social constructionist account.

There are various other conditions for which it is an open question whether the involvement of medicine is all-in a good thing for justice and human flourishing. Female sexual dysfunction and ADHD are two examples upon which it seems to me the jury is out. Whether these are properly categorized as health conditions depends on contingent, complex, socially embedded facts that are not yet fully known or even fully determined—but that are also not simply up to us to decide.

Conclusions

In the early parts of this paper, I argued that dominant approaches to defining health had difficulty making a normatively fecund distinction between health conditions and other sorts of conditions. I claimed that they appeared to do so only by ignoring one or more basic facts about human embodiment: (1) That there is no way that the body functions outside of a particular material context; (2) that not all health conditions can be traced to a particular part or subsystem of the body; and (3) that everything that we do, we do with our body.

I claim that the institutional definition of health manages to carve out a normatively relevant concept of health that does not stumble over these three facts, because it does not make the reality of a health condition depend on finding a stable or underlying bodily function or part on which it can be pinned. This account lets the concept of health play a substantive role in a theory of justice (whose details are up for grabs, as far as what I have said here goes). Unlike in scientistic or social constructionist accounts of health, the connection to justice is *built in* to my account from the start, through its appeal to empirical facts about what furthers our collective well-being.

Related Topics

Chapter 42, "Transgender," Jamie Lindemann Nelson
Chapter 44, "Body Integrity Identity Disorder (BIID) and the Matter of Ethics," Nikki Sullivan

Notes

1 At 4' 10.5", I am not sure I agree. But I will grant the claim for the sake of argument.
2 In fact I am not sure why Daniels does not count the child whose shortness is genetic as having a pathological condition, by his own definition. Why is a statistically atypical and (by assumption) harmful gene structure any less pathological, on his definition, than a statistically atypical hormonal structure—especially given that the latter is probably genetically caused anyhow? The example seems to me to raise the first problem; I am not sure how Daniels can put meaningful boundaries around the notion of pathology. But this is a side point in the context of this second argument.
3 Many philosophers, including me, are suspicious of the idea of purely natural kinds. But I will grant their existence for the purposes of this chapter, since I am about to argue that health is *not* such a kind anyhow.
4 Health and various health conditions are kinds that have what Ian Hacking (1995, 1999) calls "looping effects": Once we identify such kinds (cancer, schizophrenia, malnutrition . . .) and sort people into them, this will affect people's self-conception, behavior, and treatment, and this in turn will change the character of the kind. Think, for example, about how the medicalization of drug and alcohol addiction has radically altered the institutional and cultural setting and meaning of addiction, along with the experienced identity and social life of many addicts.
5 "Trans*" is a relatively new notational term designed to designate not just male to female and female to male transgender folks, but anyone who does not identify with the sex they were assigned at birth, including those who identify as genderqueer, non-gendered, or any other variant. The asterisk is designed to mark that this is a covering term that can include those who identify as transgender, transsexual, transvestite, or any other variation, without the need for us to lock down these possibilities in advance.

References

Boorse, C. (1977) "Health as a Theoretical Concept," *Philosophy of Science* 44: 542–73.
Conrad, P. (1992) *Deviance and Medicalization: From Badness to Sickness*, Philadelphia, PA: Temple University Press.
Cooper, R. (2002) "Disease," *Studies in the History and Philosophy of Biology and the Biological Sciences* 33: 263–82.
D'Amico, R. (1995) "Is Disease a Natural Kind," *Journal of Medicine and Philosophy* 20: 551–69.
Daniels, N. (1992) "Growth Hormone Therapy for Short Stature: Can We Support the Treatment/Enhancement Distinction," *Growth and Growth Hormone* 8: 46–8.
Daniels, N. (2007) *Just Health: Meeting Health Needs Fairly*, New York: Cambridge University Press.
Engelhardt, T. (1996) *The Foundations of Bioethics*, New York: Oxford University Press.
Godfrey-Smith (1993) "Functions: Consensus Without Unity," *Pacific Philosophical Quarterly* 74: 196–208.
Hacking, I. (1995) "The Looping Effects of Human Kinds," in D. Sperber, D. Premack and A.J. Premack (eds.) *Causal Cognition*, Oxford: Oxford University Press, pp. 351–94.
Hacking, I. (1999) *The Social Construction of What?* Cambridge, MA: Harvard University Press.
Powers, M. and Faden, R. (2006) *Social Justice: The Moral Foundations of Public Health and Health Policy*, New York: Oxford University Press.
Schaffner, K.F. (1993) *Discovery and Explanation in Biology and Medicine*, Chicago: University of Chicago Press.
Wakefield, J.C. (1997) "Normal Inability Versus Pathological Inability," *Clinical Psychology: Science and Practice* 4: 249–58.
Weiskopf, D. (2011) "The Functional Unity of Special Science Kinds," *British Journal for the Philosophy of Science* 62: 233–58.

40
HUMAN ENHANCEMENT

Nicholas Agar and Felice Marshall

Introduction

Human enhancement is the focus of an intensifying philosophical interest. Partly this is a consequence of advances in technology that promise to realize possibilities once considered the stuff of science fiction.

To examine the moral implications of human enhancement, we first require a definition of what it is to enhance a human being. We present a conceptual pluralism that acknowledges two ways to define human enhancement. These concepts highlight different moral problems and opportunities that emerge from the application of powerful genetic and environmental technologies to human beings. Distinct moral issues arise in respect of different means, degrees, and targets of enhancement. We begin by describing various *means* by which humans may be enhanced. Philosophical interest in human enhancement has tended to focus on enhancement by the modification or selection of human genetic material. This focus risks overlooking a variety of other ways in which humans may be enhanced. Enhancement can also occur through environmental means. Cochlear implants, electronic hippocampi, prosthetic legs, and traditional methods of education all involve the modification of human brains or bodies, and thus are all examples of environmental enhancements.

Next we examine the significance of different *degrees* of enhancement. Enhancement encompasses interventions many would be reluctant to consider enhancement at all, for example formal education, something that results in the improvement of cognitive capacities. More obvious cases of enhancement include injecting synthetic erythropoietin (EPO) to win the Tour de France, which results in improved physical endurance, as well as radical human enhancements: Imagine someone who lives for thousands of years and can instantly memorize the complete works of Shakespeare. Opponents of human enhancement offer a range of objections often in relation to the moral significance of the degree of enhancement undertaken. Francis Fukuyama objects that genetic enhancement of too great a degree poses a threat to human nature. Jürgen Habermas contends that genetic enhancement beyond human norms infringes on the autonomy of its subjects. Meanwhile, the most ardent proponents of human enhancement advocate enhancement of so great a degree that recipients should no longer be considered human. We will discuss these positions (and others) with a view to assessing the moral significance of varying degrees of enhancement.

We conclude the chapter with a discussion of the debate that has arisen in respect of a particular *target* of enhancement—human moral capacities. Moral disposition enhancement has the goal of improving the moral value of an individual's actions or character. Another variety of moral enhancement, moral status enhancement, improves an individual's moral priority—their moral entitlement to beneficial treatment and protection against harm.

We do not aspire to cover the debate about human enhancement in its entirety. The following should be taken as a broadly representative, philosophically interesting sample of themes from the contemporary debate.

What Does It Mean to Enhance a Human Being?

There are two ways in which we can understand human enhancement. The broader of the two accounts defines enhancement as improvement. One enhances whenever one improves. If a genetic alteration improves cognitive powers then it is a genetic enhancement. We call this *enhancement as improvement*. A narrower account limits the range of improvements properly considered to be enhancements. According to the concept of *enhancement beyond human norms* a cognitive improvement counts as an enhancement if it shifts an individual's cognitive powers from a point within the range properly considered normal for humans either to a higher point within that range or to a point beyond it.

An example serves to illustrate one significant difference between the two concepts. Injections of synthetic EPO boost the body's supply of red blood cells. Consider two circumstances in which you might inject EPO. You might be suffering from severe anemia resulting from a shortage of red blood cells. You inject EPO to make good that shortage in order to avoid compromised organ function. Alternatively, you might be a competitor in a long-distance cycling event. Your body's supply of red blood cells is normal. You inject EPO to gain a competitive advantage.

Both are examples of enhancement as improvement. Both improve capacities. But the purpose of the first is not enhancement beyond human norms. The appeal to norms in this account divides improvements into therapies and enhancements. When someone with anemia is given synthetic EPO the purpose is to restore the supply of red blood cells to a level properly considered normal for human beings. This is therapy. Proponents of this account reserve the label "enhancement" for the second case. We can suppose that the competitor enters the event with a normal supply of red blood cells. In this case the injection is not therapy. Its purpose is to increase physical endurance. The enhancing injections of EPO shifts the supply of red blood cells from a point within the spectrum of normal either to a higher point on that spectrum or to a point beyond it. Here we can consider "human norms" to refer to the capacities prior to the injection of EPO. It boosts the supply of red blood cells beyond a normal level even if the destination level lies within the normal range rather than outside of it. Many performance-enhancing Tour de France cyclists have used EPO to achieve levels of red blood cells toward the high end of the normal range rather than beyond it.

We should expect some vagueness when employing the concept of normality. The normal range of human capacities lacks precise boundaries. Other distinctions also exist along a continuum and admit borderline cases. For example, the division between the bald and the hirsute is vague, but this vagueness does not prevent us from understanding and utilizing the distinction. There are cases that lie on the boundary between therapy and enhancement. They pose practical problems for those who seek to use the therapy/enhancement distinction. But their existence does not invalidate the distinction or undermine its usefulness.

How should we understand the concept of normality? One way is statistical. This seems to carry little or no normative weight. It is statistically "normal" for humans to be right-handed, but that does not imply that it is bad to be abnormal in this respect; one is not worse off for being left-handed simply because this attribute is statistically abnormal. Another way to understand normality appeals to biology. When a heart pumps in a way that is biologically normal it performs at the level selected for by natural selection. Levels of cardiac function below biological norms tend to have bad consequences for the wellbeing of the organism of which the heart is a part.

There is no necessary connection between biologically abnormal function and reduced wellbeing. Suppose that neuro-anatomists were to discover that some cases of non-heterosexual sexual orientation resulted from a common functional abnormality in the development of the brain. It would be absurd to present this obscure biological fact as trumping the claims of non-heterosexual people to be living fully contented lives. Our understanding of the moral relevance of abnormal biological functioning must be contextual. We understand that certain varieties of abnormal biological functioning—for example, levels of red blood cells that result in anemia—tend to reduce likely wellbeing. It's clear that others do not.

There is more than one way in which we can make the distinction between therapy and enhancement morally significant. Some philosophers—for example Habermas and Fukuyama—present it as marking the difference between genetic interventions that are permissible and those that are impermissible. They say that gene therapies are permissible but genetic enhancements are not. As we shall see, there are a variety of attempts to explain why it might be impermissible to use genetic technologies to shift someone from within the normal range of human capacities either to a higher point within that range or to a point beyond that range.

Other philosophers make different uses of the distinction between therapy and enhancement. According to Buchanan et al. (2000), the category of therapy corresponds approximately to those genetic interventions that the liberal state should seek to provide to its citizens. These enable normal participation in society. A liberal state is subject to no obligation to commit resources to make enhancements available. This does not imply a requirement to ban them. It does seem that people who have traits that fall below human norms can claim greater priority for provisions to raise them up to human norms than people whose capacities are currently normal. For example, people who have hearing loss face barriers to normal participation in society. We make cochlear implants and hearing aids available to the hearing impaired. We should also make available gene therapies for deafness. Analogous reasoning does not apply to genetic modifications that would permit super-normal hearing—having super-normal hearing is not a prerequisite for normal participation in society.

We have two concepts of human enhancement that may enable us to recognize different moral problems and prospects. We offer the following guideline in making these judgments.

> A *human enhancement consistency test*: Suppose that we decide a given human enhancement is morally permissible, impermissible, or obligatory. We should say the same of comparable enhancements. If not, we need to explain why the difference makes a difference in moral assessment.

There are three ways in which we might apply the human enhancement consistency test. These correspond to three ways in which enhancements can vary. The test may be applied in respect of differences in the *means* by which humans are enhanced, the *capacities* that are the targets of enhancement, and the *degrees* to which they are enhanced.

Different Means of Enhancement

Much of the philosophical debate about human enhancement has focused on means that involve the selection or modification of genetic material. The most opportune time to attempt genetic enhancement is very early in development. A change to the DNA of a single cell human zygote will be transferred to every cell in the resulting human being. Suppose that the intention is to genetically enhance cognition. A change to the DNA of a very early embryo will manifest itself in every brain cell.

One genetic modification that presented as a candidate for human enhancement involves the NR2B gene (Tang et al. 1999). Although the function of this gene remains to be fully clarified, it is thought to be especially active during the brain's development. Mice who have had an additional copy of the gene introduced into their genomes—so called Doogie mice, named for the 1980s TV boy genius Doogie Howser MD—significantly outperform controls at a variety of cognitive tasks. The gene exists in humans, so it's possible that the introduction of an additional copy of NR2B into human genomes would have corresponding effects on intelligence.

Enhancement by the selection of genetic material has an ugly history. It is how Francis Galton, the nineteenth century founder of eugenics, imagined humans being enhanced. Galton was ignorant of DNA, but he presumed to see the effects of good hereditary factors in the successes and virtues of some individuals and bad hereditary factors in the perceived failings and vices of others. He envisaged a program of human selective breeding in which the hereditarily "good" would be encouraged to maximize their reproductive outputs. People assessed as having poor quality hereditary material would be discouraged or prevented from reproducing.

The faults of Galtonian eugenics were many (see Kevles 1998; Paul 1995). There were scientific errors. It is simply false that racial and social class groupings sort hereditary material according to quality. Galtonian eugenics also involved errors in moral reasoning. There were abuses of reproductive liberty. Galtonian eugenicists would foist on some an obligation to have children while preventing others from doing so. Eugenicists tended to assume monistic views about human flourishing. They denied the widely held pluralism according to which there are many different versions of the good life, none of which deserves primacy over all the others. Contemporary defenders of enhancement by selecting or modifying genetic material should sharply distinguish their goals from those of Galtonian eugenics.

A focus on enhancement by genetic modification underrepresents the diversity of ways in which humans might be enhanced. Human enhancement may be achieved by methods other than the modification or selection of genes. For example, the power of education to bring about enhancement as improvement is established. Given its ubiquity, education may seem an odd thing to consider as an enhancement. But it is straightforwardly a case of enhancement as improvement.

A prominent liberal argument for genetic enhancement urges consistent treatment of genetic and environmental means of human enhancement (Harris 1998). This argument draws support from a modern understanding of human development. It firmly rejects widely held beliefs in genetic determinism. According to this common misunderstanding of development, many human traits are causally fixed by genes. Genetic determinism seems to license talk of intelligence genes and genes for conservative political beliefs. It makes sense to describe traits as genetic or environmental only when addressing variation in a population. When we say that eye color is genetic we are saying that variation in eye color in a population is predominantly a consequence of variation in genes. It is simply wrong to apply language properly used to describe variation in populations to individuals. When described in a population sense, eye color is a genetic trait. But this doesn't mean that the brown color of an individual's eyes is determined or fixed by his or her genes. Environmental contributions are essential. What is true of eye color is also true of the ability to play chess. Alterations to either trait can result from changes to genetic influences. They can also result from changes to environmental influences.

This interactionist model has implications for the enhancement choices of parents. Parents in liberal societies already make choices about education that they hope may enhance their children. For example, some choose to send their children to private schools. This is a case of enhancement as improvement: Parents hope elite educational opportunities will improve their children's capacities. According to the liberal argument they should be able to make choices about their children's genomes. There are limits. Many states prohibit educational choices deemed incompatible with a child's welfare—it is illegal to refuse to provide your child with an education. Similar restrictions should apply to the genetic choices of prospective parents.

For some indication of the potential power of education to enhance beyond human norms, consider the work of the psychologist K. Anders Ericsson on the acquisition of skills by "deliberate practice" (Ericsson *et al.* 1993). Those who undertake deliberate practice do more than practice hard or a lot. They practice in a way designed to extend their skills. They thereby avoid some of the plateaus in achievement that many of us experience when we, or our teachers, decide that we can perform a skill well enough. Perhaps the most striking examples of the power of deliberate practice to produce enhancement beyond human norms are the three chess champion sisters, Susan, Sofia, and Judit Polgár. Their father insists that the girls showed no particular aptitude for chess. He subjected them to a program of extended deliberate practice—thousands of hours of highly structured instruction in the game—that turned the sisters into some of the world's strongest players.

Deliberate practice is a means of enhancement that differs from genetic modifications that have the same stated aim. The human enhancement consistency test suggests an obligation for those who find a moral difference between the enhancement of chess skills by deliberate practice and their enhancement by genetic modification to justify this difference. The liberal argument in favor of enhancement provides a *prima facie* reason to believe there is none.

Some of the issues that arise with respect to genetic enhancement may not arise with environmental enhancement. Genetic enhancement is still a comparatively new technology; the possibility of unintended side effects of genetic interventions is one reason to be more cautious when pursuing genetic enhancements than when pursuing equivalent enhancements via environmental means. Even where there are differences, the enhancement consistency test should lead us to acknowledge some issues shared by both genetic and environmental enhancements. For example, there is a concern about the distributive justice of human enhancement of both kinds. If the wealthy are permitted to fit out their children's genomes with enhancements, then we seem faced with an exacerbation of current social inequalities. The same concerns are pertinent to enhancements resulting from deliberate practice. Suppose wealthy parents identify enhancements leading to social success. They provide their children with programs of deliberate practice that enhance beyond human norms. Parents working hard to feed and clothe children are unlikely to have the means to implement such programs. Children enhanced beyond human norms by programs of deliberate practice may enjoy the same unfair advantages over the unenhanced as would genetically enhanced children.

The (possibly near) future may bring more extreme environmental enhancements. For example, the inventor and futurologist Ray Kurzweil advocates enhancement by grafting cybernetic implants and prostheses to our brains and bodies. As he sees it, the early stages of this merger between human and machine will be motivated by a desire to fix parts of our brains and bodies that have become diseased. Some profoundly deaf people are now fitted with cochlear implants that directly stimulate their auditory nerves. There is work on a prosthetic hippocampus that may someday restore memories ravaged by Alzheimer's disease. These examples can be considered both as improvements and as therapies. According to Kurzweil the integration of technology into our brains and bodies is the first significant step toward radical human enhancement. These enhancements (or therapies) can be seen as precursors to more radical human enhancement. The procedures that introduce these devices into human brains fall on the environmental side of the distinction between genetic and environmental enhancement. They involve no modification or selection of human genetic material, yet their effects could result in beings enhanced to much greater degrees than are possible via purely genetic means.

Is It Impermissible to Genetically Enhance Beyond Human Norms?

A number of philosophers, including Habermas and Fukuyama, have argued that genetic enhancement beyond human norms is impermissible. These philosophers argue for the moral relevance of both the degree of enhancement and the means by which it is obtained. They allow that some non-genetic means of enhancement beyond human norms are acceptable, as well as therapeutic genetic interventions.

Fukuyama (2002) argues that genetic enhancement is wrong because it corrupts human nature. He presents an account of human nature as fixed by human genes. It is, according to him, "the sum of the behavior and characteristics that are typical of the human species, arising from genetic rather than environmental factors" (Fukuyama 2002: 130). Fukuyama views those who aspire to genetically enhance beyond human norms as seeking to alter what has hitherto remained relatively invariant throughout human history and across the full gamut of human cultures. Fukuyama offers an explanation of the importance of his genetic conception of human nature. He connects it to a property of humans he calls Factor X. Factor X is not constituted by "the possession of moral choice, or reason, or language, or sociability, or sentience, or emotions, or consciousness, or any other quality that has been put forth as a ground for human dignity" (Fukuyama 2002: 171). Rather it is all of these attributes together. Factor X is supposed to capture "something unique about the human race that entitles every member of the species to higher moral status than the rest of the natural world" (Fukuyama 2002: 160). The shared human genome is what joins them and therefore entitles us to respect. According to Fukuyama, enhancement threatens to undermine our human dignity by intruding on its genetic foundations.

Fukuyama seems to be relying on a genetic determinist model of human development. Yet, there is a tension between his emphasis on genes and the interactionist model of development. It is mistaken to present the characteristics typical of human species as more strongly connected with human genes than with human environments. Embedding a cybernetic device in a brain could result in dramatic cognitive improvements without altering genes. Fukuyama's implicit reliance on genetic determinism, as well as being unsupported by empirical findings, fails to appreciate the magnitude of enhancements that are possible via purely environmental interventions.

There is however a deeper reason to think that appeals to human nature fail to gain traction in the debate about human enhancement. When we speculate about the harms potentially inflicted by extreme cybernetic or genetic enhancement, we are thinking of human nature as an essential property of human individuals. Norman Daniels (2009) challenges this way of thinking by arguing that we should acknowledge human nature as a population concept. Viewed this way, human nature does not describe any relatively invariant property of human individuals, which could be under threat from the wrong kind of modification. Human nature encompasses a very wide range of genetic variability and diverse gene–environment interactions. Daniels says of a modification that might push an individual human outside of the range of traits properly encompassed by human nature: "By itself, this does not alter human nature. It creates freaks." Daniels continues that "If it operated on a population level, we might well . . . count it as a change in human nature" (Daniels 2009: 37). So long as enhanced beings remain rare then enhancement cannot alter human nature. The concept of human nature seems, therefore, oriented at the wrong level of explanation to explain any harms to individuals that may follow from too much enhancement.

Earlier we described the liberal suggestion that attempts to enhance by altering genetic influences deserve similar treatment to attempts to enhance by environmental means. Habermas (2003) thinks he has found a moral difference between the two types of developmental influence. He proposes that there is something problematic in the manner of the intervention required to enhance a child-to-be. Prospective parents who presume to genetically enhance their children illegitimately present themselves as co-authors of their children's lives. "The programming intentions of parents who are ambitious and given to experimentation . . . have the peculiar status of a one-sided and unchallengeable expectation" (Habermas 2003: 51). Habermas claims this is the difference between genetic and environmental enhancement. Children confronted with a parental plan to enhance by means of an educational program can rebel. Had the Polgár sisters taken every opportunity to hurl chess pieces at daddy's head, doubtless he would have given up on his plan to manufacture chess geniuses. A particularly determined parent may quash any resistance, but they cannot rule out its very possibility. According to Habermas, genetic enhancement differs in this respect. There is simply no possibility of having a say over how your early embryo is genetically modified. There is, according to Habermas, an asymmetry between genetic enhancers and the genetically enhanced, an asymmetry in tension with the egalitarian aspirations of liberal societies. Tomorrow's citizens would become "defenseless objects of prior choices made by the planners of today" (Habermas 2003: 48). Habermas does not object to therapeutic uses of genetic selection or modification. He claims these interventions do not impose specific or idiosyncratic plans on the lives of future citizens; they do not constrain the child's future choices about the course his or her life will follow.

This challenge has drawn responses from defenders of liberal views about genetic enhancement. If important human traits emerge through the interaction of environmental and genetic factors, then it is simply impossible to make a football star by selecting or modifying embryonic DNA. If you discover, as a young teenager, that your parents have sought to replicate in your genome what they deem to be the relevant parts of Pelé's genome, then you must live with the fact that your embryonic DNA was modified. But it still remains possible for you to prevent those genetic modifications from having the effects on your development sought by your enhancers. You can choose to play badminton instead of football. Your parents' enhancement agenda does not prevent you from making uses of your genetic advantages that run counter to their plans.

The Lure of Radical Enhancement

How far should we pursue human enhancement? Transhumanism is a social and intellectual movement that "affirms the possibility and desirability of fundamentally improving the human condition through applied reason, especially by developing and making widely available technologies to eliminate aging and to greatly enhance human intellectual, physical, and psychological capacities" (The Transhumanist FAQ). Some transhumanists argue that we should enhance beyond the point where we are no longer human. We should become "posthuman." Far from seeing our humanity and human natures as warranting protection from enhancement technologies, human nature is something that we should readily abandon if in doing so we can attain more valuable lives. For transhumanists, the notion of human nature implies a collection of limitations on how long we can live and how intelligent we can be. Contrary to Fukuyama's claims, in this age of rapidly advancing technology transhumanists consider retaining our human nature as an obstacle to flourishing rather than a necessary condition for it.

Some allies of the transhumanists have offered concrete proposals not only for how we can enhance beyond human norms, but how we can achieve radical human enhancement. Here radical enhancement involves improving significant attributes and abilities to levels that *greatly exceed* what is currently possible for human beings. The contrast here is with moderate enhancement which aims to improve significant attributes and abilities to levels *within or close to* what is currently possible for human beings. Ray Kurzweil (2005) hopes to radically enhance human cognitive powers. He looks to accelerating the pace of improvement of information technologies. According to Kurzweil, humans will soon be benefiting from these advances, swapping out computationally inefficient disease-prone biological brain tissue for electronic chips. Kurzweil expects that the exponential improvement of information technologies will soon bring into existence a mind "about one billion times more powerful than all human intelligence today" (Kurzweil 2005: 136).

Nicholas Agar (2010) challenges the wisdom of radical enhancement. He questions the value to human beings of billion-fold enhancements of our cognitive powers and millennial lifespans. Agar advances an account of the valuing of future experiences or achievements that requires that we currently have some capacity to identify with them. This is a prudential claim. Radical enhancements may make us worse off by replacing valuable distinctively human experiences with radically enhanced experiences. These enhanced experiences can be considered objectively more valuable than our current experiences, but they are nonetheless of reduced value to us from our current human perspective.

There is one way we could imaginatively engage with radically enhanced experiences and therefore properly value them. We could undergo radical enhancement. Beings whose intellects are thousands of times more powerful than ours have their own distinctively valuable experiences. If we became them then we would value these radically enhanced experiences. Agar (2014) presents these as transformative changes akin to changes presented in the movie *Invasion of the Body Snatchers*. A human who is body snatched and survives the process would acquire new kinds of experience that she is likely to view as extremely valuable. Radical human enhancement involves a less extreme transformative change. But we should acknowledge that it has some of the same consequences for our values. Radical human enhancement is likely to cut us off from many of the ways we currently value our lives and experiences. Many of our most significant achievements are judged relative to explicitly anthropocentric standards. Running a four-minute mile or sending humans into space can be impressive achievements relative to anthropocentric standards. There are degrees of enhancement that will make such achievements seem trivial. Agar endorses moderate enhancements—those that fall within or just beyond the limits of current human variation. A gain of 15 IQ points that results from a genetic modification enhances in a way that does not rule out imaginative engagement. Such enhancements are compatible with the way humans are currently able to value their experiences.

The Possibility of Moral Enhancement

Recently there has been some discussion about the possibility of moral enhancement. There are two kind of moral enhancement. The aim of moral *disposition* enhancement is to increase the moral value of an agent's actions or character. Humans whose moral dispositions are enhanced may be more likely to do good deeds or to act from motives that we judge to be moral or virtuous.

Thomas Douglas (2008) argues that the moral permissibility of moral disposition enhancement is a challenge to the bioconservative thesis. This is the claim that enhancement by biomedical means is always impermissible. Douglas offers examples of what he claims are permissible moral enhancements through biomedical means. These moral bioenhancements could give us morally better motives by reducing the influence of counter-moral emotions—emotions that interfere with what we view as good moral thinking. These emotions include triggers of impulsive violent aggression and of racial prejudice. Douglas argues that if moral bioenhancement is permissible then it follows that an unqualified bioconservative thesis must be false.

Julian Savulescu and Ingmar Persson (2012) have a more practical interest in moral disposition enhancement. They appeal for urgent enhancement of human moral dispositions so that we may muster an adequate response to the problem of climate change. This problem seems to be exacerbated by a human inability to work together to properly address what is now widely appreciated as a threat to the entire human species. Savulescu and Persson think that making humans more moral will increase the likelihood that humans can look beyond their many disagreements and successfully cooperate to address the problem. They tentatively propose some candidate biomedical moral enhancers. There is some evidence that oxytocin can boost trust and gratitude, and that members of the selective serotonin reuptake inhibitors class of drugs increase cooperativeness (Savulescu and Persson 2012: 118–20). Both the proposals of Douglas and Persson and Savulescu fit best within the conception of enhancement as improvement. An increase in human cooperation could be conducive to the end of avoiding catastrophic climate change. This is true no matter where any individual is currently situated, whether it is within or below the spectrum of normal human dispositions to cooperate.

John Harris (2011) challenges this view on the grounds that moral enhancement via biomedical means undermines autonomy and the value of moral agency. Harris claims that without the "freedom to fall" our moral actions lack the intrinsic value that comes with having the choice to act immorally. He endorses the use of traditional means of moral improvement such as education and moral instruction, both of which can be considered as commonplace moral enhancements. The key difference is traditional means of moral enhancement are deliberative; they involve cognitive reasoning processes and coming to form beliefs that we can articulate and defend. According to Harris, moral enhancement by biomedical means bypasses our reasoning processes and directly affects our behavior without being subject to rational review. This is problematic in two ways. It may prevent us from performing certain moral good actions. For example, reducing impulses towards violence is not morally valuable if it results in failure to defend those unjustly threatened with harm. In addition, Harris points out that "ethical expertise is not 'being better at being good', rather it is being better at knowing the good" (Harris 2011: 104). According to Harris, morally good action must originate in the right kind of way from an agent's moral judgments.

Moral disposition enhancement is supposed to increase the moral value of an agent's actions or character. Moral *status* enhancement improves an individual's entitlement to beneficial treatment and reduces eligibility for certain forms of harmful treatment. In discussions of moral status, there is typically a distinction made between persons, beings capable of practical rationality, and non-persons, beings capable of suffering, but which lack these more complex cognitive capacities. Might a significant increase in the morally relevant capacities of persons result in beings with a moral status higher than persons, i.e., post-persons?

Allen Buchanan (2011) rejects this inference. He argues that personhood is a threshold concept. A certain level of practical rationality is required to satisfy the criteria for personhood. However, once this point is reached, no quantitative increase of the relevant capacities can result in an improvement in a being's moral status. This means that no matter what degree of enhancement humans undergo, we cannot obtain a higher moral status than personhood. With a large enough degree of enhancement we may become post-human, but there will never be post-persons.

Some philosophers have accepted Buchanan's challenge and offered accounts of beings with status superior to persons. For example, Jeff McMahan (2009) offers examples of beings that might have moral statuses superior to persons. McMahan observes that many people think that we have a moral status higher than animals because we are capable of free action and they are not. He offers a hypothesis about beings with moral statuses superior to our own that makes sense on the assumption that robust libertarian freewill is philosophically coherent. Suppose that beings whose free acts are not causally determined are metaphysically possible and furthermore that humans are not free in this strong sense. We are free only in a weaker compatibilist sense compatible with the operation of deterministic laws. McMahan suggests that we might credit beings free in the libertarian sense with a status superior to our own. "They would have a psychological capacity that we lack but that most people have believed that we have and that is what distinguishes us morally from animals" (McMahan 2009: 604). David DeGrazia (2012) describes a "Future with Post-persons" scenario set in the year 2145. DeGrazia's putative post-persons are better than current human persons in a variety of ways—they reason better than us, have far superior moral dispositions, and so on. He contends that "post-persons have about as much justification in believing that they have higher moral status than persons as persons have in believing that they have higher moral status than animals" (DeGrazia 2012: 138).

Agar (2012) takes a different approach. He proposes that we may be unable to conceive of beings with status higher than our own. The ability to fully understand the criteria for post-personhood may be beyond current human cognitive capacities. For example, giving a non-person the ability to fully grasp why the capacity for practical reason grants a superior moral status may lead it to actually satisfy these criteria. It is therefore to be expected that we will struggle to fully grasp the criteria for possessing a moral status higher than our own. Agar offers an inductive inference for the possibility of post-persons. We currently acknowledge differences in moral status in virtue of differences in properties possessed by different categories of things. Inanimate objects such as rocks have zero moral status. Sentient non-persons have an intermediate moral status. Persons currently possess the highest moral status. We therefore have good inductive grounds to believe in the possibility of beings with moral statuses superior to our own.

Conclusion

Two concepts of enhancement are required to cover the complexities of differing means, degrees, and targets of enhancement. We have outlined moral considerations that arise from pursuing enhancements through different means, and suggested a consistency test for morally evaluating different enhancements. We applied the consistency test to a variety of different means, degrees, and targets of human enhancement. Our discussion of different means of enhancement included the modification of genetic influences and the modification of environmental influences. We surveyed different degrees of enhancement ranging from those within human norms to those far beyond them. We discussed enhancement that takes as its target human moral capacities.

This chapter has sampled lines of argument from what is an exciting and increasingly thematically diverse philosophical debate. The debate is fast moving. A philosophical snapshot of the human enhancement debate 10 years hence is likely to reveal new dangers and opportunities. These questions will become increasingly important to consider as the pace of technological progress opens new avenues for human enhancement. We ought to consider them before it is too late for our answers to contribute to shaping the future trajectory of humanity.

Related Topics

Chapter 20, "The Ethics of Biomedical Research Involving Animals," Tom L. Beauchamp
Chapter 39, "Medicalization, 'Normal Function,' and the Definition of Health," Rebecca Kukla

References

Agar, N. (2010) *Humanity's End: Why We Should Reject Radical Enhancement*, Cambridge: MIT Press.

Agar, N. (2013) "Why Is It Possible to Enhance Moral Status and Why Doing So Is Wrong?" *Journal of Medical Ethics* 39: 67–74.

Agar, N. (2014) *Truly Human Enhancement: A Philosophical Defense of Limits*, Cambridge: MIT Press.

Buchanan, A. (2011) *Beyond Humanity: The Ethics of Biomedical Enhancement*, New York: Oxford University Press.

Buchanan, A., Brock, D., Daniels, N. and Wikler, D. (2000) *From Chance to Choice: Genetics and Justice*, Cambridge: Cambridge University Press.

Daniels, N. (2009) "Can Anyone Really be Talking about Ethically Modifying Human Nature," in J. Savulescu and N. Bostrom (eds.) *Human Enhancement*, Oxford: Oxford University Press.
DeGrazia, D. (2012) "Genetic Enhancement, Post-persons, and Moral Status: A Reply to Buchanan," *Journal of Medical Ethics* 38: 135–9.
Douglas, T. (2008) "Moral Enhancement," *Journal of Applied Philosophy* 25: 228–45.
Ericsson, K., Krampe, R. and Tesch-Romer. C., (1993) "The Role of Deliberate Practice in the Acquisition of Expert Performance," *Psychological Review* 100: 363–406.
Fukuyama, F. (2002) *Our Posthuman Future: Consequences of the Biotechnology Revolution*, New York: Farrar, Straus & Giroux.
Habermas, J. (2003) *The Future of Human Nature*, Cambridge: Polity.
Harris, J. (1998) *Clones, Genes, and Immortality: Ethics and the Genetic Revolution*, New York: Oxford University Press.
Harris, J. (2011) "Moral Enhancement and Freedom," *Bioethics* 25: 102–11.
Kevles, D. (1998) *In the Name of Eugenics: Genetics and the Uses of Human Heredity*, Cambridge: Harvard University Press.
Kurzweil, R. (2005) *The Singularity Is Near: When Humans Transcend Biology*, London: Penguin.
McMahan, J. (2009) "Cognitive Disability and Cognitive Enhancement," *Metaphilosophy* 40: 582–605.
Paul, D. (1995) *Controlling Human Heredity: 1865 to the Present*, Atlantic Highlands: Humanity Books.
Savulescu, J. and Persson, I. (2012) *Unfit for the Future? Modern Technology, Liberal Democracy and the Need for Moral Enhancement*, Oxford: Oxford University Press.
Tang, Y., Shimizu, E., Dube, G.R., Rampon, C., Kerchner, G.A., Zhuo, M. *et al.* (1999) "Genetic Enhancement of Learning and Memory in Mice," *Nature* 401: 63–9.
The Transhumanist FAQ. Available at: http://humanityplus.org/philosophy/transhumanist-faq/ (accessed August 2, 2014).

41
RACE AND BIOETHICS

Alexis Shotwell and Ami Harbin

Racial difference has been of central concern in many canonical cases in bioethics. Consider two historical cases: Nazi medical experimentation and the now-infamous Tuskegee Syphilis Study. It was in response to revelations about Nazi experiments on human subjects that the Nuremberg Code was formulated. The Code sets out standards for informed consent, treatment of research subjects, and the necessity of predictable benefit from any given experiment. Nazi experimentation was based on an explicitly racializing notion: That Jews were a separate, and lesser, racial group and therefore appropriate subjects for experimentation. The Tuskegee Study of Untreated Syphilis (or "the Study") was a 40-year (1932–72) clinical study that observed the progression of (mostly) untreated syphilis in a group of black men living in poverty in the U.S. These men were told that they were receiving free health care, when in fact they were not given effective treatment for syphilis even after such treatments were medically established. The Study was ended only when journalist Jean Heller broke the story. Responses to Tuskegee included the establishment in the U.S. of an Office for Human Research Protections, which aims to curtail the kinds of research abuses evident in the Tuskegee Study. In this chapter, we will use the Tuskegee Study as a touchstone for considering how racialization and bioethics matter to one another.

Racialization may be an unfamiliar word—it is less common, certainly, than *race*, or *racism*. We follow sociologists like Michael Omi and Howard Winant in thinking of race as "racial formation," which they define as "the process by which social, economic and political forces determine the content and importance of racial categories, and by which they are in turn shaped by racial meanings" (Omi and Winant 1994: 61). This means that what we think of as "race" arises out of social relations, instead of coming from some biological reality "underneath" those social meanings. Racial formation is a way to understand the way that physical, social, and material things in the world are classified as racial—things like people's hair, bodies, ways of speaking, and so on. This sort of conception of race as a dynamic, in-process social effect is also often termed "racialization."

The Study is a useful starting point for thinking about racialization and bioethics for several reasons. First, reference to the Study has been important in formulating critical conceptions of the importance of informed consent in medical research and clinical treatment; talk of it circulates widely. Second, invocations of the Study within bioethics may well be deficient precisely in their considerations of race, and so extending the considerations of race in bioethics using the example of the Study may be instructive. As Susan Reverby writes in her exhaustive history of Tuskegee:

> Bioethicists kept knowledge of the Study alive in research publications and teaching, but only in narrow ways . . . A survey of the key bioethics encyclopedias in their multiple editions and the major edited collections and texts reveals that the Study came in and out of use, primarily named as an example of the lack of informed consent and the ability of researchers to take advantage of the vulnerable. It provided a way to say that race matters and then to never really interrogate in what ways.
>
> (Reverby 2009: 193)

So, centering on the Study can help us interrogate *in what ways* race matters to bioethics. In particular, the Study opens more adequate ways to understand the racial content of our bioethical judgments than can be encompassed by talk of consent in situations of inequality.

Yet taking the Syphilis Study as a touchstone for a discussion of bioethics and racialization may also problematically limit understanding. Much of the time, discussions of race focus primarily or exclusively on the U.S., and within that context, narrowing to a near-complete focus on black/white racial inequalities. For example, the promisingly titled but ultimately limited article "Why Bioethics Cannot Figure Out What to Do with Race" concludes that the main problem with the discipline of bioethics' failure to adequately treat race is a failure to decide whether to include the (U.S.) Black Church in bioethical debates (Burton 2007: 10). While the specific historical context of the U.S. is very important for understanding the relation of race and bioethics, it would be a serious mistake to accept that the only forms of racialization relevant to bioethics arise from the U.S. black/white context. Our hope is that in taking the Tuskegee Study as a key example, the discussion below provides multi-use conceptual tools for thinking about racialization in many contexts, even while it skirts these dangers.

In looking at these early cases, we can see that some of the legal and cultural norms that established the professional and academic field of bioethics are entangled with race. And though it is not obvious that race is at work in every bioethical question we face, we will argue that race is intimately bound up in even the most everyday bioethical judgments.

Race and Racisms

Although this chapter focuses on the question of how race matters to bioethics, from the start we need to think more clearly about the central concepts—"race" and "racism." As described above, a commonsense way to think about race is as biological differences between people—and, indeed, historically this has been one way of understanding what race is. In this chapter, we reject the idea that there are bright lines of biological difference between groups that could delineate one race from another. When we say that we hold a racial formation or racialization view of race we don't mean that there's no such thing as race, or that race has no effects. We mean, though, that bioethicists should understand the effects and material realities of race as not biologically determined. Indeed, we agree with writers like Anne Fausto-Sterling, who argue that biology itself takes shape through and with social formations (see Fausto-Sterling 2005, 2008).

For its part, racism is often understood as the direct, explicit expression of interpersonal ill will, which can take the form of explicitly discriminatory policies or hateful speech (Garcia 2004). It is also seen as ignorance, whether actively shaped or passively absorbed (Mills 1998, 2007; Outlaw 2007; Sullivan and Tuana 2007; Types 2007). Of course, even people with the best intentions can be racist. There are other sorts of racism that are not formulated in words. There is another sense altogether in which we might understand racism as not thoroughly described by explicit expressions of personal ill will or prejudice. Structural or systemic racism may never take the form of racist expression; indeed, perhaps more racial wrongdoing is effected by seemingly bloodless bureaucracy than self-proclaimed or subtle individual racist people (Arendt 2006).

Interlocking Systems of Oppression

Whenever discussing the process of racial formation, we do best to also remember that other markers of social identity change the experience and meaning of the social dynamic we call "race." Individuals' experiences of gender, sexuality, class, disability, religious orientation, and more will shape their experience of race—and, indeed, attending to any of those axes of oppression and liberation requires concurrently attending to race. This mode of taking complex social relations into account in our theorizing and understanding is known as having an "interlocking oppressions" or "intersectional" analysis (see Collins 1998; Crenshaw 1991; Razack 1998). Because different forms of oppression and privilege are bound up with each other, we cannot think effectively about only one bit of the whole picture as though it is disconnected from others. In this chapter, we will for the most part use the phrase "interlocking oppressions" to name the relational co-production of social relations of inequality. This is a departure from some of the ways such analysis has been codified and made part of a feminist intellectual canon (see Carastathis 2008).

There are (at least) three levels on which we can see the importance of taking racialization into account in bioethics: Individual, group/collective, and systemic. At each level, many different social relations come together to shape the particular experience or problem under consideration. In thinking about racialization and bioethics it is particularly useful to note the ways someone may be harmed or oppressed in some ways while being benefitted or privileged in others. For example, someone may be harmed—or even oppressed—because of their gender, while receiving social goods because they are not disabled. Thus, people can be simultaneously, unevenly, oppressed and benefitting from oppression.

Individual Experiences of Racialization

On an individual level, racialization matters to bioethics. Individual physicians and researchers may have responses and make medical decisions based on their and their patients' racial position. After controlling for socioeconomic and access-related discrepancies between individuals belonging to different racialized groups, there remain significant disparities in health care across racial and ethnic lines. The Institute of Medicine (of the U.S. National Academy of Sciences) investigated these disparities and concluded that "racial or ethnic differences in the quality of health care" resulted at least in part from physician bias, stereotyping, or prejudice (Smedley et al. 2003; Balsa and McGuire 2003; Brody 2009). Current work on the concept of "implicit bias" indicates that even—and perhaps especially—people who do not believe they are discriminating based on race and other social identities actually do respond differently relative to these social categories (Wear 2003; Jost et al. 2009; Stivers and Majid 2007; Penner et al. 2010). More fundamentally, when discrimination based on race arises in health contexts, whether treatment or research, it always manifests in individual people's actual bodies and experience. So we must think about racialization on what Brody et al. call the "micro-level," at the scale of people experiencing illness in part because of how they are racialized (Brody et al. 2012: 309). Although the force of racialization may be more obvious as it manifests itself in the lives of people of color, we could see every experience of health or illness as racialized—people who hold the social position of whiteness will have a different interaction with their doctor than will people of color. And other things being equal, a white patient's interaction will have more dignity and show more respect for patient autonomy (Cooper et al. 2012). A white patient's interaction will also likely produce better health outcomes. The U.S. Department of Health and Human Services' (2012) *National Healthcare Disparities Report* tracks specific disparities in acute preventive care for numerous conditions, by race and other markers. Of course, other things are rarely equal, and white people living in poverty, white people with disabilities, queer white people, will almost certainly have health outcomes worse than, for example, higher class, non-disabled, straight white people based on their entanglement with the harmful aspects of interlocking systems of privilege and oppression.

In the Tuskegee Study, recall, doctors followed a group of African-American men who had untreated syphilis in order to study the progression of the untreated disease. Participants in the Study were told they were signing up to receive free health care, and they were also guaranteed a funeral paid for by the Study. We can see that individual-scale racialization was manifest most obviously in the interactions between the doctors running the Study and the people participating in it. The black men enrolled in the Study were told that they were being treated, though not what for, when in fact they were being given merely aspirin and iron supplements. Most damningly for the doctors overseeing the Study from the Public Health Service (PHS), in cases when the men could have received effective treatment, they were not informed of these possibilities. For example, a number of the men enrolled in the Study pursued enlistment in the U.S. armed forces. Unbeknownst to them, the PHS had provided a list of their names to the Army with an explanation of their participation in a valuable medical study (Jonsen 2003: 148; Reverby 2009: 61). The U.S. Army had a policy of treating incoming recruits for syphilis, so when it rejected men from the Study we can see that they were directly denied treatment. Far more of the participants, along with their sexual partners, were indirectly denied proper treatment through relations of omission.

Race shaped the Study in terms of who was enrolled, how they were denied treatment, and how physicians, nurses, and researchers interacted with the participants. On an individual level, particular black men enrolled in the study were not treated for syphilis. The men who participated in the PHS Tuskegee Study were never provided with the opportunity to give anything like informed consent because they were not told that they had syphilis, or that they were not being treated for a disease they had, or that treatment was available, or a host of other salient facts. This failure to secure informed consent has been the central focus of much of the response in bioethics. The doctors, nurses, and researchers who participated in the Study were ignoring the broadest duty to provide a clear account of what facts were known, possible treatment options, and likely future results of engaging in the Study. In some cases their behavior exhibited disbelief that study participants were capable of understanding their situation (Reverby 2009: 55, 60, 116, 128; Brandt 1978).

How race and racism were involved in these ethical failures is not, however, as simple as it might seem. There were now-obvious problems with the failure to allow for informed consent and with the exploitation of a vulnerable population for research purposes. There has been a temptation to tell the story of the Study as though the racial dynamics were simple: Bad, racist white doctors lied to and took advantage of illiterate Black sharecroppers to secure their careers (see Brandt (1978) for an early and important intervention in the racial dynamics of the Study). This story is accurate, but it is not complete. Not only was the Study hosted at the pre-eminent black research institution in the U.S. South, and not only were there black medical personnel involved all the way through, but the participants and practitioners were working within the constant background of everyday, unacknowledged racism. If, as we hope to show, health care and health research always function within the context of racialization, it will not be enough for medical ethics to ask about the intentional actions and omissions of "bad racist" practitioners. Bioethicists must consider the broader questions of ethical action in relation to group identity as well as in relation to systems of inequality.

The Implications of Racialization for Groups

On a group or collective level, medical practice may be informed by racialization in harmful ways. In virtue of their group membership, and perhaps also in ways that define their group membership, racialized people can be picked out for differential treatment. For example, historically, racialization was involved in group-level decision-making in the form of eugenicist medical practices. Forced sterilization—and a concomitant valuing and encouragement of white women to have children—interact with racialization in the medical domain, and not only in terms of the individual-level effects to the women sterilized (Silliman et al. 2004; Smith 2005). Other invasions of women of color's reproductive health include research informed by racialization, as in the case of Dr J. Marion Sims (1813–83), an Alabama surgeon who conducted experimental surgeries on black slave women in his development of treatment for vesicovaginal fistula (Axelson 1985; Wall 2006).

In much bioethics training today the way that students and clinicians are taught to engage with group differentiation uses the language of cultural competency for working with multicultural populations in health situations (Carrese and Sugarman 2006; Paasche-Orlow 2004; Washington 2009; Wear 2003). Although often there is some commitment to think about cultural competency as relevant to queer, disabled, non-majority language-speaking, or elderly patients, the term "culture" frequently supplements and, often, actually stands in for "race." Although it is important for medical practitioners to be competent to treat people who come from various backgrounds, there is a difference between racialization and culture (or ethnicity). This is particularly the case in medical contexts in which researchers and medical practitioners believe that there are biological differences between races (Kahn 2012). An early, and still-important, definition set out cultural competency as "a set of congruent behaviors, attitudes, and policies that come together in a system, agency or amongst professionals and enables that system, agency or those professionals to work effectively in cross-cultural situations" (Cross et al. 1989; cited in Brach and Fraserirector 2000: 182). Much racial grouping, even when it is framed as cultural, takes the form of treating people as though racial identity were a biologically determinable reality. Given this, it is striking that much clinical practice focuses on better managing the interpersonal manifestation of racialized group identities through increasing cultural competence in the medical professional. The PHS Syphilis Study should not be seen as primarily a failure of cultural competence.

As a paradigm of racialized wrongdoing, "Tuskegee" grouped black people in a particular place into a racialized group that was then understood as biologically distinct. A danger is that such clumping solidifies an implicit or explicit belief that there are biological differences between races. This was certainly a dynamic at the outset of the Study—researchers believed that African Americans had different (deficient) brains, and thus that the neurological effects of late-stage syphilis would be different by race (Reverby 2009: 45; see also Crenner 2012). Further, at least some of the individual wrong-doings on the level of consent and exploitation were the result of a perception that it was acceptable to sacrifice the interests of the men involved in the Study to the interests of black people in the U.S. more generally. At the time of the study, there was a belief that black people were biologically categorically different than white people, and therefore that it was medically beneficial to others to follow the progression of the disease (Reverby 2009: 159–61). Presumed group identity can, in cases like these, degrade the care individuals receive. The Study serves, in the present, as a short hand for talking about group-differentiated distrust of medical authority; racialized people in the U.S., especially black people, are represented as holding Tuskegee in mind (Brandon et al. 2005; Gamble 1997; Freimuth et al. 2001; W. King 2003). Some writers argue that medical practitioners should be knowledgeable about Tuskegee specifically in order to show knowledge of why race matters to medicine (i.e., as part of cultural competence) (Chiu and Katz 2011; Corbie-Smith 1999).

A perhaps surprising example of this is marked by the first drug approved by the U.S. Food and Drug Administration (FDA) for race-specific administration in the U.S., BiDil (two previously approved generic drugs, hydralazine and isosorbide dinitrate, which when combined are meant to treat heart failure in African Americans). As Johnathan Kahn has argued (see Kahn 2005, 2007), the specification of this drug as effective for, and only for, African-American patients with cardiac disorders has dubious beginnings and some pernicious effects. The dubious beginnings help us think about the difficulties in grouping people by racial group. The researcher who patented the BiDil combination re-examined past data, theorizing from a small (53-person) sample that the drug was more effective for African Americans. A second study was conducted with 1,050 self-identified African-American participants, and based on those data, the drug was approved for use in only African Americans. BiDil costs nearly six times its generic equivalents, leading some to believe that the re-patenting did not arise primarily out of a desire to benefit black patients with heart conditions. The pernicious effects of the approval include the medical reification of social groupings based on self-identification (Lee et al. 2001). Since there is no scientific definition of who, in BiDil's terms, counts as "black people," it is difficult to say who would be appropriate subjects for its administration. Since there is no biological test for racialization, there can be no biological ground for prescribing BiDil—leaving anyone from the patient's doctors to their insurance company to the FDA responsible for their racial classification for medical purposes. As Kahn argues:

> Researchers using race to develop drugs may be motivated by good intentions, but such efforts are also driven by the dictates of an increasingly competitive medical marketplace. The example of BiDil indicates that researchers and regulators alike have not fully appreciated that race is a powerful and volatile category. When used to bolster the commercial value of a drug, it can lead to haphazard regulation, sub-standard medical treatment and other unfortunate

> unintended consequences. The FDA should not grant race-specific approvals without clear and convincing evidence of a genetic or biological basis for any observed racial differences in safety or efficacy. Approving more drugs such as BiDil will not alleviate the very serious health disparities between races in the U.S. We need social and political will, not mislabeled medicines, to redress that injustice.
>
> (Kahn 2007: 45)

Kahn here points to a third way in which we can understand racialization as significant for bioethics: Health disparities arising out of systemic or structural inequality.

Racialization and Systems of Oppression

Systemically, race, in concert with other systems of privilege and oppression, is one of the most significant determinants of health or illness. As Ruth Wilson Gilmore has argued, we can track racialization in part by examining the statistical likelihood of dying young; this political point is underlined by the now vast public health literature addressing health disparities (see Institute of Medicine 2002; Fiscella et al. 2002; Lasser et al. 2006). Racial and socio-economic status differentially shape the health of children (Chen et al. 2006), making it necessary to track both race/ethnicity and class status in giving an account of health inequalities (Kawachi et al. 2005; LaVeist 2005). As such, further close attention must be paid in bioethics to how multiple systems of inequality function together to affect health, with care to not neglect the importance of race in such processes.

We mentioned the U.S. Institute of Medicine's report on health disparities (*Unequal Treatment: Confronting Racial and Ethnic Disparities in Health Care*) above; as Alan Nelson, a member of the committee that prepared the report said, the committee "finished its work convinced that the real challenge lies not in debating whether disparities exist, because the evidence is overwhelming, but in the developing and implementing of strategies to reduce and eliminate them" (Institute of Medicine 2002: 667). However, the recommendations the committee makes remain at the level of improving doctor–patient communication, patient empowerment, allocating more resources for civil rights investigations about health wrongs, with relatively scant mention of changing the U.S. health system. To address the health disparities created and sustained by racialization, bioethics must take into account the complexities of racism at individual, group, and systemic levels.

Future Directions

Encouragingly, bioethicists have begun to examine the impact of social and racial inequality on health. They have begun to highlight how the following kinds of questions must be asked in order to develop anti-racist approaches to bioethics.

How Can Bioethicists Address Racism Beyond Concerns about Informed Consent, Self-determination, and Autonomy?

Patricia King (1998, 2004, 2007) argues that despite widespread recognition in U.S. bioethics that the Tuskegee Syphilis Study stands as a common trope for recognizing racism in medical research:

> There has been inadequate attention paid to race, either in the sense of negative and differential treatment or in terms of pervasive scientific racism, in the construction of bioethics in the United States. American bioethics, from its inception, has resisted taking account of social context. In American bioethics, individualism, self-determination, and autonomy are paramount. Other values, and other ethical issues, have historically enjoyed lesser status. Even today, the failure to obtain consent from the Tuskegee subjects continues to receive greater attention than the social and economic conditions in which the subjects found themselves.
>
> (P. King 2004: 149–50)

The central insight here is that all our ethical decision-making happens in a context of relations with other people and longstanding social realities (e.g., racism). Aiming to correct racism in health care practice by focusing only on the one-to-one level of interpersonal interaction (e.g., making sure that a physician is trained not to say anything racist) fails to attend to this broader social and historical context. In situations of systemic inequality, systems of oppression and benefit, all parties involved in health care practice would do well to take the social and historical context into account. Take the case of the Study, seen from a health equity perspective (and see Braveman (2006) on terminology). As even some doctors involved reflected, while they were not providing care to the men they studied, in some real ways focusing on their own individual wrong-doing is a red herring. Most, and perhaps all, of the men who participated in the Study lacked access to basic health care. With the exception of the men who could have joined the military, they would not have received care for syphilis even if they weren't enrolled in the Study. Would it have been better to not study (and not treat) people who were not being treated anyhow? (This argument fails at the point at which penicillin was available in public health clinics, from which many of the men seem to have been turned away.) Focusing on the ethical wrongdoing of the doctors and nurses leaves the ethical wrongs of an inequitable system uninterrogated. A focus on issues of informed consent and vulnerable populations obfuscates the bigger ethical problem, which is not seen as ethical at all: How can we have bioethical reasoning in a situation of fundamental inequity distributed by race?

How Might Bioethicists be Well Positioned to Investigate the Ways Health Care, Economic, Educational, Criminal Justice, Carceral, and Other Systems Work Together to Harm Racialized Individuals?

Bioethics might be well positioned to take a quite expansive role in redefining the meaning of race. We can think about race as a social fiction with material effects—a construct that becomes social reality. When we say "race" from this point of view, we mean "racialization." Recall that *racialization* names the social process through which individuals and groups of people come to be defined as a racial group. This is a process that brings together ways of talking about people (or discursive practices) with material conditions in order to define a group of people as a race. Such ways of talking have used, for example, biological explanations (there are real biological differences between races); geographical explanations (where a group of people live shapes their racial ontology); phenotypic explanations (physical morphology makes someone "really" one race or another); social or cultural explanations (how people live either comes from or produces their racial identity). To use the concept of racialization is to see the production of race *not* as a biological or cultural given, but rather as a social process through which people's bodies, cultural practices, and social/geographical locations come to carry and hold particular racial meanings. Bioethicists have the potential to be able to think relationally and holistically about how multiple social systems work together to harm racialized individuals—and about how multiple systems would need to coordinate to prevent harms or meaningfully benefit such groups.

How Can Public Health Ethics Correct Narrow Understanding of Health Disparities and the Harms of Racialization in Health Care Practice, Research, and Theory?

Many bioethicists write persuasively in the field of public health, some arguing compellingly for the need for bioethical accounts that focus on the way power dynamics shape relationships at all levels in health care (Fagan 2004; Baylis et al. 2008). Madison Powers and Ruth Faden argue that the health inequalities arising from "systemic patterns of disadvantage are the inequalities that are most morally urgent to address. Justice here demands aggressive public health intervention to document and help remedy existing patterns of systemic disadvantage and their detrimental consequences" (Powers and Faden 2006: 87). Annette Dula and Sara Goering's *It Just Ain't Fair: The Ethics of Health Care for African Americans* (1993) offers a sustained consideration of race and health disparities in the U.S. context, including discussions of infant mortality, HIV, rural health care, homelessness, black medical students, and surrogacy (see also Dula 2003, 2007). With increased focus on narrative medicine (Gotlib 2009), further attention should be paid to how narratives of experiences of racialization and racism could be important parts of improved health care. For example, when medical practitioners started listening to the people affected by the Tuskegee Study, they better understood the severity of harms experienced and could better anticipate where similar harms might be experienced in the future. The hope for public health ethics approaches is that they will begin already at a group level of understanding oppression in health care ethics, and so may be more able to resist reducing questions of race in health care practice to the imperative that individual racist health care providers become more racially competent.

How Can Race and Racism Shape Diagnostic Categories, Including (and not only) in Domains of Mental Health and Illness?

Bioethicists have worked from insights in science studies, biology, philosophy, and other domains to offer critical reflections on how classification systems can shape the health and lives of individuals subject to them. Of particular interest have been contentious diagnostic systems (e.g., classifications for sexual and reproductive illnesses; the Diagnostic and Statistical Manual of Mental Disorders). Bioethicists have highlighted the ways in which categorization and diagnosis have the power to shape not only the kind of treatment individuals receive, but the ways individuals perceive their own experience, and the possibility of individuals receiving care for conditions at all. Some bioethicists have investigated, for example, the ways perceptions of gender, class, and sexuality shape diagnoses of mental illness and the likelihood that individuals will be harmed by diagnostic categories. For example, bioethicists now know to be concerned about how readily characteristics of "sexual deviance" have been made diagnosable as mental illness (Martin 2001; Nissim-Sabat 2001; Potter 2004, 2005). New directions in bioethics will further attend to the ways racialization has shaped diagnostic categories in ways that harm individuals subject to them.

How Do Questions of Race and Racism Arise in the Development and Use of Medical Technologies?

Bioethicists have become able to appraise technological advancements in medicine and health research with a critical eye to what drives the development of technologies, what populations they are meant to aid, and how they can be used for goals beyond those for which they were intended (Gillis and de Melo Martín 2010). Attention to racialization could be productive in further considerations of all these questions. For example, how do genetic technologies intersect with racialization (Braun 2002)? How can practices of "biobanking" biological samples for research harm racialized groups in ways not obvious to those whose specimens are taken (Halverson and Ross 2012; Tutton 2009)? If researchers discover differences in how diseases and illnesses affect people by ethnic group, will health insurance coverage for different groups be affected? How do reproductive technologies reinforce racialization (Russell 2010)? In the domain of public health, area-based research and technologies of "geo-coding" can investigate the ways location/place intersects with race, gender, and socio-economic status to lead to health disparities (Kreiger et al. 2003). Engaging further with the extensive literature on how medical technologies affect populations could facilitate future bioethical investigations of race and medical technologies.

How Does Racialization Limit Communities' Ability to Direct and Conduct Research to Reflect Their Needs?

In questions of research ethics in medicine, bioethicists have been deeply critical of research conducted on communities that are not likely to benefit from the research, and of strategic neglect of the research questions of communities that are not likely to be profitable or universally relevant. Racialized communities have been harmed by both of these phenomena, and bioethicists could offer directions for highlighting the particular needs and vulnerabilities of racialized communities within public and private medical research agendas. How does racial grouping by researchers affect an individual participant's willingness to participate in a given study (Goldenberg et al. 2011)? How can bioethics help clarify the successes and challenges of research directed by racialized communities themselves?

Are Models Based on "Cultural Competence" Adequate for Understanding Race and Racism?

There are numerous problems with "cultural competency" approaches as a way to engage group differentiation by race. (For critical assessments, see Kumagai and Lypson (2009); Beagan and Kumas-Tan 2009.) One problem is that in attempting to describe medically salient features of different cultures the full heterogeneity of those cultures is occluded; it can become received wisdom that all Native Americans prefer to not have end-of-life decisions talked about explicitly, when in fact that preference may be specific to one tribe or nation, or to non-Christian first peoples. Another problem arises from the documented prevalence of implicit bias and stereotyping among white, Christian, Anglo nurses and doctors (Cooper et al. 2012) and how difficult it is to overcome bias even once it is made explicit. As we have discussed, perhaps the most significant problem with focusing primarily or exclusively on cultural competency training as a solution to the harms of racism in health care is when such a focus eclipses broader structures and systems that perpetuate inequality.

In sum, the challenge for bioethicists committed to developing anti-racist approaches in all domains of bioethics is to see racial inequities as a problem both perpetuated and partly addressable by clinical and theoretical bioethics. Bioethical thinking and practice can be improved, particularly with regard to the complex manifestation of race and racialization as health and illness. Doing justice to the individual, group, and systemic levels of racialization is difficult work, but both bioethics as a field and the lives of the people about whom bioethicists think and care would be better for it.

Related Topics

Chapter 2, "Social Determinants of Health and Health Inequalities," Michael Marmot and Sridhar Venkatapuram

Chapter 14, "Biomedical Research Ethics: Landmark Cases, Scandals, and Conceptual Shifts," Jonathan D. Moreno and Dominic Sisti

Chapter 18, "Research Involving 'Vulnerable Populations': A Critical Analysis," Toby Schonfeld

References

Arendt, H. (2006) *Eichmann in Jerusalem: A Report on the Banality of Evil*, London: Penguin Classics.

Axelson, D.E. (1985) "Women as Victims of Medical Experimentation: J Marion Sims's Surgery on Slave Women, 1845–1850," *Sage* 2 (2): 10–13.

Balsa, A.I. and McGuire, T.G. (2003) "Prejudice, Clinical Uncertainty and Stereotyping as Sources of Health Disparities," *Journal of Health Economics* 22 (1): 89–116.

Baylis, F., Kenny, N.P. and Sherwin, S. (2008) "A Relational Account of Public Health Ethics," *Public Health Ethics* 1 (3): 196.

Beagan, B. and Kumas-Tan, Z. (2009) "Approaches to Diversity in Family Medicine: 'I Have Always Tried to be Colour Blind,'" *Canadian Family Physician* 55: e21–8.

Brach, C. and Fraserirector, I. (2000) "Can Cultural Competency Reduce Racial and Ethnic Health Disparities? A Review and Conceptual Model," *Medical Care Research and Review* 57 (4 Suppl.): 181–217.

Brandon, D.T., Isaac, L.A. and LaVeist, T.A. (2005) "The Legacy of Tuskegee and Trust in Medical Care: Is Tuskegee Responsible for Race Differences in Mistrust of Medical Care?" *Journal of the National Medical Association* 97 (7): 951.

Brandt, A.M. (1978) "Racism and Research: The Case of the Tuskegee Syphilis Study," *Hastings Center Report* 8 (6): 21–9.

Braun, L. (2002) "Race, Ethnicity, and Health: Can Genetics Explain Disparities?" *Perspectives in Biology and Medicine* 45 (2): 159–74.

Braveman, P. (2006) "Health Disparities and Health Equity: Concepts and Measurement," *Annual Review of Public Health* 27: 167–94.

Brody, H. (2009) *Race and Health Disparities in the Future of Bioethics*, New York: Oxford University Press, 138–41.

Brody, H., Glenn, J. and Hermer, L. (2012) "Racial/Ethnic Health Disparities and Ethics: The Need for a Multilevel Approach," *Cambridge Quarterly of Healthcare Ethics* 21: 309–19.

Burton, O. (2007) "Why Bioethics Cannot Figure Out What to Do with Race," *The American Journal of Bioethics* 7 (2): 6–12.

Carastathis, A. (2008): "The Invisibility of Privilege: A Critique of Intersectional Models of Identity," *Les ateliers de l'éthique* 3 (2): 23–38.

Carrese, J.A. and Sugarman, J. (2006) "The Inescapable Relevance of Bioethics for the Practicing Clinician," *CHEST Journal* 130 (6): 1864–72.

Chen, E., Martin, A.D. and Matthews, K.A. (2006) "Understanding Health Disparities: The Role of Race and Socioeconomic Status in Children's Health," *Journal Information* 96 (4): 702–8.

Chiu, C.T. and Katz, R.V. (2011) "Identifying the 'Vulnerables' in Biomedical Research: The Vox Populis from the Tuskegee Legacy Project," *Journal of Public Health Dentistry* 71 (3): 220–8.

Collins, P.H. (1998) "It's All in the Family: Intersections of Gender, Race, and Nation," *Hypatia* 13(3): 62–82.

Cooper, L., Roter, D., Carson, K., Beach, M.C., Sabin, J., Greenwald, A. and Inui, T. (2012) "The Associations of Clinicians' Implicit Attitudes About Race With Medical Visit Communication and Patient Ratings of Interpersonal Care," *American Journal of Public Health* 102 (5): 979–87.

Corbie-Smith, G. (1999) "The Continuing Legacy of the Tuskegee Syphilis Study: Considerations for Clinical Investigation," *American Journal of the Medical Sciences* 317 (1): 5–8.

Crenner, C. (2012) "The Tuskegee Syphilis Study and the Scientific Concept of Racial Nervous Resistance," *Journal of the History of Medicine and Allied Sciences* 67 (2): 244–80.

Crenshaw, K. (1991) "Mapping the Margins: Intersectionality, Identity Politics, and Violence against Women of Color," *Stanford Law Review* 43 (6): 1241–99.

Cross, T.L., Bazron, B.J., Dennis, K.W. and Isaacs, M.R. (1989) *Towards a Culturally Competent System of Care: A Monograph on Effective Services for Minority Children Who Are Severely Emotionally Disturbed*, Washington, DC: CASSP Technical Assistance Center, Georgetown University Child Development Center.

Dula, A. (2003) "Racism and Health Care: A Medical Ethics Issue," in Lott, T.L. and Pittman, J.P. (eds.) *A Companion to African-American Philosophy*, Oxford: Blackwell Publishing.

Dula, A. (2007) "Whitewashing Black Health: Lies, Deceptions, Assumptions, and Assertions—and the Disparities Continue," in Prograis, L.J. and Pellegrino, E.D. (eds.) *African American Bioethics: Culture, Race, and Identity*, Washington DC: Georgetown University Press.

Dula, A. and Goering, S. (eds.) (1993) *It Just Ain't Fair: The Ethics of Health Care for African Americans*, Westport, CT: Praeger.

Fagan, A. (2004) "Challenging the Bioethical Application of the Autonomy Principle Within Multicultural Societies," *Journal of Applied Philosophy* 21 (1): 15–31.

Fausto-Sterling, A. (2005) "The Bare Bones of Sex," *Signs* 30 (2): 1491–528.

Fausto-Sterling, A. (2008) "The Bare Bones of Race," *Social Studies of Science* 38: 657–94.

Fine, M.J., Ibrahim, S.A. and Thomas, S.B. (2005) "The Role of Race and Genetics in Health Disparities Research," *American Journal of Public Health* 95 (12): 2125.

Fiscella, K., Franks, P., Doescher, M.P. and Saver, B.G. (2002) "Disparities in Health Care by Race, Ethnicity, and Language Among the Insured: Findings from a National Sample," *Medical Care* 40 (1): 52.

Freimuth, V.S., Quinn, S.C., Thomas, S.B., Cole, G., Zook, E. and Duncan, T. (2001) "African Americans' Views on Research and the Tuskegee Syphilis Study," *Social Science and Medicine* 52: 797–808.

Gamble, V.N. (1997) "Under the Shadow of Tuskegee: African Americans and Health Care," *American Journal of Public Health* 87 (11): 1773–8.

Garcia, J.L.A. (2004) "Three Sites for Racism: Social Structures, Valuings and Vice," in Levine, M.P. and Pataki, T. (eds.) *Racism in Mind*, Ithaca, NY: Cornell University Press.

Gillis, M. and de Melo Martín, I. (2010) "Editors' Introduction: Biomedical Technologies," *Hypatia* 25 (3): 497–503.

Gilmore, R.W. (2007) *Golden Gulag: Prisons, Surplus, Crisis, and Opposition in Globalizing California*, Volume 21, Oakland, CA: University of California Press.

Goldenberg, A.J., Hull, S.C., Wilfond, B.S. and Sharp, R.R. (2011) "Patient Perspectives on Group Benefits and Harms in Genetic Research," *Public Health Genomics* 14 (3): 135–42.

Gotlib, A. (2009) "Stories from the Margins: Immigrant Patients, Health Care, and Narrative Medicine," *International Journal of Feminist Approaches to Bioethics* 2 (2): 51–74.

Halverson, C. and Ross, L. (2012) "Engaging African-Americans about Biobanks and the Return of Research Results," *Journal of Community Genetics* 3 (4): 275–83.

Institute of Medicine (2002) *Unequal Treatment: Confronting Racial and Ethnic Disparities in Health Care*, London.

Jonsen, A.R. (2003) *The Birth of Bioethics*, Oxford: Oxford University Press.

Jost, J.T., Rudman, L.A., Blair, I.V., Carney, D.R., Dasgupta, N., Glaser, J. et al. (2009) "The Existence of Implicit Bias Is Beyond Reasonable Doubt: A Refutation of Ideological and Methodological Objections and Executive Summary of Ten Studies That No Manager Should Ignore," *Research in Organizational Behavior* 29: 39–69.

Kahn, J. (2005) "From Disparity to Difference: How Race Specific Medicines May Undermine Policies to Address Inequalities in Health Care," *Southern California Interdisciplinary Law Journal* 15: 105–29.

Kahn, J. (2007) "Race in a Bottle," *Scientific American* 297: 40–5.

Kahn, J. (2012) *Race in a Bottle: The Story of BiDil and Racialized Medicine in a Post-Genomic Age*, New York: Columbia University Press.

Kawachi, I., Daniels, N. and Robinson, D.E. (2005) "Health Disparities by Race and Class: Why Both Matter," *Health Affairs* 24 (2): 343–52.

King, P.A. (1998) "Race, Justice and Research," in Kahn, J.P., Mastroianni, A.C. and Sugarman J. (eds.) *Beyond Consent: Seeking Justice in Research*, New York: Oxford University Press, pp. 88–110.

King, P.A. (2004) "Reflections on Race and Bioethics in the United States," *Health Matrix* 14: 149.

King, P.A. (2007) "Race, Equity, Health Policy, and the African American Community," in Prograis, L.J. and Pellegrino, E.D. (eds.) *African American Bioethics: Culture, Race, and Identity*, Washington DC: Georgetown University Press.

King, W.D. (2003) "Examining African Americans' Mistrust of the Health Care System: Expanding the Research Question. Commentary on 'Race and Trust in the Health Care System,'" *Public Health Reports* 118 (4): 366.

Krieger, N., Chen, J.T., Waterman, P.D., Rehkopf, D.H. and Subramanian, S.V. (2003) "Race/Ethnicity, Gender, and Monitoring Socioeconomic Gradients in Health: A Comparison of Area-Based Socioeconomic Measures—the Public Health Disparities Geocoding Project," *Journal Information* 93 (10): 1655–71.

Kumagai, A.K. and Lypson, M.L. (2009) "Beyond Cultural Competence: Critical Consciousness, Social Justice, and Multicultural Education," *Academic Medicine* 84 (6): 782–7.

Lasser, K.E., Himmelstein, D.U. and Woolhandler, S. (2006) "Access to Care, Health Status, and Health Disparities in the United States and Canada: Results of a Cross-National Population-Based Survey," *Journal Information* 96 (7): 1300–7.

LaVeist, T.A. (2005) "Disentangling Race and Socioeconomic Status: a Key to Understanding Health Inequalities," *Journal of Urban Health* 82: iii26–34.

Lee, S.S.J., Mountain, J. and Koenig, B.A. (2001) "Meanings of Race in the New Genomics: Implications for Health Disparities Research," *Yale Journal of Health Policy Law & Ethics* 1: 33.

Martin, N. (2001) "Feminist Bioethics and Psychiatry," *Journal of Medical Philosophy* 26 (4): 431–41.

Mills, C.W. (1998) *Blackness Visible: Essays on Philosophy and Race*, Ithaca, NY: Cornell University Press.

Mills, C.W. (2007) "White Ignorance," in Sullivan, S. and Tuana, N. (eds.) *Race and Epistemologies of Ignorance*, New York: State University of New York Press, pp. 11–38.

Nissim-Sabat, M. (2001) "Review Article: Psychiatry, Psychoanalysis, and Race," *Philosophy, Psychiatry & Psychology* 8 (1): 45–59.

Omi, M. and Winant, H. (1994) *Racial Formation in the United States: From the 1960s to the 1990s*, New York: Routledge.

Outlaw, L.T. (2007) "Social Ordering and the Systematic Production of Ignorance," in Sullivan, S. and Tuana, N. (eds.) *Race and Epistemologies of Ignorance*, New York: State University of New York Press.

Paasche-Orlow, M. (2004) "The Ethics of Cultural Competence," *Academic Medicine* 79 (4): 347–50.

Penner, L., Dovidio, J.F., West, T.V., Gaertner, S.L., Albrecht, T.L., Dailey, R.K. et al. (2010) "Aversive Racism and Medical Interactions with Black Patients: A Field Study," *Journal of Experimental Social Psychology* 46 (2): 436–40.

Potter, N. (2004) "Gender," in J. Radden (ed.) *The Philosophy of Psychiatry: A Companion*, Oxford: Oxford University Press.

Potter, N. (2005) "Liberatory Psychiatry and an Ethics of the In-Between," in Shildrick, M. and Mykituik, R. (eds.) *Ethics of the Body: Postconventional Challenges*, Cambridge, MA: MIT Press, pp. 113–33.

Powers, M. and Faden, R. (2006) *Social Justice: The Moral Foundations of Public Health and Health Policy*, Oxford: Oxford University Press.

Razack, S. (1998) *Looking White People in the Eye: Gender, Race, and Culture in Courtrooms and Classrooms*, Toronto: University of Toronto Press, Scholarly Publishing Division.

Reverby, S. (2009) *Examining Tuskegee: The Infamous Syphilis Study and Its Legacy*, Chapel Hill, NC: University of North Carolina Press.

Russell, C. (2010) "The Limits of Liberal Choice: Racial Selection and Reprogenetics," *The Southern Journal of Philosophy* 48 (Suppl.): 97–108.

Silliman, J., Fried, M., Ross, L. and Gutierrez, E. (2004) *Undivided Rights: Women of Color Organizing for Reproductive Justice*, New York: South End Press.

Smedley, B.D., Stith, A.Y. and Nelson, A. (eds.) (2003) *Unequal Treatment: Confronting Racial and Ethnic Disparities in Health Care*, Washington, DC: National Academies Press.

Smith, A. (2005) *Conquest: Sexual Violence and American Indian Genocide*, New York: South End Press.
Stivers, T. and Majid, A. (2007) "Questioning Children: Interactional Evidence of Implicit Bias in Medical Interviews," *Social Psychology Quarterly* 70 (4): 424–41.
Sullivan, S. and Tuana, N. (2007) *Race and Epistemologies of Ignorance*, New York: State University of New York Press.
Tutton, R. (2009) "Biobanks and the Inclusion of Racial/Ethnic Minorities," *Race/Ethnicity: Multidisciplinary Global Contexts* 3 (1): 75–95.
Types, T. (2007) "Epistemologies of Ignorance," in Sullivan, S. and Tuana, N. (eds.) *Race and Epistemologies of Ignorance*, New York: State University of New York Press.
U.S. Department of Health and Human Services (2012) *2012 National Healthcare Disparities Report*. Available at: www.ahrq.gov/research/findings/nhqrdr/index.html (accessed July 22, 2013).
Wall, L.L. (2006) "The Medical Ethics of Dr J Marion Sims: A Fresh Look at the Historical Record," *Journal of Medical Ethics* 32 (6): 346–50.
Washington, D.A. (2009) "Critical Race Feminist Bioethics: Telling Stories in Law School and Medical School in Pursuit of Cultural Competence," *Albany Law Review* 72: 961.
Wear, D. (2003) "Insurgent Multiculturalism: Rethinking How and Why We Teach Culture in Medical Education," *Academic Medicine* 78 (6): 549.

42
TRANSGENDER

Jamie Lindemann Nelson

A recently coined term that has already developed a somewhat complicated and controversial history of meanings, "transgender" will be used in this chapter to characterize people who are uncomfortable—sometimes deeply so—with the gender to which they've been assigned at birth, as well as a loose collection of ways in which some of those people express that discomfort.

For some transgender people, medicine plays a significant role in how they deal with their unwelcome identities as women or as men—as it has in Karl's life. On the basis of the standard indications that are so carefully noted at birth, Karl was identified as female, and raised in one of the many ways that are more or less distinctive for girls. As life went on, however, Karl found that he could not find a rewarding or even coherent way of living as a woman, and that it made much more sense to see himself, and be seen by others, as male. Eventually, he obtained some rather invasive medical interventions—in his case, his ovaries and uterus were removed, his chest re-contoured and he was started on a regular regimen of testosterone—that helped him to do so.

Carrie has lived out an analogous story. Identified and reared as a boy from the start, growing up into what almost everyone thought of as just one guy among others, Carrie had a private but powerful conviction that life as a man simply could not be made to fit with her own grasp of who she was and wanted to be. As part of finding a way of living that seemed more in keeping with her feelings and hopes, she also turned to medicine: Carrie started taking estrogen and a medication that reduced the effects of testosterone. She later underwent a number of surgical procedures that reshaped her genitals and otherwise provided her with physical traits associated with women, and rid her of those associated with men.

For present purposes, then, "transgender" will be taken to include people like Karl and Carrie, who are also often referred to as "transsexuals," and in whose experience medicine plays a special role. Yet there are also people who, while rejecting (or at least revising) the gender identities thought to be determined by their bodies, don't look to medicine to provide physical changes, perhaps because they have no access to the kind of intensive interventions required, or possibly because they don't like the balance of risks and benefits involved, or maybe because they don't accept that a person's genitals, hormones or other "sex characteristics" necessarily determine gender. They use medicine largely for more ordinary kinds of health care, although they can face some extraordinary barriers to getting it.

Some transgender people take themselves to have permanently "migrated" from one gender to another, using clothing and accessories, verbal and non-verbal forms of expression, and self-ascription, rather than hormones and surgery, to help provide passage. Others cross back and forth between gendered presentations, perhaps because the ways in which they most value their lives overall won't accommodate permanent moves, or perhaps because they don't see gender as a deep identity-determining fact about who they are, but as something that should be treated less seriously, as a set of tools for access to different experiences, for personal growth, for amusement, even for profit. Still others are resistant to the seemingly relentless drive, at least in contemporary Western societies, to fix everyone as female or male. Rather than "migrating" from femaleness to maleness, or "visiting" femaleness from maleness, they tend to be suspicious about whether those very categories are good places for them—or perhaps for anyone—to inhabit. Some such people might selectively use surgery or hormones; many do not.

These people often identify themselves as transgender, too—in fact, in some uses of the term, they occupy the center of the concept, while people who are transsexual are admitted to the term by courtesy, if at all. So, while all transgender people will have health care needs like anyone else—and perhaps more so on average than people who confront less stigma (Institute of Medicine (IOM) 2011)—there is not a necessary connection between transgender and scalpels or syringes.

Yet, while some transgender or otherwise gender-variant people have tried to dismantle or at least substantially reconfigure gender, and some theorists have recommended people adopt skeptical or ironic attitudes towards it, gender remains a gravely important status socially as well as subjectively. Transgender people often strenuously try to understand themselves and be understood by others as women or as men as these notions are typically used. Success can be vital to transgender people, in part because being seen as gender ambiguous or non-conforming can make a person vulnerable to various harms: Harassment, vocational insecurity, and violence, including deadly violence (Beemyn and Rankin 2011). Further, the disharmony between how some transgender people feel, how their bodies are shaped, and how others see them can threaten their ability to live lives they see as authentic. For some of those people, medicine does play a centrally important role.

Yet if medicine is not a necessary means for expressing transgender objections to some of the standard ways gender is understood and enacted, neither are all objections to gender's operations necessarily examples of transgender. Feminism, for example, might also be a name for some people's deep discomfort with how the gender to which they have been assigned plays itself out in their lives. It may be tempting to say that many feminists' objections to gender are inherently political, whereas transgender people's dissent tends to be fundamentally personal. Yet feminist theories and practices themselves have made the "personal/political" distinction difficult to see as very helpful. It might be more accurate to suggest that feminism's range of complaints against how gender is practiced is broader than those typically pressed by people insofar as they are transgender.

Further, some feminists see these forms of objection to standard gender practices as operating at cross purposes. They have complained that transgender practices and understandings don't really grasp how deeply gender structures lives—one's identity as a woman or a man, so the complaint goes, is not something that decisions, or desires, or dress, or even surgery and hormones, can change. This line of thought has led to general critiques of medicine's involvement in gender reassignment procedures as exploitive of those who seek them out, and as disrespectful to women generally (most notably, Raymond 1979). Some feminists have worried that forms of transgender expression reinforce what's objectionable about gender categories: A transgender woman's concern about high heels, for example, may end with the fact that she can be punished for wearing them, while a feminist's objection may start with the fact that they can be punishing to wear. The tendency to construe genital surgery as the heart of gender reassignment strikes some feminists as reducing gender from a complex, encompassing social phenomenon to mere bits of biology that are themselves quite inoffensive; an authoritative social institution, medicine, that provides the interventions and the mental health screening that "justifies" access to the operating room, has been charged with reinforcing such naïve and politically retrogressive attitudes (see, for instance, Hausman 1995).

Yet it may not do to press too hard the notion that the scope of feminist objections to gender is wider than those of transgender people. Transgender individuals who see themselves as demonstrating with their lives that gender is as porous as it is problematic have also criticized many of the uses made of gender categories. Some transgender people are themselves explicit feminists: Transgender-based dissatisfaction with how gender is practiced may be influenced by feminist convictions (e.g., Aragon 2006; Bettcher 2009); some feminists have written sympathetically and insightfully about transgender and its possibilities for enriching feminist thought. (e.g., Scheman 1997; Salamon 2008). Despite the many ways that gender can limit and damage human lives, many transgender people's experiences testify to how vital a habitable gender identity can be to a rewarding or even merely tolerable life.

At the same time, transgender desires and actions may help undermine what some writers have identified as fundamental "natural attitudes" about gender: That being male or female is given, exclusive, and immutable. Everybody gets one and only one gender, and the one they get is unchangeable. Medicine contains a wealth of experience with various disorders of sexual development that put enormous pressure on this "natural attitude"—as do the lives of people with intersex conditions. The interest in medical and surgical interventions on the part of some transgendered people, however, in part perhaps because such interventions are often sought by people whose bodies seem perfectly "normal" physically, may make it harder to ignore just how much social stage setting and personal effort is required to maintain gender distinctions in their familiar forms. In light of what's been done by people such as Carrie and Karl (and the health care professionals helping them), any effort to insist that gender distinctions, roles, identities, or practices are as natural as breathing, rather than complicated and carefully monitored social practices, becomes much harder to defend (Kessler and McKenna 1985).

Medical Practices, Transgender Goals, and Bioethics

While some transgender people, then, do not take medicine to be a special ally in how they express their genders, others do want substantial interventions: Surgeries on genitals and reproductive organs, and procedures aimed at changing body contours or rendering faces more typically feminine or masculine; the use of hormones and hormone blockers to suppress menstrual cycles or erections, or to stimulate mammary growth or facial hair. Some physicians were providing some such services as early as the 1920s (Meyerowitz 2002; Ebersoff 2000). More recently, medicine in many parts of the world has largely regularized how it responds to such requests; there are diagnostic criteria and treatment protocols that are widely accepted as constituting good practice. There is, further, at least some ongoing research into the social and physical impact of transgender interventions, as well as into just why some people are so powerfully convinced that their given gender assignment is so profoundly wrong for them.

Bioethicists, it seems, should find these ways in which medicine so dramatically connects with such a central and problematic organizing concept of human life a rich source of fascinating moral and philosophical questions. Is "gender reassignment surgery" a paradigm of problematic "medicalization" of a social problem? Is it an effective treatment for a bona fide disease? Or, rather, might it best be seen as a way of reducing unhappiness and releasing human potential? Might medicine's response actually increase the incidence of the condition, channeling various forms of intense discomfort with gender norms that might be expressed politically into a single diagnosis–treatment pair? Or is gender reassignment itself a kind of social and political action against prevalent understandings of gender? Do people who ask for medical help with their gender crossing show themselves by that very request to be mentally ill? Or are they exhibiting a valuable form of human diversity that ought to be respected and facilitated, rather than tolerated and treated?

Oddly enough, although other scholars have raised questions of this sort, bioethicists for the most part have not (Nelson 1998, 2012). Academic efforts to come to grips with medicalized gender transitions were readily available through the 1980s—in addition to work by feminists, cultural theorists interested in gender and social scientists interested in health care made contributions (e.g., Billings and Urban's (1982) sharp skepticism about the motives of professionals involved in gender identity clinics)—but the amount of bioethical attention to the issue was meager in quantity if not quality. (Lavin's (1987) critique of the idea that "sex change" procedures were inherently mutilating or deceptive stands out for its thoughtfulness, but also for its simple presence.) In the early 1990s, an interdisciplinary field of transgender studies started to emerge (touched on by Stone's (1996) reply to Raymond), and social trends started to make transgender a less outlandish topic generally. Yet bioethicists still showed little interest. While some attention focused on a related area—"gender normalization" procedures performed on children born with disorders of sexual development (Dreger 1999; Chase 1998)—bioethics failed to keep pace with other bodies of scholarship. Until very recently, such bioethical literature that did specifically address transgender issues often relied on older theoretical understandings, rather than trying to develop or even question them (e.g., Draper and Evans (2006), drawing importantly on Raymond (1979)). Well into the first decade of the twenty-first century, it would not have taken long—certainly the inside of a non-taxing fortnight, more likely a moderately paced week—to read with due care all the literature on transgender-related themes contained in the twenty or so most prominent journals publishing bioethics.

There are, however, signs that bioethics is finally starting to take a closer, more considered look at medicine's efforts to help transgender people to achieve or consolidate their desired gender identities, and about health care's broader interactions with transgender people as well. An initiative started in 2010, "Bioethics, Sexuality, and Gender Identity," spearheaded by Autumn Fiester and Lance Wahlert from the University of Pennsylvania, aims to enrich bioethics with research from queer studies, an interdisciplinary field that includes the study of lesbian, gay, transgender, and related forms of sexual or gender expression (see http://www.queerbioethics.org). The initiative now involves a large number of bioethicists from many centers and programs, some of whose work includes an interest in transgender. In 2012, it sponsored a conference, and has organized special issues of bioethics journals around its themes. Further, at the national meeting of the American Society for Bioethics and Humanities (ASBH) held in Washington, DC in October 2012, there were for the first time several presentations explicitly addressing bioethics and transgender.

Then, of course, there is this very entry in the *Routledge Companion to Bioethics*—apparently the first general discussion of the issue to appear in an anthology designed for a general readership in the field. Essays of this sort often provide something of a critical summary of the leading issues and contributions of a given field to a particular issue. Yet this strategy hardly fits bioethics and transgender, precisely because the record of engagement is so sparse. If there could be said to be a standard topic for bioethics and transgender, it most likely has been whether it is legitimate to use medicine to facilitate gender reassignment, either at all, or for special populations, such as children. Against this background, however, new issues are starting to emerge.

For example, Alison Reiheld's American Society for Bioethics and Humanities paper (2012) reminds the field that transgender people have "ordinary" health needs too, and that some have faced serious obstacles in the way of getting quite standard kinds of care; track records of disrespect or rejection by health care professionals, or even the anticipation that a bad experience may be in store when a person's gender non-conformity is revealed, can delay or derail needed treatment (see also Harbin et al. 2012). Reiheld argues that some of those obstacles may not be just plainly poor practice, but ethically more complex: A provider may understand her refusal to care for transgender people as a matter of "conscientious objection," the result of a considered ethical judgment that transgender is sinful or otherwise immoral and that providers ought not to be compelled to support such forms of life by providing health care.

At another session of the same meeting, Cameron Waldman in effect argued against seeing any such objection as an ethically complex issue; he maintained that it ought to get no more hearing than would a professional's claim that he or she could not in good conscience treat people of color. Waldman also was skeptical about whether bioethics had anything of substance to contribute to society's achieving the sort of moral progress that would be marked by such questions about the treatment of transgender or otherwise queer people being simply placed off the table (Waldman 2012).

This exchange hints at the rich payoff bioethics might expect to gain from taking on transgender issues more fully; consideration of what might seem a straightforward issue—abandoning patients—quickly develops into deeper questions about tensions between personal integrity and professional values, about what moral issues decent societies ought to regard as definitively settled, and about what bioethics' role might be in *constricting* the set of open moral questions.

Research that focuses on transgender people also poses ethical issues that are starting to attract notice. The IOM's recent report on the health care needs of lesbian, gay, bisexual, and transgender people called for further investigation of relevant topics—for example on the long-term health impacts of continued hormone use by transgender people (IOM 2011). To aid research on such relatively small populations, the IOM report recommended that transgender people be routinely identified in their medical records; this proposal raises questions about how to define such a fluid and contestable term, about who has the authority to use or withhold the label, and about privacy and safety for a group of people whose gender identities put them at risk for suffering from just the kinds of stigma the IOM report itself carefully notes.

Perhaps a more fundamental issue is whether the "causes" of people's understanding themselves as transgender is an appropriate target of research at all. Such investigations have gone on, often generating considerable controversy, although not typically among bioethicists. Some transgender scholars and activists for example have expressed vehement opposition to investigations supporting the view that the desire to change gender is a form of paraphilia—i.e., what is sometime called by lay people a "perversion," a phenomenon driven by fundamentally erotic desires, targeted at an unconventional object.

A substantial part of the criticism in that particular case surrounded issues of research methods and research ethics used by Michael Bailey in his defense of his paraphiliac analysis of transgender (Bailey 2003); apart from a 2008 article by Alice Dreger, the dispute did not generate much attention in the bioethics literature. Yet the deeper research ethics issue may lie simply in seeing transgender desires and behaviors as inherently more puzzling than why our gender identities have the shape and significance that they do to people in general. Singling out transgender as a kind of gender identity particularly in need of explanation can convey the thought that there is something problematic with transgender ways of making sense of oneself—for example, that transgender is, or may be in some of its forms, a kind of mental disorder (cf. Wahlert and Fiester 2012).

Transgender and Mental Disorder

Whether transgender identities as such, or some ways of expressing those identities, should count as an illness or a disorder (terms that are used as rough synonyms) is a question that falls properly to the philosophy of medicine. It has ethical implications, though, perhaps chiefly for what was earlier identified as the basic question that bioethicists have tended to ask when transgender has been considered: Is gender reassignment an ethically defensible use of medicine? The "illness or not" issue also has some significant personal implications for transgender people. As the passionate debate that surrounded the de-listing of homosexuality from the American Psychiatric Association's (APA) *Diagnostic and Statistical Manual* (*DSM*) testifies, the difference between being considered mentally ill and being thought of as simply part of life's rich pageant can matter deeply to people (Bayer 1981).

Karl and Carrie, along with several tens of thousands of other people (Olyslager and Conway 2007), chose to undergo extensive surgeries on biologically healthy tissue that at least compromised their reproductive abilities, and subjected them to the standard dangers of surgery, including the possibility of death. They elected hormone treatments that may increase long-term risks of certain serious illnesses. They were well informed about the possible consequences. Were their informed choices sufficient to authorize professionals to provide the desired interventions?

Not if those professionals are guided by standard treatment protocols. The accepted standards of care pivot on a condition—"gender identity disorder," or, in more recent diagnostic manuals and clinical guidelines, "gender dysphoria" (APA 2013; Coleman et al. 2011)—as diagnosed by mental health professionals. According to the guidelines, then, a person's own reflective and informed choice is not sufficient to authorize gender reassignment interventions. What is perhaps more troubling is the hint that, if a person wants such interventions, her choice may not be a *necessary* part of the authorizing conditions either.

The problem is that the idea of being mentally disordered is often associated with the notion that your ability to make good decisions is doubtful, at least in areas affected by the illness, if not globally. Having a mental disorder does not mean that a person cannot make authoritative choices about her life. Yet a psychiatric diagnosis, and the insistence on using mental health professionals as gatekeepers to hormonal treatment and genital surgeries, can carry powerful stigmas. The transgender desires and choices of people in Karl or Carrie's position, then, might not be regarded as authentic expressions of who they most fundamentally and rationally take themselves to be, authorizing willing providers to intervene. Rather, they might be seen as symptoms of an illness, whose appropriate therapy is to be determined by professionals.

If mental health professionals involved in gender reassignment thought their job were to help people make a complicated and consequential decision well, that would probably not prompt great controversy. If they took themselves to be determining whether people requesting transgender medical procedures were suffering from serious depression, or another mental disorder that might impair decision-making, that might seem somewhat less contestable. Yet as things stand, if a candidate completes the screening with the authorization for surgery in hand, she or he hasn't emerged with a clean bill of mental health. What the candidate gets is a potentially stigmatizing psychiatric diagnosis.

Yet incorporating the desire to "change sex" into medicine's list of pathologies also came with advantages to both providers and recipients. Physicians and other health professionals could feel that their efforts were not merely glorified plastic surgery, serving idiosyncratic desires. Rather, their aim was to ameliorate a very serious mental disorder that, untreated, was extremely painful, correlated with serious depression and even suicidal behavior. Further, practicing under a recognized diagnosis, secured via official criteria applied by mental health professionals, reduced anxiety that a person who had received surgery might change her or his mind about whether the interventions had really been beneficial.

For their part, transgender people in search of medical interventions could feel that they weren't merely in the grip of some private perversion. Rather, they could understand themselves as ill with a recognized disorder, for which medicine had reliable responses. They were not "bad," then, merely sick. In principle, at least, they could approach physicians, not as supplicants, but as sufferers, for whom appropriate treatment could be regarded as a reasonable expectation built into the social contract between physicians and the public—at least for those who could afford it. And a recognized diagnosis could help there, too. Even though some insurance plans explicitly rule out coverage for transgender interventions, some have covered hormones, and even surgery—as the American Medical Association (AMA) explicitly advocates (AMA 2012).

Yet many transgender people do not see their discomfort with their assigned genders as warranting a psychiatric diagnosis and are not particularly keen to be seen as mentally diagnosable by others. The stresses in dealing with social stigmas and expectations surrounding what is normal for women and for men to be, to do, and to appear—like many forms of stress—may make someone prone to illness; various forms of gender transition may bring medical problems in their wake—surgical complications, for instance, or the impact of long-term use of hormones. Yet, at most, these considerations suggest that being transgender can be a health risk, not that it is itself an illness. The thought that people seeking transgender interventions were simply delusional—"this person with a penis thinks that he is *really* a woman"—have become less plausible, as understandings of what constitutes "reality" in this area have become more sophisticated, and as the ways available to transgender people to understand their own experience have also developed. While transgender desires can cause intense discomfort, this may not be diagnostic of an illness, but simply reflect that people typically are hardly indifferent to their gender. It seems reasonable to imagine that many non-transgender people would find life quite difficult if they found themselves having to live out a gender role that felt thoroughly alien to them.

Can bioethics—aided, perhaps, by the philosophy of medicine—help resolve this issue? Not conclusively, or at any rate, not so far. Consider, for example, Jerome Wakefield's "harmful dysfunction" analysis. Wakefield's account is attractive in that it incorporates biological and social elements in its understanding of disorder, rather than trying to assimilate disorder to one or the other of these categories, as earlier theories have attempted (e.g., Boorse 1977; Englehardt 1975). His thought is that for a person to count as having a mental disorder, two conditions must be fulfilled: At least one of the person's physical or mental systems must not be operating according to its naturally selected function, and the effects of that failure to operate are generally regarded as harmful, in the disordered person's social context (1992). As Wakefield sees it, then, both biological and social considerations must be met for a condition to count as a mental disorder.

Transgender desires and feelings can clearly meet the social condition. In ways of life that make so much of gender distinctions as do contemporary societies, many people who feel that the gender they were assigned at birth does not fit them experience pain and other substantial limits to their ability to form and pursue their interests. It is, however, at least unclear whether Wakefield's biological clause holds. Gender identity is such a socially shaped, varied, and—in particular—such a heavily monitored status, that it is curious to see it as a natural result of a well-functioning biological mechanism emerging from evolutionary processes. The amount of social pressure that is exerted to police gender norms, punishing those who stray too far, seems peculiar if gender identity reliably emerges from some properly functioning neural structure.

The case that transgender desires, even if they are intense enough to prompt people to seek medical interventions, constitute a mental disorder, then, is under some strain. It might seem in the interests of transgender people, simply as a pragmatic matter, to let the current situation stand, if it keeps open the possibilities for receiving desired interventions—and maybe even having their costs reduced. Yet taking such a wholly strategic approach, the diagnosis and treatment enterprise may be experienced by some transgender people as damaging to their integrity; some health care professionals might feel something of the same sort themselves.

Consider the "clinically correct story"—the kind of transgender life story that many gatekeeping mental health professionals have seen as diagnostic for bona fide gender dysphoria (Nelson 2001). According to classic versions of the story, the desire to change sex emerges early and enduringly; it concerns identity rather than sexuality, involves revulsion at discordant body parts, includes cross-dressing and cross-living, and comes complete with a set of plausible accounts of the teller's actions and decisions that might not seem to fit in to a narrative of life-long conviction that down deep, where it mattered, one was *really* a man or a woman (e.g., "Joining the Marines/Getting pregnant was part of my struggle to suppress the truth about myself").

Unsurprisingly, many transgender people came to be able to relate this narrative by heart, whether or not the story accurately captured their own experience. Equally unsurprisingly, canny professionals knew that the narrative was no secret, and had strategies to detect the overly glib (Stone 1996). Those who were focused on getting medical interventions might then anticipate and counter the detection strategies. And so on. The problem, however, was not only staying ahead of the game. The deeper problem is that there is something deeply dissonant in having to falsify the story of one's life in order to obtain medical interventions, when for many the drive to obtain those interventions is rooted in a powerful commitment to authenticity.

Requiring strict adherence to the clinically correct story may have eased as people's notion of what behavior is acceptable in women and men, and thus transgender people, became more accommodating. Still, as Judith Butler noted:

> It won't do, for instance, to walk into a clinic and say that it was only after you read a book . . . that you realized what you wanted to do, but that it wasn't really conscious for you until that time. It can't be that cultural life changes, that words were written and exchanged, that you went to events and to clubs, and saw that certain ways of living were really possible and desirable, and that something about your own possibilities became clear to you in ways that they had not been before. You would be ill-advised to say that you believe that the norms that govern what is a recognizable and livable life are changing, and that within your lifetime, new cultural efforts were made to broaden those norms, so that people like yourself might well live in supportive communities as a transsexual, and that it was precisely this shift in public norms, and the presence of a supportive community, that allowed you to feel that transitioning had become possible and desirable.
>
> (Butler 2004: 80–1)

Yet this *may* be the kind of narrative that most adequately does capture a given transgendered person's experience and sense of self.

The most recent edition of the *Standards of Care* of the leading organization of medical professionals involved in transgender care, the World Professional Association for Transgender Health (WPATH), is sensitive to the stigmas associated with mental disorder, and reads very much as if it is trying to split the difference between the benefits and the liabilities of diagnosis (Coleman et al. 2011). That edition—the seventh—states clearly that transgender self-understandings are not, simply as such, to be regarded as symptoms of mental disorder. It is eloquent about how transgender and analogous phenomena are human variations widely distributed among cultures and throughout history, and are to be respected. However, it retains the idea that when a person's transgender feelings make surgery or hormone treatments seem like a good way to live better, that person has gone from being (merely) "gender noncomforming" to "gender dysphoric," in the terms WPATH borrows from the fifth edition of the APA's *DSM* (APA 2012, 2013). And when a person becomes gender dysphoric, then their unhappiness with their bodies and/or their lives has crossed the threshold from a human variation to be respected, to a medical problem that requires the services of mental health professionals and the confirmation of a diagnostic category before surgery or hormones would be deemed appropriate.

The WPATH standards are clear that a diagnosis of this kind should not be thought of as grounds for taking away anyone's rights or diminishing their dignity: "A disorder is a description of something with which a person might struggle, not a description of a person or a person's identity" (Coleman et al. 2011: 169). Yet there remains the danger that in continuing to assert that the desire to obtain medical interventions for gender transitions constitutes a mental disorder, the authoritative professional group will undermine transgender people's sense of acceptance of their own identities, and may delay fuller measures of social respect.

Further, there are available alternatives for how medical professionals and transgender people might see their relationship. Jacob Hale has argued that the gatekeeping position assigned to mental health providers by the WPATH standards violates "the dominant principles of bioethics in the contemporary United States"—in particularly, nonmaleficence, beneficence, and respect for autonomy (Hale 2007: 493).

There are, as Hale acknowledges, risks to long-term hormone use as well as to invasive surgery, including the possibility of regret (Pfäfflin and Junge, in their 1998 article relied on by Hale, report an incidence of postoperative regret of less than 1 percent for people obtaining female-to-male procedures, and of 1–1.5 percent for those undergoing male-to-female procedures). Yet he suggests that health care professionals who have developed and enforced these standards overstress the risks, while underplaying the value of the potential benefits, and that properly weighed, the risks do not justify curtailing respect for the autonomous choices of patients. Hale notes that other decisions people make carry serious risks as well, offering the example of vasectomy, to which might be added the decision to bear and rear a child. It is also worth noting that although neither unwanted fertility nor pregnancies count as diseases, physicians are involved in how people respond to them, and insurance plans, both private and social, very often cover them.

Since the publication of Hale's article, the newest WPATH *Standards of Care* have relaxed the requirement that surgical candidates undergo extensive psychotherapy, which is a significant alteration. However, the Standards still require mental health screening, particularly when genital or gonadal surgery are in prospect. Portraying the difference between gender non-conformity and gender dysphoria as a difference between healthy and disordered states remains a controversial feature of the relationship between transgender people and health care providers, and a live topic for bioethics. Arguments for understanding the difference in this fashion drawn from the philosophy of medicine appear at best to be inconclusive, and the possibility of reinforcing stigma cannot be taken lightly. At the same time, the low levels of postoperative regret cited by Hale himself might be understood as strong evidence that the current procedures, relying on mental health screening for surgical candidates, are working very well to avoid bad outcomes.

Further, there are cases where reasons separate from the very desire to transition prompt concern about some people's ability to make self-regarding decisions. In principle, this includes transgender people who uncontroversially suffer from certain forms of mental illness, or who are cognitively or emotionally handicapped. In practice—or at least in the literature—the brunt of bioethical attention has fallen on gender-variant children.

Some young people, including pre-pubertal children, report strong and persistent transgender desires; sometimes those desires persist into adulthood, and sometimes they do not (Meyer 2012). In such cases some clinicians have advocated the use of puberty-delaying drugs (e.g., Spack et al. 2012). The effects of such drugs are reversible if suspended, and they buy time for children to mature and for their sense of their gender identity to consolidate, without their having to deal with physical changes that are deeply unwelcome, and whose impact they might have to try to reverse if they did elect gender reassignment. Some bioethicists (e.g., Giordano 2008) have defended this response, and called for it to become a more widely available option for transgender children.

Both the clinical and the bioethical justifications offered in the literature concerning puberty suppression hinge on the claim that such children have a serious problem that is made worse by social forces, but is at base medical. As such, they have a substantial claim to available medical care. It seems quite possible that any successful effort to de-pathologize gender dysphoria could make it harder for them to get hold of that resource. The main alternative justification pressed on behalf of transgender adults, stressing their right to make informed and free choices about their lives, is less clearly applicable to children.

Bioethics and Transgender: Coming Out from Behind the Curve?

The founding of university-based gender identity clinics began during the mid to late 1960s—roughly speaking, the same historical moment that saw the founding of research centers dedicated to the development of bioethics as a distinctive, interdisciplinary approach to understanding and guiding the growing power of medicine (Meyerowitz 2002; Jonsen 1998). While there was always a regulatory strain in its practice, bioethics was from the first interested in medicine's impact on how people understood and dealt with questions posed by our embodiment: What constitutes life, and what signals death; what distinguishes health and illness. Unlike questions concerning the nature and value of natality, mortality, and morbidity, gender stayed off the bioethics map for a long time. It is interesting to speculate on how contemporary discussions in transgender health care, but perhaps more generally about gender and social life as well, might have gone on had bioethics risen to that particular occasion, and interesting too, to speculate on why it did not.

It seems plain, however, that whatever thicket surrounded the topic and kept it insulated from bioethics is down now. Bioethicists are starting to take on a number of pertinent questions—e.g., about the authorization and financing of transgender-focused medical interventions, about the stigmas that may be inherent in transgender-oriented research agendas, as well as about the relationship between disorder and health. Newer issues are starting to come to light, too. For example, there is a small but growing literature concerning the interest of people undergoing gender reassignment in preserving their fertility and becoming parents (e.g., Hembree et al. 2009; Murphy 2012). There is reason to expect theoretically significant and practically helpful results from such work.

However, bioethics may now be less likely on its own to make as big an impact on how transgender is understood by medicine and society generally as it once might have done. In the past decade or so, many people looking to medicine for help with achieving a more desirable gender identity have started to develop a political consciousness that resembles how many people with disabilities or with intersex histories think of themselves. Many transgender people now regard themselves more as agents empowered by their identification with a social group, than as individuals significantly defined by their connection with surgeons and endocrinologists.

Bioethics has much to contribute to responsible thinking about the uses of medical power in connection with gender transitions; its contributions may well grow. However, the future relationships of transgender people with health care providers may be affected more by the political clout of a LGBT movement that is successfully transforming other central features of social life than by academic or clinical reflection.

For example, whether or not future editions of the *DSM* or the WPATH *Standards of Care* include "gender dysphoria" as a psychiatric diagnosis, the advantages and disadvantages of doing so as weighed by bioethicists may be less important than how transgender people themselves respond to the question. Insofar as they and their allies refuse to see health care concepts or practices as stigmatizing, forge their self-understandings chiefly from their own shared experiences, and assert the legitimacy of their own place in social life, bioethical thinking about transgender will need to go on with transgender people not merely as subjects of analysis, but as partners in conversation.

Related Topics

Chapter 39, "Medicalization, 'Normal Function,' and the Definition of Health," Rebecca Kukla
Chapter 44, "Body Integrity Identity Disorder (BIID) and the Matter of Ethics," Nikki Sullivan

References

American Medical Association (2012) AMA Policies on GLBT Issues. Available at: http://www.ama-assn.org/ama/pub/about-ama/our-people/member-groups-sections/glbt-advisory-committee/ama-policy-regarding-sexual-orientation.page? (accessed November 1, 2012).

American Psychiatric Association (2012) *DSM-5 Development*. Available at: http://www.dsm5.org/ProposedRevision/Pages/GenderDysphoria.aspx (accessed November 5, 2012).

American Psychiatric Association (2013) *Diagnostic and Statistical Manual of Mental Disorders* (5th edition), Arlington, VA: American Psychiatric Publishing.

Aragon, A.P. (2006) *Challenging Lesbian Norms: Intersex, Transgender, Intersectional, and Queer Perspectives*, Binghampton, NY: Harrington Park Press.

Bailey, M. (2003) *The Man Who Would Be Queen*, Washington, DC: Joseph Henry Press.

Bayer, R. (1981) *Homosexuality and American Psychiatry*, New York: Basic Books.

Beemyn, G. and Rankin, S. (2011) *The Lives of Transgender People*, New York: Columbia University Press.

Bettcher, T. (2009) "Feminist Perspectives on Trans Issues," *Stanford Encyclopedia of Philosophy*. Available at: http://plato.stanford.edu/entries/feminism-trans/ (accessed November 8, 2012).

Billings, D. and Urban, T. (1982) "The Socio-Medical Construction of Transsexualism: An Interpretation and Critique," *Social Problems* 29 (3): 266–82.

Boorse, C. (1977) "Health as a Theoretical Concept," *Philosophy of Science* 44: 542–73.

Butler, J. (2004) *Undoing Gender*, London: Routledge.

Chase, C. (1998) "Hermaphrodites with Attitude: Mapping the Emergence of Intersex Political Activism," *GLQ: A Journal of Lesbian and Gay Studies* 4 (2): 198–211.

Coleman, E., Bockting, W., Botzer, M., Cohen-Kettenis, P., DeCuypere, G., Feldman, J. et al. (2011) "Standards of Care for the Health of Transsexual, Transgender, and Gender Non-Conforming People, Version Seven," *International Journal of Transgenderism* 13: 163–232.

Draper, H. and Evans, N. (2006) "Transsexualism and Gender Reassignment Surgery," in D. Benatar (ed.) *Cutting to the Core: Exploring the Ethics of Contested Surgeries*, Lanham, MD: Rowman & Littlefield, pp. 97–110.

Dreger, A. (1999) *Intersex in the Age of Ethics*, Fredrick, MD: University Publishing Group.

Dreger, A. (2008) "The Controversy Over *The Man Who Would Be Queen*," *Archives of Sexual Behavior* 37 (3): 366–421.

Ebersoff, D. (2000) *The Danish Girl*, New York: Viking Penguin.

Englehardt, H.T. (1975) "The Concepts of Health and Disease," in H.T. Englehardt and S. Spicker (eds.) *Evaluation and Explanation in the Biological Sciences*, Dordrecht and Boston, MA: Reidel.

Giordano, S. (2008) "Lives in a Chiaroscuro: Should We Suspend the Puberty of Children with Gender Identity Disorder?" *Journal of Medical Ethics* 34 (8): 580–4.

Hale, C.J. (2007) "Ethical Problems with the Mental Health Evaluation Standard of Care for Adult Gender Variant Prospective Patients," *Perspectives in Biology and Medicine* 50 (4): 491–505.

Harbin, A., Beagan, B. and Golberg, L. (2012) "Discomfort, Judgment, and Health Care for Queers," *Journal of Bioethical Inquiry* 9: 149–60.

Hausman, B. (1995) *Changing Sex: Transsexualism, Technology, and the Idea of Gender*, Durham, NC: Duke University Press.

Hembree, W.C., Cohen-Kettenis, P., Determarre-van de Wall, H.A., Gooren, L.J., Meryer, W.J., III, Spack, N.P. et al. (2009) "Endocrine Treatment of Transsexual Persons: An Endocrine Society Clinical Practice Guideline," *Journal of Clinical Endocrinology and Metabolism* 94 (9): 3132–54.

Institute of Medicine (IOM) (2011) *The Health of Lesbian, Gay, Bisexual, and Transgender People: Building a Foundation for Better Understanding*, Washington, DC: National Academies Press.

Jonsen, A. (1998) *The Birth of Bioethics*, New York: Oxford University Press.

Kessler, S. and McKenna, W. (1985) *Gender: An Ethnomethodological Account*, Chicago, IL: University of Chicago Press.

Lavin, M. (1987) "Mutilation, Deception, and Sex Changes," *Journal of Medical Ethics* 13: 86–91.

Meyer, W. (2012) "Gender Identity Disorder: An Emerging Problem for Pediatricians," *Pediatrics* 129 (3): 571–3.

Meyerowitz, J. (2002) *How Sex Changed: A History of Transsexuality*, Boston, MA: Harvard University Press.

Murphy, T. (2012) "The Ethics of Fertility Preservation in Transgender Body Modification," *Journal of Bioethical Inquiry* 9 (3): 311–16.

Nelson, H.L. (2001) *Damaged Identities, Narrative Repair*, Ithaca, NY: Cornell.

Nelson, J. (1998) "The Silence of the Bioethicists: Ethical and Political Aspects of Managing Gender Dysphoria," *GLQ: A Journal of Lesbian and Gay Studies* 4 (2): 213–30.

Nelson, J. (2012) "Still Quiet After All These Years: Revisiting 'The Silence of the Bioethicists,'" *Journal of Bioethical Inquiry* 9: 249–59.

Olyslager, F. and Conway, L. (2007) "On the Calculation of the Prevalence of Transsexualism," Presented to the World Professional Association for Transgender Health Symposium, Chicago, IL.

Pfällin, F. and Junge, A. (1998) *Sex Reassignment: Thirty Years of Follow-Up Studies after Sex Reassignment Surgery. A Comprehensive Review, 1961–1991*, trans. R.B. Jacobson and A.B. Meier, Dusseldorf: Symposium Publishing.

Raymond, J. (1979) *The Transsexual Empire: The Making of the She-Male*, Boston, MA: Beacon Press.

Reiheld, A. (2012) "'She Walked Out of the Room and Never Came Back': Is Provider Refusal to Treat Transgender Patients a Legitimate Case of Conscientious Objection, or a Betrayal of the Patient–Provider Relationship?" Presented at the American Society for Bioethics and Humanities National Meeting, Washington, DC, October 18.

Salamon, G. (2008) "Transfeminism and the Future of Gender," in J.W. Scott (ed.) *Women's Studies on the Edge*, Durham, NC: Duke University Press.

Scheman, N. (1997) "Queering the Center by Centering the Queer: Reflections on Transsexuals and Secular Jews," in D. Meyers (ed.) *Feminists Rethink the Self*, Boulder, CO: Westview.

Spack, N., Edwards-Leeper, L., Feldman, H.A., Leibowitz, S., Mandel, F., Diamond, D.A. et al. (2012) "Children and Adolescents With Gender Identity Disorder Referred to a Pediatric Medical Center," *Pediatrics*, published online February 20, 2012; DOI: 10.1542/peds.2011-0907.

Stone, A. (1996) "The Empire Strikes Back: A Posttranssexual Manifesto," in K. Staub and J. Epstein (eds.) *Body Guards: The Cultural Politics of Sexual Ambiguity*, New York: Routledge.

Wahlert, L. and Fiester, A. (2012) "Questioning Scrutiny: Bioethics, Sexuality, and Gender Identity," *Journal of Bioethical Inquiry* 9: 243–8.

Wakefield, J. (1992) "The Concept of Mental Disorder: On The Boundary Between Biological Facts and Social Values," *American Psychologist* 47 (3): 373–88.

Waldman, C. (2012) Presentation, "What Is Progress for Lesbian-Gay-Bisexual-Transgendered Health in Bioethics?" Panel, American Society for Bioethics and Humanities National Meeting, Washington, DC, October 20.

43

ORGAN TRANSPLANTATION ETHICS FROM THE PERSPECTIVE OF EMBODIED PERSONHOOD

Fredrik Svenaeus

Transplantation Ethics

Organ transplantation is a medical procedure that presents stunning possibilities in saving and improving the lives of people who are ill and suffering (Tilney 2003). Although organ transplantations in this sense are ethically commendable things to do, the procedure has presented doctors, the law, and policy makers with a series of problems that have engaged medical ethics ever since the first transplants were carried out about half a century ago (Munson 2002). The ethical issues can roughly be grouped under four headings.

First, there are questions about the form of consent required from donors of organs. These questions regard both living donation—primarily kidney transplantations—and donation after death. Should consent be explicit or may it in cases of dead donation be presumed? What say should relatives have in the case of dead donation? How well informed must a donor be and what risks should he or she be allowed to take in the case of living donation? Should any form of compensation for the gift of organs be permitted?

The issue of compensation brings us to the second heading, namely questions regarding the buying and selling of organs. Should trade in human body parts be permitted? In nearly all countries of the world it is forbidden to buy or sell human organs, but the black market is large and growing. Kidney trafficking is a big business and the reason for this is the shortage of organs available for transplantation in rich parts of the world. Those in favor of lifting the ban on organ trade point out that legalization would improve the situation of vendors in poor parts of the world (Radcliffe-Richards et al. 1998). Under a legal organ trade vendors would receive a bigger share of the money that now ends up in the hands of organ brokers and they would presumably receive better medical treatment if selling was made legal. In addition to this, legalization would increase the supply of kidneys for transplantation in the world to a point at which the present lack would possibly cease. Costs for dialysis and other health care measures for people with kidney failure could be reduced, and the patients in question could live much better lives with a new organ in their body. In many cases a new organ would mean life rather than death to these patients (Tilney 2003).

Arguments against a legal organ trade can be made in different ways. The claims that trade would lead to better consequences for everybody involved can be challenged. Would donation rates not fall if people expected to get paid for their organs instead of giving them away for free? Will poor people not be forced to sell their organs, having no better options to relieve their present misery, especially if they are in debt to unscrupulous profiteers who could now make use of this new opportunity of income (Wilkinson 2003)? Another way of defending a prohibition on selling and buying body parts is to point towards ways in which legalization of an organ trade would expand market behavior into yet another zone of human interaction (Waldby and Mitchell 2006). To give an organ—or several organs if we are talking about posthumous donation—is a way to contribute to the life and welfare of other human beings without profiting from it. It is a commendable act that serves as a model for how we should live together in a society (Campbell 2009).

The third heading involves questions about when persons are dead and/or when they have any interests that could be violated by letting them die by way of removing their organs. Most countries in the world have changed their legal definition of death (primarily, though, admittedly, not only) as a consequence of the new opportunities of treatment with which organ transplantation presents us. The brain has succeeded the heart as the organ that needs to be functioning if the person should be considered to be alive. Presently it is the functions of the whole brain that should be determined absent and beyond chances of recovery for the person to be proclaimed dead in the legal definitions of most countries (Russell 2000). But the possibilities of keeping patients alive (or dead) on respirators have also raised the question of whether persons who are beyond hope of regaining consciousness (although parts of their brains are still functioning) should not be considered to lack any interests to be kept alive, whereas their organs could be used to favor the interests of many other persons who are presently conscious and suffering (Singer 1995).

The fourth heading concerns what we *owe* to people who are ill and suffering. The concept of justice is, indeed, central to all questions of organ transplant ethics, since the question of whether anybody *deserves* to be in need of a new organ (being ill and facing death) is a pressing one. Does the principle of justice not oblige us all to give the needy organs we could dispense with and still go on living a good life (i.e., one kidney)? Does it not oblige us to give them that which we do not need ourselves once we are dead (i.e., all our viable organs)? Whether people are obliged to become organ donors as a matter of justice is a central ethical question in the organ transplant literature (Fabre 2006).

Embodiment and Selfhood

The ethical questions grouped under the headings above all touch upon the relationship a person (a self) has to his or her body. It seems to be presumed by most philosophers that organs are something that *belong* to each person respectively. That is presumably why the persons must always consent to their organs being removed, although they may not be allowed to do *anything* they like with their organs for various reasons—consider the prohibition against selling. The two latter headings—the questions regarding when a person is dead and if we are obliged to give away our organs when we do not need them anymore—also concern issues of what belongs to the self. Can ownership rights be overruled in certain situations when the person is no longer there and/or parts of his or her body can be used to save the lives of others? These are the fundamental questions of transplantation ethics as it is currently pursued.

But what if our organs—kidneys and hearts will be my main examples in what follows—are not things that belong to us as commodities, but instead are to be looked upon as something that we *are*? How would such a *phenomenological* view upon selfhood, as fundamentally embodied, change our views on the ethics of organ transplantation? This is the question I will explore in this chapter, introducing some concepts from phenomenological philosophy and giving detailed descriptions of two cases of kidney and heart transplantation, respectively. Phenomenologists take their starting point in the first-person perspective when exploring an issue and I will try to stay true to this ideal in what follows (Zahavi 2005). This first-person perspective includes the second-person perspective (the dialogue with other persons), but it is to be contrasted with taking an impersonal third-person perspective of science as our philosophical starting point.

At first it may look as if the phenomenological view on the body would weaken the incentive or duty to give away one's organs when one can dispense with them, because it would equal giving away something of one's *self* instead of merely giving away one or several *things* that belong to you. However, as I will attempt to show, an embodied account of organ transplantation will rather make apparent that although different organs contribute to our embodied selfhood in various ways, this essential belonging of the person to his or her organs—rather than the other way around—shows us that our embodiment *connects* us to the lives and sufferings of other people in a fundamental way (Leder 1999).

The connectedness by way of the body goes back to the way we are delivered to the world as fundamentally *dependent* on other persons, a predicament made obvious in situations in which we become ill or disabled in various ways and need the support of others (Mackenzie 2010). We share the same fundamental needs and desires as human beings because we are embodied in similar ways. This does not mean that we are unable to, or should not, care about other embodied creatures than humans, but our particular form of embodiment is an essential part of the life form in which we develop an ethics of human interaction. The "face of the other," as the phenomenologist Emmanuel Levinas puts it, is the basic source of ethical obligation, and it is not by accident that this metaphor is connected to embodiment (Diprose 2002). I encounter the other person by seeing, hearing, touching, even smelling him or her, and by this bodily encounter our belonging together is made possible. If not embodied, we would not desire and fear things that may happen to us; as a matter of fact, in order to have any kinds of feelings at all, we need to be embodied (and not just "embrained") (Damasio 1999). It is doubtful whether radically enhanced, post human persons, who have left the current limitations of human embodiment behind, will ever come into being, but if they do, they will probably not have an ethics that is similar to ours (Agar 2010).

Kidneys, hearts, and other types of organs, according to such an embodied view, are not just functional parts of the biological body; they are parts of what the phenomenologist calls "the lived body" (Zahavi 2005). The lived body is the body as it appears from the first-person perspective of the person *being* it, enabling the person to encounter and understand things around her in the world as meaningful for her in various ways. Our "being-in-the-world," as the phenomenologist Martin Heidegger puts it (1996), is consequently basically a bodily phenomenon, an insight elaborated by yet another influential phenomenologist, Maurice Merleau-Ponty (1962). The body to a large extent organizes my experiences already on a preconscious level by way of neurological systems centered in the brain that coordinate my movements and perceptions (Gallagher 2005). To the ways of the lived body also belong the processes of my biological organism: Breath, digestion, blood flow, etc., which are mostly absent from my awareness but nevertheless provide the backdrop for my intentionality—my being directed towards different things that I engage with (Leder 1990).

Normally, when we engage in the world, busy doing various things, we do not pay much attention to our own bodies. They perform their duties inconspicuously in the background and make it possible for us to encounter things and other persons in the world around us, a world that we share as embodied, human beings. Sometimes, however, the lived body *shows up* in resisting and disturbing our efforts to do things. It "dysappears," rather than disappears, to use a term coined by Drew Leder (1990). The body plagues us and demands our attention by revealing itself, not only as our home, but as an *alien* creature. Organ transplantation, and also the process of falling ill, which in most cases (if one does not end up in the operating room because of an accident) precedes the transplantation, to a large extent inflicts such changes in self-being when our bodies display an unhomelike character. As phenomenologist Richard Zaner writes in his study *The Context of Self*:

> If there is a sense in which my own-body is "intimately mine," there is furthermore, an equally decisive sense in which *I belong to it*—in which I am at its disposal or mercy, if you will. My body, like the world in which I live, has its own nature, functions, structures, and biological conditions; since it embodies me, I thus *experience myself as implicated* by my body and these various conditions, functions, etc. *I* am exposed to whatever can influence, threaten, inhibit, alter, or benefit my biological organism. Under certain conditions, it can fail me (more or less), not be capable of fulfilling my wants or desires, or even thoughts, forcing me to turn away from what I may want to do and attend to my own body: because of fatigue, hunger, thirst, disease, injury, pain . . . .
>
> (Zaner 1981: 52)

I will now proceed to a more direct phenomenological analysis of organ transplantation in developing examples of what it is like to have a kidney and a heart transplant, respectively. In the examples, I will attend to the ways the body shows up as "other" (unhomelike, alien) in situations preceding and following transplantation and the way these different types of otherness should be understood. The phenomenological analysis of organ transplantation situations will then be reconnected to the ethical issues concerning the relationship to one's body and the bodies of others surveyed above.

The Kidney Transplant

In the book *Holograms of Fear*, Slavenka Drakulić tells the story of her first kidney transplantation, which takes place in Boston in 1986 (Drakulić 1993). Drakulić has left her homeland of Yugoslavia, her family, friends, and even her young daughter, in order to live in New York as a journalist. This radical decision is forced upon her not by political oppression but by a genetic disorder affecting her kidneys: Polycystic kidney disease. The medical care she is getting in Yugoslavia is not sufficient (she watches her fellow patients in the dialysis ward deteriorate and die), and she has poor chances in Yugoslavia of getting the transplant she needs to survive. In the book she tells how the disease and her dysfunctional kidneys force her to undergo dialysis every second day in the hospital for several hours:

> I had no choice. Every other morning at five o'clock I went for my dialysis at the hospital on 72nd Street. I didn't consider the possibility of not going. The healthy can choose. Life is simple when you're sick, as it is for people in jail or in the army. There are rules that are more than rules because breaking them can only mean one thing. At first this is non-freedom but later, it is just certainty . . . Here the blood flows in streams: in veins, capillaries, pumps, rubber hoses, in clear plastic tubes, in cylindrical dishes with filters. As if the white room was woven with a red web. Everyone is quiet, deathly tired. They communicate in code, in subdued tones.
>
> (Drakulić 1993: 3–4)

To be in dialysis treatment means that your life becomes *regimented* in a new way. This concerns not only the hours you have to spend connected to the dialysis machine but also the way you have to watch and regulate your body, considering diet, how much to drink, sleep, exercise, etc. to keep the disease under control. But the most thoroughgoing effect of the kidney disease is that the body shows up in new and disconcerting ways that become central to your everyday experience, self-reflection, and life story:

> The thing moved from person to person like bad luck. No one could tell who it would attack. It attacked my father. It attacked me. It left my brother unharmed. We almost thought that it had skipped us, too, that those ancestors who had died in the past had nothing to do with us. But at the first signs—nausea, vomiting, tiredness—I knew that it had come. The doctors didn't tell me right away although they suspected it. I was already pale, my pulse was fast and every time I lay down I thought I might not be able to get up. Later my father came down with it as well. They told us that these days it was possible to live with it, that there were machines, kidney transplants. Various deals could be struck with the sickness, negotiating with bad luck.
>
> (Drakulić 1993: 6–7)

The uncanniness of such experiences is hard to deny. The body reveals itself as incorporating alien, unhomelike elements in illness (Svenaeus 2000). The uncanniness concerns the way the body becomes an obstacle and a threat, instead of my home territory and basic affordance, but in this (and most other severe) case(s) of illness it also concerns the ways I address the meaning of my life and my relationship to others. Bodily connectedness is made even stronger in cases of inherited diseases in which the family bonds are not only the source of security, joy or annoyance, but of a possible deadly curse.

Waiting for the transplant, knowing that you are on the waiting list but with no knowing when, if ever, the doctors will find a suitable kidney for you, is a vexing experience in itself. So is the fear of pain or dying as a result of the operation. You long desperately for a life with more freedom and fewer symptoms, but at the same time, the regime of dialysis might become a habit and a kind of security you are afraid of leaving for the uncertainty of the operation, which is, certainly, a dramatic event:

> "Breathe, breathe." An English voice penetrates the darkness in which I'm floating . . . Terrified I try to suck in air, catch it with my open mouth, but something is inside, something is inside. It is smothering me, I have to retch it out. They are pulling out a long tube with a sudden jerk from my throat, tearing the membranes. A deep sigh. Then a sharp pain under my stomach cuts me in half. "Your kidney is functioning."
>
> (Drakulić 1993: 42)

Only slowly does Drakulić recover after the operation; it takes hard exercise and a lot of time to be able to sit up, stand, walk, eat, etc. Even the routine of going to the toilet is an effort and, in the specific case of kidney transplants, also a new and remarkable experience for the patient, since the kidneys have not been producing any urine for a long time.

Even in the successful cases, when the new kidney works properly and is not rejected by the immune system, life after a transplant is not like life before the onset of disease. To suffer from a disease that destroys your kidneys and to get a new kidney means that life becomes prolonged and normalized, but it does not mean that life becomes the way it was before the onset of the disease, since you are at constant risk of renewed kidney failure. To live with a foreign kidney in your body means to lead a life that is extremely regimented regarding the relationship to your body. It often means a more anxious life, in the sense that the basic trust in the body is gone, but it could also mean a more self-reflected life, in the sense that the finitude of your life and the question of what is of real importance in it have come to the surface (Frank 1995). Finally, it will lead to thoughts about the life of others and how they are connected to you, particularly the person whose death (in the case of cadaveric transplant) and generous gift means life for you:

> "Her kidney came from a woman," the doctor said to someone. He was leaving the room. He thought I was asleep . . . I don't care who it belonged to, I am not curious. I think of it as an organ, not as part of a person. I must not be sentimental. My life is on the line. But the picture reappears. Her smiling face, gone forever. A lot of time will pass, then in a subway somewhere, a tall man will stop me . . . "Excuse me, I couldn't help myself, but you look so much like my late wife." I'll stare at him, indifferent at first. I'll pretend that I have no idea what he is talking about. Perhaps I'll say I don't know any English. But something will force me to change my mind and I'll say: "Yes. Yes, I probably do look like her. We are sisters, almost twins—you didn't know that she had a sister? You see this thin scar? It has almost disappeared, but this is where she moved in. We live well together, the two of us. Sometimes she gets a little obstinate. I can't keep her from spreading. Sometimes she chooses a smile, other times a gesture, or a walk—to show that she is here, that I am in her power. I think perhaps she wants to make me feel grateful. It's not my fault that she was killed."
>
> (Drakulić 1993: 73–4)

To sum up, already the kidney *disease* leads to experiences of bodily alienation—the body behaving in painful ways that I cannot control—which have implications for the way I think about myself and my life in relationship to others. However, the otherness displayed by my own body in severe disease has repercussions for my entire life, making it hard, sometimes impossible, to be at home in the world in carrying out everyday activities. It also affects my relationship to other persons and sometimes the way I think about my entire life and its purpose. Why did this happen to me? What kind of a person am I and who do I want to be? After having the transplant this reflection in many cases leads to feelings and thoughts about the origin of the new kidney I now bear in my body (Sharp 2006). The scientific attitude to my new organ as a thing among other things, an attitude that will be encouraged by the doctors, can easily be conquered by an attitude in which the kidney of the other person harbors his or her identity in some way that has now been transposed to me. It might also lead to a thankfulness that becomes transformed into guilt. (How have I earned this life that was made possible by the other person's death?)

The Heart Transplant

In the case of the heart, things are slightly different, not only when it comes to the symbolic character of the heart (life, love, goodness) in comparison to the kidney (what, really, is a kidney symbolic of?) but also regarding the extent to which the heart *shows up* to me, in illness, and also in health. In contrast to the case of the kidney, it is possible to direct one's attention to the activity of one's heart at any time, and in situations that make us react strongly emotionally it is almost impossible *not* to notice one's heart pounding in association with other bodily processes, such as blushing or sweating. In exercise, the heart (together with the rest of the body, of course) sets the limit for what we are able to accomplish, and these limits are clearly *felt* on the embodied level as intense heart and lung activity or pain and weakness of muscles when, for example, I run fast for a long time.

Heart disease does not always make itself known through the experience of pain in the heart itself; a heart attack is experienced as a chest pain radiating out through chest and arms, for example. But the possible irregularity in the rhythm of the heart's beating, which can be a very powerful and frightening experience, nevertheless marks out the heart as something that appears in a more singular manner than the kidney does, in at least some cases of heart disease.

Human hearts have been transplanted since the late 1960s while the history of kidney transplantation dates back to the 1950s. A heart transplant is an even more dramatic and difficult operation than a kidney transplant, and it was not until the 1980s that surgical techniques and new immunosuppressive medications made it possible for patients to survive a heart transplant for a longer time (Tilney 2003). To find a new heart for a dying patient is even harder than finding a new kidney, for two simple reasons. Each person only has one heart, which makes living donation impossible (as long as we do not allow killing one person to let another live). Furthermore, hearts deteriorate much faster than kidneys outside the body, which means that we have only a very limited time in which to carry out the transplant (kidneys last much longer if they are kept the right way). Hearts for donation will most often come from patients who have been put on respirators as the result of accidents or sudden occurrences of disease (stroke) and have then been declared brain dead while they are still connected to the machine that assists the breathing and the circulation of the blood that keep the organs of the deceased person fresh.

In the early 1990s, the French philosopher Jean-Luc Nancy underwent a heart transplant after a period of severe illness. He wrote about this event and the cancer that he was subsequently taken with—probably as a result of the heavy doses of immunosuppressive medicines that post-transplantation patients have to take to prevent rejection of their grafts—in the essay "The Intruder," which I will make use of in what follows

(Nancy 2008). Nancy's main figure for understanding the process he is undergoing is found in the title of his essay:

> The intruder introduces himself forcefully, by surprise or ruse, not, in any case, by right or by being admitted beforehand. Something of the stranger has to intrude, or else he loses his strangeness. If he already has the right to enter and stay, if he is awaited and received, no part of him being unexpected or unwelcome, then he is not an intruder any more, but neither is he any longer a stranger . . . To welcome a stranger, moreover, is necessarily to experience his intrusion.
>
> (Nancy 2008: 161)

This way of conceptualizing the *intruder* (as a person, but also, as we will see, as a thing that intrudes in me, such as an organ) is very similar in structure to the analysis of bodily *alienation* I have developed above. When Nancy's analysis is coupled to the experience of illness and transplantation, the overlap becomes almost total:

> If my own heart was failing me, to what degree was it "mine," my "own" organ? Was it even an organ? For some years I had already felt a fluttering, some breaks in the rhythm, really not much of anything: not an organ, not the dark red muscular mass loaded with tubes that I now had to suddenly imagine. Not "my heart" beating endlessly, hitherto as absent as the soles of my feet while walking. It became strange to me, intruding by defection: almost by rejection, if not by dejection. I had this heart at the tip of my tongue, like improper food. Rather like heartburn, but gently. A gentle sliding separated me from myself.
>
> (Nancy 2008: 162–3)

In comparison with the kidney failure experienced by Drakulić, we can see that the failing heart penetrates the experiences of Nancy to a far greater extent regarding the perception of the organ itself. But the alienation is also driven by the unique symbolic quality of the heart as the essence of life, goodness, and personal identity (Lakoff and Johnson 2003). Despite living in a scientific age, it is almost impossible to view the heart as a pure biological entity among others, a "pump" only, rather than the center of our emotional life. The heart is loaded with meaning and identity; therefore the intruding heart (still his old one) separates him from himself.

A new heart (the transplanted heart) is certainly also an intruder, but it is an intruder that we would like to welcome. This is possible, however, only by "experiencing his intrusion," as Nancy writes (2008: 161). This means the pains and plagues following the procedure of having the sternum cracked and the chest cut wide open in an operation that lasts for several hours and during which the blood is circulated and oxygenated by way of an external device, a heart–lung machine. It also means suppressing the body's immune system to prevent it from attacking and rejecting the graft, something that will otherwise happen immediately after the operation or in due time. The graft is foreign, an "intruder" in the body, which we have difficulties welcoming. But the immunosuppressive actions taken mean that other intruders (bacteria, viruses), lying dormant in the body or entering from outside, become a major threat. It also means that the regular outbreaks of uncontrolled cell division in the body, which otherwise are dealt with by the immune system before they grow and spread, can now lead to cancer diseases. Nancy describes this multiple intrusion by organs, viruses, and cancerous cells, but also by medical technology and therapies. The latter make him *objectify* his own body, and in this way he becomes alienated from it in a way that aggravates the physical suffering (Nancy 2008: 169).

To sum up, the heart is "mine" in a way that the kidney is not, despite their both being hidden under the skin, rarely visible, except in the extreme situations of accidents, operations, and autopsies. This is probably due to the heart's being an organ that can be *felt* to a greater extent than the kidney can, and also due to the symbolic connotations of the heart in comparison with the kidney. Heart transplants may therefore evoke questions of identity in an even stronger way than kidney transplants will sometimes do (as in the case of Drakulić). Two good illustrations of how such questions of identity surface and lead to new bonds being formed between people as the result of heart transplants are the movies *All About My Mother* by Pedro Almodovar (1999), and *21 Grams* by Alejandro Gonzales Innarritu (2003). In both movies, stories are told about heart transplants and the attempts made by patients and family members of donors to find out more about the identity of donors and recipients of hearts, respectively. In these interactions new connections and relationships between persons are formed as a result of the transplant.

Embodied Selfhood and Transplant Ethics

Getting a new organ—a kidney, a heart, a lung, a liver, a pancreas, a hand, a face, or some other part of the body that the doctors are able to transplant—will help a patient to a better life in most cases, at least when the new body part is installed in the patterns of the lived body in a successful way. It follows from the phenomenology of organ transplantation, unsurprisingly, that donating organs is a good thing to do because it will help other persons to be more at home with their bodies, enabling them to live a richer life (and survive). To donate posthumously may even be an obligatory thing to do, at least in situations when the transfer of organs can be brought about without violating the dignity of the embodied self (Campbell 2009). To what extent a body with an irreversibly damaged brain, kept "alive" through artificial measures, can be violated depends on the cultural practices of caring for and taking leave of the dying (Lock 2002). Dignity is a tricky concept (The President's Council on Bioethics 2008), but in the situations of organ transplantation, to violate dignity would primarily mean to treat brain dead bodies as entities that are first and foremost useful things—or collections of things—instead of bodily traces of persons that are connected to family members and friends by histories of life-long interaction. Dead bodies, however, have been treated in various ways in different cultures throughout human history, all found respectful in their particular contexts, and it should not be impossible to successfully install practices that can be combined with donation of organs. Indeed, this is already happening in many parts of the world, but the issue of how and why the dead body is more than an organ bank needs to be addressed in bioethics rather than being hidden or dismissed as bad metaphysics or religious superstition (Svenaeus 2010).

The phenomenological idea that we in a fundamental way belong to our own bodies, rather than the other way around, can work as an antidote to the influential organ-commodity paradigm in contemporary bioethics. The phenomenological account can deliver an argument explaining why body parts are not just yet another type of things to be traded, but rather fundamental parts of our self-being. We are born *as* a body coming from *another* body. The body makes our existence and appearance as persons possible and it does so in a way that is related to how we depend on each other as finite human beings fated to die. This explains why organs are not things that belong to us in the same way as outer things in the world do. Organs are identity bearing in the sense that they belong to the *processes* of selfhood—the lived body—rather than being things that the self (the brain) controls and makes decisions about. Therefore, according to an embodied, phenomenological view, organs should not be traded in, even though they can and should be shared by way of transplants. "Giving life," as the slogan for encouraging organ donation goes, is a *sharing* of life, not an offer of a valuable commodity. Rather than fearing that a view upon grafts as anything but useful biological material will create confusion and feelings of guilt in patients who receive new organs, health care professionals should perhaps to a greater extent acknowledge the bonds that are created between people and families by organ transplantation, also in cases of posthumous transplantation (Sharp 2006).

My attempt above to develop a phenomenological framework in which to place the ethics of organ transplantation is far from complete and the theses put forward here may not be directly applicable to the writing of ethical codes or guidelines. Many questions about the implications of a phenomenology of the embodied, interconnected self for bioethics in the case of organ transplantation have been left unanswered in this chapter. They concern the exact responsibilities embodied bonds put on individuals in different situations. Do I have the same obligations to all human beings in need? Are the obligations stronger in cases of people I connect to in my everyday life and meet face to face than in cases of people far away whom I hear of or watch on television? The phenomenological ethics to guide organ transplantation certainly remains to be worked out in more detail. Nevertheless, I hope to have shown that phenomenology is a viable way to go in searching for theories in bioethics to complement autonomy, welfare, and virtue-based approaches in an interesting way.

Related Topics

Chapter 8, "Medical Tourism," I. Glenn Cohen
Chapter 21, "Autonomy," Catriona Mackenzie
Chapter 35, "Brain Death," Winston Chiong
Chapter 44, "Body Integrity Identity Disorder (BIID) and the Matter of Ethics," Nikki Sullivan

References

Agar, N. (2010) *Humanity's End: Why We Should Reject Radical Enhancement*, Cambridge, MA: MIT Press.

Campbell, A.V. (2009) *The Body in Bioethics*, London: Routledge.

Damasio, A.R. (1999) *The Feeling of What Happens: Body and Emotion in the Making of Consciousness*, New York: Harcourt Brace.

Diprose, R. (2002) *Corporeal Generosity: On Giving with Nietzsche, Merleau-Ponty, and Levinas*, Albany, NY: State University of New York Press.

Drakulić, S. (1993) *Holograms of Fear*, London: The Women's Press.

Fabre, C. (2006) *Whose Body Is It Anyway? Justice and the Integrity of the Person*, Oxford: Oxford University Press.

Frank, A.W. (1995) *The Wounded Storyteller: Body, Illness and Ethics*, Chicago, IL: University of Chicago Press.

Gallagher, S. (2005) *How the Body Shapes the Mind*, Oxford: Oxford University Press.

Heidegger, M. (1996) *Being and Time*, trans, J. Stambaugh, Albany, NY: State University of New York Press (original work published 1927).

Lakoff, G. and Johnson, M. (2003) *Metaphors We Live By* (2nd edition with a new afterword), Chicago, IL: University of Chicago Press.

Leder, D. (1990) *The Absent Body*, Chicago, IL: Chicago University Press.
Leder, D. (1999) "Whose Body? What Body? The Metaphysics of Organ Transplantation," in M.J. Cherry (ed.) *Persons and Their Bodies: Rights, Responsibilities, Relationships*, Dordrecht: Kluwer Academic Publishers, pp. 233–64.
Lock, M. (2002) *Twice Dead: Organ Transplants and the Reinvention of Death*, Berkeley, CA: University of California Press.
Mackenzie, C. (2010) "Conceptions of Autonomy and Conceptions of the Body in Bioethics," in J.L. Scully, L.E. Baldwin-Ragaven and P. Fitzpatrick (eds.) *Feminist Bioethics: At the Center, on the Margins*, Baltimore, MD: Johns Hopkins University Press, pp. 71–90.
Merleau-Ponty, M. (1962) *Phenomenology of Perception*, trans. C. Smith, London: Routledge (original work published 1945).
Munson, R. (2002) *Raising the Dead: Organ Transplants, Ethics and Society*, Oxford: Oxford University Press.
Nancy, J.-L. (2008) "The Intruder," in *Corpus*, trans. R. Rand, New York: Fordham University Press (original work published 2000), pp. 161–70.
Radcliffe-Richards, J., Daar, A.S., Guttmann, R.D., Hoffenberg, R., Kennedy, I., Lock, M. et al. (1998) "The Case for Allowing Kidney Sales," *The Lancet* 351: 1950–2.
Russell, T. (2000) *Brain Death: Philosophical Concepts and Problems*, Aldershot: Ashgate Publishing.
Sharp, L. (2006) *Strange Harvest: Organ Transplants, Denatured Bodies, and the Transformed Self*, Berkeley, CA: University of California Press.
Singer, P. (1995) "Is the Sanctity of Life Ethic Terminally Ill?" *Bioethics* 9: 307–43.
Svenaeus, F. (2000) *The Hermeneutics of Medicine and the Phenomenology of Health: Steps Towards a Philosophy of Medical Practice*, Dordrecht: Kluwer Academic Publishers.
Svenaeus, F. (2010) "The Body as Gift, Resource, or Commodity: Heidegger and the Ethics of Organ Transplantation," *Journal of Bioethical Inquiry* 7: 163–72.
The President's Council on Bioethics (2008) *Human Dignity and Bioethics*, Washington, DC: Essays Commissioned by the President's Council on Bioethics.
Tilney, N.L. (2003) *Transplant: From Myth to Reality*, New Haven, CT: Yale University Press.
Waldby, C. and Mitchell, R. (2006) *Tissue Economics: Blood, Organs and Cell Lines in Late Capitalism*, Durham, NC: Duke University Press.
Wilkinson, S. (2003) *Bodies for Sale: Ethics and Exploitation in the Human Body Trade*, London: Routledge.
Zahavi, D. (2005) *Subjectivity and Selfhood: Investigating the First-Person Perspective*, Cambridge, MA: MIT Press.
Zaner, R. M. (1981) *The Context of Self: A Phenomenological Inquiry Using Medicine as a Clue*, Athens, OH: Ohio University Press.

44

BODY INTEGRITY IDENTITY DISORDER (BIID) AND THE MATTER OF ETHICS

Nikki Sullivan

Over the past decade or so there has been increasing interest amongst psychiatrists, psychologists, philosophers, medical ethicists, cultural theorists, neurologists, and others in a range of desires for what we might think of as "non-normative" forms of embodiment, that is, for bodies with less than a "full complement" of limbs, for bodies that are, to varying degrees, paralyzed, deaf, blind, and so on. Such desires are now widely regarded as symptomatic of what psychiatrist Michael Fine calls body integrity identity disorder (BIID), a condition defined primarily by a consistent sense of non-contiguity between body and self. The vast majority of people who identify with the phenomenological sense of bodily being that defines BIID call for access to surgery in order that their desired mode of corporeality be realized, and the dysphoria from which they suffer overcome. Such calls raise a range of questions about the ethics of amputating a healthy limb, injuring a healthy spinal cord, producing deafness, and so on, or, alternately, of refusing to conceive surgery as a viable treatment protocol. This chapter will consider current debates regarding the ethics of "elective amputation"—since this is the procedure which has garnered most interest to date—and at the same time, will attempt to critically interrogate the constitutive effects of the (bio)ethical principles brought to bear on BIID. In other words, rather than simply applying ethical principles to BIID, this chapter strategically deploys the (desire for) "non-normative forms of embodiment" associated with BIID in an attempt to problematize some of the assumptions that underpin what Margrit Shildrick refers to as "conventional bioethics."

Shifting Conceptions of the Desire for Amputation

The desire for the amputation of a healthy limb or limbs has been understood historically as symptomatic of one of a range of pathological conditions.[1] For example, in a 1977 publication John Money et al. conceived the desire for amputation as primarily sexual and thus coined the term apotemnophilia.[2] In the late 1990s Richard Bruno proposed that those who desire amputation, "pretend" to be amputees, and/or are sexually attracted to amputees, constitute a diagnostic grouping that could be called factitious disability disorder (1997: 257). By the early twenty-first century such desires came to be understood as disorders of identity: Robert Smith and Greg Furth introduced the term amputee identity disorder in a 2000 publication, and in 2005 Michael First coined the now widely used term body integrity identity disorder. More recently, Paul McGeoch and his colleagues at the Centre for Brain Cognition, University of California, have formulated the term xenomelia to refer to a neurological "disorder of body image" which they associate with right parietal lobe damage and/or dysfunction (2011).[3]

Whilst the naming of desires for non-normative forms of embodiment may seem somewhat trivial in the face of the suffering experienced by those whose access to surgeries which may give them the bodies they feel themselves to be is currently blocked, diagnostic nomenclature is inextricably bound up with ideas about what causes such desires, and how they might be appropriately treated. Currently, as Christopher Ryan notes, there "is no consensus on what constitutes BIID, nor even that BIID exists as an independent entity" (2009: 22).[4] But despite this, Sabine Müller asserts that "understanding . . . the causes for BIID is crucial for the development of an appropriate treatment" (2009: 109), and Ronald Pies agrees, arguing that an effective treatment protocol can only be determined on the basis of a clear understanding of disease process (2009: 179). Before examining in more detail competing accounts of desires for and treatment of non-normative morphologies, it is perhaps worth noting here that despite their differences each of the authors cited thus far embrace the assumption that such desires are "abnormal" and/or in need of explanation. Such an assumption has, as will become apparent in due course, been problematized by analyses that draw attention to the discursive character of desires and their regulation, and to the generative effects of naming.

BIID

In his first published study of the desire for limb amputation, First set out to determine whether such desires are paraphilic, symptomatic of psychosis, or indicative of a "new type of identity disorder" (2005: 919). The data gathered during interviews with 52 "wannabes"[5] led him to conclude that the desire for amputation is not primarily sexual, nor is it, in the vast majority of cases, an effect of psychosis.[6] Rather, it is most often motivated by the desire for wholeness, for a sense of contiguity between the self and the body (which is experienced as "wrong"). First also reported that most of the interviewees had desired amputation since an early age; that the location of the amputation is often extremely specific and unchanging; that 92 percent of those interviewed had been involved in "rehearsal" activities; and that in the majority of cases the respondents' present bodily state is experienced as disabling. In terms of treatment, First, like many others who have worked directly with those desiring non-normative morphologies, claimed that whilst therapy and psychotropic drugs may, in some cases, have some positive effect on general wellbeing, both have proven to have no impact on the desires themselves, or the associated feelings of dysphoria, or a disjunction between body and self.

On the basis of these findings, First argued that whilst the clinical profile that emerges does not fit any of the existing diagnostic categories found in the fourth edition of the *Diagnostic and Statistical Manual of Mental Disorders* (DSM-IV-TR), it closely resembles the phenomenology of gender identity disorder (GID), a "condition" whose key diagnostic features include discomfort with an aspect of anatomy; onset in childhood or early adolescence; frequent mimicking of the desired identity; sexual fantasies and/or arousal around the image of a post-surgical self; and successful treatment by surgery (2005: 926). Like the desire for amputation, GID has no known etiology, and whilst the standard treatment for those meeting the criteria is now surgery, such treatment was once held to be highly contentious.[7] These parallels lead First to formulate the diagnostic category BIID, to suggest that BIID should perhaps be included in the DSM-V and the ICD-II, and to note that that such inclusion may facilitate the development of treatments including, for some, amputation (2005: 927).

In a 2012 paper co-authored with Carl E. Fisher, First reiterates these claims regarding classificatory nomenclature and treatment, and develops diagnostic criteria for BIID which include "an intense and persistent desire to become physically disabled in a significant way" and "persistent discomfort or intense feelings of inappropriateness concerning current nondisabled body configuration" (2012: 12). This shift in First's conception of BIID from a desire for "wholeness" to "a persistent desire to acquire a disability" (2012: 3) may be useful insofar as it poses a challenge to neurological accounts of the etiology of desires for non-normative morphologies.[8] However, at the same time, it is troubling in its reiteration of normative perceptions of dis/ability and ab/normalcy which ultimately work against the desires of which First speaks, and more particularly, against their safe surgical realization, as will become apparent as my discussion of the deep-seated association of "disability" with "undesirability" unfolds.

Desiring the Undesirable

Having researched and taught courses on a wide range of modificatory technologies for a number of years, it has become clear to me that most people's initial response to desires for amputation, blindness, paraplegia, and the like, is one of horror and disbelief. Such responses are tellingly different from those elicited by, for example, the desire for and practice of breast enhancement, labiaplasty, or procedures associated with gender confirmation (or sex reassignment as it is sometimes known). This differential response is particularly interesting given that the desires—or perhaps more accurately, the need—for non-normative corporealities and access to the surgical procedures that may enable their realization, are more often than not articulated, as John Jordan notes, in terms "that are nearly identical to mainstream plastic surgery applicants, but they are not granted the same legitimacy" (2004: 329). The same could be said of the asymmetrical responses by medical practitioners to the use of the "wrong body" narrative by wannabes and by those experiencing so-called gender dysphoria (Sullivan 2008): Whilst the feeling that one is or has the "wrong body" is taken as symptomatic of transsexualism, the claim that the body of the person desiring amputation is wrong is largely understood as indicative of wrong headedness rather than as a recognized symptom of a clinical disorder that can, or perhaps even should, be treated surgically. One might argue that what these asymmetries demonstrate is that the surgical transformation of individual bodies is regulated by idea(l)s about what constitutes desirability and/or normalcy, and that rather than being objective, such idea(l)s are culturally constructed and contextually specific: It is highly unlikely, for example, that our great, great grandparents would perceive the elective insertion of sacks of saline or silicone into subpectoral or subglandular pockets for aesthetic purposes as rational or unremarkable.

Whilst the logic of analogy is central to First's account of BIID, Dan Patrone is critical of "the master argument" which he associates with the work of First and others, and which, he claims, is reliant on "imperfect analogies" that lead to medically unethical conclusions regarding treatment. His critique consists of two claims regarding the principles of non-maleficence and autonomy: First, that "no disability follows from the putatively non-problematic case of cosmetic surgery" (Patrone 2009: 542),[9] and second, that "those who have a disorder that causes them to desire to maim and disable their bodies cannot meet [the required] standard of voluntarily accepting the burdens of choice that makes the practice of respecting autonomy acceptable" (2009: 545). In short, then, as Patrone sees it, since amputation unquestioningly results in disability, and disability is by definition undesirable,[10] then the desire for amputation is necessarily irrational, and the expression of a disorder which compromises the capacity of the person thus affected to make a well informed, autonomous, choice about what, at least in this regard, is in his or her best interests. Further, since "elective" amputation is disabling and medically unnecessary, its practice is, as Patrone sees it, unethical. Interestingly, Patrone's critique of "imperfect analogies" makes no mention of the analogy most commonly posited in discussions of desires for non-normative morphologies, and central to First's conception of BIID, namely the analogy with GID and gender confirmation surgeries. This oversight is perhaps not accidental since in the case of GID the association of a (relatively uncommon, long-held, and compelling) desire for a particular anatomy with a clinical disorder is not seen as compromising the patient's competency to make an informed decision about treatment, or the reputation of the surgeon who performs the desired surgery.[11]

Richard Bruno explicitly dismisses the analogy between "GID" and the desire for amputation in his articulation of what Chris Partridge refers to as "the insanity objection.[12] He writes, "the notion that a [wannabe] is a 'disabled person trapped in a nondisabled body' is difficult to justify, there being no 'naturally-occurring' state of disability that would correspond to the two naturally-occurring genders" (1997: 251).[13] There are a number of assumptions that Bruno makes that call for further consideration. First, he implies that gender is an empirical fact, that it is a natural, and therefore naturally desirable bodily state. Hence the desire for and practice of "gender confirmation" surgeries is, from his perspective, intelligible (that is, understandable and therefore rational), and justifiable. The determinist model of gender on which Bruno's argument relies has long been challenged by writers as diverse as John Money, Betty Friedan, and Judith Butler, all of whom have convincingly argued that gender is, in large part, a social phenomenon.[14] Whilst I do not have time to rehearse these arguments here, it is my contention, following Butler, that gender is the performative effect of repeated, culturally learned actions which, over time, come to feel, and to appear to others as, "natural," as the expression of an innate interiority. Gender, on this model, is simultaneously an idea(l), a practice (a set of everyday labors aimed—often less-than-consciously—at attaining an ideal),[15] and a discursive effect, rather than something we (naturally) have.

And what of disability? Bruno claims that whilst gender is "naturally-occurring," there is "no 'naturally-occurring' state of disability that would correspond to the two naturally-occurring genders" (1997: 251). Disability, in Bruno's schema is, then, the antithesis of able-bodiedness (as a natural developmental state) rather than its complement. Disability is unnatural insofar as it is the result of an accident (whether congenital or social): It is, by definition, both an aberration and an abomination and as such, is literally undesirable. Bruno's understanding of disability is one that is widely shared in the contemporary west in which, as Jordan notes, "even suggesting that an amputated body would be preferable to a healthy, full-limbed body would seem to contradict every tenet of cultural body logic" (2004: 341). And this is clearly illustrated by

Wesley J. Smith's presumptuous assertion that obviously no one "but a severely mentally disturbed person would want a healthy leg, arm, hand, or foot cut off" and that "such people need treatment, not amputation" (cited in Ryan 2009: 23).

Critical disability theorists such as Rosemarie Garland-Thomson (2002) and Lennard Davis (1995) have convincingly argued that there is nothing natural about the pervasive view of disability as unnatural and undesirable: For such writers this problematic construction of disability is symptomatic of a way of knowing/seeing that is particular to Western modernity and is itself disabling. However, in making this claim, such theorists do not reproduce the logic deployed by Bruno by arguing that in fact disability is natural and therefore, presumably, desirable. Davis, for example, argues that disability is a regulatory fiction, "a function of the concept of normalcy" (1995: 2) which shapes not only the lived bodies of those it purports to merely describe, but also those deemed able-bodied. In making such claims Davis does not, as some might suspect, negate bodily differences, but rather, focuses a spotlight on the way in which difference comes to matter. In short, Davis's insights challenge Bruno's construction of disability as the antithesis of able-bodiedness, showing that the former is integral to the latter as well as to the psycho-social imaginary that sustains dichotomous conceptions of being, and, invariably, shapes the practice of ethics.

I will return to the matter of disability and its constitution in the work of those who deploy the insanity objection in their depiction of amputation surgery as unethical throughout this paper. Now, however, I want to focus on the notion of autonomy since this has loomed large in debates about desires for non-normative morphologies and their possible realization through surgery.

Autonomy

One of the most vocal critics of "elective" amputation is Sabine Müller, who perceives desires for non-normative morphologies currently associated with BIID as symptomatic of an underlying neuropsychological problem which, she asserts, will not (indeed, cannot) be "cured" by the removal of a limb. Consequently, she argues that amputation is unethical because the desire for such is not autonomous, and because "it leads to disability" (2009: 116) thereby producing more harm than benefit. She writes: "[t]o fulfill the desire for a bodily harm of a patient with a substantial lack of autonomy is a severe violation of the medical fiduciary duty and of the principle of non-maleficence" (2009: 117). Whilst there are at least four ethical principles implicated here—autonomy, utility, duty, and non-maleficence—the principle of autonomy seems to most concern Müller: She argues, for example, that if a patient's desire for such could be shown to be autonomous, then amputation would be ethical. However, close examination of Müller's attempts to substantiate her claim that wannabes lack autonomy reveals that her perception of wannabes (and their desires) is underpinned and shaped by an obvious prejudice which links amputation with "disability," and the desire for "disability" (as, by definition, undesirable) with "madness." Let me explain. First, Müller claims that "[i]n all cases of BIID which have been investigated by psychiatrists, the diagnosis states that the amputation desire is obsessive[16] or results from a monothematic delusion,[17] comparable to anorexia, [and] Capgras' syndrome"[18] (2009: 117). For anyone who has read the existing literature on BIID, such a claim is, to say the least, questionable. Studies such as those carried out by First (2005), First and Fisher (2012), and Blom et al. (2012) explicitly deny that wannabes are delusional, and in fact, as Neil Levy notes in his response to

Müller, having delusional beliefs about the limb that a wannabe desires to have removed would necessarily disqualify him or her from the classification of BIID (2009: 50).

The second aspect of Müller's argument that requires critical attention is her account of free and unfree will. Following Kant, Müller argues that autonomy depends on a coherence of will, or of what Harry Frankfurt describes as first- and second-order mental states. An agent lacks autonomy when there is a contradiction between a first-order and a second-order desire: Imagine, for example, that I am sexually attracted to other women, and yet I desire for this not to be the case. As Müller sees it:

> in BIID patients the amputation desire is a first-order volition, whereas their wish to have no amputation desire is a second-order volition. The latter could be filled in principle in two different ways: First by amputation, second by eliminating the amputation desire.
>
> (2009: 117)

Like Levy (2009) and Craimer (2009), I find Müller's universalizing characterization of wannabes as embodying a contradiction of will unconvincing. In many, if not most, of the first-person accounts of desires for non-normative morphologies that are available on activist websites and/or cited in scholarly studies, wannabes do not express a desire *not* to desire amputation, but rather, desire that their desire for amputation, paraplegia, for deafness, for "wholeness," be satisfied.[19] Thus, as Levy notes, on Frankfurt's account wannabes demonstrate a coherence of will and thus satisfy the criteria for autonomy (2009: 50). Müller's interpretation of amputation as the fulfillment of the desire *not* to desire amputation is, then, not simply out of keeping with first-person accounts of wannabes; it is, more particularly, symptomatic of a total inability to comprehend the fact that a desire for amputation (which Müller reads as disability) is possible. And this lack of intelligibility is a direct effect of the perception of "disability" as, by definition, undesirable—a perception which is shaped by social norms (as opposed to being objective), and which produces disabling effects.

This becomes clearer still if we turn to Müller's assertion that:

> [b]ecause a mere coincidence of first-order volitions and second-order volitions is not sufficient for autonomy, it is important to refer to Kant's . . . demand for the rationality of higher-order volitions. Because the amputation desire is conflicting with many rational desires of the BIID sufferers, especially with those for health, painlessness, mobility, and social acceptance, the second-order volition to get rid of the amputation desire is rational, whereas the first-order volition to fulfill the amputation desire is irrational.
>
> (2009: 117–8)

Tellingly, Müller makes no attempt to substantiate this claim by discussing how one might determine irrationality, nor does she reference those who she alleges (rationally) desire painlessness, mobility, and so on. Given this, it seems safe to assume that Müller presumes irrationality to be self-evident and universal; an assumption which is, of course, highly questionable.

Incompetency and Irrationality

There has been much criticism in the literature on BIID of the conflation of desires for non-normative embodiment with an *a priori* inability to make an informed decision about treatment (or, more particularly, about amputation: Those who articulate the insanity objection do not claim that wannabes are incapable of choosing "non-disabling" treatments such as cognitive behavioral therapy). For example, writers such as Savulescu (2006), Levy (2009), Dua (2010), Partridge (n.d.), Ryan (2009), Jotkowitz and Zivotofsky (2009), Bryant (2011), and Swindell (2009) argue either that the question of autonomy is, as Levy puts it, largely irrelevant (2009: 50), or that the particular conception of autonomy that informs Müller's thesis is problematic. Perhaps the most compelling critique of Müller's position is that even if:

> the BIID sufferer is not making an autonomous choice (in the philosophical sense) when she requests amputation . . . all that is needed for her choice to be respected in the medical context is 1) that she is informed and has decision-making capacity; and 2) that her choice is among the medically reasonable alternatives.
>
> (Swindell 2009: 53)

Decision-making capacity is not, argue Slatman and Widdershoven, something that can be accorded or denied BIID patients *a priori* (2009: 49). Rather, as Swindell asserts "in order to argue that BIID patients lack decision-making capacity, formal assessments of capacity should be performed by psychiatrists with the assistance of tools such as the MACCAT-T [MacArthur Competence Assessment Tool for Treatment]" (2009: 53). Indeed, individual assessment (in terms of diagnosis and competency) is central to the protocols developed by First who draws on those established in relation to GID.

Building on the view that individuals have different desires and values, and that difference should be encouraged not least because it contributes to the richness of life, Julian Savulescu likewise argues that the question of whether or not a particular practice is ethical can never be answered in any absolute or universal sense since value judgments are inherently contextual. Using the verb "to hump" as a placeholder for whatever contentious activity one might be interrogating, Savulescu writes:

> [w]hile there may be reasons in general not to hump, an individual may have most reason to hump, given a particular history and set of circumstances . . . Some individuals might have *most reason* to seek amputation. Thus not only might amputation be permissible in some situations, it might be desirable.
>
> (2006: 8–9)

This is in keeping with calls made by Slatman and Widdershoven (2009), De Preester (2011), and Sullivan (2005) for the development of phenomenological accounts of the lived embodiments of those desiring non-normative morphologies. Such analyses would, these authors argue, acknowledge that the relationship between an individual's corporeality, his or her experience of integrity (or its lack), and his or her life-world is simultaneously singular and social: It is an effect of his or her particular embodied history as well as of the cultural context in which s/he comes to be. Such an approach would have, at its heart, an emphasis on "the constitutive and always incomplete nature of embodiment, the transformatory potential of the body itself and of embodied identity," as well as an awareness of "the [(re)productive] operation[s] of a bioscientific imaginary in both professional and lay discourse" (Shildrick 2004: 150).

Elsewhere (2005) I have argued, for example, that rather than being a thing-in-itself, "integrity" (or its lack) is an embodied experience that may be difficult to discern from "the outside."[20] Those who claim that elective amputation is unethical because it disables a heretofore "normal" body overlook this, presuming instead that integrity is visibly self-evident (the full-limbed, fully functioning body being emblematic of this), and that since the wannabe does not feel what is "true" then s/he is in some sense deluded. Such delusion is, on this model, both a symptom and an effect of an underlying pathology that is psychological, neurological, or both. In and through this constitutive perception/interpretation (of the other and his or her desires) the wannabe's bodily-being-in-the-world, his or her lived embodiment, is rendered inauthentic, as are his or her desires. At the same time, the experience of integrity of the one who perceives/evaluates is reproduced as natural, as normal, and the continual labor that is required to achieve and/or maintain a coherent embodied identity (as, for example, a cissexual[21] woman, "able-bodied," and so on) is veiled over. From this normative position, the desire for the removal of a limb, for deafness, blindness, paraplegia, for what in short appears in the normative imaginary as "disability" can only be figured as unintelligible, abnormal, and harmful. And conceding to such desires, rather than curing the pathology of which they are a symptom, can only be figured as at best misguided, and at worst, morally wrong.

If, however, we move away from universalizing assumptions about dis/ability, un/desirability, ir/rationality, in/competence, bodily integrity, and so on, and instead acknowledge that such concepts and their perception are culturally constructed and situated, we may be better equipped to concede that what may be good for one person may not be appropriate for another: We might then be able to more effectively evaluate the benefits and harms of different forms of treatment,[22] and their capacity to restore "wholeness" to different individuals. For example, deep brain stimulation (DBS), which is one of the treatments proposed by some who regard the desire for amputation as a symptom of right parietal lobe dysfunction, may be something that some individuals whose desired morphologies are currently unrealizable are prepared to try. For others, however, such treatment may appear antithetical to their needs, or even medically and/or politically spurious: Imagine, for example, a person who has, in the past, been subjected to electro-shock therapy to cure them of homosexual desires, or even a person who is aware that invasive practices like this one have occurred and who has a long-held political (and therefore affective) aversion to the continuation of such (potentially dangerous) curative measures. To propose that such a person should undergo DBS is no less ethically problematic than suggesting that a person who experiences sexual desires for people of the so-called same sex should submit to electro-shock therapy, or that people desiring EE breasts should only and ever be treated with cold-water vestibular caloric stimulation, another treatment which, it has been suggested, may temporarily relieve feelings of body dysphoria.

Accepting that amputation (for patients with BIID) may not be a universally unethical practice does not mean that amputations should or would be performed without due care, nor does it mean that surgeons opposed to such a practice would be required to perform it.[23] What it would require is, as in the case of "GID," the formulation of widely agreed-upon diagnostic criteria (such as those developed by First) and guidelines for clinical practice. If we accept that it is possible to develop such criteria and guidelines, and agree that the claim that desires for amputation constitute, *a priori*, a lack of autonomy and impaired decision-making capacity is both unsound and the effect of a profound prejudice against "disability," then is it any longer possible to argue that amputation is ethically wrong? One of the most common objections found in popular cultural discussions of BIID is the idea that amputation will result in significant costs (economic and otherwise) that society cannot be justly expected to bear. This argument is also made by

Müller who claims that not only is medical treatment and rehabilitation expensive—an argument that could similarly be made against gender affirmation surgeries, but rarely is—but, more particularly, amputation will result in diminished capacity, and increased dependence (financial, physical, and emotional) on loved ones and on the state (2009: 120), and as such, it contravenes the principle of distributive justice.

One counter to this position might be to argue for a rights-based conception of justice which would give due consideration to the individual's right to self-determination, and to the cost of denying that right, or at least a particular manifestation of that right. Whilst such a position is not without its merits, it nevertheless assumes (and reaffirms) a humanist model of the subject, the social, and the relation between them which, as I have attempted to demonstrate throughout this paper, is integral to the "problem" of "disability" as it is currently conceived/constructed. An alternative approach would be to "lay bare the psycho-social imaginary that sustains modernist" projects (Shildrick 2009: 2), and shapes the perception of difference in disabling, dichotomous terms (i.e., able/disabled, normal/abnormal, desirable/undesirable, healthy/unhealthy, and so on). Such an approach would first involve acknowledging that:

> Where physical and mental autonomy, the ability to think rationally and impartially, and interpersonal separation and distinction are valued attributes of western subjectivity, then any compromise of control over one's own body, any indication of interdependency and connectivity, or of corporeal instability, are the occasion—for the normative majority—of a deep seated anxiety that devalues difference.
>
> (2009: 2)

It would also require a rethinking of justice beyond the limits of the associative and rights-based model that I have identified above.

Conclusion

This chapter has offered an overview of the various ways in which ethical principles have been deployed in debates about how best to respond to the desires for bodily transformation associated with BIID. At the same time, it has critically engaged with the practice(s) of ethics and the effects such practice(s) produce. Whilst I have evaluated some of the claims made and positions taken by the various writers discussed, my aim has not been to develop a definitive ethical position on how to best treat such desires. Rather, I have attempted to draw attention to the ways in which debates about bodies and about ethics (as well as the assumptions that inform them) are themselves constitutive: Despite a focus on abstract concepts (such as autonomy, rights, beneficence, and so on) ethical principles shape the objects, the subjects, the desires, they claim merely to respond to, as well as the being-in-the-world of those who debate their application. Acknowledging this jams the machinery of naturalization/normalization, calling on those who practice (in the name of) ethics to give serious consideration not only to the effects of the ways in which we see, but also, to the onto-political forces that shape our perceptions. Such an approach demands that rather than repeating well-rehearsed conceptual moves, we ask how particular ways of seeing and knowing orient us such that some conceptual associations become naturalized whereas others remain unrealized and unrealizable. We might, for example, ask why the conflation of amputation with "disability" is such an easy perceptual/conceptual/constitutive move to make. And why it is that "disability" is so widely seen as, by definition, undesirable. We also need to consider what such perceptions fail to see, what psycho-social operations they render invisible, and what ethico-cultural imaginaries they sustain. In fostering "an ethics of encounter without a commitment to resolution or closure" (Campbell and Shapiro 1999: xi, xvii) we would, I contend, be better equipped to respond sensitively and with respect to the matter of BIID.

Related Topics

Chapter 21, "Autonomy," Catriona Mackenzie
Chapter 39, "Medicalization, 'Normal Function,' and the Definition of Health," Rebecca Kukla
Chapter 42, "Transgender," Jamie Lindemann Nelson

Notes

1 See Sullivan (2009) for a discussion of the problematics of pathologization.
2 Whilst the conception of the desire for amputation as primarily sexual has fallen out of favor, there are still a small number of writers who argue for this particular interpretation. See, for example, Lawrence (2006). The separation of "the sexual" from other aspects of lived embodiment has been challenged by De Preester (2011).
3 See also Aoyama et al. (2012). Whilst not deploying the term xenomelia, the following writers argue that the desire for amputation is caused by a neurological disorder: Brang et al. (2008); Blanke et al. (2009); Giummarra et al. (2011); and Seda (2011).
4 See also Bryant (2011).
5 This is a term that those desiring amputation often use. The term is often used in conjunction with two other terms, namely "pretender," which refers to those who participate in what might be called rehearsal activities, and devotee, which is used to refer to someone who desires amputees.
6 Whilst First acknowledges that (a desire for) amputation may be associated with psychoses—for example, self-amputation has been known to be performed by psychotic individuals in response to command auditory hallucinations (see First 2005: 920)—his use of questions about general psychopathology, adapted from the *Structured Clinical Interview for DSM-IV*, suggested that none of those interviewed and evaluated were delusional (2005: 926). In cases in which (the desire for) amputation was shown to be associated with somatoform disorders, body dysmorphic disorder, panic disorder, obsessive–compulsive disorder, or psychosis, the individual would not be diagnosed as suffering from BIID.
7 See Sullivan (2008) and Stryker and Sullivan (2009).
8 By broadening the category of BIID to include amputation for non-normative morphologies that do not require amputation—for example, bodies that do not see—First troubles the idea that BIID (or xenomelia) is caused by a mismatch between anatomy and one's neurological body map due to right parietal lobe dysfunction. Whilst it is relatively easy to explain the desire for amputation (or the feeling that a limb is extraneous) in this way, desires for blindness, paraplegia, deafness, and so on do not easily fit with such an explanation.
9 Ryan et al. (2010) challenge this claim.
10 This assumption could be said to constitute what Robert McRuer refers to as "compulsory able-bodiedness" (2002: 88).
11 This was not always the case. See Sullivan (2008).
12 No date or page numbers provided for this online, unpublished article.
13 In a discussion of amputation as a possible treatment option, Ray Blanchard makes a similar claim. He states: "I can't see society in general accepting it, [a]nd I can't see medicine accepting it. Medicine is going to see it as conferring a disability on a patient. In that sense it's different from sex-reassignment surgery. Being a man or woman is not a disability" (cited in Ellison 2008: n.p.).
14 I do not mean to suggest here that these theorists share a singular position, in fact, quite the opposite is true. The models of gender (acquisition) that these writers have developed are significantly different at the same time that they are each informed by the belief that gender is never simply an empirical, biological fact.
15 Margrit Shildrick puts this well when she argues that "the so-called normal and natural body is . . . an achievement . . . a body that requires unceasing maintenance . . . to hold off the constant threat of disruption: extra digits are excised at birth, tongues are shortened in Down's syndrome children, noses

are reshaped, warts removed, prosthetic limbs fitted, HRT prescribed. In short, the normal body is materialized through a set of reiterative practices that speak of the instability of the singular standard" (1999: 80).

16 Williamson (2010) argues that the "intense and obsessive urge for amputation" that BIID sufferers allegedly experience is likely to impair their autonomy. Interestingly, no account is given of the fact that similarly intense feelings of discomfort with one's morphology, and an intense and longstanding desire for a sense of "wholeness" or congruity that can seemingly only be attained through surgery are key diagnostic criteria for GID.

17 This is the name given to a delusional state that concerns only one particular topic. Such delusions have been associated in the clinical literature with schizophrenia and dementia and also with organic dysfunction caused by brain injury, stroke, or neurological illness.

18 This is the clinical name given to the delusional belief that a close relative or spouse has been replaced by an identical-looking impostor.

19 See, for example, first person accounts by Sebastian Schmidt, Nelson, Sean O'Conner, Michael Gheen, and Andrew Becker, all in Stirn et al. (2009).

20 Similarly, Slatman and Widdershoven claim that "Bodily integrity or wholeness does not simply refer to biological, functional, or neurological intactness, but rather involves a positive identification with the body one has" (2009: 48).

21 Cissexual is a critical term developed to name an individual's self-perception of his or her body and his or her gender as congruent. For Jessica Cadwallader, *cissexual* is "a way of drawing attention to the unmarked norm against which trans* is identified, in which a person feels that their gender identity matches their body/sex" (2009: 17).

22 Bayne and Levy (2005) argue that if a person requesting amputation is shown to be competent in his or her request, then amputation may be justified on the basis that it minimizes the harm that wannabes may inflict on themselves in an attempt to achieve the bodies they feel themselves to be. In this sense, amputation would be beneficial rather than contravening the principle of non-maleficence.

23 If amputation was established as a viable treatment protocol, then Ryan (2009) contends that as is the case in the termination of pregnancy, dissenting doctors would be under no obligation to perform an amputation, but they would be under an obligation to refer the patient to another doctor whom they believe might proceed with the surgery.

References

Aoyama, A., Krummenacher, P., Palla, A., Hilti, L.M. and Brugger, P. (2012) "Impaired Spatial-Temporal Integration of Touch in Xenomelia (Body Integrity Identity Disorder)," *Spatial Cognition & Computation: An Interdisciplinary Journal* 12: 96–110.

Bayne, T. and Levy, N. (2005) "Amputees by Choice: Body Integrity Identity Disorder and the Ethics of Amputation," *Journal of Applied Philosophy* 22: 75–86.

Blanke, O., Morgenthaler, F.D., Brugger, P. and Overney, L.S. (2009) "Preliminary Evidence for Front-Parietal Dysfunction in Able-Bodied Participants with a Desire for Limb Amputation," *Journal of Neuropsychology* 3: 181–200.

Blom, R.M., Hennekam, R.C. and Denys, D. (2012) "Body Integrity Identity Disorder," *Plos One* 7: 1–6.

Brang, D., McGeoch, P.D. and Ramachandran, V.S. (2008) "Apotemnophilia: a neurological disorder," *Cognitive Neuroscience and Neuropsychology* 19: 1305–6.

Bruno, R.L. (1997) "Devotees, Pretenders, and Wannabes: Two Cases of Factitious Disability Disorder," *Sexuality & Disability* 15: 243–60.

Bryant, A.L. (2011) "Consent, Autonomy, and the Benefits of Healthy Limb Amputation: Examining the Legality of Surgically Managing Body Integrity Identity Disorder in New Zealand," *Bioethical Inquiry* 8: 281–8.

Cadwallader, J. (2009) "Diseased States: The Role of Pathology in the (Re)production of the Body Politic," in N. Sullivan and S. Murray (eds.) *Somatechnics: Queering the Technologisation of Bodies*, Aldershot: Ashgate, pp. 13–28.

Campbell, D. and Shapiro, M. (1999) "Introduction: From Ethical Theory to the Ethical Relation," in D. Campbell and M. Shapiro (eds.) *Moral Spaces: Rethinking Ethics and World Politics*, Minneapolis: University of Minnesota Press, pp. vii–xx.

Craimer, A. (2009) "The Relevance of Identity in Responding to BIID and the Misuse of Causal Explanation," *The American Journal of Bioethics* 9: 53–5.

Davis, L. (1995) *Enforcing Normalcy: Disability, Deafness and the Body*, New York: Verso.

De Preester, H. (2011) "Merleau-Ponty's Sexual Schema and the Sexual Component of *Body Integrity Identity Disorder*," *Medicine, Healthcare and Philosophy*. Available at: http://rd.springer.com/article/10.1007/s11019-011-9367-3 (accessed March 15, 2012).

Dua, A. (2010) "Apotemnophilia: Ethical Considerations of Amputating a Healthy Limb," *Journal of Medical Ethics* 36: 75–8.

Ellison, J. (2008) "Cutting Desire," *The Daily Beast*. Available at: http://www.thedailybeast.com/newsweek/2008/05/28/cutting-desire.html (accessed January 20, 2010).

First, M. (2005) "Desire for Amputation of a Limb: Paraphilia, Psychosis, or a New Type of Identity Disorder," *Psychological Medicine* 35: 919–28.

First, M. and Fisher, C.E. (2012) "Body Integrity Identity Disorder: The Persistent Desire to Acquire a Physical Disability," *Psychopathology* 45: 3–14.

Garland-Thomson, R. (2002) "Integrating Disability, Transforming Feminist Theory," *NWSA Journal* 14: 1–32.

Giummarra, M.J., Bradshaw, J.L., Nicholls, M.E.R., Hilti, L.M. and Brugger, P. (2011) "Body Integrity Identity Disorder: Deranged Body Processing, Right Fronto-Parietal Dysfunction, and Phenomenological Experience of Body Incongruity," *Neuropsychology Review* 21: 320–33.

Jordan, J. (2004) "The Rhetorical Limits of the 'Plastic Body,'" *Quarterly Journal of Speech* 90: 327–58.

Jotkowitz, A. and Zivotofsky, A. (2009) "Body Integrity Identity Disorder (BIID) and the Limits of Autonomy," *The American Journal of Bioethics* 9: 55–6.

Lawrence, A. (2006) "Clinical and Theoretical Parallels Between Desire for Limb Amputation and Gender Identity Disorder," *Archives of Sexual Behavior* 35: 263–78.

Levy, N. (2009) "Autonomy Is (Largely) Irrelevant," *The American Journal of Bioethics* 9: 50–1.

McGeoch, P.D., Brang, D., Aong, T., Lee, R.R., Huang, M. and Ramachandran, V.S. (2011) "Xenomelia: A New Right Parietal Lobe Syndrome," *Journal of Neurology, Neurosurgery & Psychiatry* 82: 1314–19.

McRuer, R. (2002) "Compulsory Able-Bodiedness and Queer/Disabled Existence," in S. Snyder, B.J. Brueggeman and R. Garland-Thomson (eds.) *Disability Studies: Enabling the Humanities*, New York: The Modern Language Association, pp. 88–99.

Money, J., Jobaris, R. and Furth, G. (1977) "Apotemnophilia: Two Cases of Self-Demand Amputation as Paraphilia," *Journal of Sex Research* 13: 115–25.

Müller, S. (2009) "BIID: Under Which Circumstances Would Amputations of Healthy Limbs be Ethically Justified?" in A. Stirn, A. Thiel and S. Oddo (eds.) *Body Integrity Identity Disorder: Psychological, Neurobiological, Ethical and Legal Aspects*, Lengerich: Pabst Science Publishers, pp. 109–23.

Partridge, Chris (n.d.) "On the Moral Permissibility of Voluntary Amputation." Available at: http://organizations.oneonta.edu/philosc/papers09/Partridge.pdf (accessed September 5, 2012).

Patrone, D. (2009) "Disfigured Anatomies and Imperfect Analogies: Body Integrity Identity Disorder and the Supposed Right to Self-Demand Amputation of Healthy Body Parts," *Journal of Medical Ethics* 35: 541–5.

Pies, R. (2009) "The Ethics of Limb Amputation and Locus of Disease," *Neuroethics* 2: 179–80.

Ryan, C.J. (2009) "Out on a Limb: The Ethical Management of Body Integrity Identity Disorder," *Neuroethics* 2: 21–33.

Ryan, C.J., Shaw, T. and Harris, A.W.F. (2010) "Body Integrity Identity Disorder: Response to Patrone," *Journal of Medical Ethics* 36: 189–90.

Savulescu, J. (2006) "Autonomy, the Good Life, and Controversial Choice," in R. Rhodes, L.P. Francis and A. Silvers (eds.) *The Blackwell Guide to Medical Ethics*, London: Wiley-Blackwell, pp. 17–37.

Seda, A (2011) "Body Integrity Identity Disorder: From a Psychological to a Neurological Syndrome," *Neuropsychology Review* 21: 334–6.

Shildrick, M. (1999) "This Body Which Is Not One: Dealing With Differences," *Body & Society* 5: 77–92.

Shildrick, M. (2004) "Genetics, Normativity and Ethics: Some Bioethical Concerns," *Feminist Theory* 5: 149–65.

Shildrick, M. (2009) *Dangerous Discourses of Disability, Subjectivity and Sexuality*, London and New York: Palgrave Macmillan.

Slatman, J. and Widdershoven, G. (2009) "Being Whole After Amputation," *The American Journal of Bioethics* 9: 48–9.

Smith, R. and Firth, G.M. (2000) *Amputee Identity Disorder: Information, Questions, Answers and Recommendations About Self-Demand Amputation*, United States: 1st Books.

Stirn, A., Thiel, A. and Oddo, S. (eds.) (2009) *Body Integrity Identity Disorder: Psychological, Neurobiological, Ethical and Legal Aspects*, Lengerich: Pabst Science Publishers.

Stryker, S. and Sullivan, N. (2009) "King's Member, Queen's Body: Transsexual Surgery, Self-Demand Amputation and the Somatechnics of Sovereign Power," in N. Sullivan and S. Murray (eds.) *Somatechnics: Queering the Technologisation of Bodies*, Farnham: Ashgate, pp. 49–64.

Sullivan, N. (2005) "Integrity, Mayhem, and the Question of Self-Demand Amputation," *Continuum: Journal of Media & Cultural Studies* 19: 325–33.
Sullivan, N. (2008) "The Role of Medicine in the (Trans)Formation of 'Wrong' Bodies," *Body & Society* 14: 105–16.
Sullivan, N. (2009) "Queering the Somatechnics of BIID," in A. Stirn, A. Thiel and S. Oddo (eds.) *Body Integrity Identity Disorder: Psychological, Neurobiological, Ethical and Legal Aspects*, Lengerich: Pabst Science Publishers, pp. 187–99.
Swindell, J.S. (2009) "Two Types of Autonomy," *The American Journal of Bioethics* 9: 52–3.
Williamson, K. (2010) "Healthy Limb Amputation, Bioethics, and Patient Autonomy," *Emergent Australian Philosophers* 3: 1–21.

INDEX

Printed by PGSTL